ESSENTIALS OF INFECTIOUS DISEASES

ESSENTIALS OF INFECTIOUS DISEASES

edited by

Lionel A. Mandell, M.D., F.R.C.P. (C)

Head, Division of Infectious Diseases, and
Associate Professor of Medicine,
McMaster University

and

Edward D. Ralph, B.Sc., M.D., F.R.C.P. (C)

Associate Professor of Medicine
Division of Infectious Diseases
Department of Medicine
University of Western Ontario

BLACKWELL SCIENTIFIC PUBLICATIONS
BOSTON OXFORD LONDON
EDINBURGH PALO ALTO MELBOURNE

Blackwell Scientific Publications

Editorial Offices:
52 Beacon Street, Boston
Masssachusetts 02108, USA
Osney Mead, Oxford, OX2 OEL
8 John Street, London, WC1N 2ES
23 Ainslie Place, Edinburgh, EH3 6AJ
667 Lytton Avenue, Palo Alto
California 94301, USA
107 Barry Street, Carlton
Victoria 3053, Australia

DISTRIBUTORS
USA
Blackwell Mosby Book Distributors
11830 Westline Industrial Drive
St Louis, Missouri 63146

Canada
Blackwell Mosby Book Distributors
120 Melford Drive, Scarborough
Ontario M1B 2X4

Australia
Blackwell Scientific Book Distributors
31 Advantage Road, Highett
Victoria 3190

Library of Congress Cataloging in Publication Data
Main entry under title:

Essentials of infectious diseases.

Includes index.
1. Communicable diseases. I. Mandell, Lionel A., 1946– . II. Ralph, Edward D., 1944– . [DNLM: 1. Communicable Diseases. WC 100 E78]
RC111.E87 1985 616.9 84-20400
ISBN 0-86542-014-9

89 88 87 86 5 4 3 2 1

Typeset by Compset, Inc.
Printed and bound by the Maple-Vail Book Manufacturing Group, Binghamton, New York.
Cover design by BEC Design.

To our families
and our teachers

CONTENTS

FOREWORD

The number of textbooks and monographs pertaining to the specialty of infectious diseases has increased considerably during the past five years. This not only reflects the relative paucity of such literature existing previously, but also demonstrates that the proper diagnosis and therapy of patients with infection is now recognized as a basic component of medical practice.

Essentials of Infectious Diseases, written by practicing infectious disease specialists with a variety of backgrounds and interests, carefully emphasizes a practical, clinical approach to patients with common infectious disease syndromes in the community or hospital setting.

Microbiological knowledge, practical laboratory techniques, and principles of the host-microbe interaction which are relevant to the clinician are clearly and concisely presented in the opening chapters. The major part of the book, however, is devoted to a syndrome approach to patients with proven or suspected infection. The syndromes are classified in this book not only by organ system involvement (e.g., cardiovascular system infection, central nervous system infection), but also by major symptoms or signs (e.g., fever of unknown origin, septic shock), and epidemiologic features (e.g., nosocomial infection, postoperative infection). Where applicable, these chapters are organized under the headings of Etiology, Epidemiology, Pathophysiology, Clinical Manifestations, Diagnosis, Treatment, Prognosis, and Prophylaxis to ensure uniformity of presentation and thereby facilitate comprehension and comparison of various disease entities. In addition, for easy reference and review purposes, separate chapters have been written to consolidate major topics such as Antibiotics and Antifungal Drugs, Immunization, and Chemoprophylaxis of Infection.

No single book can meet the requirements of everyone interested in a subject area as diverse as Infectious Diseases. However, *Essentials of Infectious Diseases* should prove a very useful and practical text for a broad cross section of individuals involved in clinical medicine including medical students, housestaff, and practicing physicians.

William M. M. Kirby, M.D.
Professor of Medicine
University of Washington
Seattle, Washington

PREFACE

Through our close association with medical students, house staff, and community- and hospital-based physicians and surgeons, it became obvious to us that there was a need for a textbook of infectious diseases aimed at the general medical practitioner. Standard medical texts do not seem to give quite enough detail and occasionally suffer from an ivory tower approach to clinical problems. Subspecialty texts, on the other hand, are far too detailed and expensive for general use. Since infections continue to be a major cause of morbidity and mortality worldwide, a rational approach to their management is needed if they are to be dealt with properly.

In planning this book, we relied on our own clinical experience as well as that of numerous colleagues across North America. It became apparent that what was needed was a systems-oriented approach presented in a clear, concise manner with emphasis on clinical features, diagnosis, and management.

The first several chapters deal with relevant basic areas such as microbiology, pathogenicity, diagnostic techniques, and therapeutic and prophylactic use of antimicrobial agents. The bulk of the book, however, is devoted to infections in each of the major organ systems of the body as well as certain special situations such as fever of unknown origin, infections in immunocompromised hosts, and postoperative infections.

We are grateful to our contributors who have put a great deal of time and effort into preparing their respective chapters. We are also appreciative of the constant input provided by our students and colleagues whose questions and criticisms helped shape this book. Richard Zorab, Elizabeth O'Neill McGuire, Patricia Sheehan Wright and Kathleen Beane of Blackwell Scientific Publications were a tremendous help, and without their support and advice, as well as that of our families, this book would not have been written.

CONTRIBUTORS

Michael R. Achong, M.B., F.R.C.P.(C), F.A.C.P.
Associate Professor, Department of Medicine, McMaster University

Marcoux J. André, M.D., C.R.C.P.(C)
Professor of Medicine and Head, Division of Infectious Diseases, Centre Hospitalier Universitaire, Quebec

Thomas W. Austin, M.D., F.R.C.P.(C)
Infectious Diseases Consultant, Victoria Hospital, and Associate Professor of Medicine, University of Western Ontario

Michel G. Bergeron, M.D., F.R.C.P.(C)
Professor of Medicine and Microbiology and Chief, Infectious Diseases Service, Le Centre Hospitalier de l'Université Laval

John M.A. Bohnen, M.D., F.R.C.S.(C)
Lecturer, Department of Surgery, University of Toronto

William R. Bowie, M.D., F.R.C.P.(C)
Associate Professor of Medicine, Division of Infectious Diseases; Department of Medicine, University of British Columbia

M. Ian Bowmer, M.D., C.M., F.R.C.P.(C)
Associate Professor of Medicine (Infectious Diseases) Memorial University of Newfoundland

L.E. Bryan, M.D., Ph.D., F.R.C.P.(C)
Professor and Head, Microbiology and Infectious Diseases, Faculty of Medicine, the University of Calgary

Max A. Chernesky, B.Sc., M.Sc., Ph.D.
Director, McMaster University Regional Virology Laboratory; Professor of Pediatrics and Pathology, McMaster University

Anthony W. Chow, M.D., F.R.C.P.(C), F.A.C.P.
Professor and Head, Division of Infectious Diseases, University of British Columbia and Vancouver General Hospital

Ronald Feld, M.D., F.R.C.P.(C), F.A.C.P.
Associate Professor of Medicine and Medical Microbiology, University of Toronto

M. John Gill, B.Sc., M.B., Ch.B., F.R.C.P.(C)
Assistant Professor, Department of Microbiology and Infectious Diseases, and Department of Medicine, Health Sciences Centre, University of Calgary

Ronald Gold, M.D.
Professor of Pediatrics and Chief, Division of Infectious Diseases, Hospital for Sick Children, Toronto

David A. Haase, M.B.B.S., B.Sc., F.R.C.P.(C)
Fellow, Infectious Diseases, Department of Infectious Diseases, St. Boniface General Hospital, Winnipeg

Ole Hammerberg, M.Sc., M.D., F.R.C.P.(C)
Assistant Professor of Pathology and Pediatrics, McMaster University

Godfrey K.M. Harding, M.D., F.R.C.P.(C)
Associate Professor of Medicine and Medical Microbiology, University of Manitoba; Head, Section of Infectious Diseases, St. Boniface General Hospital, Winnipeg

Daryl J. Hoban, Ph.D., RM (CCM)
Assistant Director, Department of Clinical Microbiology, Health Sciences Center, Assistant Professor, Department of Medical Microbiology, Faculty of Medicine, University of Manitoba

Jay S. Keystone, M.D., M.Sc. (CTM), F.R.C.P.(C)
Director, Tropical Disease Unit, Toronto General Hospital; Associate Professor of Medicine and Medical Microbiology, University of Toronto

Stephan J. Landis, M.D., F.R.C.P.(C)
Assistant Professor of Medicine, Division of Infectious Diseases, McMaster University

Thomas J. Louie, M.D., F.R.C.P.(C)
Assistant Professor of Medicine and Medical Microbiology, University of Manitoba

Lionel A. Mandell, M.D., F.R.C.P. (C)
Head, Division of Infectious Diseases, and Associate Professor of Medicine, McMaster University

Thomas J. Marrie, M.D., F.R.C.P.(C)
Program Director in Infectious Diseases, Associate Professor of Medicine, Dalhousie University

David J. McNeely, M.D., F.R.C.P.(C)
Director, Division of Infectious Diseases, Toronto Western Hospital; Assistant Professor of Medicine and Microbiology, University of Toronto

Jonathan L. Meakins, M.D., D.Sc., F.R.C.S.(C), F.A.C.S.
Associate Professor of Surgery and Microbiology, McGill University; Associate Surgeon, Royal Victoria Hospital

Lindsay E. Nicolle, M.D., F.R.C.P.(C)
Assistant Professor, Department of Medicine, Department of Medical Microbiology and Infectious Diseases Calgary General Hospital

Peter Phillips, M.D., F.R.C.P.(C)
Fellow, Division of Infectious Diseases, University of British Columbia and Vancouver General Hospital

Harvey R. Rabin, M.D., F.R.C.P.(C)
Associate Professor of Medicine and Division Head, Infectious Diseases, and Associate Professor of Microbiology and Infectious Diseases, Health Sciences Centre, University of Calgary

Edward D. Ralph, B.Sc., F.R.C.D. (C)
Associate Professor of Medicine, Division of Infectious Diseases, Department of Medicine, University of Western Ontario

Stanley E. Read, M.D., Ph.D., F.R.C.P.(C)
Associate Professor of Pediatrics and Microbiology, Division of Infectious Diseases, Department of Pediatrics Hospital for Sick Children and the University of Toronto

Allan R. Ronald, M.D., F.R.C.P.(C), F.A.C.P.
Professor and Head, Department of Medical Microbiology, University of Manitoba

H. Grant Stiver, M.D., F.R.C.P.(C)
Associate Professor, Division of Infectious Diseases, Department of Medicine, University of British Columbia and Vancouver General Hospital

D. Lorne J. Tyrrell, M.D., Ph.D., F.R.C.P.(C)
Professor of Medicine and Biochemistry, Departments of Medicine and Biochemistry, University of Alberta

Hillar Vellend, M.D.
Head, Division of Infectious Diseases, Toronto General Hospital and Mount Sinai Hospital; Associate Professor, Department of Medicine and Microbiology, Faculty of Medicine, University of Toronto

I GENERAL PRINCIPLES

1 MICROBIOLOGY FOR THE CLINICIAN

Allan R. Ronald and Daryl Hoban

Agents that cause infectious disease processes have the ability to exist independently in the environment or in parasitic association with the host, and provoke responses that may be inflammatory, immunologic, or destructive. Microbial organisms that are involved in such processes are organized according to varying degrees of complexity. The range is from subcellular particles, for example viruses, which are incapable of multiplication or function outside the host cell, to wholly saprophytic bacteria and fungi with the necessary energy-producing and biosynthetic processes for fully independent existence and multiplication. In between are the chlamydias, mycoplasmas, and rickettsias, which possess some biosynthetic functions but are still dependent upon intracellular existence in a host cell for their multiplication and survival.

CLASSIFICATION

Many classifications of infectious agents that cause human disease have been proposed. These are modified as more knowledge is acquired for defining genera and species. In considering the extremely varied biologic complexity and heterogeneity of pathogenic microorganisms, the most rational classification is based on anatomic and functional complexity, and the range is from acellular particles to multicellular parasites (Table 1.1).

Acellular Organisms

Viruses are examples of acellular infective agents that vary in size from 20 to 200 nm. Composed of a central core of either DNA or RNA, they are surrounded by a protein coat and sometimes an outer lipoprotein layer. Table 1.2 shows some of the viruses pathogenic for humans. Even smaller subcellular infectious agents composed of low-molecular-weight protein units less than 5 nm in size and resistant to nucleic acid-modifying procedures are also known. The word *prion* has been proposed to describe these infectious units, such as the scrapie agent of sheep and possibly also the agents implicated in such atypical virus like diseases as kuru and Jakob-Creutzfeldt disease in humans.

Unicellular Organisms

Unicellular microorganisms can be divided into two types according to their basic structural arrangement and complexity — prokaryotic and eukaryotic cells. The former are simpler in structure than the latter with one exception: the cell wall of the prokaryotic cell may be composed of several layers and is often complex. Bacteria in particular usually possess rigid cell walls that are responsible for their constant shape. In most other respects the prokaryotic cell is simpler; it lacks a nuclear membrane and the cytoplasm does not contain mitochondria. The cytochrome enzymes are located instead on the cell membrane. By contrast, the eukaryotic cell has a nucleus bounded by a nuclear membrane with an associated endoplasmic reticulum, and undergoes a chromosomal mitotic phase of nuclear division. The cytoplasm contains mitochondria and is surrounded by a lipoprotein cell membrane. Eukaryotic cell walls are relatively simple and are composed of either chitin or cellulose, as is found in fungi. Table 1.3 compares eukaryotic and prokaryotic cell structures.

Chlamydiae have cell particle sizes of 200- to 300-nm diameter, are obligate intracellular parasites, and

TABLE 1.1. A Simple Schema of Infectious Agents Related to Cell Type and Size

Organism Cell Type and Size	*Agents*
Acellular (less than 5–200 nm diameter)	Prions Viruses
Unicellular (200–2000 nm diameter)	
Prokaryotic cells	Chlamydiae, mycoplasmas, rickettsiae, bacteria
Eukaryotic cells	Fungi (yeasts), protozoa
Multicellular eukaryotic parasites	Fungi (mycelial), helminths

TABLE 1.2. Animal Viruses Pathogenic to Humans

Virus	*Examples*
RNA	
Picornavirus	Poliovirus, coxsackievirus, rhinovirus
Togavirus	Eastern/western encephalitis, yellow fever
Paramyxovirus	Mumps, measles, respiratory syncytial virus
Orthomyxovirus	Influenza A, B, C
Rhabdovirus	Rabies
Reovirus	Human reovirus
Retrovirus	Visna virus, leukosis group
Bunyavirus	Bunyamwera viruses
Coronavirus	Human strains
Arenavirus	Lassa virus
DNA	
Parvovirus	Adeno-associated virus
Papovavirus	Human wart virus
Adenovirus	Human adenovirus
Herpes virus	Herpes simplex types 1 and 2, Epstein-Barr, zoster, cytomegalovirus
Poxvirus	Variola, vaccinia

TABLE 1.3. Functional and Structural Differences Between Eukaryotes and Prokaryotes

Characteristic	*Eukaryotes*	*Prokaryotes*
Presence of nuclear membrane	+	−
Chromosomes contain histone protein	+	−
Presence of		
Nucleolus	+	−
Endoplasmic reticulum	+	−
Golgi apparatus	+	−
Lysosomes	+	−
Chloroplasts	+/−	−
Ribosomes	80S and 70S	70S
Microtubules	+	−
Peptidoglycan in cell wall	−	+/−
Phagocytosis	+	−
Pinocytosis	+	−
Cytoplasmic streaming	+	−
Intracellular digestion	+	−

have distinctive life cycles involving the production of cytoplasmic inclusion bodies in susceptible eukaryotic host cells. Unlike viruses, chlamydiae are susceptible to antimicrobial agents such as chloramphenicol, tetracycline, and sulfonamides. The acids DNA and RNA, proteins, carbohydrates, lipids, and peptidoglycans may be demonstrated, thereby relating these organisms more closely with bacteria than with viruses. Chlamydiae are devoid of energy-producing processes and therefore are dependent on the host cell for the energy necessary to complete biosynthetic activities. These organisms are responsible for such infections in humans as trachoma, lymphogranuloma venereum, and nongonococcal urethritis.

Mycoplasmas are pleomorphic organisms that lack cell walls. They are generally not much larger than the largest viruses, and range from 150 to 500 nm or larger. The absence of a cell wall renders these organisms particularly susceptible to the osmotic pressure of their surroundings. They are resistant to the β-lactam group of antibiotics that affect cell wall synthesis. Mycoplasmas are capable of growth on artificial media and are thus the smallest infective agents that can do so. *Mycoplasma pneumoniae* is the principle human pathogen of this group and is an etiologic agent of atypical pneumonia. *Ureaplasma urealyticum,* a related species, has been implicated as a cause of urethritis.

Rickettsiae are obligate intracellular parasites with a marked inability to survive outside a host. Diseases associated with these organisms are characterized by severe exanthematous rashes and are transmitted by ar-

TABLE 1.4. Major Bacterial Groupings

Shape	Morphology	Genera
	Gram-positive	
Cocci	Round, in clusters or tetrads	*Staphylococcus* *Micrococcus* *Peptococcus**
	Oval/round, in chains	*Streptococcus* *Peptostreptococcus**
Bacilli	Club-shaped, palisading	*Corynebacterium* *Listeria* *Erysipelothrix* *Mycobacterium* (rapid growers) *Propionibacterium**
	Acid-fast, filamentous	*Mycobacterium* *Lactobacillus** *Eubacterium** *Actinomyces** *Arachnia** *Streptomyces* *Nocardia*
	Spore forming	*Bacillus* *Clostridium**
	Gram-negative	
Cocci	Round, kidney-shaped	*Neisseria* *Veillonella**
Bacilli	Coccobacillary	*Acinetobacter* *Moraxella* *Brucella* *Bordetella* *Bacteroides**
	Pleomorphic coccobacillary	*Hemophilus* *Pasteurella* *Francisella* *Actinobacillus* *Eikenella* *Cardiobacterium* *Flavobacterium*
	Pointed ends	*Fusobacterium** *Streptobacillus*
	Curved	*Vibrio* *Campylobacter*
	Uniform	Enterobacteriacea *Pseudomonas* *Aeromonas* *Alcaligenes* *Chromobacterium*
	Others	
Spiral	Spiral, motile	*Treponema** *Borrelia** *Leptospira*
Pleomorphic	Lack cell wall	*Mycoplasma*
?Round	Intracellular parasite	*Rickettsia* *Coxiella* *Chlamydia*

* = anaerobes.

thropod vectors. The group is responsible for the various typhus diseases and Rocky Mountain spotted fever. A related species, *Coxiella burnetii,* differs in not requiring an arthropod vector, in not producing an exanthematous eruption, and in being able to survive outside the host for long periods.

Bacteria are unicellular organisms with rigid cell walls composed of peptidoglycans, proteins, and lipoproteins. In addition to rigid shape, the cell wall provides the bacterium with increased resistance to osmotic destruction and some protection from the environment that is not afforded the eukaryotic cell. This relative rigidity of structure permits a morphologic grouping of medically important bacteria by shape. Bacteria may be rod-shaped bacilli, spherical cocci, or spiral-shaped spirochetes. Table 1.4 shows the major groupings.

Electron microscopy reveals two types of bacterial cell wall structures that are related to their Gram's staining reaction. Gram-negative bacteria have a layered cell wall with a narrow peptidoglycan basal layer linked to lipoprotein, with an outer layer of phospholipids, lipoproteins, and lipopolysaccharides. Gram-positive cells have a thick peptidoglycan layer with no polysaccharide component, but which includes polymers of ribitol or glycerol known as teichoic acids.

Other structural differences that contribute to the identification of bacteria include presence of flagella, capsulation, and endospore formation. Complete identification to species level may be very time consuming and depend on a complex investigation of biochemical activities and growth requirements of an isolate. Size, morphology, motility, staining reaction, presence of spores, and oxygen requirements, however, are important in the initial assessment of isolates from clinical specimens.

Fungi have a eukaryotic cell structure; are capable of sexual and asexual reproduction; may exist as unicellular yeasts, cenocytic, or multicellular mycelia from 2 to 10 μm in diameter; or may even be dimorphic, growing as yeasts or mycelia depending on growth conditions. Many fungi that cause human mycoses exist and reproduce as asexual forms and for this reason are referred to as fungi imperfecti. The true classification of fungi depends on the type of sexual reproduction and the form of the diploid phase. As more is known about the generation and growth phases of fungi imperfecti, they are reassigned to their appropriate classes. They are subdivided as follows:

Class 1 Phycomycetes — nonseptate hyphae, asexual spores born in a structure, called a sporangium. Sexual fusion produces a zygote; example, *Aspergillus fumigatus*.

Class 2 Ascomycetes — sexual fusion results in a sac or ascus containing spores. Asexual spores are borne at tips of hyphae; example, *Trichophyton rubrum*.

Class 3 Basidiomycetes — sexual fusion produces a basidium that bears basidiospores. Asexual spores are borne at the tips of hyphae; example, the common mushroom.

Class 4 Imperfect fungi — forms in which a sexual process has not been demonstrated. Many resemble the ascomycetes; example, *Candida albicans*.

Some common human mycoses are as follows:

1. Deep mycoses
   - *Blastomyces dermatitidis*
   - *Histoplasma capsulatum*
   - *Paracoccidioides brasiliensis*
   - *Cryptococcus neoformans*
   - *Coccidioides immitis*
2. Opportunistic mycoses
   - *Aspergillus* sp.
   - *Candida* sp.
   - *Geotrichium* sp.
   - *Torulopsis glabrata*
3. Subcutaneous mycoses
   - *Fonsecaea* sp., *Wangiella* sp., *Phialophora* sp., *Exophila* sp., *Cladosporium* sp. } Chromoblastomycosis
   - *Pseudoallescheria* sp., *Madurella* sp., *Exophila* sp., *Sporothrix schenckii* } Mycetoma
4. Superficial mycoses
   - *Trichophyton* sp., *Microsporum* sp., *Epidermophyton floccosum* } Dermatomycosis

Protozoa of importance in human infections are unicellular, eukaryotic cells that have no cell walls and may vary in size from 2 to 50 μm in diameter. Classification of these organisms depends on their morphology and in particular, nuclear morphology and locomotor structures as shown below where the phylum Protozoa is divided into four main groups:

Class 1 Flagellates — possess locomotor structures called flagella. Some are free living, others are parasitic; example, *Giardia lamblia*.

Class 2 Amebas — move by pseudopodia, may be free living or parasitic; example, *Entamoeba histolytica*.

Class 3 Sporozoa — no specialized locomotor organelles. All members are parasitic; example, *Isospora belli*.

Class 4 Ciliates — possess cilia that aid locomotion. Both free-living and parasitic forms exist; example, *Balantidium coli*.

Multicellular parasites of medical importance predominantly belong to one of two phyla comprising three classes. They are identified on the basis of the morphology of the adult worm, the larval form, and the ovum. These are trematodes (flukes); cestodes (flat worms), which are exclusively parasitic for all of the predominant part of their life; and nematodes (round worms), which may be free living for a considerable period of their life cycle. Examples of these classes are as follows:

Class 1 Trematodes (flukes) — adult flukes live in blood vessels such as the venous plexus; example *Schistosoma haematobium*. The ova stimulate severe host reactions in tissue. There is one intermediate host, a fresh-water snail and a free-living infective stage that enters through the skin and later develops into the adult fluke.

Class 2 Cestodes (tapeworms) — transmitted as the intermediate stage in infected beef. The adult worm inhabits the intestine; example *Taenia saginata*.

Class 3 Nematodes (round worms) — the skin is penetrated by the intermediate larval stages that pass through the blood stream and lungs to the intestine where the adult worm exists; example *Necator americanus*.

SPECIMEN COLLECTION

When an infectious process is suspected, it is the responsibility of the physician to initiate studies and cultures either to confirm or reject this diagnosis. Proper specimen collection is essential if the etiologic agent is to be recovered from submitted material. Poorly collected specimens may fail to yield a true causative agent or may even lead to isolation of other flora that could confuse the diagnosis and result in incorrect therapy or diagnostic decisions. Several basic concepts of specimen collection must be emphasized.

1. The specimen that is sent for culture must be from the actual site of infection and should be as free of contamination from adjacent areas as possible. For example, improperly collected sputum that is heavily contaminated with saliva will grow contaminating mouth organisms and may not yield the true causative agent in a patient with clinical pneumonia. The depths of wounds should be cultured without touching adjacent skin, periurethral skin must be cleansed prior to a midstream urine collection, and abscesses should be aspirated using a sterile needle.
2. The optimal times for specimen collection must be followed. Early morning sputum and urine contain high concentrations of infecting organisms, making this the best time for collection; 24-hour collections are inadequate due to growth of contaminating organisms. Knowledge of the natural history of infectious diseases in many cases will help determine the type of specimen and time of collection.
3. A sufficient quantity of the specimen must be submitted to enable the laboratory to culture a variety of potential pathogens. It is often difficult to obtain adequate amounts of material.
4. It is essential that the correct collection device and appropriate containers or transport devices are used. Sterile containers should be used for all specimens. Synthetic-fiber swabs are preferable to cotton swabs in that fatty acids on cotton may inhibit growth of fastidious organisms. All swabs and specimens should be transported immediately to the laboratory, and transport media for swabs are recommended. Swabs are poor collection devices for the recovery of anaerobic bacteria; material aspirated with a syringe is preferred. All specimens to be cultured anaerobically must be protected from oxygen if culture is delayed more than one or two hours. Several types of transport systems are available.
5. If possible, material for culture should be obtained before antimicrobial agents are administered. Several organisms such as *Neisseria gonorrhoeae, Streptococcus pyogenes, Hemophilus influenzae,* and *N. meningitidis* are very susceptible to injury from antibacterial treatment. Culture results on specimens submitted after the administration of these drugs must be interpreted accordingly.
6. All specimen containers and accompanying requisitions should be properly labeled and filled out. Special requests or instructions should be indicated or discussed directly with the laboratory.

In addition to these general rules, specific guidelines are important for specimen collection from various body sites. Table 1.5 lists some of the sites or body fluids commonly cultured, frequently encountered pathogens, and the appropriate media.

Blood

Except in patients with endocarditis, endarteritis, brucellosis, and typhoid fever, bacteremia is intermittent, and thus timing of cultures is important. Bacteremia classically precedes fever or chills by 30 to 60 minutes. In patients with endocarditis (continuous bacteremia), three blood cultures are sufficient to isolate the etiologic agent in almost all patients. If initial cultures are negative at 24 hours, special cultural techniques to identify more fastidious organisms should be reviewed with a microbiologist. This is particularly important if patients have been treated with antimicrobial agents. In patients with a febrile illness and a focus of infection, a pair of blood cultures drawn before initiation of antimicrobial therapy is usually adequate.

Skin antisepsis is essential to ensure that cutaneous contamination of the blood culture does not occur. Cleansing the skin with 70% alcohol followed by 2% iodine left on for one minute before removal with alcohol is acceptable. The rate of false positive results of blood cultures should be less than 3%. In general, a set of blood cultures refers to two separate samples (aerobic

TABLE 1.5. Specimen Source, Potential Bacterial Pathogens, and Isolation Media

Source	*Pathogens*	*Media**
Throat	*S. pyogenes*	Blood agar
Sputum	*S. pneumoniae, S. aureus,* gram-negative rods, *Legionella*	Blood agar, chocolate agar Charcoal yeast extract, Feeley-Gorman
Transtracheal aspirate	*H. influenzae, S. aureus,* gram-negative rods, anaerobes	Chocolate agar, blood agar
Urine	Gram-negative rods, streptococci, staphylococci	Blood agar, MacConkey agar
Wounds, abscesses	*S. aureus, S. pyogenes,* gram-negative rods, anaerobes	Blood agar, chocolate agar, cooked meat
Stool	*Salmonella, Shigella, Yersinia, Campylobacter, Aeromonas*	Deoxycholate citrate agar, MacConkey agar, Skirrow media
Urethra, cervix	*N. gonorrhoeae*	Thayer-Martin and chocolate
Spinal fluid	*N. meningitidis, H. influenzae, S. aureus, S. pneumoniae,* gram-negative rods	Chocolate agar, enriched liquid media
Blood	*H. influenzae, Staphylococcus* sp., gram-negative rods, *Streptococcus* sp.	Blood agar, chocolate agar
Eye and ear	*H. influenzae, Psuedomonas, S. aureus, S. pyogenes, N. gonorrhoeae*	Chocolate agar, blood agar
Joint fluids	*N. gonorrhoeae,* gram-negative rods	Chocolate agar, blood agar, cooked meat

*A number of enriched, selective, or inhibitory media may be used. These may vary from one laboratory to another.

and anaerobic). At least 10 ml of blood should be collected for each sample since smaller amounts will decrease the recovery rate of organisms. In infants, 1 to 5 ml is satisfactory since children and infants have a higher level of bacteremia than adults. Blood is inoculated into the culture medium in use at each institution and submitted to the laboratory for incubation. Specialized media for culturing fungal pathogens may be required occasionally.

Cerebrospinal Fluid

If meningitis is suspected, a lumbar puncture becomes an urgent procedure; however, contraindications to the procedure in a particular patient should always be ruled out. In the absence of contraindications, as much cerebrospinal fluid (CSF) as possible should be collected, especially if several examinations are required, such as culture for fungi or mycobacteria. Aseptic technique is essential. The fluid should be delivered to the laboratory by a responsible individual as soon as it is obtained. Most laboratories will immediately perform a cell count and Gram's stain to aid in the differential diagnosis.

Other Fluids

Aspiration of body spaces and joints must be carried out aseptically and the material aspirated should be submitted as quickly as possible, preferably in a syringe with all air expelled or in a sterile container. Various types of transport tubes are available if desired when anaerobes are suspected.

Respiratory Tract

Interpretation of culture results from respiratory specimens is fraught with error. Many potential pathogens are normal flora of the respiratory tract and many patients are colonized with these organisms. It is particularly important when nasopharyngeal swabs are submitted that physicians list the diagnoses under consideration. For instance, *Bordetella pertussis* will not be cultured unless specimens are inoculated on special media. When throat swabs are performed, an effort must be made to minimize oral contamination. For example, tongue depressors are essential to minimize swab contact with heavily colonized sites (particularly the tongue).

Sputum cultures often give confusing results. To minimize these, samples ideally should be produced by a deep cough and must be transported quickly to the laboratory. Admixture with oropharyngeal flora inevitably occurs. This can make it difficult to determine which of perhaps many potential pathogens isolated is the etiologic agent of pneumonia. It is standard practice in most laboratories now to check sputum samples for presence of epithelial cells. If many epithelial cells but few polymorphonuclear neutrophils are present, this suggests that the sample is not appropriate for culture. Specimens from the lower respiratory tract collected by transtracheal aspiration, bronchial washings, or brushings are generally preferable to expectorated sputum samples since oropharyngeal contamination is greatly reduced. Anaerobic cultures of sputum are probably of little or no value. Again, rapid transport of all respiratory specimens to the laboratory is essential to reduce overgrowth of normal flora.

Biopsy specimens obtained by transthoracic needle or open lung procedure are superior to other specimens, but are only required under certain circumstances.

Skin

Except where a superficial lesion is present, skin cultures are of no value. Requests for dermatophytes should be stated, and in these instances, skin scrapings are preferred. Specimens from subcutaneous lesions should be obtained by aspiration or incision after the skin has been disinfected.

Urine

Generally the clean-voided midstream urine specimen is satisfactory. Patients or staff collecting the urine must ensure that proper cleansing has taken place. Urine is an excellent culture medium and a small number of contaminating organisms can quickly reach significant numbers. To avoid this, urine should be transported to the laboratory and cultured within one hour of collection or if this is not possible, it should be refrigerated. Urine obtained by urethral catheterization, by suprapubic aspiration, or from patients with indwelling catheters provides better specimens. Again, adherence to aseptic technique is important.

Stool

Feces are preferred to a rectal swab for isolation of enteric pathogens. They should be transported to the laboratory promptly since many organisms, including some shigellae, die quickly in feces as the temperature drops after collection. If this is not possible, several buffering transport agents are available. One gram of stool (a piece approximately the size of a pea) is sufficient. If a rectal swab is obtained, it must be inserted past the rectal sphincter, rotated, and withdrawn. Swabs should be sent directly to the laboratory, preferably in a screw-capped tube containing preservative. If a specific organism such as *Clostridium difficile* is suspected, the microbiologist should be informed. A single stool specimen may not identify the pathogen, and where disease persists and initial cultures are negative, repeat cultures are indicated.

Eye

Patients in whom conjunctivitis and, more important, keratitis is diagnosed pose special problems. Swabs provide a minimal specimen and should be obtained before topical anesthetics are used, as the anesthetics are generally bactericidal. Corneal scrapings are necessary if fungal or viral keratitis is suspected. Inoculation of media and preparation of slides for Gram's and Giemsa staining should be carried out immediately.

Genital Cultures

In symptomatic males, a Gram's stain of urethral discharge in which diplococci resembling gonococci are seen is as sensitive as a culture. In asymptomatic males and in females, a culture is indicated. Oropharyngeal and rectal cultures are important to obtain if sexual contact involving these areas is suspected, or in women, in whom cross-contamination from the vagina to the rectal area can occur. All specimens should be planted as soon as possible. In the investigation of genital ulcers, the laboratory should be advised so that a darkfield examination can be set up properly.

Wounds and Abscesses

Material should be collected from undrained abscesses with a syringe and needle since swab specimens usually contain inadequate material. Swabs collected from a draining sinus may be nonproductive because open wounds are invariably contaminated with skin or mucosal organisms. Intravenous catheter tips may be submitted for culture. Skin entry sites must be disinfected prior to catheter removal and the tip of the catheter cut off aseptically and sent to the laboratory in a sterile container.

Burn wounds are unique. Quantitative cultures may be of value as well as culture of draining material. Gram's stains may be beneficial in some instances.

INDIGENOUS MICROORGANISMS OF HUMANS

Knowledge of both resident and transient human flora is essential to appreciate the microbial ecology of health and disease states.

Two varieties of organisms are always present on the skin and mucous membranes. These consist first of a normal resident flora, usually of limited variety, that is rarely pathogenic in the normal host, and second, of a transient flora that may often harbor pathogens. The transient flora is usually derived from the environment and under most circumstances does not produce disease, especially if the resident flora is not disturbed.

The resident flora is made up of commensal organisms. It is not essential to life but it does play an important role in maintaining health. For example, resident flora in the intestine synthesizes vitamin K; on skin surfaces and on mucous membranes, it helps prevent colonization of pathogens. Under certain conditions, however, the resident flora itself can cause disease. If these organisms are removed from their natural environment and gain admittance to the blood stream or tissues, they can become pathogens. Usually in the absence of tissue damage, nutritional, or immunologic deficiencies, the flora is harmless.

Intestinal Tract

Diet is the most important factor in determining the composition of intestinal and fecal flora. Bowel flora changes dramatically, from lactic acid streptococci and lactobacilli in breast-fed babies to a varied flora in adults. The oral mucosal membranes are very heavily colonized with both aerobes and anaerobes. The esophagus is also colonized with these organisms but total numbers drop dramatically in the normal stomach (10^1 to 10^3/gm of stomach contents) due to low pH. If the pH rises, the concentration of microflora also rises. In the duodenum, the normal flora numbers 10^3 to 10^6 organisms per gram, in the jejunum and ileum 10^5 to 10^8, and in the cecum and transverse colon 10^8 to 10^{10} per gram. Lactobacilli and enterococci are most prominent in the upper intestine, while aerobic and anaerobic gram-negative rods are present in the lower ileum and cecum. The sigmoid colon and rectum harbor about 10^{11} bacteria per gram contents. The resident flora in the colon is predominantly anaerobes (95% to 99%), especially *Bacteroides fragilis,* lactobacilli, streptococci, and clostridia. Aerobes comprise only about 1% to 5% of the total flora and can include up to 100 species of organisms, including gram-negatives, facultative anaerobes, enterococci, candidae, and others. Colonic flora help to maintain normal health by producing vitamin K, resisting colonization by pathogens, and converting bile acids. Many aerobic organisms are transitory and persist for brief time periods. Oral antimicrobial agents eliminate drug-susceptible organisms, which are quickly replaced by resistant organisms.

Skin

The skin has a variety of transient organisms but has a fairly steady and well-defined resident flora that varies according to anatomic site and is influenced by presence of clothes, secretions, and relationship to mucous membranes.

The predominant organisms are *Corynebacterium, Propionibacterium, Staphylococcus epidermidis, Peptococcus, Bacillus* sp., *S. viridans, S. faecalis,* and *Acinetobacter.* Fungi, yeasts, and nonpathogenic mycobacteria can be found in certain skin folds or areas of concentrated sebaceous secretions. Nonresident organisms are removed by lysozyme, low pH, and desquamation. Simple washing does not alter the resident flora and surgical scrubbing has only a transient effect.

Upper Respiratory Tract

The mucous membranes of the mouth and pharynx are colonized by viridans streptococci within 12 hours of birth. Also, during the first few weeks of life aerobic and anaerobic staphylococci, neisseriae, branhamellae, diphtheroids, and some lactobacilli establish resident status. Only when teeth erupt do the anaerobes such as spirochetes, bacteroides (*B. melaninogenicus*), fusobacteria, and lactobacilli establish themselves. In many adults, *Actinomyces* sp. and yeasts reside in the gingivae, mouth, and tonsillar tissues. The pharynx and trachea contain nonhemolytic and alpha-hemolytic streptococci and neisseriae. Hemophili, staphylococci, diphtheroids, and pneumococci may be encountered in the pharynx as normal flora.

Urethra and Vagina

In both males and females the anterior urethra contain small numbers of organisms similar to those resident on the nearby skin or mucous membranes.

Aerobic lactobacilli are present in the vagina soon after birth. As the pH rises during infancy, a mixture of flora is established. At puberty, as the pH once again becomes acidic, lactobacilli reestablish residence and maintain this acidic pH. This prevents colonization by pathogenic organisms. After menopause, lactobacilli diminish and a mixed flora is reestablished. Often present in the vagina along with lactobacilli are anaerobic streptococci, clostridia, and occasionally group B streptococci.

Eye

Diphtheroids, coagulase-negative staphylococci, *Neisseria, Hemophilus*-like organisms, and *Moraxella* sp. are the most common organisms of the conjunctival surfaces. This flora is held in check by lysozyme present in tears.

IMPORTANCE OF PLASMIDS

Plasmids are a large, broad group of extrachromosomal genetic elements. They may replicate autonomously, independent of the host chromosome, and are not essential for cell viability. They are cyclic, double-stranded DNA molecules. The F agent was the first plasmid described, and it transfers chromosomal genes from one bacterium to another during conjugation (simple contact). Other plasmids have specific functions such as antimicrobial resistance, synthesis of proteins called bacteriocins that kill other bacteria, resistance to metals, and metabolism of various compounds. Most known functions permit the bacterial host to survive an adverse environment or to compete more effectively.

TABLE 1.6. Effects of Plasmids

Plasmid Characteristic	*Bacterial Species*
Antimicrobial resistance	Widespread
Metal ion resistance	Widespread
UV light resistance	*E. coli*
Bacteriocin production	Widespread
Exotoxin production	*C. botulinum*
Enterotoxin production	*E. coli, S. aureus*
Exfoliatin production	*S. aureus*
Sugar metabolism	Widespread
Degradation of unusual hydrocarbons	Pseudomonas

Two main classes of plasmids exist. Large plasmids are usually conjugative; that is, they are self-transmissible because they possess the genetic information necessary to generate their own transfer to another cell during contact. The second group are small plasmids, which are nonconjugative but can be transferred if a second plasmid is present to effect mobilization.

In recent years plasmid classification strictly on the basis of observable phenotypic effects has decreased in importance. It is now known that plasmids can specify a wide range of functions or properties (Table 1.6). Also, many small plasmids are described as cryptic; that is, they have no known phenotypic effects. Recently the biology and taxonomy of plasmids has been an important epidemiologic tool for tracing resistance genes in organisms.

Resistance plasmids were first described in clinical isolates of shigellae in Japan during the 1950s after it was recognized that resistance patterns to two or more drugs could be transferred to other bacteria maintaining the same resistance pattern. Random mutation was excluded as the mechanism by which this pattern of resistance was acquired. It quickly became apparent that these drug-resistance traits were inherited by an infectious process. By the early 1970s the majority of shigellae in Japan were resistant to many drugs. This phenomenon was also observed in many other bacteria of medical importance. The DNA that specified antibiotic resistance was shown to be plasmid DNA. Plasmids coding for drug resistance were called R factors and are now commonly called R plasmids. Plasmid-mediated resistance has been documented against many antimicrobial agents, such as β-lactam antibiotics, aminoglycosides, spectinomycin, chloramphenicol, erythromycin, lincomycin, tetracycline, sulfonamides, and trimethoprim. Mechanisms of resistance are usually the result of drug-inactivating enzymes. Antibacterial agents have not induced resistance plasmids but have selected for them. This has been documented by finding R plasmids in organisms isolated prior to the use of the antibiotic.

The genetic mobility of plasmids is further enhanced by the presence of transposons or transposition elements. These discrete DNA segments have the capacity to move from plasmid to plasmid as well as between plasmids and chromosomes, rearranging genetic material. Transposons are responsible for most of the determinants of antimicrobial resistance.

With the widespread use of antimicrobial agents, R plasmids are being selected for in populations of bacteria. This, combined with their ability to transfer from one species to another, presents a threat to the treatment of many bacterial diseases. These plasmids are widespread, not only in Enterobacteriaceae but in many other species of organisms such as *Bacteroides* and *N. gonorrhoeae*.

Perhaps plasmids and viruses evolved together from bacterial chromosomes. Viruses developed the ability to spread from cell to cell but usually killed their host. Plasmids developed a greater symbiotic relationship with their host. Genetic recombination events occurring with plasmids have shown us that this is not restricted to classic homology-dependent mechanisms. Bacterial plasmids are now widely used for recombinant DNA biology and have been developed as vectors for cloning human genes for the production of biologic products such as insulin.

Microbiology is a discipline undergoing rapid transition. Although physicians who care for patients with infections must continually add to their knowledge of the clinical features and management of microbial diseases, this alone is inadequate. Continuing review of the fundamentals of microbiology and of the advances occurring in the discipline are essential if patients are to receive optimal care.

ANNOTATED BIBLIOGRAPHY

David BD, Dulbeco R, Eisen HN, Ginsberg HS. Microbiology, 3rd edition. New York: Harper & Row, 1980.

A text designed for both students and investigators in medicine and related disciplines. In-depth discussions of metabolism, genetics, immunology, bacterial and mycotic infections, and virology.

Koneman EW, Allen SD, Dowell VR Jr, Sommers HM. Color atlas and textbook of diagnostic microbiology, 2nd edition. Philadelphia: JB Lippincott, 1983.

Text is an up-to-date, practical introduction to clinical microbiology. It provides a foundation on which current clinical microbiology literature can be analyzed.

Lennette EH, Balows A, Hausler WJ Jr, Truant JP, eds. Manual of clinical microbiology, 3rd edition. American Society for Microbiology, 1980.

Designed for clinical, medical, and public health microbiologists. Information is presented in a manual format and covers the characterization and identification of most bacteria, fungi, parasites, and viruses encountered clinically. Also includes in-depth discussions of laboratory tests used in chemotherapy.

Rippon JW. Medical mycology. The pathogenic fungi and the pathogenic actinomycetes, 2nd edition. Philadelphia: WB Saunders, 1982.

Basic information on medical mycology, including clinical disease, pathology, serology, and laboratory diagnosis. It is also an overview of current fungal research and provides excellent historical perspectives in the field.

2 DISEASE MECHANISMS AND HOST DEFENSES

Lionel A. Mandell

GENERAL CONSIDERATIONS

The host-parasite relationship is a common and fundamental biologic phenomenon. A basic understanding of this relationship is essential before one can fully appreciate pathogenetic mechanisms involved in infectious diseases.

As outlined in Chapter 1, a multitude of organisms comprise the normal flora found in various parts of the body. Organisms in the oropharynx, lower gastrointestinal tract, and on skin surfaces are classic examples. In most cases, the flora consist of commensal organisms and do not cause disease. Overt infection, however, may result if the defense mechanisms of the host are impaired, allowing either some of the normal flora or new pathogens to which the host is exposed to gain access to tissues. Examples of infections caused by one's own flora are aspiration pneumonia and infection due to the introduction of new pathogens that might be found at the site of a compound fracture.

Essentially, we can think of the host-parasite relationship as a continuum. At either extreme are colonization and overt infection respectively, with subclinical infection somewhere in the middle. Subclinical infection, although obviously not as spectacular as overt infection, is extremely important from an immunologic point of view. Repeated subclinical infections are likely responsible for continuing immunity to such diseases as rubeola (measles) and pertussis (whooping cough), thereby providing the host with lifelong protection.

PATHOGENICITY, VIRULENCE, AND DISEASE MECHANISMS

As mentioned above, if the defense mechanisms of the host are absent, impaired, or overwhelmed by microorganisms, infection may result. Organisms capable of causing disease, e.g., pathogens — bacteria, fungi, viruses, and so on — vary greatly in their pathogenicity. In cases where host defenses are severely impaired, infection may be caused by organisms usually considered to be nonpathogens. This is typically seen in patients with cancer who are undergoing intensive myelosuppressive therapy or in transplant recipients. In such cases, "opportunistic" infections are said to occur (this is discussed in detail in Chapter 22).

Virulence refers to the degree of pathogenicity of a particular organism. Highly virulent bacteria are more likely to infect a host and cause disease than are their less virulent counterparts. Virulence itself is determined by factors that essentially either protect the organism from ingestion by phagocytes or allow it to adhere to cells so that infection can be established.

Once infection is established, disease may be caused by any or all of the following mechanisms:

1. Invasion of host tissues by the pathogen
2. Intoxication of certain host cells by toxins produced by the pathogens
3. Immunologic reactions initiated by the pathogens

The steps involved in the establishment of infection are not completely understood; however, it appears that attachment of a potential pathogen to host cells is a necessary first step in establishing consistent colonization. Attachment is dependent upon surface macromolecules of the organisms that potentiate adherence to receptors on certain host cells. Specificity of various pathogens for particular tissue sites is referred to as tropism, and examples are adherence of shigellae and gonococci to intestinal and urethral epithelium respectively. Once adherence to cells occurs, several factors come into play that determine whether overt infection will develop.

TABLE 2.1. Selected Examples of Organisms and Toxins

Organism	*Toxins*	*Effects of Toxins*
S. aureus	α-Toxin, staphylokinase, leukocidin, hyaluronidase	Hemolysis, dermonecrosis, fibrinolysis, kills phagocytes, dissolves connective tissue
S. pyogenes	Streptolysin S, streptodornase, streptokinase, erythrogenic toxin	Hemolysis, deoxyribonuclease, fibrinolysis, vasodilatation
C. botulinum	Neurotoxin	Blocks release of acetylcholine
C. tetani	Neurotoxin	Blocks action of inhibitory neurons
C. diphtheriae	Schick toxin	Dermonecrosis
V. cholerae	Enterotoxin	Activates adenyl cyclase

Invasion

Invasion of host cells in a given site is obviously dependent upon local proliferation of pathogens. Multiplication of the organisms may interfere with local cell function by producing waste products injurious to the cells, by inducing cytotoxins, and by competing for nutrients. Local spread and invasion of bacteria may also be facilitated by extracellular enzymes produced by the pathogens. Enzymes such as collagenase, for example, can weaken the structural integrity of collagen, thereby allowing the invading organisms to spread more readily. Extracellular enzymes elaborated by the invading pathogens are types of exotoxins. Some of these exotoxins facilitate invasion and local spread, whereas others may act at remote sites, resulting in a state of intoxication.

Intoxication

As mentioned, exotoxins may aid in local invasion and may also act on tissues not directly involved by the organisms. Toxins in and of themselves are rarely the sole determinants of disease, although there are instances in which true intoxication occurs. Some classic examples of disease manifestations due to such toxins are botulism, diphtheria, tetanus, and cholera. Immunologic proof of this is seen by the fact that if one is given inactivated diphtheria toxin in the form of a toxoid, the host is then immune to the disease despite the fact that subsequent colonization with diphtheria can be documented. Table 2.1 lists a few of the exotoxins elaborated by various organisms.

Although they are not responsible for intoxication per se, endotoxins are appropriately considered at this point. As opposed to exotoxins, which are heat-labile proteins, endotoxins are heat-stable lipopolysaccharides and are associated with the outer membranes of gram-negative bacteria. The endotoxin molecule itself consists of three parts: the lipid moiety, which is the active component; the R core, which contains the common enterobacterial antigens; and the O polysaccharide, which determines the O-antigenic specificity of the organism. Lipopolysaccharide has a number of biologic properties, including activation of complement, of kalikrein, and the coagulation cascade. These assume clinical relevance in the shock syndrome seen with certain gram-negative infections (see Chapter 25).

Immunologic Reactions

Activation and expression of the immune response to invasion by pathogens results in inflammation and humoral and cell-mediated reactions that can cause tissue damage. The degree and severity of the response can vary and although often mild, may at times lead to extensive tissue damage and even death. The inflammatory response, which is discussed later, results in local warmth, redness, swelling, and pain. This is of little or no consequence in many infections but, for example, in purulent meningitis, the sequelae can be lethal.

The standard immunopathologic reactions, anaphylaxis, cytotoxic, immune-complex, and cell-mediated, may also result in damage to the host. With respect to infectious disease, the reactions likely to cause damage are the last three. Cytotoxic mechanisms depend on interaction of antibody with antigen and subsequent activation of complement. The antibody-mediated destruction of infected cells, if extensive, may result in damage to the host. Immune-complex reactions also result in activation of complement and can cause tissue damage. Examples are the immune-complex glomerulonephritis seen in subacute bacterial endocarditis and the arthritis seen in cases of meningococcemia.

Cell-mediated immunity is discussed in some detail in the last section of this chapter. Suffice it to say that occasionally this form of immunity can result in extensive tissue damage, as seen in some cases of tuberculosis.

Having briefly considered some of the general principles involved in disease causation by microorganisms, we must also examine how pathogens are able to spread throughout the body. Spread can occur in the following ways:

1. Direct route
2. Lymphatic route
3. Blood-borne route
4. Miscellaneous routes — cerebrospinal fluid, neural route, serous surfaces

Direct Route

Direct spread can occur in a number of ways. One of the simplest is spread of pathogens over epithelial surfaces in the lung and gastrointestinal tract. An example of this is the patient with a sinus infection and postnasal drip who subsequently develops a lower respiratory tract infection due to surface spread of pathogens from the sinuses. Another simple but effective way of spreading pathogens is by direct inoculation from one site to another. The patient with a staphylococcal infection on his arm might pick at the lesion and then transfer the organisms to his face, thereby helping to establish a second site of infection.

At a particular site of infection, for example, the staphylococcal infection mentioned above, the bacteria are able to advance locally with the aid of certain exotoxins elaborated by the pathogens. Viruses are also capable of local spread by successive cycles of infection of and release from host cells.

Lymphatic Route

Once pathogens have reached epithelial surfaces and have gained access to the subepithelial tissues, they enter lymphatic capillaries and are carried to local lymph nodes. If they are not trapped and inactivated within the nodes, they are further transported along the lymphatic route to the thoracic duct and ultimately reach the blood. Within the nodes, phagocytosis of organisms by the resident macrophages lining the sinusoids results in activation of antibody and cell-mediated responses. Local inflammatory responses also result in the recruitment of polymorphonuclear neutrophils that aid in ingestion and killing of pathogens.

Blood-Borne Route

Access to the bloodstream is by way of the lymphatic route first or directly, either by damage to small vessel walls by pathogens or by introduction of organisms into blood vessels secondary to a local injury, such as a bite or stab wound. Pathogens can be carried along in the blood in one of two ways: free in the plasma or in association with cellular components of blood.

Free in Plasma

Numerous pathogens can be transported free in plasma, but while being carried along they are exposed to antimicrobial factors that may be present in plasma. Once they have arrived at a particular focus, they can then infect that site only by first adhering to local vascular endothelial cells or by being engulfed by local reticuloendothelial cells.

Associated with Cellular Components

Red cells. The classic example of a red cell-associated pathogen is the malaria parasite. Viruses can be transported while adsorbed to the surface of erythrocytes, as can rickettsiae.

White cells. A number of viruses, (e.g., cytomegalovirus), can be transported either on or inside lymphocytes and monocytes. Bacterial pathogens, such as tubercle bacilli, that are able to survive within monocytes are essentially afforded a protected environment as well as a free ride to various organ systems.

Platelets. To date, platelet transport does not appear to be clinically important in humans despite the fact that these cells are capable of phagocytosis.

Miscellaneous Routes

Organisms that have reached the cerebrospinal fluid (CSF) either by direct or hematogenous routes can

TABLE 2.2. Surface Factors Involved in Host Defense

Skin	*Respiratory Tract*	*Gastrointestinal Tract*	*Urinary Tract*
Stratified, cornified epithelial covering	Nasal hairs	Gastric acid	Flushing action
Desquamation of surface cells	Mucous secretions	Peristalsis	Low pH
Acid pH	Ciliary movement	Mucous covering of intestinal epithelium	Bladder mucosa
Medium-chain fatty acids	Cough reflex	Secretory IgA	Prostatic fluid
Resident microflora	Epiglottis	Resident microflora	Polymorphonuclear neutrophils
	Respiratory secretions		
	Lysozyme		
	Interferon		
	Alpha$_1$-antitrypsin		
	Secretory IgA		
	Alveolar macrophages		
	Polymorphonuclear neutrophils		

readily spread throughout the neuraxis simply by being suspended within the CSF as it flows from the ventricles to the subarachnoid space. In the case of peripheral nerves, pathways are provided for the transport of exotoxins such as tetanus toxin and viruses such as rabies and herpes simplex. Spread of infection along serous surfaces is really a form of direct spread; a typical example is local infection in the peritoneal cavity after rupture of an intraabdominal viscus, resulting ultimately in diffuse peritonitis.

HOST DEFENSE MECHANISMS

The many forces involved in protecting the host against infection represent a complex and fascinating interplay between natural and acquired mechanisms. The former can be subdivided into surface factors and inflammation and the latter into immunologic mechanisms which include humoral and cellular-immune responses.

Surface Factors

Surface factors represent a mixture of physiologic, biochemical, mechanical, and anatomic factors. It is easiest to consider these according to the specific anatomic site or organ system involved (Table 2.2).

Skin

The skin covers almost the entire body and provides a mechanical barrier against infection. Unless the integrity of the skin is interrupted, most organisms are unable to penetrate the stratified, cornified epithelial covering. In addition to this bulwark against microbial invasion, desquamation of the surface layer of keratinized cells rids the skin of colonizing organisms.

Further protection is afforded by the acid pH on the skin surface, medium-chain unsaturated fatty acids created by the sebaceous glands, and the normal resident microflora of the skin that produce antibacterial substance and retard colonization by new organisms.

Respiratory Tract

Pathogens can gain access to the lower respiratory tract by inhalation, aspiration, or hematogenous spread. An elaborate defense network protects this vital area by several means. The first is by anatomic barriers. Nasal hairs trap large particles and also create turbulence in the airstream, making it easier for particles to be trapped by mucous secretions lining the membranes of the upper respiratory tract. Above the level of the terminal bronchioles, mucus-covered ciliated epithelium lines the respiratory tract. The cilia, which beat at the rate of approximately 1000 times per minute, maintain the flow of mucus and the entrapped particles are moved upward toward the pharynx where either expectoration or swallowing may ensue. Only particles under 10 μm in diameter can traverse these obstacles and reach the alveoli.

In the lower regions of the respiratory tree, the normal secretions also contain varying quantities of lysozyme, interferon, lactoferrin, alpha$_1$-antitrypsin, and immunoglobulins. The major immunoglobulin both here and in the gastrointestinal tract is immunoglobulin A (IgA). Secretory IgA is thought to play a role in aggregating foreign particles and interferes with binding of pathogens to host cells.

Particles and organisms that manage to bypass these defenses and reach the alveoli are handled by the alveolar macrophages. These phagocytic cells, aided by prior opsonization of the pathogens by antibodies, readily ingest invading microorganisms.

Another effective means of expelling bacteria is the cough reflex. With a cough, tremendous linear velocity is imparted to the air so that organisms trapped by the mucus secretions are readily expelled.

In the event of hematogenous spread of infection to the lung, the above mechanisms are essentially bypassed and defense depends upon the opsonizing activity of serum opsonins and the chemotactic, phagocytic, and microbicidal activity of polymorphonuclear neutrophils.

Gastrointestinal Tract

Despite the fact that organisms colonize the skin and oropharynx, neither of these is exposed to the tremendous quantity and variety of organisms and potential pathogens that form part of the normal flora of the gastrointestinal tract. In addition to this, bacteria are constantly introduced to this area in the food that we eat. If we consider that a gram of feces contains in the order of 10^{10} bacteria, it is clear that defense mechanisms are necessary to protect against infection. It is not at all surprising that in the immunocompromised host, the most common site of origin for bacteremias is the lower gastrointestinal tract.

Organisms ingested in food are killed by stomach acids. The importance of gastric acidity is attested to by the fact that patients with achlorhydria have a significant likelihood of contracting a number of enteric infections such as salmonellosis, shigellosis, and strongyloidiasis. Pathogens that manage to survive the gastric acid are propelled along the intestine by peristaltic action. This continuous movement reduces their chances of adhering to intestinal epithelial cells, thereby lessening the risk of infection. Contact is also impeded by the mucus that lines the intestinal epithelial cells.

As in the respiratory tract, secretory IgA causes agglutination of bacteria and inhibits adherence to the intestinal epithelial cells. The IgA can also neutralize certain viruses and bacterial toxins.

The normal bacterial flora of the gastrointestinal tract serves a number of functions. In addition to synthesizing certain required nutrients such as vitamin K, thiamine, and folic acid, it also maintains the ecologic balance and prevents infection by new pathogens. The ability of the normal bacterial flora to prevent colonization with new organisms may be due to colonization resistance factors elaborated by certain organisms within the gut. It was demonstrated that 10^7 organisms are required to establish intestinal colonization in animals with their microbial flora intact, but only 10^2 organisms are needed in germ-free animals. If the animals are allowed to maintain their anaerobic flora, however, 10^5 organisms are required to establish colonization, implying that anaerobes play a major role in colonization resistance.

Urinary Tract

Unlike the skin, upper respiratory tract, and gastrointestinal tract, in healthy hosts the bladder, ureters, and kidneys are sterile. Several mechanisms act in concert to maintain this state, including the flushing action that accompanies micturition and the low pH of normal urine, which can be bacteriostatic. The bladder mucosa itself also has antibacterial properties.

Prostatic fluid has antibacterial activity, and it has been suggested that this coupled with the longer male urethra may be responsible at least partially for the low prevalence of urinary tract infection in men. Infection in the kidney usually arises as a result of ascending spread of infection from the lower urinary tract or by hematogenous spread. Defense mechanisms here rely mainly upon antibody production and recruitment of polymorphonuclear neutrophils.

Inflammation

When pathogens have breached the surface defense mechanisms, the inflammatory response is activated. Inflammation plays a critical role in host defense, particularly in the acute stages of infection, although chronic and granulomatous inflammatory reactions are important as well.

Very simply, inflammation can be thought of as a nonspecific response of the microcirculation and its contents to tissue injury. The objective of this response is to localize infection by bringing phagocytic cells and plasma containing immunoglobulins and complement to the site of injury. When host tissues are damaged by infection, humoral mediators such as histamine, serotonin, leukotrienes, kinins, and prostaglandins are released, causing local changes in microcirculation. Vessels dilate and become more permeable, the vascular endothelium becomes "sticky," and lymphatic capillaries dilate. Vascular dilatation and enhanced permeability allow leakage of protein-rich fluid into the tissues. In this fluid are immunoglobulins that can act as opsonins, and complement that once activated, provides chemoattractants and opsonins and mediates the immune reactions. Fibrinogen is also present and when converted to fibrin, provides a fibrillar network that helps in containing infection. The stickiness of the vascular endothelial cells makes it easier for polymorphonuclear neutrophils to adhere to them, and the phagocytes can then exit into the tissues by the process of diapedesis.

Lymphatic vessels also dilate and the rate of lymph flow is increased during inflammation, so that inflammatory fluids as well as pathogens are taken up more readily and transported to the local lymph nodes. Organisms reaching the nodes are then exposed to macrophages, which not only are phagocytes but are involved in initiation of the immune response, as described in further detail below.

The classic manifestations of acute inflammation reflect the changes described. The affected site becomes warm, red, swollen, and painful due to vasodilatation, exudation of fluid and cells into tissues, and tissue distension.

As mentioned earlier, one of the main objectives of the inflammatory response is to provide phagocytic cells capable of ingesting and killing the invading pathogens. There are two main types of specialized phagocytic cells: polymorphonuclear neutrophils and cells of the monocyte-macrophage series. In acute inflammation, the former are principally involved. These cells develop from undifferentiated hematopoietic stem cells in the marrow. When mature, they leave the marrow to circulate in blood for approximately six hours, then exit through endothelial cell junctions into the tissue spaces. These are end cells in the sense that they are incapable of further development and their primary function is to ingest and kill invading pathogens.

Cells from the monocyte-macrophage series also develop from a myeloid stem cell and in fact, there is considerable evidence to suggest that monocytes and granulocytes derive from a common progenitor cell. The mononuclear phagocyte system is made up of circulating monocytes and tissue macrophages. The latter exist in several forms, including the Kupffer cells of the liver, pulmonary alveolar macrophage, and peritoneal and pleural macrophages. These cells constitute part of the reticuloendothelial system. Unlike polymorphonuclear neutrophils, mononuclear phagocytes have a number of functions. They not only are capable of ingesting pathogens, but remove senescent or dying cells, and are important from an immunologic point of view since they participate in bidirectional cellular interactions with lymphocytes. They also play a role in providing factors that regulate other cellular functions, including prostaglandins, pyrogen, and complement components.

Since the principles involved in phagocytosis are essentially similar for both polymorphs and macrophages, the following description focuses on the former.

Chemotaxis

For the ingestion and killing of microorganisms to take place, polymorphonuclear leukocytes must first come into contact with the invaders. The neutrophils exit from the vascular system by diapedesis, and once in the tissues, chemotaxis ensues. This is a directed movement of the neutrophil along a concentration gradient of specific molecules capable of stimulating cell movement. Neutrophils have specific receptor sites on their membrane that allow chemotactic agents to bind to the cell, thereby initiating the chemotactic response.

Several factors act as chemoattractants: products secreted by stimulated phagocytes and lymphocytes, bacterial and viral products, cleaved fragments of certain components of complement, and members of the coagulation and kinin pathways, to name a few.

Culture filtrates from numerous bacterial pathogens have chemotactic activity independent of any interaction with serum. Some bacteria produce proteinases capable of cleaving C3 and C5, thereby yielding the chemoattractants C3a and C5a. The other two methods by which chemotactic factors are produced depend upon the interaction of bacteria with either the classic complement sequence or the alternative pathway, both resulting ultimately in the production of C3a, C5a, and C567.

It is evident that many mechanisms are available by which chemotactic factors are produced, thereby ensuring that polymorphonuclear neutrophils are directed to the site of infection.

Opsonization

Having arrived at the focus of infection by chemotactic mechanisms, polymorphonuclear leukocytes must then

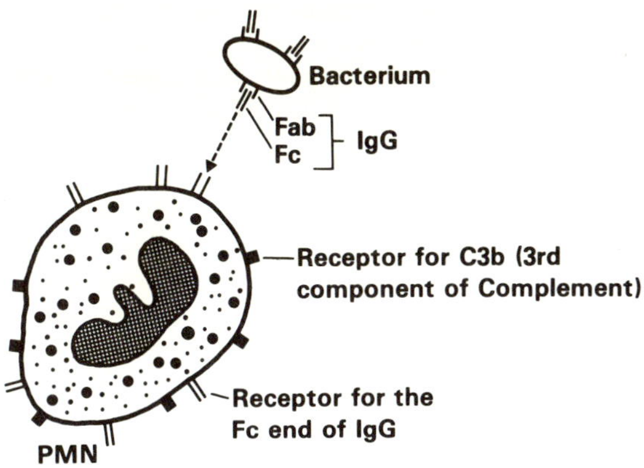

FIGURE 2.1. Opsonization and recognition.

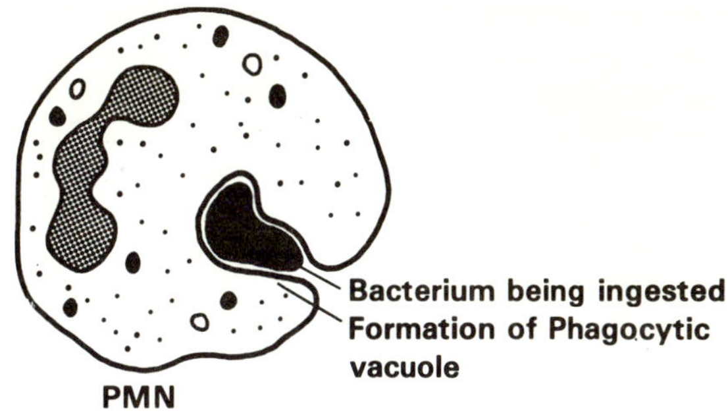

FIGURE 2.2. Phagocytosis.

be able to recognize and attach themselves to the bacteria if the processes of ingestion and killing are to take place. Substances in serum, collectively referred to as opsonins, coat the bacterial surface, thereby rendering the organisms more palatable to the phagocytic cells.

In humans, both heat-stable and heat-labile serum factors are capable of opsonizing bacteria. The former are made up of the first and third subclasses of IgG (IgG_1 and IgG3), while the latter is predominantly the third component of complement (C3b). There is also some support for the role of C5 as an opsonin in humans, but this is still somewhat controversial.

The antigen-combining sites in the $F(ab)_2$ part of the IgG molecule allow it to bind to antigen on the surface of the bacteria (Figure 2.1). Binding of IgG molecules to bacteria, then interaction of the Fc ends of these molecules with C1, and subsequent activation of the complement cascade lead to the cleavage of C3 into the chemotactic factor C3a and the opsonizing factor C3b that also binds to the surface of the bacteria. In the nonimmune state, since little or no specific antibody is available for activation of the classic complement pathway, the properdin system, or alternate pathway, is capable of generating the required C3b fragment.

Ingestion

By means of the receptors on the surface of the polymorphonuclear leukocyte for the Fc end of the IgG molecule and C3b, a mechanism for attachment of the opsonized bacteria to the neutrophil is provided (Figure 2.1). Once this contact is established, a signal triggers the formation of pseudopodia, which extend out from the polymorphonuclear leukocyte, gradually surround, and eventually completely encircle the organism (Figure 2.2). This process depends upon the sequential interaction of the Fc or C3b receptors on the polymorphonuclear leukocyte with ligands distributed over the surface of the particle about to be ingested, and has been referred to as the "zipper" mechanism of phagocytosis.

Another mechanism whereby phagocytosis can proceed in the absence of opsonization is referred to as surface phagocytosis. The bacteria may be trapped against a surface by the polymorphonuclear leukocyte and then ingested. In inflammatory exudates where the cell concentration is sufficiently high, a polymorphonuclear leukocyte may trap a bacterium against the surface of another cell. In the lung, bacteria may be trapped against alveolar walls. Phagocytosis is an energy-requiring process, and the adenosine triphosphate (ATP), which ultimately supplies this energy, is derived from glycolytic mechanisms rather than from oxidative phosphorylation.

Intracellular Killing

When the pseudopods have completely encircled the organism, a phagocytic vacuole or phagosome is formed. Two postphagocytic events then take place that provide the mechanisms whereby the internalized bacteria are killed. These are the respiratory burst and degranulation, and they are both related to membrane stimulation. One hypothesis is that their initiation is related to depolarization of the neutrophil membrane and calcium fluxes.

Respiratory Burst

The respiratory burst is a series of reactions that results in the two-electron reduction of oxygen, thereby providing a number of highly reactive agents that, either singly or in combination, are microbicidal. The metabolic events constituting the respiratory burst result in the following: (1) increased oxygen uptake; (2) increased superoxide anion production; (3) increased hydrogen peroxide production; and (4) increased hexose monophosphate shunt activity (HMP).

The primary reaction is the one-electron reduction of oxygen to superoxide anion catalyzed by nicotinamine-adenine dinucleotide phosphate (NADP) oxidase:

$$2O_2 + NADP \rightarrow 2O_2^- + NADPH^+ + H^+.$$

The superoxide anion is a free radical and undergoes spontaneous dismutation, resulting in the formation of hydrogen peroxide:

$$2O_2^- + 2H^+ \rightarrow {}^1O_2 + H_2O_2.$$

The HMP shunt, normally relatively inactive in nonphagocytosing cells, provides a mechanism of refurbishing the supply of NADP.

Through a series of reactions, two other reactive agents, singlet oxygen and hydroxyl radical, are produced. These plus superoxide anion and hydrogen peroxide account for part of the oxygen-dependent microbicidal mechanisms of the cell and are discussed later.

Degranulation

The other major postphagocytic event is degranulation. Polymorphonuclear leukocytes contain two distinct types of granules: primary granules, or lysosomes, and secondary, or so-called specific, granules. The former contain myeloperoxidase, acid hydrolases, and cationic proteins, while the latter contain alkaline phosphatase, lactoferrin, and lysozyme. The aim of the process of degranulation is to deliver the contents of the granules into the phagosomes. By fusion of the granule membrane with the membrane of the phagocytic vacuole, the granular contents that play a role in bacterial killing are delivered directly into the vacuole without leaking into the cytoplasm of the polymorphonuclear leukocyte.

The microbicidal mechanisms of the polymorphonuclear leukocyte can be considered as oxygen dependent and oxygen independent. Oxygen-dependent microbicidal activity can be further divided into myeloperoxidase-dependent and -independent reactions (Table 2.3). The former depends upon the interactions of myeloperoxidase, hydrogen peroxide, and a halide ion such as chloride or iodide. The activated halide is incorporated into the bacterial cell wall, resulting in structural and functional derangements and ultimately leading to the death of the organism. Another mechanism of action of the myeloperoxidase system is the decarboxylation of amino acids to aldehydes by the activated halide.

TABLE 2.3. Oxygen-dependent Microbicidal System

Myeloperoxidase-dependent	*Myeloperoxidase-independent*
MPO + H_2O_2 + halide*	Respiratory Burst
Halogenation of organisms	Superoxide anion
Amino acids, aldehydes	Hydrogen peroxide
Singlet oxygen	Singlet oxygen
	Hydroxyl radical

*MPO = myeloperonidase.

Singlet oxygen can also be produced by the interaction of the chloride, hydrogen peroxide, myeloperoxidase system or by interaction between the superoxide anion and hydrogen peroxide — the Haber-Weiss reaction. It can therefore be part of either the myeloperoxidase-dependent or -independent mechanism. Singlet oxygen itself may be bactericidal.

Oxygen-dependent myeloperoxidase-independent mechanisms include superoxide anion, hydrogen peroxide, singlet oxygen, and the hydroxyl radical. The Haber-Weiss reaction, which yields singlet oxygen, also produces the hydroxyl radical. Although the superoxide anion in itself is probably not directly toxic to the cell, the singlet oxygen and the hydroxyl radical may well be.

Oxygen-independent mechanisms rely on a decrease in intraphagosomal pH and the granular contents: lysozyme, lactoferrin, and cationic proteins. The decrease in pH in itself is harmful to some microorganisms, but its main purpose is to provide an optimal milieu for the enzyme activity necessary for bacterial killing. Lysozyme acts on bacterial cell walls, lactoferrin binds iron necessary for bacterial growth, and the cationic proteins react with bacterial surfaces, thereby inhibiting growth.

With macrophages, some of the chemotactic mediators are different from those that act on polymorphs, and with respect to intracellular killing, macrophages lack the cationic proteins found in polymorph granules and they do not have the same oxygen-dependent microbicidal system.

Immunologic Mechanisms

The immune response differs significantly from the nonspecific phagocytic response in two ways. First, it is specific for a particular antigen and second, it is an acquired response. The immune response itself can be broken down into antibody (or humoral), and cell-mediated components. With respect to infection, although not absolutely correct, the humoral arm can be considered to function primarily against pyogenic encapsulated bacteria and certain viruses, and the cell-mediated arm against facultative bacteria, fungi, and most viruses.

Initiation of the immune responses depends upon immunologically reactive lymphocytes, the B and T cells. These cells originate from the same precursor stem cells but subsequently develop along separate lines. One group of stem cells is processed in fetal liver and adult marrow and differentiates into mature B cells. The other group, influenced by factors in the thymus, differentiates into T cells. The B and T cells have surface receptors that enable them to interact with antigen, thereby initiating subsequent events.

Another subpopulation of lymphocytes is referred to as non-T, non-B cells. These include natural cytotoxic (natural killer, NK) cells and may play a role in immune surveillance against virus-infected cells and possibly tumor cells.

Plasma proteins and leukocytes constantly pass from capillaries into tissues and then into lymphatic capillaries, creating an ongoing recirculation of lymphocytes. During this process, lymphocytes come in contact with microbial antigens and provide the body with a sensitive surveillance mechanism: the cells primarily involved are T lymphocytes.

Central to this process is the macrophage. As described earlier, macrophages are capable of ingesting and killing invading pathogens, but in addition to this they are able to "process" microbial antigens and by presenting these foreign antigens to T cells, are able to initiate cell-mediated immunity. A subset of T cells (T helper cells) is able to provide a signal to reactive B cells to begin antibody production.

Humoral Immunity

Once stimulated, B cells undergo successive divisions until a clone of mature plasma cells is formed. A clone is then capable of producing immunoglobulin molecules of the same class with specificity for a single antigen. Some of the clone will persist as memory cells that are able to respond much more rapidly on reexposure to the same antigen.

The immunoglobulin IgM is produced first in response to infection and is then replaced by IgG. Although the half-life of IgG antibody is only approximately 25 days, one can often detect antibodies against a particular microbial antigen years later. This is probably achieved in one of two ways. In some cases, the host is repeatedly reexposed to that particular microbial antigen during subclinical infections. In other cases, certain organisms, such as Mycobacteria, can persist in the body and provide continual stimulation of the immune system.

In the case of newborn infants, antibody protection is provided by IgG that crosses the placenta and secretory IgA in breast milk.

There are five classes of immunoglobulins in humans: G, M, A, D, and E. Of these, the first three are important from the point of view of antibody. The basic structure of immunoglobulins consists of four polypeptide chains, two heavy and two light, in the shape of a Y. The Fab arms of the Y contain the sites that interact with antigen while the Fc end is used for complement activation and interaction with receptors on the surface of polymorphonuclear neutrophils and macrophages.

Immunoglobulin G (IgG) consists of four subclasses and is the major circulating type of antibody, although it can be found in lesser amounts in tissues. Immunoglobulin M (IgM) is a much larger molecule and is a pentamer consisting of five subunits. Because of its large size, IgM is virtually completely contained within the vascular compartment and does not cross the placenta. Since IgM is produced first in response to infection, it is generally only found during acute stages or in the recovery period.

Immunoglobulin A exists as a serum immunoglobulin and as secretory IgA. In its latter form, it is found on the mucosal surfaces of the gastrointestinal, respiratory, and urinary tracts and in human milk. Secretory IgA differs structurally from serum IgA in two important ways. It is a dimer rather than a monomer and it contains two additional polypeptide chains, the J chain and the secretory piece. The exact roles of these polypeptides are uncertain, but they probably stabilize the dimeric molecule and make it more resistant to proteolytic degradation. Secretory IgA appears to act by preventing pathogens from adhering to mucosal epithelium.

Immunoglobulin E is important in immediate hypersensitivity reactions. The functional significance of IgD is not yet known.

Antibodies can confer protection in a number of different ways.

1. Opsonizing activity — this has already been discussed in this chapter in the section dealing with phagocytosis. In addition to the standard method of opsonization, however, free antibody can combine with phagocytes, thereby acting as a cytophilic antibody and providing a measure of immunologic specificity to the phagocytic response.
2. Lysis of organisms — antibody in concert with complement can cause lysis of certain organisms. Immune lysis is due to binding of the antibody to the surface of the organism and activation of complement. This can be seen with certain gram-negative bacteria, viruses, protozoa, leptospiras, and spirochetes. It is not seen with gram-positive organisms.

   The complement system refers to a complex interaction of protein components that serve to mediate as well as to amplify immune reactions. Two major pathways have been described — classic and alternate. Activation of these pathways initiates a series of reactions that result in the production of chemoattractants, opsonins, anaphylotoxins, and a membrane attack complex that is capable of damaging various cells including certain pathogens.
3. Preventing attachment of organisms — antibodies such as secretory IgA probably protect against infection by bacterial and viral pathogens by preventing adherence to and penetration of host epithelial cells.
4. Neutralization of toxins — the first part of this chapter discussed how organisms may produce disease by elaborating exotoxins. In cases where exotoxin is produced in large enough quantities to be antigenic (e.g., diphtheria), antibody production to the toxin is stimulated thereby protecting the host by blocking attachment of the toxin to cells. In cases where very powerful exotoxins are elaborated in quantities too small to be antigenic (e.g., tetanus), active immunity can be acquired by injection of inactivated toxin (toxoid).

Cell-Mediated Immunity

With respect to infectious diseases, cell-mediated immunity (CMI) can be considered very simply as that resistance to infection provided by T lymphocytes and macrophages working in concert. Other areas where CMI plays a major role are tumor and transplantation immunology. These, however, are beyond the scope of this text.

The T-cell subpopulations can be defined in a number of ways such as by surface differentiation antigens and IgG receptors. From a functional point of view, however, there are essentially two subpopulations: regulatory and effector lymphocytes. The former can be further subdivided into helper and suppressor cells and the latter into those concerned with delayed hypersensitivity (DTH-reactive cells), cytotoxic T lymphocytes (killer cells), and mixed lymphocyte reactivity cells. Again, considering only infectious disease, the effector T cell functions of concern are the DTH-reactive cells since they are involved in infections such as tuberculosis, and the killer cells since they play a role in control of virus-infected cells. The final group, those involved in mixed lymphocyte reactivity reactions, are of more interest to tumor and transplantation immunologists.

As mentioned previously, macrophages play a key role in initiation of the immune response. Macrophages ingest pathogens and then in a manner not yet fully understood, present microbial antigens in such a way that they are recognized by the T lymphocytes. This antigen presentation provides the first of two signals necessary to activate either helper or DTH-reactive T cells. The second signal is provided by a soluble substance called interleukin 1. This is synthesized and released by the macrophage and acts on the T cell, stimulating it to produce another mediator called interleukin 2. This then acts on activated T cells causing them to proliferate.

The production of interleukins 1 and 2 illustrates two very important principles necessary for regulation of the immune response:

1. The production of biologically active molecules
2. The concept of cell to cell communication

Soluble mediators are produced by lymphocytes and cells of the monocyte-macrophage series. Those produced by lymphocytes are referred to as lymphokines and those by monocytes as monokines.

Lymphokines are produced by sensitized T cells after stimulation by antigen. Their primary function is to mediate and amplify cell-mediated immune reactions, but some are also able to affect B cells, thereby playing a role in regulating antibody production. The lymphokines that specifically affect cell-mediated reactions include a number of substances known to affect monocytes and macrophages. Examples of some of these are macrophage-activating factor, migration-inhibitory factor, as well as chemotactic factors for macrophages, neutrophils, eosinophils, and basophils.

Interleukin 1 is an example of a monokine, as are interferons, although these are also lymphokines. Interferons, in fact, represent a family of glycoproteins of which three types have been described to date: alpha, beta, and gamma. These are produced by leukocytes, fibroblasts, and lymphocytes respectively.

Interferons play a role in defense against viral infection. Several agents are known to induce their production, including viruses, bacteria, chlamydiae, rickettsias, and fungi. Protection does not depend on a direct effect upon the infecting virus, but rather on derepression of the host cell gene for viral translation-inhibitory protein, resulting in inhibition of messenger RNA translation. Interferons may also activate natural killer cells.

It is quite clear that an elaborate system of defenses protects the host against infection. Regulation and maintenance of this system are still not yet well understood, but the consequences of its breakdown are unfortunately usually all too obvious. Problems with infection in patients with impaired host defenses are discussed in Chapter 22.

ANNOTATED BIBLIOGRAPHY

Densen P, Mandell GL. Phagocyte strategy vs microbial tactics. Rev Infect Dis 1980;2:817–838.

An excellent review of how microorganisms developed ways of avoiding the host's phagocytic cells.

Dinarello CA. Interleukin 1. Rev Infect Dis 1984;6(1):51–95.

A detailed review of experimental and clinical data linking mediation of host responses to infection and inflammation with the activity of interleukin 1.

Gallin JI, Fauci AS, eds. Phagocytic cells. Advances in host defense mechanisms. Vol. 1. New York: Raven Press, 1982.

A collection of papers dealing with various aspects of phagocyte function. Emphasis is on basic science aspects of cell function but where appropriate, clinical relevance is discussed.

Mims CA, ed. The pathogenesis of infectious disease, 2nd edition. London: Academic Press, 1982.

An excellent overview of the entire area of pathogenetic mechanisms in microbiology and infectious disease. Concise, well written, and easy to follow.

Rubenstein E, Federman DD. Scientific American medicine. Vol. 7.

An up-to-date section on virtually all aspects of immunology. Easy to read with excellent diagrams.

Swanson J, Sparling PF, Puziss M, eds. Bacterial virulence and pathogenicity. Rev Infect Dis 1983; September-October (suppl).

The entire issue is devoted to papers dealing with bacterial virulence and pathogenicity. The selected topics fall into two broad categories: mechanisms of bacterial virulence and host resistance and defense.

3 METHODS OF RAPID DIAGNOSIS OF INFECTIOUS DISEASES

Ole Hammerberg and Max A. Chernesky

Diagnosis of an infectious disease generally depends upon cultivating and identifying incriminating microorganisms. For rapidly growing aerobic or facultatively anaerobic bacteria, final identification by conventional methodology takes at least 48 to 72 hours, although in many instances, microorganisms are fastidious and grow slowly in vitro or cannot be cultivated at all. In such instances, diagnosis often depends upon seroconversion of the host to similar or related antigens, and thus it can only be made retrospectively. Therefore the time required to diagnose infections in the laboratory often falls short of clinical requirements.

There has evolved an interest in the development of rapid diagnostic methods in infectious diseases. Such methods are defined as diagnostic techniques that establish a diagnosis definitively or presumptively in sufficiently short a period to influence patient management. This chapter outlines such methods, some of which are currently investigational, but most are already used widely in the diagnosis of infectious diseases. These methods have been applied in the areas of bacteriology, virology, mycology, and serology. In the future, clinicians will increasingly discover that diseases that used to take weeks or even months to diagnose can be identified in much shorter periods.

Some of the advantages of prompt diagnosis include the following:

1. A rapid, specific, etiologic diagnosis of severely ill patients is highly desirable. For example, rapid detection of antigen in cerebrospinal fluid of patients with bacterial meningitis can result in early and appropriate management.
2. Inappropriate administration of antimicrobial agents is minimized by early knowledge of the etiologic diagnosis. This in turn results in fewer adverse reactions to such drugs and reduces selection for resistant bacteria.
3. Sample sizes required for rapid diagnosis techniques are often smaller than those required for conventional cultivation. This may enhance the diagnostic yield in certain groups of patients such as small children and infants, from whom large sample sizes are difficult to obtain.
4. Certain microorganisms can only be identified by rapid methods and cannot be cultivated by conventional methods, for example, hepatitis B and rotaviruses.
5. Rapid diagnostic methods are usually less labor intensive and are amenable to automation, thus decreasing the cost of laboratory tests.

STAINS

Many stains have been described for use in medical practice. Those used most commonly to detect microorganisms in clinical material are Gram's, acid-fast, Giemsa, silver, India ink (negative), and iodine stains (Table 3.1).

In general, positive stains of bacteria and fungi in body fluids only provide a provisional diagnosis, but when considering the clinical context this can be extremely useful. For example, gram-negative diplococci in cerebrospinal fluid (CSF) from a patient with puru-

TABLE 3.1. Types of Microorganisms Detected in Clinical Specimens with Commonly Used Stains

Stain	*Microorganisms Identified*
Gram's	Bacteria, yeasts
Acid-fast	*Mycobacteria, nocardia*
Giemsa	*Chlamydia, plasmodia* (malaria), other blood and tissue protozoa
Silver	Tissue protozoa, yeasts, filamentous fungi
India	*Cryptococcus neoformans* (negative stain of capsule)
Iodine	Stool protozoa and helminths

lent meningitis would almost invariably indicate a diagnosis of meningococcal meningitis. This would be specific enough to initiate therapy with penicillin without the need for chloramphenicol, which is usually combined with penicillin to treat purulent meningitis when the Gram's stain is negative or not available.

When the microorganism cannot be cultured, a stain of the clinical specimen may provide the only means of diagnosis. Thus a Giemsa stain of a blood film is the definitive method used to diagnose malaria and the silver stain of lung tissue or aspirate is the definitive method used to diagnose *Pneumocystis carinii* (tissue protozoa) pneumonia.

The Gram's and acid-fast stains, in particular the Kinyoun method, are simple enough that they can be performed by clinical personnel. It must be remembered, however, that appropriately concentrated body fluids (e.g., CSF) may increase the sensitivity, and thus interpretation of the stains is best accomplished by the experienced. Staining should also be quality controlled by the inclusion of known positive and negative smears. It is easy for the inexperienced observer to confuse crystal violet sediment for gram-positive cocci or inadequately decolorized bacteria as acid-fast organisms.

Gram's Stain

Not only is the Gram's stain used to examine bacteria in clinical specimens, it also serves as a basis for the taxonomic classification of bacteria.

It was described by the Danish microbiologist Gram in 1884. Although this procedure has been widely performed for almost a century, its mechanism of action remains largely unknown. It has been speculated that the difference between gram-positive and gram-negative bacteria is based on the composition of the cell wall. This appears unlikely, since yeasts, which possess a very different cell wall composition from bacteria, stain gram-positive and mechanically traumatized gram-positive bacteria stain gram-negative. The difference is now postulated to be based on cell wall permeability. Gram-positive bacteria are believed to possess a cell wall barrier to the elution of the dye-iodine complex by alcohol.

Method

1. On a precleaned, dry microscope slide place a drop of specimen. If it is quite purulent, spread with a sterile cotton swab or bacteriology loop to prevent too thick a smear.
2. Allow smear to dry completely, and heat-fix without overheating the glass (one should be able to touch slide).
3. Place slide on a stain rack in a sink and apply crystal violet solution for approximately one minute, *after* filtering the solution to remove stain particles.
4. Wash with tap water. Apply Gram's iodine for approximately one minute.
5. Wash with tap water and decolorize with 95% ethyl alcohol or acetone alcohol until the stain appears to have been removed (approximately 5 to 10 seconds, longer if smear is thick).
6. Wash with tap water. Counterstain with safranine for approximately 30 seconds. Wash one final time with tap water and allow smear to dry (this can be done quickly by blotting).

Although ideally, control smears should be done when performing Gram's stains, an experienced person may not routinely need to include such smears since the appearance of the neutrophils and bacteria will reveal the adequacy of the stain and the staining technique. Gram-positive bacteria appear dark blue and gram-negative pink. The smear should quickly be screened under the high dry lens for an area abundant in neutrophils and bacteria. If the neutrophils do not appear as distinctly polymorphonuclear, the slide was probably overheated during heat fixation. The pattern (gram-positive or -negative), bacterial morphology (rods vs. cocci, chains vs. clusters), and relationship to the neutrophils should be observed under oil immersion.

Acid-Fast Stain

Mycobacteria are difficult to stain due to their highly lipid nature. Once stained, however, the color is difficult to remove even by using acid alcohol, hence the term acid-fast. Conventionally, carbolfuchsin is heated to accomplish staining, but with the Kinyoun method (described here) this is unnecessary, which simplifies the procedure.

Method

1. Prepare smear and heat-fix as above. Note that *M. tuberculosis* is highly contagious, and one should handle specimens only when using an appropriate biologic safety hood.
2. Always prepare positive and negative control smears to evaluate whether staining procedure is satisfactory.
3. On a staining rack in a sink, flood slides with Kinyoun carbolfuchsin and leave for two minutes.
4. Wash with tap water and decolorize by applying 3% acid alcohol until all the stain has been removed from slide.
5. Wash with tap water and counterstain by flooding slide with methylene blue (0.3%) for approximately 30 seconds. Wash with tap water and blot dry.

Mycobacteria appear as slender pink rods against a light blue background. Since they are small and often scarce in clinical specimens, the whole smear must be examined under oil immersion. Recently, fluorescent dyes have been used to screen specimens more easily by fluorescence microscopy.

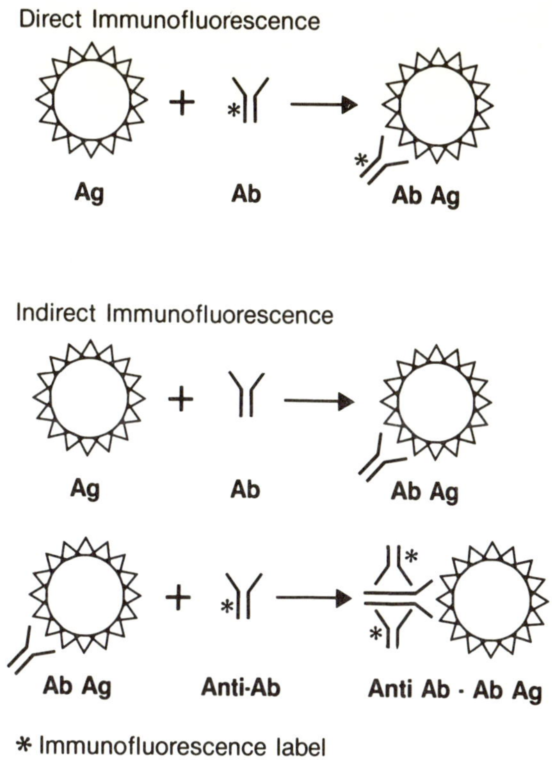

FIGURE 3.1. Direct and indirect immunofluorescence.

IMMUNOFLUORESCENCE

Immunofluorescence (IF) is based on tagging antibodies with a fluorescent conjugate such as fluorescein, which allows them to be visualized by fluorescence microscopy. The fluorescent antibody can either be specific for a particular antigen (direct IF) or nonspecifically directed against antibody (indirect IF). The antigen to be detected must be attached to a particle or organisms that can be fixed onto a slide. Thus the procedure is used to detect fixed rather than soluble antigen.

Direct immunofluorescence is essentially a one-stage procedure (Figure 3.1). For each antigen to be detected, a specific immunofluorescent antibody must be used. This procedure has proved to be highly specific and sensitive in detecting several bacterial and viral antigens. Such antigens can be detected in smears of body fluids, sections of tissue, or smears from cultures of clinical materials.

Indirect immunofluorescence is a two-stage procedure (Figure 3.1). An antiimmunoglobulin fluorescent antibody is added to the antibody-antigen complex previously prepared. Hence, unlike direct immunofluorescence, the immunofluorescent antibody is not specifically aimed against a particular antigen and only one fluorescent antibody is required for any number of tests. Additionally, this method is not restricted to detection of antigen, but can also be used to measure serum antibodies.

As in the case of nonimmunologic staining procedures, expertise is required to interpret an immunofluorescent smear or tissue section. In particular, it is easy to confuse fluorescent microorganisms with nonspecific fluorescence. Therefore positive and negative controls should always be included to determine the ade-

TABLE 3.2. Immunofluorescent Tests Currently Used in Diagnostic Microbiology

Immunofluorescent Assay	*Comment*
Group A streptococci	Organisms can be rapidly and reliably detected from throat swabs by IF following brief incubation in broth.
L. pneumophila	IF is used to detect *Legionella* in sputum or lung tissue. Several serotypes exist.
B. pertussis	IF has been applied for detection of this organism in nasopharyngeal aspirates after brief incubation in broth. This method is less sensitive than conventional cultures.
Herpes simplex virus	Virus can be rapidly detected by IF in brain tissue or corneal scrapings. This should not replace viral cultures.
Rocky Mountain spotted fever	IF can be performed on skin biopsy tissue of lesions to provide a rapid diagnosis.
Respiratory viruses	IF on nasal epithelial cell washings can rapidly indicate the presence of respiratory viruses. Some of these viruses may not be readily propagated in vitro.

quacy of the specimen. Major factors that also determine the specificity of this procedure, as in all immunologic assays, are the quality of the antiserum, its specificity for the antigen and well conjugated antisera. Antisera that cross-react with either related or nonspecific antigens are obviously likely to produce false positive assays. Examples of currently used IF tests in diagnostic microbiology are summarized in Table 3.2.

COUNTERIMMUNOELECTROPHORESIS, LATEX AGGLUTINATION, AND COAGGLUTINATION

Unlike immunofluorescence, which is used to detect antigens that are fixed to the microorganisms, counterimmunoelectrophoresis (CIE), latex agglutination

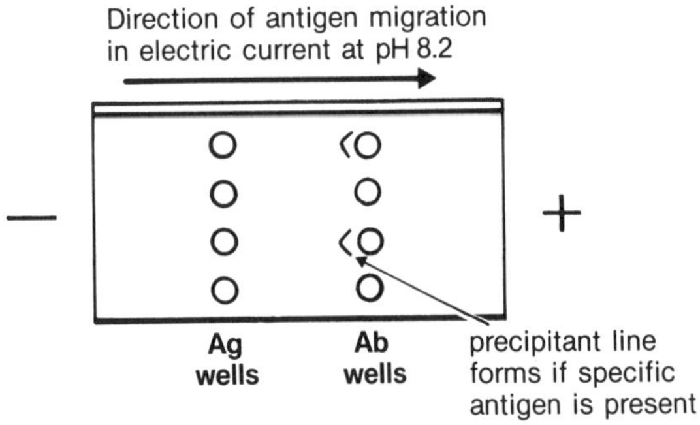

FIGURE 3.2. Schematic illustration of a CIE agarose gel-coated slide with antigen and antibody wells.

(LA), and coagglutination (CoA) can be used to detect antigens that are not fixed but occur freely in body fluids, referred to as soluble antigens.

The principle of immunodiffusion assays, including CIE, is that antigen-antibody complexes precipitate in gelled media. At a basic pH of 8.2 to 8.6, antigens are negatively charged and thus migrate electrophoretically toward the anode by a process called electroendosmosis. Wells containing antibody and antigen are cut to oppose each other on agarose gel-coated slides. When a current is applied, the antigen migrates toward the antibody-containing wells in the direction of the anode. This technique is especially suited for antigen detection since it is performed in the presence of antibody excess and since minimal dilution of antigen occurs in the gel due to prevention of lateral diffusion. When the antigen meets a specific antibody near the antibody-containing wells, a precipitation line forms (Figure 3.2).

CIE has been used in a variety of clinical settings. It has been applied most widely to the rapid detection of bacterial antigens in body fluids in cases of meningitis. It has also been applied to the detection of *Cryptococcus neoformans*, hepatitis B, and *Pneumocystis carinii* antigen in body fluids. Much of the application of CIE for rapid diagnosis has largely been replaced by LA and CoA, however.

LA for antigen detection is based on the principles of the indirect passive agglutination assays. Antigen or antibody can be bound to inert particles that serve as passive carriers and act as agglutinogens, indicating specific antigen-antibody reactions by the appearance of agglutination. One of the most widely used substances is latex, a polystyrene polymer. In the case of antigen assay, specific antibody is absorbed onto latex particles of uniform diameter. This preparation can be applied to detect soluble antigen directly from body fluids. The major advantages of this test, especially in comparison with CIE, are simplicity of performance, enhanced sensitivity, and no requirements for expensive equipment. Commercial LA kits tend to be expensive, however.

In addition, the method detects smaller amounts of antigen than CIE. In instances where the LA reagents are prepared in reference laboratories or commercially, the clinical laboratory simply mixes the antibody-coated latex particles with a preparation of body fluids or other antigen-containing solution and observes if an agglutination of the particles occur. The importance of appropriate positive and negative controls cannot be overemphasized, however, including controls containing nonsensitized latex particles. Rheumatoid factor, an anti-IgG immmunoglobulin, which is present in some patients' sera, and cross-reacting antigens may produce false positive agglutinations.

The agglutinogen in coagglutination is a strain of *Staphylococcus aureus* that has protein A on the outer surface (Cowan strain). The Fab fragment of IgG is bound to staphylococci and is thus free to bind to the homologous antigen. Agglutination occurs when antibody-coated *S. aureus* organisms are incubated with material containing homologous antigen. There are several commercial coagglutination kits that can be used to detect rapidly the presence of various bacterial antigens in body fluids. As with LA, no equipment is necessary for CoA, as these agglutination reactions are detected on a slide by simply mixing the appropriate reagents with the clinical material. It must be emphasized that whenever these tests are performed, appropriate positive and negative controls must be used. Also, there is always a concern regarding agglutination with related antigens that may yield false positive results. There also exists the possibility that some patients may have antibody directed against *S. aureus* and that this could result in false positive agglutination.

Recently, many LA and CoA kits have been introduced commercially. These have been developed primarily for the rapid detection of bacterial antigens in body fluids in meningitis. They are generally highly specific and sensitive. The introduction of monoclonal antisera for preparation of such kits will likely further enhance their sensitivity and specificity as well as broaden their clinical application.

SOLID-PHASE IMMUNOASSAYS

Solid-phase immunoassays (SPIA) for the detection of antigens or antibodies use as indicators a radioactive label for the radioimmunoassay (RIA) or the action of an enzyme on a substrate as a label for the enzyme-linked immunosorbent assay (ELISA). Most SPIAs for the detection of antigen employ one of three methods: (1) competitive, (2) direct (double-antibody sandwich method), or (3) indirect (double-antibody sandwich-antiglobulin method) (Figure 3.3).

In competitive assays, labeled antigen is mixed with the test sample that contains antigen and they compete for a limited amount of antibody attached to the solid phase. A negative control sample containing only labeled antigen is included. Unbound antigen is washed away and the difference in indicator activity between the specimen and control is measured (Figure 3.3A).

A direct SPIA for detection of antigen involves adding the clinical specimen to a capture antibody (CA) attached to the solid phase (Figure 3.3B). Unbound antigen is washed away before the addition of a labeled detector antibody (DA). The DA is measured spectrophotometrically or visually (ELISA) or in a radioactive counter (RIA). The more labeled substrate detected, the more antigen present in the sample.

The indirect test is similar to the direct assay employing a CA and DA, but the DA is not labeled. Instead, a third indicator antibody (IA) that is antispecies to DA is labeled; the remainder of the assay is similar to the direct procedure (Figure 3.3C). This approach has become the most popular because of the availability of IA conjugates from commercial sources. The indirect test provides some amplification of the binding reactions, similar to that experienced in indirect IF. They may create some problems, however, as they are very sensitive and antispecies antisera may cross-react nonspecifically.

Several solid phases have been used, including test tubes, microtiter plates, beads, filter paper, discs, and resins. Immunoglobulins adhere to many plastics by hydrogen bonding. Therefore covalent bonding of CA to the solid phase by reagents such as gluteraldehyde or cyanogen bromide is usually not necessary. The type of solid phase will dictate the kinds of instrumentation to be used for the steps in the procedure.

If polyclonal antibodies are used in these tests they should be prepared by the inoculation of purified antigen into animals. The immunoglobulins may be used in

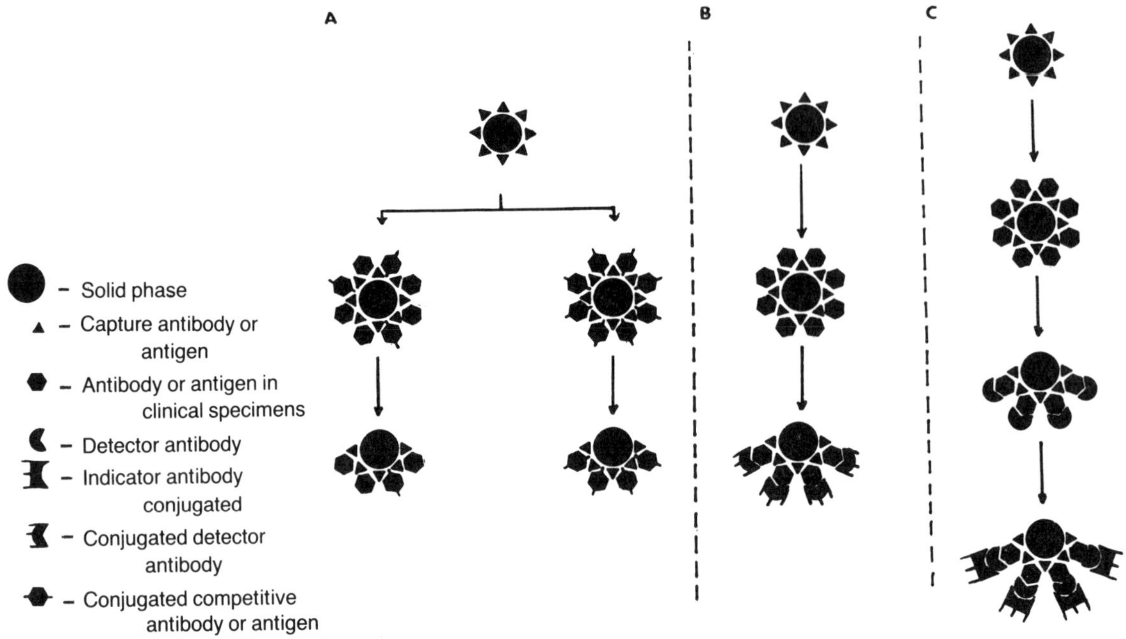

FIGURE 3.3. Solid-phase immunoassays. (A) Competitive. (B) Direct. (C) Indirect.

serum or after precipitation. Different species antibodies should be used in double-antibody systems and they should be predominantly of the IgG class. Optimal dilutions of CA, DA, and IA are determined by checkerboard titrations and optimal incubation conditions (time and temperature) must be determined. In ELISA, optimal conditions for enzyme-substrate reactions must also be achieved. The two most widely used enzymes are peroxidase and alkaline phosphatase, and iodine 125 has become a convenient label for RIA. Monoclonal antibodies are becoming increasingly popular as highly specific reagents for SPIA purposes.

The ELISAs may be designed to observe qualitative or quantitative color changes that indicate the presence or absence of an antigen or antibodies in a clinical specimen. In the qualitative type of test, a positive specimen is determined by comparing the reaction to that in a predetermined positive. In a quantitative assay a spectrophotometer (ELISA) or gamma counter (RIA) is used, and several control specimens with known quantities of reagent are included to construct a reaction curve to determine the positivity or negativity of an unknown. Results are expressed as optical density or radioactive counts, then reported as positive or negative after necessary calculations with the mean of a suitable number of controls. The specificity of each test result can be controlled by testing each specimen in duplicate. Thus the second test is performed with a control solid phase. Alternatively, all positives should be confirmed using a blocking technique in which the known is incubated with immune serum before it is added to the CA, or blocked with an unlabeled IA before adding the appropriate conjugate. Elimination or significant depression of the positive reaction should be observed.

The SPIA techniques have been successfully applied to detect many microorganisms or antibody responses. Commercial kits are available for the detection of hepatitis B markers as well as other infections. Fluid specimens are most appropriate to detect viral antigens by ELISA. Serum may be used directly in these tests, whereas urine and feces may need homogenization with saline and preliminary clarification by centrifugation before they are suitable. Nasopharyngeal or sputum specimens should be collected into appropriate transport media, then diluted in 20% *N*-acetyl cysteine before use in the test.

The ELISA assays offer two main advantages: reagents are relatively stable and nonradioactive, and the results can be either qualitative or quantitative. They are usually more sensitive than all other assays, except

RIA. The equipment necessary for these tests can be quite simple and objective. Inherent disadvantages include the variability of solid-phase carriers and the possible carcinogenicity of certain chromogenic substrates and radioactive labels. Most SPIAs require a day or overnight incubation with several washing procedures. For the optimal use of SPIA in rapid viral diagnosis, several specimens should be examined for antigen in a given run. Thus SPIA techniques are best suited for diseases such as viral gastroenteritis, viral hepatitis, or respiratory infections where many specimens are submitted to the laboratory at a given time. Although a single specimen could be analyzed, quite often an alternative assay (IF, EM, etc.) might be more appropriate.

IgM IMMUNOASSAYS

Another approach to identifying a microorganism or antigen in a clinical specimen is to detect early antibody responses in the serum or body fluids (IgM). Techniques have been described using solid-phase assays and several forms of indicator systems (immunofluorescence, radioactivity, ELISA, and erythrocytes). One method (Figure 3.4) has been to use a capture antigen immunoassay in which specific IgM in the specimen is sandwiched in between antigen on the solid phase and a tagged antibody (direct technique). This can be modified into an indirect technique by using a labeled antispecies indicator. A second method is a capture antibody system that uses antihuman IgM antibody attached to a solid phase (Figure 3.4). Trapped IgM from the clinical specimen can be sandwiched first with labeled or unlabeled antigen and then a labeled antibody to this antigen. Capture antigen immunoassays using anti-IgM conjugates may result in false positive results if the serum being tested contains rheumatoid factor (RF) and IgG. The RF is an IgM antibody binding to Fc portions of IgG. If positive, the specimen must be treated by a procedure such as latex agglutination to remove rheumatoid factor. The IgG antibody may inhibit the binding of specific IgM, particularly when high titers of IgG yield false negative results. The IgG may have to be removed by SPA. Solid-phase IgM systems have been described and successfully used to measure early antibody responses in hepatitis A, cytomegalovirus, toxoplasmosis, Coxsackie B virus, Japanese B encephalitis, and rubella, and some are available as commercial kits.

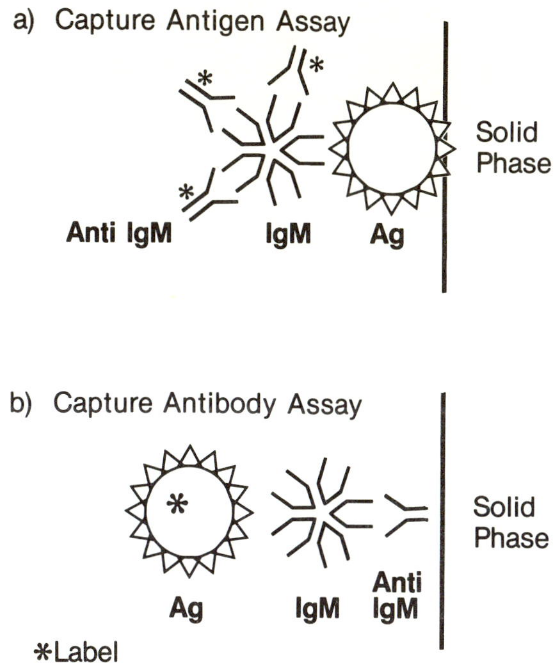

FIGURE 3.4. Schematic illustration of IgM immunoassays.

A solid-phase immunosorbent test (SPIT) employs erythrocytes as an indicator system. Microtiter wells are coated with antihuman IgM and the test serum is added, then followed by a series of reagents similar to a solid-phase hemagglutination inhibition assay. The test has been described to detect rubella IgM and modified according to the concentration of erythrocytes added into a hemadsorption inhibition test (HIT). Thus with the use of solid-phase technology and a variety of novel indicator systems, serologic procedures performed on single early sera may often be the best approach for rapid diagnosis, especially when brisk IgM antibody responses are manifested (hepatitis A, rubella, toxoplasmosis, etc.).

ELECTRON MICROSCOPY

Diseases for which electron microscopy (EM) has played a role in rapid diagnosis include gastroenteritis, herpes simplex infections, varicella zoster, variola, vaccinia, congenital cytomegalovirus infection, viral hepatitis, pustular contagious dermatitis, molluscum contagiosum, and warts.

Specimens should be collected and transported at ambient temperature in sealed containers to prevent drying. Depending upon the type of clinical specimen, centrifugation may help to prepare it better. Feces can be prepared by making a 10% to 20% suspension in distilled water and then clarifying with a bench centrifuge if necessary. Vesicle fluid should be collected from unbroken lesions using a tuberculin syringe containing a small amount of distilled water. A sheath should be placed over the needle and tape applied to the plunger and sheath before the instrument is transported to the laboratory inside an appropriate container. Urine should be centrifuged at 2500g for 30 minutes. The supernatant fluid will usually yield virus more readily if as large a volume as possible is used. Serum contains many low-molecular-weight proteins that must be washed out by diluting with an equal volume of distilled water. As with urine, centrifugation for one hour at 1500 g is necessary, and the serum may even require recentrifugation to provide a cleaner preparation. Biopsy or autopsy tissue should be frozen and thawed, or mechanically homogenized using a mortar and pestle or homogenizer. After this, a relatively smooth suspension can be achieved by mixing the homogenate in small amounts of distilled water using a fine-bore Pasteur pipette. Other less commonly examined specimens such as conjunctival scrapings or cerebrospinal fluid should be examined directly without centrifugation. Sputum specimens should be diluted in saline, then homogenized or treated with 20% *N*-acetyl cysteine.

The most appropriate laboratory technique for EM examination of clinical specimens is negative staining, and the most commonly used stain is phosphotungstic acid (PTA) as a 2% to 4% solution adjusted to a pH of 6 to 8 with 1 normal potassium hydroxide and stored as a working solution at 4°C. Formvar and carbon-coated, 400-mesh copper grids provide the most versatile carriers for specimen viewing. The technique involves placing a drop of the specimen on a drop of sterile distilled water that has been placed on a waxed surface (Figure 3.5). A grid held by fine forceps is touched to the drop, held upright, and stained with a drop of PTA. Excess fluid is removed by blotting with a strip of filter paper, after which the specimen is dried before EM examination. The total process takes about five minutes.

Because many specimens contain too few virus particles to enable viewing ($<10^6$ particles per ml), techniques to enhance visualization may be appropriate.

Ultracentrifugation should be performed on all negative specimens when those results might affect management of an ill patient or of a person exposed to disease. The specimen is spun to deposit bacteria and other large contaminants before pelleting. The supernatant is pelleted and then resuspended in phosphate buffer or distilled water before being stained and examined.

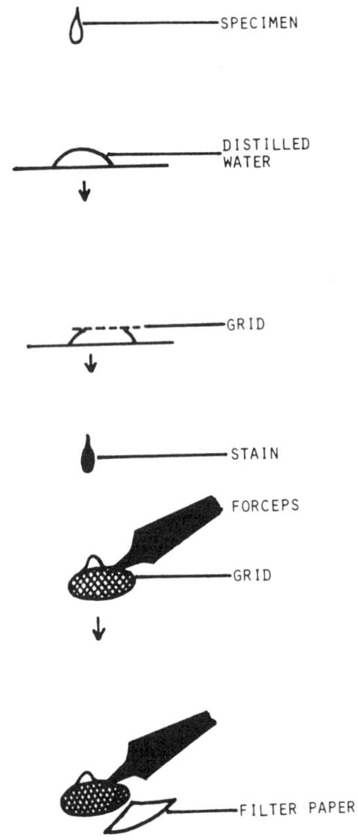

FIGURE 3.5. Schematic illustration of specimen preparation for electron microscopy.

The techniques of pseudoreplication and agar gel diffusion employ the principle of diffusing the liquid phase of the specimen into an agar substrate and concentrating virus particles on the surface. These techniques can be used successfully on clinical specimens such as urine or feces, but require a preliminary centrifugation step to remove larger debris from the specimen. A modification of these techniques incorporates antibodies into the agar (serum-in-agar technique). Immune electron microscopy (IEM) is becoming increasingly popular as a method for rescuing microorganisms from clinical specimens. Specific antibody is used to create aggregates of viral particles, thereby enhancing detection. This technique has been used to detect rubella virus, the Norwalk agent, and hepatitis A virus. Solid-phase IEM techniques have emerged that use staphylococcal protein A to stick virus-specific capture antibody onto formvar-carbon-coated grids. These highly specific immunosorbent grids have been shown to increase the sensitivity of electron microscopy for certain viruses 100- to 1000-fold. Thus, solid-phase techniques similar to those described employing enzymes or radioactive tags as indicators have been devised for the electron microscope.

RADIOMETRIC CULTURES

Radiometric detection of radioactive carbon dioxide, which is generated by bacterial metabolism of carbon 14-labeled precursors in culture media, serves the basis of a new approach to automated detection of growth of bacteria in vitro. This technique is now widely employed to detect growth in blood cultures and of mycobacteria. Instruments and culture media are commercially available from Johnston Laboratories, Cockeysville, Maryland, and are known as the BACTEC system. Culture bottles are analyzed for growth of bacteria by an instrument that flushes out the air overlying the broth and detects the level of radioactive carbon dioxide. This level is translated by the instrument to a growth index. A growth index of 30 or above indicates a positive blood culture, and a significant increase of the index indicates a positive mycobacterial culture.

In the case of blood cultures, the BACTEC system does not necessarily result in more rapid detection of growth than manually performed methods in which simply the turbidity of broth is observed. The ability of a clinical laboratory to process blood cultures by automated methods allows for more frequent determinations per day of growth, and this occasionally results in more rapid detection. The most up-to-date BACTEC instrument can process bottles 24 hours per day since an incubator is included. This enables cultures to be processed during hours the laboratory is closed and results in earlier reporting of some specimens.

The BACTEC system has been recently applied to the radiometric recording of mycobacterial growth. The average time for *M. tuberculosis* to be detected on agar slants inoculated with clinical specimens is three weeks. The average duration of time for this organism to be detected from sputum specimens cultured in BACTEC bottles is seven to ten days. In addition, antimicrobic susceptibility tests of mycobacteria can be performed using radiometric techniques, which may also result in considerable saving of time.

Most of the methods discussed in this chapter are used routinely in laboratories. Because the pathogenesis of each infection varies, the approach to diagnosis often requires several of these techniques. Thus it is important to emphasize that the appropriateness of collection and transportation of specimens will influence the outcome of the rapid diagnostic technique.

ANNOTATED BIBLIOGRAPHY

Balows A, Tilton R, eds. Body fluids and infectious diseases — clinical and microbiological advances. Am J Med 1983; (suppl): 75;1–148.

Many authors contributed to this symposium and summarized most aspects of rapid diagnosis.

Freedman AD, Gray CG. Rapid diagnosis of infection. Pediatr Infect Dis 1982;1:366–373.

Brief, well-referenced review of clinical applications of various mainly immunologic methods of rapid diagnosis. Bacterial and viral infections are discussed.

Koneman EW, Allen SD, Dowell VR Jr, Sommers HM. Color atlas and textbook of diagnostic microbiology, 2nd edition. Philadelphia: JB Lippincott, 1983.

Excellent clinical microbiology textbook for medical students and practitioners. Many illustrations and tables, and concise text. Especially useful for further reading regarding collection and transportation of specimens, staining, and direct microscopy.

Lennette EH, Schmidt NJ. Diagnostic procedures for viral, rickettsial, and chlamydial infections, 5th edition. Washington, DC: American Public Health Association, 1979.

A major reference manual for virological laboratory procedures. Many procedures discussed in the preceding chapter are presented in detail.

Tilton RC, ed. Rapid methods and automation in microbiology. Proceedings of the Third International Symposium on Rapid Methods and Automation in Microbiology, Washington DC, May 1981. Washington DC: American Society for Microbiology, 1982.

Summary of the state of the art of many aspects of rapid bacterial, viral, and chlamydial diagnosis. A large number of authors, all experts in their respective fields, contributed.

4 SEROLOGY AND SKIN TESTING

H. Grant Stiver

Serologic testing for the diagnosis of infection determines the presence of antibody or antigen in body fluids, usually serum, urine, or cerebrospinal fluid (CSF). Serologic methods are particularly useful in situations in which specimens for culture are difficult to obtain or when the potential pathogens are difficult or impossible to culture.

Although identification of antigen is determined by the presence or absence of components of the infectious agent, the detection of antibody depends upon the ability of the host to recognize the invading pathogen and then to produce the appropriate antibody. Usually one looks for a fourfold rise in antibody titer between sera taken from those who are acutely ill and persons who are convalescent, although in some cases a single high titer may be diagnostic. Obviously, various clinical conditions could interfere with this response, for example, dysproteinemias such as multiple myeloma, administration of cancer chemotherapy or immunosuppressive therapy, or severe malnutrition. Making an accurate diagnosis also depends greatly on the sensitivity and specificity of the test itself. Many tests are associated with a high frequency of cross-reactions with related organisms, resulting in false positive results (low specificity) and false negative results (low sensitivity). A good practice is to consult the director of the serology or microbiology laboratory if one has questions about which tests to order or how to interpret results.

Finally, partly because of the limitations of serology as described, one should always attempt to identify infectious agents by smear and/or culture whenever possible. These techniques are often more rapid and specific than serologic results.

INFECTIONS IN WHICH SEROLOGIC TESTS CONSTITUTE THE MAIN METHOD OF DIAGNOSIS

Mycoplasmal Pneumonia

Identification of *Mycoplasma pneumoniae* can be suspected on clinical grounds but confirmation depends upon either positive cultures or serology. Cultures require special hypertonic media and identifiable growth may take up to three weeks. A rapid but nonspecific serologic test is one for cold agglutinins, positive in about 50% of *M. pneumoniae* infections. A quick bedside screen can be done by taking heparinized blood from the patient and from a control, cooling the tubes in a paper cup with ice, and looking for granularity of the blood (agglutinating red cells) on the sides of the tube. The granularity should disappear on rewarming the tubes in one's hands. A positive bedside test correlates with a quantitative titer of 1:64, and should be confirmed by laboratory titration. Cold agglutinins may be positive in other infections such as mononucleosis, adenoviral infections, and rubella, but titers are usually less than 1:64. High titers may occur in certain hematologic malignancies and paraproteinemias.

The most specific method is the complement fixation test for *M. pneumoniae* antibodies. One may sometimes get a fourfold rise in 10 days. Single titers are difficult to interpret unless they are very high ($\geq$ 1:128) in a patient with a compatible clinical illness.

Viral Infections

Most practicing physicians do not order viral cultures unless a virus laboratory is readily available or an efficient system for transporting specimens exists. Recent advances in rapid tests, such as enzyme-linked immunosorbent assay (ELISA) and fluorescent antibody kits, may make viral diagnoses more readily available to family physicians, even in rural areas. At the present time, however, they are usually made through serologic testing of serum. There are two commonly recognized problems from the laboratory's point of view: (1) acute-phase serum is received, but only in 10% to 20% of cases does a convalescent sample arrive, and (2) the physician often writes "blood for viral studies" on the requisition, thus preventing the laboratory from being able to direct the serologic investigation in a discriminating manner. Details of serologic testing for viruses are listed in Table 4.1.

TABLE 4.1. Serodiagnosis of Viral Diseases

Suspected Problem	*Serologic Test*	*Interpretation*
Respiratory infection (non-immunosuppressed patient)	Respiratory battery, usually includes influenza A and B; adenovirus, parainfluenza 1, 2, and 3; respiratory syncytial virus; *M. pneumoniae* and coxsackievirus A and B	A single titer is very difficult to irfterpret. Complement fixation (CF) titers usually rise and fall over several months, whereas hemagglutination inhibition titers may be high for more than a year. Paired sera 2 weeks apart showing 4-fold rise is the only sure way to make a positive diagnosis.
Respiratory infection (immunosuppressed patient)	Above tests plus cytomegalovirus CF and herpes simplex titers	4-fold rise in titer is diagnostic; should be accompanied by efforts to demonstrate virus in urine, bone marrow, buffy coat leukocytes and biopsy material.
Diarrhea		
Norwalk agent	Not available	
Rotavirus	Complement fixation, fluorescent antibody*	4-fold rise.
Enteroviruses	Neutralization test*	Useful if serum can be tested against a positive viral isolate from the stool, or in an epidemic known to be due to a certain serotype. There are too many serotypes to make neutralization testing on all reference strains practical.
	Complement fixation	CF titers may be higher with other enteroviruses than with the actual infecting strain. Therefore as an indicator of the infecting serotype, the test has limited usefulness.
Hepatitis		
A	Anti-HA IgM antibodies (ELISA)	Present at the time of clinical illness, and in any titer indicates active or very recent infection.

TABLE 4.1. *(continued)*

Suspected Problem	*Serologic Test*	*Interpretation*
	Anti-HA IgG antibodies	Appear later than IgM, persist for life, and indicate immunity. 4-fold rise is diagnostic of acute infection.
B	HB surface antigen (HBsAg)	Presence in serum indicates infection, either as the asymptomatic carrier state or clinical hepatitis, depending on results of liver function tests.
	Anti-HBs antibodies (HBsAb)	4-fold rise indicates recent infection and a static titer correlates with immunity due to a previous HBV infection (which may have been asymptomatic), provided the patient has not received gamma globulin.
	Anti-HB core antibodies (HBcAb)	Antibodies directed against the core antigen of HBV. They rise earlier in the course of hepatitis than surface antibodies. If HBcAb is present in high titer in the face of a negative HBsAb, this in many cases correlates with active infection or the HBV carrier state. Early in convalescence, when HBsAg has disappeared, one can still have positive titers for HBcAb and negative HBsAb, as the latter are slower to rise. If HBsAb are present as well as HBcAb, this correlates with later stages of convalescence or remote previous HBV infection (see text).
	e Antigen (not available in all laboratories)	Presence of this viral antigen correlates with high serum titers of virus particles ($\geq$1:10,000 by CF test), and increased likelihood of transmission of infection.
Mononucleosis syndrome		
Epstein-Barr virus (EBV)	Heterophile antibodies	The conventional Paul-Bunnell test is not used as frequently as the monospot or slide tests. These tests are 96% sensitive (85% in the first week), and if done properly, their specificity is also high (98%). These antibodies may persist for more than a year but this does not correlate with disease activity. Only 40% of children with infectious mononucleosis will have a positive heterophile test.

TABLE 4.1. *(continued)*

Suspected Problem	*Serologic Test*	*Interpretation*
	Antibodies against the EBV capsid antigen (VCA), fluorescent antibody test	These antibodies are often near peak titer at the onset of illness and one may not see a 4-fold rise (10–20% of patients). Presence of VCA antibodies correlates with immunity to EB virus.
	Antibodies against EBV early antigen (EA), fluorescent antibody test	Antibodies to the EA appear early in the acute infection and disappear early in convalescence. Therefore positive EA test, especially with negative NA test, indicates recent EBV infection.
	Antibodies against EBV nuclear antigen (NA), fluorescent antibody test	These antibodies appear later in convalescence and persist for years.
CMV	Complement fixation test	4-fold rise required for diagnosis.
T. gondii	See Table 4.4	
Viral exanthems		
Measles	Hemagglutination inhibition	Single titers not very useful. 4-fold rise may be demonstrated using paired sera drawn within a week of onset of rash.
Rubella	Hemagglutination inhibition, passive hemagglutination (PHA)	Both tests are useful in screening for immunity to rubella in women before pregnancy. Women with titers ≤1:8 should receive rubella vaccine if they are not pregnant.
	Complement fixation, hemagglutination inhibition	4-fold rise indicates active rubella. IgM antibodies can be measured on single serum specimens if rubella is strongly suspected in a pregnant patient or in a newborn, and their presence indicates active infection.
Chickenpox, zoster	Complement fixation	4-fold rise often within the first week after onset of rash demonstrates infection, although the striking clinical appearance rarely makes this necessary. Diagnostic rise may take 3 weeks or more in an immunosuppressed patient.
	Fluorescent antibody against membrane antigen (FAMA)	Negative test indicates susceptibility to varicella.

* = best test(s).

Hepatitis

The hepatitis A and B viruses cannot be cultured in vitro and thus serology, together with clinical findings, must be relied upon for diagnosis. Acute hepatitis A (HA) is confirmed by finding any titer of immunoglobulin M (IgM) anti-HA antibodies in the patient's serum, and a single positive specimen is sufficient. Immunoglobulin G (IgG) antibodies may be present from a much earlier infection and therefore a fourfold rise in IgG titer must be found, requiring paired specimens several weeks apart. Single positive IgG titers are useless for diagnosis but do signify immunity.

Hepatitis B (HB) infection is confirmed by finding hepatitis B virus surface antigen (HBsAg) in the serum. This confirms infection with the virus, but the clinical phase, be it carrier, acute (which can be anicteric), or chronic, must be determined by clinical signs and symptoms and results of liver function tests and/or biopsy of liver tissue. The degree of relative infectivity correlates with the presence of the e antigen, which can now be detected with commercially available kits. The presence of HBs antibody in serum means that the patient has had hepatitis B and is immune to the disease.

Infectious Mononucleosis Syndrome

To diagnose the infectious mononucleosis syndrome, three agents are commonly sought by means of serologic testing: (1) Epstein-Barr virus (EBV), (2) cytomegalovirus (CMV), and (3) toxoplasmosis. Serologic tests should be ordered in the following clinical situations: lymphocytosis with or without atypical lymphocytes, obscure illness with lassitude, not necessarily with fever; illness accompanied by posterior cervical lymphadenopathy; hepatitis with negative HAV and HBV serology; fever of unknown origin (FUO); splenomegaly of uncertain cause; a general work-up of fever in an immunosuppressed patient; and investigation of a patient with multisystem findings, especially if febrile.

Fungal Meningitis

In addition to many other fungal infections (Table 4.2), the two most common types of fungal meningitis, cryptococcosis and coccidioidomycosis, are best diagnosed by serologic tests.

In cryptococcosis, the organisms are often difficult to detect in the cerebrospinal fluid (CSF) by the conventional India ink test unless very large numbers of organisms are present. Similarly, the culture may yield false negative results. The most sensitive evaluation is the latex agglutination test that detects the capsular antigen of *Cryptococcus neoformans*. Not only do positive titers make the diagnosis, but a fall in titer in serial CSF samples, once appropriate antifungal therapy has been instituted, correlates with chances of cure. Treatment failure is likely if there is a high CSF antigen titer (1:8) at the end of therapy, or if the titers do not become negative or at least fall more than fourfold during therapy.

In coccidioidal meningitis, there are no satisfactory stains that can be done on CSF, and the cultures may be falsely negative. The best diagnostic method is to order CSF coccidioides antibody titers. The diagnosis can be made by a positive complement fixation test at any titer, and these can be followed serially (usually biweekly, then monthly) over many months to assess cure.

Bacteriologic Diseases

Some additional serologic tests that are worth mentioning are those used to detect certain *Salmonella* infections, brucellae, and streptococci (Table 4.3).

Widal Test

The Widal test measures antibodies to *Salmonella* somatic O and flagellar H antigens. In general, it is an ancillary test for the diagnosis of typhoid fever, cultures of blood, urine, and stool being far superior and easier. There are sometimes false positive reactions to nontyphoidal group D salmonellae. The test is decidedly unhelpful in patients who have received typhoid vaccine (in whom test results are usually positive), and it has not proved useful in investigating enteric fever-like disease or diarrhea. It is sometimes ordered during the investigation of FUO where the symptoms and signs suggest typhoid, but again has not been very useful.

Antibody Tests for Brucella

The Widal test is often accompanied by a request for *Brucella* agglutinins. *Brucella* antibodies are very useful in diagnosing brucellosis. A titer of 1:160 or over in a person who does not work in an abattoir strongly suggests the diagnosis, and blood and bone marrow cultures for *Brucella* should be done. In an abattoir worker, one usually likes to see an agglutinin titer over 1:320. If the illness is of recent onset, acute and convalescent titers may show a diagnostic fourfold rise.

TABLE 4.2. Serodiagnosis of Fungal Infections

Suspected Problem	*Serologic Test*	*Interpretation*
Histoplasmosis	Complement fixation (CF) + immunodiffusion (ID) test to yeast-phase antigen* of *H. capsulatum* or to mycelial-phase antigen (histoplasmin)	4-fold rise (usually within 4 weeks) is diagnostic. A single titer to yeast antigen (early antibody response) ⩾1:32 suggests recent infection. In chronic illness both yeast and mycelial CF titers are high and should decline at a variable rate after cure. Cross-reaction occurs frequently with *Blastomyces dermatitidis.*
Coccidioidomycosis	Tube precipitin	80% positive within 2 weeks of infection, but antibodies do not usually persist longer than a few months.
	CF test on serum or CSF against the mycelial antigen coccidioidin*	Positive test even in low titers of 1:2 or 1:4 indicates recent infection. Titers in CSF become negative with effective therapy and should be followed serially. Serum CF titers ⩾1:32 usually indicate disseminated infection.
Blastomycosis	Immunodiffusion against yeast antigen*	Positive lines of identification with reference antiserum indicate blastomycosis. Precipitin lines disappear with follow-up sera when disease is responding to treatment.
	Complement fixation against yeast antigen	Not very sensitive nor specific.
Sporotrichosis	Tube agglutination*, latex slide agglutination*, complement fixation, immunodiffusion	Best used to diagnose systemic sporotrichosis, the latex agglutination (LA) slide test is rapid and 94% sensitive. For unknown reasons, patients with leishmaniasis may show cross-reactive false positive titers up to 1:16, otherwise a ⩾1:16 titer by LA is diagnostic of previous or present sporotrichosis. 4-fold rise confirms acute infection. Unlike some tests, the titers do not consistently fall with effective treatment and cannot be used as an index of cure.
Candidiasis	Immunodiffusion, Crossed immunoelectrophoresis (XIE)*, latex agglutination	The difficulty with interpretation of these tests is that patients with mucosal candidiasis, as well as patients with invasive systemic candidiasis, often have positive results. 100% of patients with invasive infection have positive XIE results, but of all tests that are positive, only 56% represent invasive disease.
Aspergillosis	Immunodiffusion, counterimmunoelectrophoresis	Positive ID test is very suggestive of invasive aspergillosis but the sensitivity is only 60%.
Cryptococcosis	Detection of *antigen* by latex agglutination	99% positive (titer ⩾1:8) in CSF of patients with cryptococcal meningitis. Titers fall with effective treatment and should be followed serially. It is the best test for diagnosing cryptococcal meningitis.

TABLE 4.2. *(continued)*

Suspected Problem	*Serologic Test*	*Interpretation*
	Detection of *antibody* by fluorescent antibody or tube agglutination	Specificity = 77% and 89% respectively; however, there may be up to 50% false negative results. These tests should therefore be done in conjunction with the antigen test, culture, and microscopy.

* = best test(s).

TABLE 4.3. Serodiagnosis of Bacterial Infections

Suspected Problem	*Serologic Tests*	*Interpretation*
Streptococcal pharyngitis, rheumatic fever	Antistreptolysin-O (ASOT)* Antideoxyribonuclease (anti-DNase-B) Antihyaluronidase (anti-Hase) Antinicotinamide adenine dinucleotidase (anti-NADase) Streptozyme test*	4-fold rise or single antibody titer ≥1:170 ASOT, ≥1:170 anti-DNase-B, ≥1:256 anti-Hase, ≥1:270 anti-NAD = recent streptococcal infection. With the streptozyme test, a positive reaction has a 90% correlation with the above single titers. With all of these tests, penicillin therapy within 5 days after onset of infection delays the 4-fold antibody response up to 90 days.
Streptococcal pyoderma and impetigo Poststreptococcal glomerulonephritis	Streptozyme test* Anti-DNase-B*	Positive streptozyme test or anti-DNase titer ≥1:256 = recent infection with group A streptococcus. ASOT, NAD titers weak.
Staphylococcal infection	Teichoic acid (TA) antibodies	Positive titers correlate with deep infections such as endocarditis, osteomyelitis, and chronic suppurative foci. Fall in TA antibodies does not consistently correlate with therapeutic cure.
Salmonellosis		
Gastroenteritis	Serology not useful	4-fold antibody rise to group D salmonellae in O or H antigens is diagnostic. Single titers not helpful by themselves (see text). Occasional false positive cross-reactions have been reported. Serologic diagnosis is no substitute for bacteriologic proof of infection.
Enteric fever	Serology not useful	
Typhoid fever	Widal test	
Yersiniosis		
Enteritis	Agglutination test to O antigen of *Y. enterocolitica* and *Y. pseudotuberculosis*	Acute enteritis often results in 4-fold rise. Single titer ≥1:160 is suggestive especially if serum is adsorbed with antigens to brucella and *F. tularensis.*
Plague	Passive hemagglutination (PHA), antibodies against *Y. pestis*	4-fold rise diagnostic. Single titer ≥1:256 suggests recent infection.

TABLE 4.3. *(continued)*

Suspected Problem	*Serologic Tests*	*Interpretation*
Tularemia	Agglutinins to *Francisella tularensis*	4-fold rise diagnostic. Single titer ⩾1:160 suggestive of recent infection. Titers ⩽1:80 may persist for years. Cross-reactions may occur in brucellosis and yersiniosis.
Brucellosis	Tube agglutinin titer*	4-fold rise is diagnostic. Single titer of ⩾1:320 = recent infection in general population, but not useful if the patient is an abbatoir worker or has received brucella vaccine. Cross-reactions may occur in cholera, tularemia, and yersiniosis.
	Slide test	Useful for screening and should be confirmed by tube agglutinin titer.
Legionnaires' disease	Indirect fluorescent antibody	Uses the patient's serum. 4-fold rise is diagnostic but may take 6 weeks. Single titer ⩾1:128 is suggestive of recent infection.
	Direct fluorescent antibody	Uses high-titer fluorescein-tagged reference serum. Lung biopsy specimens and transtracheal aspirates are more frequently positive than sputum. Positive test is diagnostic of the presence of *Legionella* sp.
Leptospirosis	Slide agglutinin test against whole organisms	Titers ⩾1:100 suggest the diagnosis. Acute and convalescent sera 3–4 weeks apart may yield a 4-fold antibody titer rise.

* = best test(s).

Antibody Tests for Streptococcal Infections

Serologic diagnosis of streptococcal infection is useful in few instances because Gram's stain and culture are so easy and accurate. In a patient who has previously had rheumatic fever and develops another streptococcal pharyngitis, the magnitude of the antistreptolysin 0 titer (ASOT) rise correlates directly with the chances of a recurrence of rheumatic fever; for example, eightfold rise is associated with four times the recurrence rate seen with a twofold rise. Single titers are difficult to interpret, especially in populations where the prevalence of streptococcal pharyngitis is high.

In patients with streptococcal pyoderma, such as impetigo, serologic testing is redundant because Gram's stain and culture readily yield the diagnosis. In acute streptococcal cellulitis where cultures, even by aspiration at the advancing edge, are not often positive, the anti-DNase or the streptozyme test may show a rise. The ASOT is not generally useful in patients with streptococcal skin infection.

Leptospirosis

Leptospirosis is an underdiagnosed zoonotic infection that can be responsible for a variety of clinical conditions including aseptic meningitis, myocarditis, jaundice, and an influenza-like illness. Most laboratories do not routinely culture for leptospires, and therefore serologic tests are most helpful. Titers should be ordered on serum from acutely ill and convalescent patients, especially if there is a history of animal exposure or con-

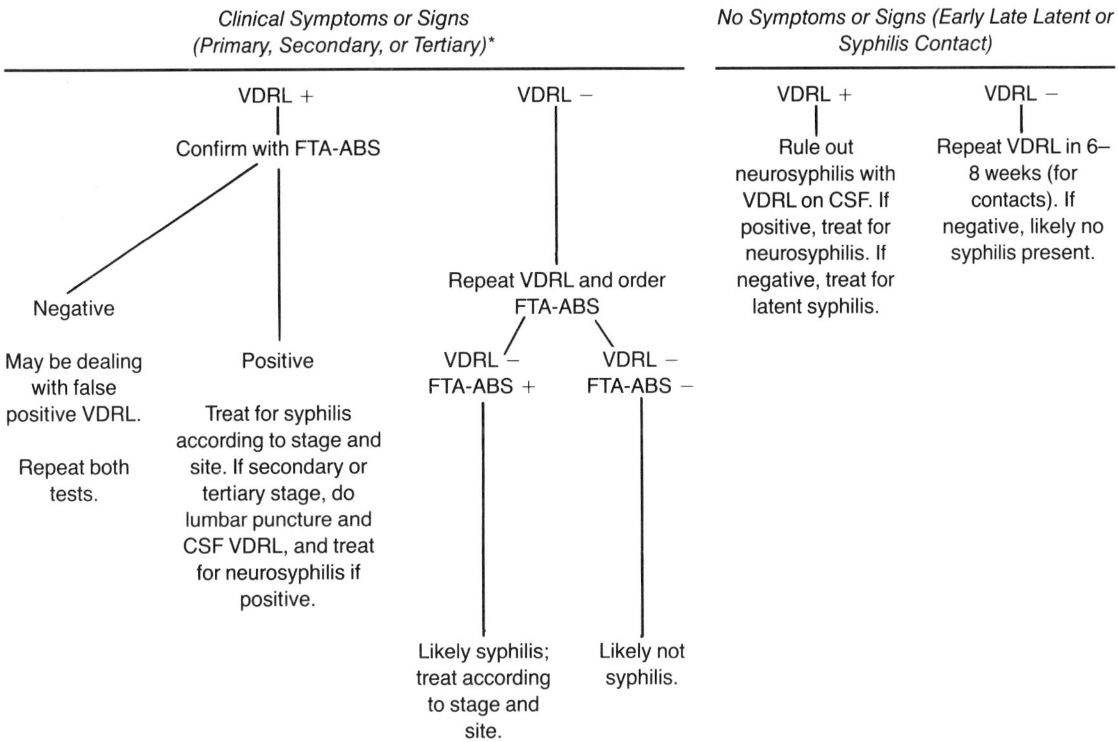

*Darkfield examination should be done whenever possible.

FIGURE 4.1. Serologic diagnosis of syphilis.

tact with water in animal drinking dugouts or farm irrigation ditches.

Syphilis

In current practice, most cases of syphilis are detected by serologic tests often done because the patient has some other sexually transmitted disease. It should be stressed, however, that one should at all times perform a darkfield examination of ulcers and of fluid from lesions characteristic of secondary syphilis or congenital syphilis. An algorithm used for the serologic diagnosis of syphilis is presented in Figure 4.1.

Nontreponemal Tests

The Venereal Disease Research Laboratories (VDRL) test, the automated reagin test (ART), and the rapid plasma reagin (RPR) card test are very sensitive but not specific tests. They detect antibodies to cardiolipin antigen present in serum of patients with syphilis and also other conditions, such as lupus and postvaccinia, although in these latter instances the antigen is usually not present in titers greater than 1:8. The VDRL is the preferred nontreponemal test for CSF, and if positive in any titer, indicates neurosyphilis. A bloody spinal tap may make the CSF VDRL give false positive results, but for this to occur, the CSF sample in the tube must be grossly bloody. The presence of only microscopic amounts of blood in the CSF is not associated with enough contamination to make the test positive.

One should keep in mind that at the time a syphilitic chancre appears, only 50% of VDRL tests will be positive, and by two weeks (the average time between onset of the chancre and visit to the doctor) only 85% will be positive. In secondary syphilis virtually 100% of patients have a positive VDRL, often in high titer, 1:16 or above. In late syphilis the results of the VDRL may fall to weakly reactive or even negative, and in these instances the specific fluorescent treponemal antibody absorption test (FTA-ABS) is the most useful. Both in neurosyphilis and non-neurosyphilis, the VDRL titer should be followed in CSF and/or serum. The titer should fall to nonreactive in early syphilis, but may remain "serofast," that is, positive at low titer, if the patient had the infection for a long time before treatment.

For example, after effective treatment of early latent syphilis (of less than one year's duration before treatment) approximately 75% of patients become seronegative within five years, 20% have a fourfold drop in the VDRL titer, and 5% have a fixed static titer. After adequate treatment of late latent syphilis, only 45% of patients become seronegative within five years. A patient with late syphilis, active or latent, and with a VDRL of 1:2 may have a fixed titer of 1:2 for years after treatment. This is probably the serofast phenomenon and should not prompt repeated courses of therapy.

Specific Treponemal Tests

The TPI (*Treponema pallidum* immobilization test) is no longer used, having been replaced by the specific and sensitive FTA-ABS. This is positive in 80% to 85% of patients at the time the chancre appears, and in almost all patients by two weeks. Once positive, it remains so for life except in the rare situation where the patient is treated within a day or so of onset of the chancre, in which case a positive test may become negative. It is a very useful test in ruling out a suspected false positive VDRL. A negative FTA-ABS would indicate that a positive result of the VDRL is indeed a false positive. Results of the FTA-ABS may be falsely positive in nonsyphilitic treponemal infections such as yaws, and in this situation the clinician often has to rely on a history of skin infection in the tropics with residual scarring, usually on the extremities, characteristic of yaws. If there is any doubt, one must treat for syphilis. The FTA-ABS may be truly false positive in certain connective tissue diseases including rheumatoid arthritis, and in hematologic malignancies and autoimmune hemolytic anemias. Fortunately, false positive results are rare.

There is still debate about the significance of a positive FTA-ABS in the CSF in the face of a nonreactive CSF VDRL. The "gold standard" for diagnosis of neurosyphilis is still a positive CSF VDRL, but in those instances where there is a history of syphilis together with neurologic signs, a positive CSF FTA-ABS, and negative CSF VDRL, the patient should be treated for neurosyphilis. The diagnosis of congenital syphilis was previously thought to be confirmed by a positive FTA-ABS IgM in the neonatal serum. Recent evidence, however, has suggested that the positive result may not detect antitreponemal IgM, but IgM against antitreponemal IgG passively transferred from the mother. Therefore the diagnosis still depends on clinical findings and the presence of syphilis in the mother. Virtually 100% of infants born of mothers with syphilis will have passively transferred reagin-like antibody and IgG, giving positive VDRL and conventional FTA-ABS tests.

Another problem that has arisen with the FTA-ABS is the interpretation of the borderline positive result, which may occur in 8% of patients on routine hospital admission testing. These patients should be retested. If the repeated test remains borderline, there is no history of syphilis or contact with the disease, and the VDRL is negative, it is probably best to follow these patients without labeling them as having syphilis.

Parasitic Infections

Many parasitic infections can be diagnosed by direct examination of blood smears, skin biopsies, or stool for ova, cysts, and trophozoites (Table 4.4). In some patients, however, the diagnosis may depend solely on the results of serologic tests. Some of the more common parasitic infections diagnosed in this way are extraintestinal amebiasis; toxoplasmosis; toxocariasis, the usual cause of the visceral larva migrans syndrome; cysticercosis, the larval stage of *Taenia solium*; trichinosis; hydatid disease; and Chagas' disease. Rather than knowing the exact test to order, it is more important to inform the serology laboratory about the suspected diagnoses and whether one thinks the problem is acute (in which case IgM antibody tests may be useful) or chronic. For some of these parasites the serum samples submitted must be sent to a central reference laboratory, and there may be significant time delay before the result is reported. In these instances one usually manages the patient on clinical grounds, the serologic test if positive, providing confirmatory evidence.

Extraintestinal Amebiasis

Serologic tests for *Entamoeba histolytica* should be ordered if one suspects an amebic liver abscess. This suspicion is usually based on a history of travel to endemic areas. There may be a history of dysentery, although

TABLE 4.4. Serodiagnosis of Parasitic Infections

Suspected Problem	*Serologic Tests*	*Interpretation*
Amebiasis	Indirect hemagglutination*, enzyme-linked immunosorbent assay (ELISA)	Serology is very sensitive for diagnosing extraintestinal disease, less so with dysentery only, and least with the intestinal carrier state. Reports of positive results in normal subjects and in other types of dysentery = 2–6%.
Giardiasis	Not available	
Toxocariasis	Bentonite flocculation	ELISA has the highest degree of sensitivity and specificity and should be ordered when there is clinical suspicion of ocular toxocariosis or visceral larva migrans with eosinophilia.
Toxoplasmosis	IgM fluorescent antibody†	Positive titer ≥1:20 confirms diagnosis of active toxoplasmosis. IgM titers fall within a few months postinfection to <1:10 (see text).
	Conventional fluorescent antibody (IgG), complement fixation, Sabin-Feldman dye test	IFA and the Sabin-Feldman dye test appear to measure the same antibodies. A 4-fold titer rise is needed for definite diagnosis. Usually titers rise to >1:1000 and may persist for a year or more (see text).
Cysticercosis	Indirect hemagglutination against larval antigen of *Taenia solium,* the pork tapeworm	85% of human cases of cysticercosis have positive sera. CSF titers are lower or negative. 2–5% of normal persons and 17% of patients with *T. saginata* tapeworm (the adult beef tapeworm) are positive. Patients with both echinococcosus and coenurosis (larval infections with dog tapeworm) may show positive cysticercus titers.
Chagas' disease	Indirect hemagglutination (IHA)*, fluorescent antibody, complement fixation, latex agglutination, ELISA*	Approximately 95% sensitive in patients with Chagas' cardiomyopathy. Titer of 1:128 positive for IHA. Some false positive results may occur in patients with leishmaniasis. With effective therapy the titers become negative in 4–24 months in 80% of patients.
Leishmaniasis Tropical sore Kala azar	Fluorescent antibody*, ELISA*, indirect hemagglutination*	Serology mainly used for diagnosing kala azar or visceral leishmaniasis, and less useful for tropical sore, where biopsy and microscopy is best. A high degree of cross-reactivity occurs in acute malaria and also in Chagas' disease.
Trichinosis	Bentonite flocculation	Larvae in muscle may remain viable for 5 years, providing a continuous stimulus for antibody production. Titers rise to detectable levels within 17 days. The test is both sensitive and specific. The titers fall with resolution of the disease and low antibody levels persist for years.
	Fluorescent antibody*	More sensitive than the BF and therefore perhaps more useful because of low parasitic loads in muscle in most patients seen today.

* = best test(s).

†Except in congenital toxoplasmosis, where the Sabin-Feldman test or the new ELISA IgM is more accurate.

this is not always the case, and diarrhea is usually not present at the time the patient is seen with fever and right upper quadrant tenderness. An indirect hemagglutination test or latex agglutination test (available in commercial kit form) yielding titers above 1:128 indicates active infection.

Toxoplasmosis

Toxoplasmosis is a common parasitic infection that is diagnosed almost exclusively by serology. The most helpful procedure is the IgM fluorescent antibody test, which indicates that the patient has had toxoplasmosis within the past several months, although in a few instances the IgM titer may persist for a year or more at or below 1:20. Titers rise within a week of infection. A titer of 1:80 or greater is considered high.

Uncertainty exists as to whether reactivated toxoplasmosis, for example, in immunosuppressed hosts, is consistently associated with an IgM antibody response. The diagnosis of active toxoplasmosis may be made by demonstrating a fourfold antibody rise, and the most common assay is the conventional (IgG) fluorescent antibody test. Usually sera are taken three weeks apart; the titer usually rises to 1:1000 or more while the patient is symptomatic.

The Sabin-Feldman dye test has largely been replaced by the fluorescent antibody test. The complement fixation (CF) test may sometimes be useful if the first serum sample is drawn late in the illness, for example, after three weeks, since complement-fixing antibodies may rise further after this time, yielding a fourfold rise. Therefore it is important for the attending physician to let the serology laboratory know how long the patient has been ill, as well as the fact that toxoplasmosis is suspected.

Suspicion of the disease in pregnancy poses a special problem because of the potential risk of congenital toxoplasmosis. A major concern arises when physicians detect a conventional IgG titer result of 1:1000 or more in a woman at 12 weeks gestation. This titer could, however, have been present for a year or more, and one should try to demonstrate IgM antibodies. If these are negative, one can be reasonably certain that the patient has not had toxoplasmosis within the past two to three months. If there is still some doubt, the complement fixation test done on paired serum samples three weeks or more apart may still detect an antibody rise, as CF antibodies rise more slowly than do antibodies measured using the fluorescent technique.

An equally difficult problem may arise in establishing the diagnosis of congenital toxoplasmosis by serology. Remington's group at Stanford University has shown that whereas the Sabin-Feldman dye test was positive in virtually 100% of newborns with proved congenital toxoplasmosis, the IgM fluorescent antibody test, which is reliable for acute infection outside the neonatal period, was positive in only 25%. A fourfold antibody rise by the CF test is reliable, but may take as long as six months. A new test, the double sandwich IgM ELISA, is much more sensitive than the IgM fluorescent antibody technique. The former is positive in approximately 80% of infants with congenital toxoplasmosis.

Toxocariasis

With the development of the ELISA test, an accurate and sensitive method has become available for diagnosing toxocariasis. In a patient with unexplained pulmonary infiltrates eosinophilia, central nervous system signs, urticaria, hepatosplenomegaly, and/or ocular involvement (endophthalmitis or retinal granuloma) visceral larva migrans should be suspected, especially if exposure to cats or dogs is documented, and serum should be sent for *Toxocara* antibodies.

Cysticercosis

Cysticercosis is a relatively uncommon infection occurring when a person ingests the ova of *Taenia solium*, the pork tapeworm, and becomes the intermediate host. Fluctuating cerebral or spinal cord symptoms as the cysticerci degenerate and calcify should prompt radiologic and serologic investigation. Serum and CSF samples should be accompanied by precise information about the illness, since samples from provincial or state laboratories will be sent off to a central reference laboratory. Samples of CSF with titers of 1:16 or greater are highly suggestive of CNS cysticercosis.

Trichinosis

Trichinosis is rarely acquired from domestic animal meat products, but has been acquired from wild game. The clinical findings of myalgia and eosinophilia suggest the diagnosis, and a fourfold antibody rise as measured by bentonite flocculation and immunofluorescent tests confirms it. Titers may remain high for months or years due to persistence of cysts in muscle.

Hydatid Disease

Hydatid disease in the cyst form is suggested by radiologic demonstration of a liver or lung cyst with eggshell calcification in its wall. The multilocular form is less easy to identify clinically. A positive epidemiologic history of contact with carnivore feces where the carnivores could have eaten wild game (sylvatic cycle) should prompt a serologic investigation. Liver involvement has been associated with higher titers than lung involvement, but the percentage of positive tests is equal, and approximately 90% of patients with echinococci will have positive titers. As mentioned later in this chapter, the Casoni intradermal test, although sensitive, lacks sufficient specificity to make it clinically reliable.

Chagas' Disease

Chagas' disease is limited to the western half of the world, and is the leading cause of cardiovascular death in South America. It is due to infection with *Trypanosoma cruzi,* with reduviid bugs as the vector. Serum from patients with cardiomyopathy, megaesophagus, or megacolon who have a history of travel to Central and South America should be tested. Roughly 95% of patients with chronic disease will have positive titers.

Rickettsial Infections

Serological diagnosis of rickettsial infection is best accomplished by demonstrating a four-fold rise in the indirect hemagglutination, indirect fluorescent antibody, or complement fixation tests. Although the Weil-Felix reaction to proteus OX-19, OX-2, and OX-K antigens may be useful, (Table 4.5) it should not be used as the sole diagnostic test.

Diagnosis of Infection by Testing for Antigens

Antigen detection has already been mentioned in connection with cryptococcal meningitis. Some bacterial infections may be diagnosed by serologic tests for antigen as well. The most commonly used ones are counterimmunoelectrophoresis (CIE) done on body fluids (serum, CSF, pleural fluid, and urine) to detect *Hemophilus influenzae,* pneumococci, and meningococci. Commercial kits for *H. influenzae* type B are available to detect this agent by latex particle agglutination, a simple test that does not require electrophoresis equipment. Urine is a particularly good fluid to test because it is easily obtained and the antigens are concentrated in proportion to the urine concentration.

Clinical situations in which these tests are useful include meningitis where the Gram's stain and culture of CSF are negative, such as partially treated bacterial meningitis; acute pneumonia where pneumococci are suspected but not seen on Gram's stain or culture; and acute fulminant septicemia where either meningococci or pneumococci (the latter in a patient with asplenia) are suspected but where previous antibiotic therapy has interfered with the cultures.

Newer developments, especially the ability to make monoclonal antibody, may make detection of antigen a much more widespread practice in the future.

SKIN TESTS

There are three major reasons for performing skin tests: to aid in diagnosing specific infections; to screen for evidence of previous exposure to certain infectious agents; and to determine whether or not a patient has cutaneous anergy (problems with cell-mediated immunity). A wide variety of skin test preparations has been evaluated, but the majority are not used in most clinical situations because of difficulty in interpretation (both false positive and false negative reactions) and lack of commercially available test antigens, and because alternative diagnostic methods are generally more precise and easier to standardize. Depending on the type of infection, the detection of delayed hypersensitivity may vary from 1 to 10 weeks.

Skin testing of patients living in an endemic area, such as the coccidiodin test in residents of southern California, is virtually useless since a positive result probably reflects remote or continuous antigenic exposure. Skin testing may be of value in travelers returning from these areas and may indicate recent exposure. If clinical manifestations are appropriate, the skin test may indicate active infection; however, the diagnosis should be confirmed by other methods before beginning therapy. Table 4.5 shows some of the more commonly employed skin tests with comments regarding their interpretation. Interpretation must be done taking into account any concurrent factors that might modify macrophage–T-cell responsiveness. For example, therapy with corticosteroids, severe malnutrition, or a recent viral infection such as measles can cause a negative result (cutaneous anergy). Physicians should also pay attention to the antigen preparation itself, being careful not to use outdated purified protein derivative (PPD) and not allowing prepared syringes to sit for

TABLE 4.5. Serologic Diagnosis of Rickettsial Diseases

	*Weil-Felix Results**
Typhus Group	
Epidemic louse-borne typhus Murine typhus	Strong OX-19 and weak or negative OX-2
Recrudescent typhus (Brill-Zinnser)	Weak or negative OX-19 and/or OX-2
Scrub typhus	Strong OX-K only
Spotted Fever Group	
Rocky Mountain Spotted Fever Tick-borne typhus	Strong OX-19 and weak OX-2
Rickettsialpox	All negative
Other	
Q-fever	All negative

*For firm diagnosis one should demonstrate a 4-fold indirect hemagglutination, fluorescent antibody, or complement fixation titer rise, any of which are much more specific and sensitive than the Weil-Felix reaction.

more than an hour at room temperature. Even though PPD is Tween-stabilized, mishandling may result in loss of antigen potency.

Care should be taken in planting the test material. The needle, with the bevel up, should be inserted intradermally on the anterior aspect of the forearm so that the bevel can be seen through the skin; 0.1 ml of antigen is then injected, creating a discrete bleb. Induration is looked for and measured 48 to 72 hours after injection of antigen, but a positive reaction may be noted earlier than this or, in some cases, not until five or more days later. To be interpreted as positive, the area of induration should be present for longer than 24 hours. Measuring the degree of induration in a reproducible way can be facilitated by using the ballpoint pen technique. The pen is run firmly along the skin toward the edge of induration at all four quadrants. The point will stop rolling when it hits the indurated edge. Both diameters can then be measured. This technique yields more consistent measurements than the palpation method.

Problems with clinical interpretation relate to the inability of skin tests to tell the clinician whether the patient has active disease now or had the disease in the past. Some skin tests are decidedly unhelpful and indeed, may confound matters by virtue of their cross-reactivity or false positivity (Table 4.6). Examples are tests for histoplasmosis and blastomycosis, the Casoni test for hydatid disease, the Frei test for lymphogranuloma venereum, and the brucellin test for brucellosis. Not only do histoplasmin and blastomycin cross-react with each other and with coccidioidin, they also cause an elevation of humoral antibodies, making subsequent serologic tests useless. The coccidioidin skin test does not alter subsequent serology and is specific for coccidioidomycosis. In the face of clear-cut epidemiologic, clinical, and microbiologic evidence for coccidioidomycosis, a negative skin test implies an anergic state secondary to disseminated disease.

Of the skin tests available for tuberculosis, the 5-TU Mantoux test is most widely used. Severe necrotizing skin reactions are rare even in patients with active tuberculosis, and for this reason the weaker 1-TU test is of little value even in children. Ten or more millimeters of induration indicates the presence of *Mycobacterium tuberculosis* somewhere in the body (whether in a dormant nonreplicating state or associated with active disease). A reaction of from 5 to 9 mm induration to 5-TU may indicate latent or active infection with atypical mycobacteria. The size of the reaction over 10 mm does not correlate with disease activity, and a large reaction by itself in the absence of any high-risk factors such as recent conversion, evidence of old healed nondrug-treated tuberculosis on chest x-ray, steroid therapy, gastrectomy, and so on, should not be interpreted as an indication for the use of prophylactic antituberculosis drugs. An exception applies in infants and young chil-

TABLE 4.6. Skin Tests Commonly Employed in Clinical Practice

Agent	*Positive Test*	*Interpretation*
5-TU PPD (intermediate strength)	⩾10 mm induration (disregard erythema)	⩾10 mm presumably indicates viable though not necessarily multiplying acid-fast bacilli (*M. tuberculosis* or bacille Calmette-Guérin) in the body. 6–9 mm may indicate infection with atypical mycobacteria.
1-TU PPD (first strength) 250-TU PPD (second strength)	⩾10 mm induration	Previous exposure to *M. tuberculosis* or BCG.
Candida, Trichophyton	⩾5 mm induration	Intact dermal cell-mediated response to this antigen.
Mumps	⩾5 mm induration	
Streptokinase-streptodornase (SK-SD)	⩾5 mm induration	
Coccidioidin, spherulin	⩾5 mm induration	Previous or current infection with *Coccidioides immitis.*

dren in whom prophylaxis is indicated if the skin test shows 10 mm or greater induration, whether the high-risk factors are present or not.

When should one employ the 250-TU skin test? Seventy-five percent of patients with active pulmonary tuberculosis will have 10 mm or more induration to 5-TU and 91% will have similar reactions to 250-TU. The 250-TU skin test is therefore of value when there is a high index of suspicion of active pulmonary tuberculosis in a patient with less than 10 mm induration to the 5-TU PPD preparation.

In acute disseminated tuberculosis, the reaction to 5-TU will be negative in 52% of patients. Twenty-five percent to 87% of these tuberculin-negative patients will also have negative skin tests to *Trichophyton,* streptokinase-streptodornase, or *Candida* antigen, thus demonstrating total anergy.

TABLE 4.7. Reasons for False Positive and Negative Results of Skin Tests

False Positive	*False Negative*
Poor technique in reading induration, e.g., measuring erythema instead of only induration.	Poor technique in injecting antigen, e.g., subcutaneously rather than intradermally.
Hematoma formation caused by faulty injection of antigen.	Low-potency antigen due to its being outdated or stored improperly.
Poor antigen giving too many cross-reactions with other organisms.	Inherently poor antigen, e.g., blastomycin.
Use of 250-TU rather than 5-TU results in increased false positive results due to cross-reaction with atypical mycobacteria.	Poor technique in reading induration.
5-TU PPD may be falsely positive for tuberculosis in a patient who has received BCG vaccine.	Skin tests for a particular infection may be falsely negative if the patient is anergic due to overwhelming infection, old age, recent vaccination with other antigens, concomitant viral infection, or immunosuppressive therapy.

ANNOTATED BIBLIOGRAPHY

Evans, AS, Niederman JC, Cenabre LC, West B, Richards VA. A prospective evaluation of heterophile and Epstein-Barr virus-specific IgM antibody tests in clinical and subclinical infectious mononucleosis: specificity and sensitivity of the tests and persistence of antibody. J Infect Dis 1975;132:546–554.
Synthesis of data concerning the relationship of disease and convalescence to the EBV antibody and to the various types of heterophile antibody tests available.

Jaffe HW. The laboratory diagnosis of syphilis. Ann Intern Med 1975;83:846–850.
Brief review of serologic tests available for the diagnosis of syphilis together with their use and interpretation in the primary, secondary, tertiary, and congenital stages.

Kaplan EL, Anthony BF, Chapman SS, Ayoub EM, Wannamaker LW. The influence of the site of infection on the immune response to group A streptococci. J Clin Invest 1970;49:1405–1414.
Clear presentation of which tests yield the most accurate results in specific types of streptococcal infections.

Krick JA, Remington JS. Toxoplasmosis in the adult — an overview. N Engl J Med 1978;298:550–553.
A valuable office reference to guide physicians' interpretation of toxoplasmosis serology.

Krugman S, Gocke DJ. Viral hepatitis. Philadelphia: WB Saunders, 1978:147.
A 140-page monograph on hepatitis A and B with examples of serologic responses and how they correlate with disease, the carrier state, and immunity.

Nash DR, Douglass JE. Anergy in active pulmonary tuberculosis. A comparison between positive and negative reactors and an evaluation of 5-TU and 250-TU skin test doses. Chest 1980;77:32–37.
Report on the incidence of negative skin tests in active pulmonary tuberculosis, together with data that aid in determining how and when to use the 5-TU and 250-TU PPD skin tests.

Rose NR, Friedman H, eds. Manual of clinical immunology, 2nd edition. Washington, DC: American Society of Microbiology, 1980:1105.
An excellent reference text on methodology and interpretation of virtually all diagnostic serology tests.

Typhoid and its serology. (Editorial) Br J Med 1978;1:389–390.
A brief review of the interpretation and reliability of serologic tests for typhoid fever.

5 ANTIBIOTICS AND ANTIFUNGAL DRUGS

Harvey R. Rabin and L. E. Bryan

Antibiotics comprise a diverse group of therapeutic agents involved in inhibiting specific and unique cellular functions of bacterial cells. Biochemical targets of individual antibiotics include biosynthetic enzymes associated with cell wall synthesis, components of cytoplasmic membrane integrity, components of nucleic acid synthesis, ribosomal subunits involved in protein synthesis, and enzymes of synthesis and reduction of dihydrofolate. A small group of miscellaneous target sites is also important for a select few antibiotics.

Certain microbiologic and pharmacologic considerations pertinent to rational and safe antibiotic administration are listed in Table 5.1. Important among these is *selective toxicity,* which is defined as follows: the detrimental effect of an antibiotic to the infecting microorganism (prokaryotic cell) must greatly exceed any detrimental effect of that antibiotic to the patient (eukaryotic cell). To appreciate fully any antibiotic's selective toxicity one must have an understanding of that drug's microbiologic mechanism(s) of action and how this correlates with its human pharmacology. Antibiotics of high selective toxicity are sufficiently unique in their antimicrobial mechanism(s) of action specifically to avoid overlapping mammalian cell cytotoxicity. Of the commonly prescribed antibiotics the majority have high selective toxicity whereby adverse effects on the host's cells are minimized and of real concern only if drug doses and/or duration of therapy exceeds published recommendations. Antibiotics of low selectivity tend to be less frequently prescribed, as pharmacologic toxicity usually limits their true beneficial effects.

How the benefit:risk ratio of antibacterial therapy might also influence the selection of an antibiotic is exemplified when one examines the *spectrum of activity* of the agent in question. A narrow spectrum of activity indicates that the antibiotic is inhibitory only to the infecting (etiologic) microorganism, without significant overlapping cytotoxicity to any other systemic organism not involved in the disease. The *antibiotic of choice* is defined as the narrowest spectrum, least toxic drug to which the infecting organism is sensitive. Broad-spectrum antibiotics have the major clinical disadvantage that they also inhibit or lyse organisms that are part of the host's normal bacterial flora. Suppression of the normal flora, those organisms not necessarily responsible for the infectious process under treatment, often leads to bacterial or fungal superinfections that further compromise the patient's safe therapeutic response to the prescribed drug. Candidal suprainfection of the mouth and oropharynx (thrush), of the vagina (candidal vaginitis), and toxigenic *Clostridium difficile* overgrowth in the colon (pseudomembranous colitis) are common examples of suprainfections associated with modern broad-spectrum antibiotics.

One important reason that beta-lactam antibiotics and aminoglycosides are preferred general-purpose agents for both hospitalized persons and outpatients with infectious disease is that they are bactericidal. That is, their mechanism of action is both to inhibit bacterial growth and lyse bacterial cells at low concentration. Bacteriostatic antibiotics inhibit bacterial growth without lysis, only kill bacteria at high concentrations, and depend heavily on the patient's normal host defenses, especially opsonophagocytosis, for their clinical efficacy. Infection that complicates the management of persons with reduced host defenses is occurring more frequently, usually in hospitalized patients who have nosocomial infection. Nosocomial pathogens tend first to colonize and subsequently infect patients whose illness or its treatment have caused reduced host defenses. Nosocomially infected patients are those whose host defenses are compromised,

TABLE 5.1. Microbiologic and Pharmacologic Considerations

Microbiologic	*Pharmacologic*
Mechanisms of action	Dose and dose interval
Selective toxicity: high or low	Route of administration and bioavailability
Spectrum of activity: broad or narrow	Absorption and distribution
	Metabolism and excretion
Quality of effect: cidal or static	Time course of drug action
	Adverse effects
Potency: MIC, MBC	Contraindications to use
Mechanisms of resistance	

whose infection gained entry through a recognized portal, and whose normally protective flora has been suppressed by prior therapy with broad-spectrum antibiotics.

Nosocomial infections are further complicated by the recognized antibiotic resistance patterns of the common hospital-acquired pathogens. In such instances, consideration of antibiotic potency is important to the successful outcome of therapy. Where one antibiotic, representative of a known pharmacologic group of antibiotics, is considered the drug of choice, the decision is usually based on the knowledge that this drug has a several times lower *minimum inhibitory concentration (MIC)* to the infecting pathogen being treated. The MIC of a single bacterial isolate to an antibiotic is defined as the lowest concentration of drug that will inhibit growth of the organism in a fixed time period as examined according to a specifically defined microbiologic in vitro method. Similarly, the *minimum bactericidal concentration (MBC)* is the lowest concentration of antibiotic necessary not only to inhibit growth but to lyse bacterial cells as defined by no growth of the organism when recultured in the absence of the test antibiotic. Sensitivity and resistance definitions of a pathogenic bacterial isolate to any one antibiotic are based on the approximate correlation of that organism's MIC to that antibiotic compared to the mean blood or tissue antibiotic levels achieved after administration of a pharmacologically safe dose. In only selected instances is this correlation further refined such that the criteria for susceptibility are examined in relation to the published record of clinical efficacy of therapy.

Physicians tend to overestimate the true in vivo susceptibility of an infecting organism to the prescribed antibiotic of choice. In vitro testing, however, usually reflects the final bacteriologic response outcome of therapy. Yet in the clinical situation where one is treating a nosocomial infection with its known resistance patterns in a patient with depressed host defenses, any disparity between true in vitro susceptibility and in vivo response is emphasized. The physician must always consider that even a twofold to fourfold lower MIC value between two antibiotics of the same pharmacologic class may be of real benefit to support a significant bacteriologic response and a full and rapid recovery from the infection.

Added to this is the responsibility to prescribe antibiotics to patients in pharmacologically effective but safe dosage schedules. Whatever the choice of therapy, the physician must always consider administration of accurate doses to avoid not only dose-related toxicity but suppressive nontherapeutic dosages that encourage the emergence of low-grade antibacterial resistance.

Resistance of any microorganism to any antimicrobial agent is due to one of three mechanisms: alteration in the target site of drug action (mutational or chromosomal resistance), chemical substitution or degradation of the drug itself (plasmid- or enzyme-mediated resistance), and inhibition of cell wall or outer membrane permeability. A good example of mutational resistance is illustrated by penicillin resistance among *Streptococcus pneumoniae* or methicillin resistance among coagulase-positive and -negative staphylococci (*S. aureus* and *S. epidermidis*). The target site alteration shared by these two examples of beta-lactam–resistant pyogenic cocci is due to the fact that a critical enzyme (one of several specific penicillin-binding proteins, see below) no longer binds the penicillin in question. Mutational resistance is limited to only a few other examples and is not as common as either the enzyme-mediated or altered-permeability types of resistance.

The classic example of an enzyme-mediated resistance mechanism is hydrolysis of the beta-lactam ring of penicillins or cephalosporins by beta-lactamases (penicillinases or cephalosporinases). These bacterial enzymes, whether of plasmid origin or from transposable DNA, are capable of degrading the central nucleus of the beta-lactam antibiotic (the beta-lactam ring), resulting in relatively profound high-level resistance. Other enzymatic antibiotic resistance is exemplified by the alteration of structure induced by plasmid-mediated enzymes. This is an important and popularly described mechanism principally because it is so sharply defined and easily recognized. Low-level resistance due to altered bacterial cell wall/outer membrane permeability of the antibiotic is even more statistically significant and clinically worrisome.

Low-level resistance, in which a twofold to fourfold increase in MIC values correlates with a significant decrease in bacteriologic response rates, is an emerging clinical problem. Permeability changes in the outer membrane of enteric gram-negative bacilli mediate a significant reduction in the amount of free antibiotic available to the drug's internal target site of action. In the case of beta-lactam antibiotic resistance, this is further aggravated by the rate of enzymatic hydrolysis whereby a sufficient reduction in permeability may allow for complete hydrolysis of all available antibiotic, thus preventing binding to penicillin binding proteins. These account for the lack of responsiveness of nosocomial gram-negative bacillary infections to antibiotic therapy and treatment failure of infections at sites slightly less accessible to full antibiotic distribution.

In addition to these bacterial causes of treatment resistance, many host determinants play an aggravating role in attempts to achieve a satisfactory clinical response. Patients whose defenses against infection are compromised by congenital or acquired defects in phagocytosis or cellular or humoral immunity, or whose mechanical barriers to infection are obstructed (such as the absence of a normal mucociliary protective effect of the lung in chronic obstructive pulmonary disease or the presence of urinary tract obstruction in pyelonephritis) are significantly at risk of aggravated infection that is less responsive to conventional antibiotic chemotherapy. These are frequent patient factors that complicate a serious underlying disease process and lead to a less than satisfactory outcome of antibiotic therapy.

Other host factors influencing susceptibility are the pharmacokinetic properties of the antibiotic that govern the distribution of the drug to the active site of infection. Before concentrating at the site of the infection, an antibiotic may be affected by the degree of bioavailability, serum protein binding, diffusion within the extracellular fluid space by virtue of its molecular size, lipid solubility and state of ionization, and the mechanism by which it is cleared from the body. These are all important when we consider active drug distribution to the cerebrospinal fluid (CSF), brain, eye, bile, joint fluid, bone, saliva, prostate, and so on — all sites to which drug access is relatively restricted. Drugs that are rapidly absorbed and excreted tend not to concentrate in specific host tissues. Advantage is taken, however, in the case of an antibiotic whose rapid elimination into the urine provides for effective management of urinary tract infections.

Important pharmacologic considerations in antibiotic chemotherapy include the route of administration for optimal absorption and patient compliance, the time for maximal absorption, the drug's distribution in the host (especially to key sites such as CSF, brain, eye, bone, joint, prostate, etc.), metabolism by the liver with biliary excretion usually of inactive metabolites, and finally, renal excretion of parent drug and metabolites. Much emphasis is placed on these factors in dosage selection, timed dose interval, route of administration, and duration of treatment.

Appropriate dose selection is mainly empiric and estimated such that attainable serum concentrations will exceed the MIC of the organism to the particular antibiotic of choice. In most situations the dosage interval is based on the principal of repeated administration to avoid low subtherapeutic serum concentrations whenever possible. This usually equates to a timed interval equal to three or four times the serum half-life of the antibiotic. The oral route of administration, the mainstay of outpatient antibiotic therapy, is probably underused in hospitalized patients. Many antibiotics with excellent bioavailability achieve satisfactory serum concentrations after oral administration. Intramuscular injections, a now less frequently prescribed route of administration, have the disadvantage of causing irritation at the site of administration. Thus intravenous antibiotic use is the widely accepted choice for seriously ill patients, especially as larger doses can be safely administered.

Duration of antibiotic therapy is also empiric, although a general rule is to continue therapy for at least 48 to 72 hours after the patient clinically responds as assessed by fever lysis, return to a normal white blood cell count and differential, resolution of symptoms, and improvement of mood, appetite, and level of activity. For selected infections, specific durations of therapy are set out. Examples are, 10 days for *S. pyogenes* pharyngitis, 4 weeks for subacute bacterial endocarditis, 2 weeks for pyelonephritis, and a minimum of 2 weeks for *S. aureus* bacteremia.

Direct adverse effects of antimicrobial drug therapy include hypersensitivity, organ toxicity, and suprainfections and are summarized as follows:

1. Hypersensitivity reactions
   All beta-lactam antibiotics
   Sulfonamides

Nitrofurantoin
2. Nephrotoxicity
   Aminoglycosides
   Sulfonamides
   Beta-lactam antibiotics
   Polymyxins
3. Ototoxicity and vestibulotoxicity
   Aminoglycosides
   Vancomycin
4. Neurotoxicity
   Nitrofurantoin
   Metronidazole
   Aminoglycosides
   Isoniazid
5. Hepatotoxicity
   Isoniazid
   Erythromycin estolate
   Clindamycin
   Intravenous tetracycline
6. Hematopoietic toxicity
   Chloramphenicol
   Sulfonamides
   Trimethoprim
7. Bleeding diathesis
   Moxalactam
   Carbenicillin, ticarcillin, piperacillin

The indirect effects of antibiotics are more subtle and include the adverse effects of therapy on both the environmental flora (including the hospital flora) and the host's own flora. Appropriate therapy helps minimize both direct and indirect effects, and elevates the specific therapeutic response to an acceptable level for the best prospect of achieving a full and satisfactory clinical and bacteriologic response.

SELECTIVE TOXICITY

The importance of selective toxicity to antibacterial efficacy is illustrated by chloramphenicol and tetracycline, both inhibitors of bacterial protein synthesis, and by sulfonamides and trimethoprim, inhibitors of the synthesis and reduction of dihydrofolate respectively.

Inhibitors of Bacterial Synthesis

Bacterial protein synthesis differs from that of mammalian cells because prokaryotic cells use 70S ribosomes. Eukaryotic cells base their cytoplasmic synthesis on their 80S ribosomal RNA with the exception that their mitochondrial protein synthesis involves prokaryotic-type ribosomes.

Chloramphenicol reversibly binds to the larger ribosomal subunit (50S), resulting in inhibition of protein synthesis and bacterial stasis. Its primary target is the aminoacyl-tRNA site (A site) of the peptidyl transferase center, although lower affinity binding to the peptidyl-tRNA site (P site) does occur. Chloramphenicol inhibits binding of aminoacyl-tRNA and formation of peptide bonds. Much of its selective toxicity to a broad spectrum of bacterial pathogens is based on its high lipid solubility and excellent permeability, achieving bacteriostatic microbial intracellular concentrations. Accumulation of chloramphenicol in high concentrations in host tissues is deleterious to normal mammalian cell functions because of the drug's overlapping inhibition of mitochondrial protein synthesis. This is a limitation to its selectivity and is responsible for its dose-related toxicities.

Tetracyclines are another group of broad-spectrum bacteriostatic antibiotics that inhibit ribosomal protein synthesis. Tetracyclines prevent enzymatic and nonenzymatic binding of aminoacyl-tRNA to the A site of the ribosome by first chelating with magnesium and then binding strongly to the 70S ribosome. If tissue concentrations of tetracycline accumulate, toxicity is manifest as antianabolic effects, probably by virtue of its overlapping inhibition of host cell protein synthesis and subsequent failure to utilize amino acids into proteins. This relatively low selective toxicity is a significant disadvantage of the tetracyclines.

Inhibitors of the Synthesis and Reduction of Dihydrofolate

Sulfonamides have an antibacterial mechanism of action specific to bacterial synthesis of dihydrofolate, with no antimetabolic effects on host cells, affording these drugs high selective toxicity. Sulfonamides inhibit dihydropteroate synthetase by competing with *p*-aminobenzoic acid. The reduced rate of synthesis of dihydrofolate explains the drug's antimetabolic bacteriostatic cellular effects.

Trimethoprim, a drug not structurally related to sulfonamides, acts as a competitive inhibitor of dihydrofolate reductase (the enzyme that converts dihydrofolate to tetrahydrofolate). The latter is used as 1-carbon cofactors in the synthesis of thymidylate and purines, conversion of homocystine to methionine, and the production of formyl-methionyl-tRNA. Trimethoprim-sensitive bacteria have dihydrofolate reductase enzyme susceptibility to inhibition by trimethoprim at therapeutic concentrations. Trimethoprim's high selective toxicity is based entirely on the fact that it has higher affinity for the dihydrofolate reductases of bacterial cells than the corresponding mammalian enzymes (50,000 times more trimethoprim is necessary to inhibit dihydrofolate reductases of mammalian cells than dihydrofolate reductase of *Escherichia coli*). Folate deficiency is therefore a most uncommon toxicity of trimethoprim therapy.

GENERAL APPROACH TO ANTIBIOTIC SELECTION

The selection of an antibiotic is complex enough without having continually to evaluate newly marketed agents with their individual microbiologic or pharmacologic advantages. By understanding the basic few drugs of each class of antibiotics, however, one gains a perspective to rational selection. Obviously, the final choice depends on knowing the in vitro antimicrobial susceptibility profile of the infecting bacterial pathogen. Yet even then the selection is confused by the long list of antibiotics to which the organism is sensitive. The critical therapeutic decisions that are usually necessary before any organism is even identified require that the clinician know if it is necessary to include pyogenic cocci, *S. aureus,* unusual or nosocomial gram-negative bacilli, *Pseudomonas aeruginosa, Hemophilus influenzae, Streptococcus faecalis,* or other antimicrobial-resistant organisms within the spectrum of initial blind therapy.

A classification (Table 5.2) of all major antibiotic groups either as general-purpose or for specific use will help simplify the initial decision of which drug is appropriate. Within the general-purpose group are drugs of sufficiently broad or narrow spectrum to apply to almost all therapeutic situations. Although this group includes only two antibiotic classes, the beta-lactams and the aminoglycosides, the list of individual agents easily exceeds the number in the category for specific indications. The specific-use drugs are only prescribed when the differential diagnosis includes bacterial pathogens known to be treated best with one of these agents. Otherwise it is usually preferable to make the selection for initial therapy from the general-purpose antibiotics.

TABLE 5.2. Classification of Antibiotics

General Purpose	*Specific Use*
First-generation beta-lactams	Sulfonamides, trimethoprim, TMP/SMZ
Penicillins, natural and semisynthetic	Chloramphenicol
Cephalosporins	Tetracyclines
Second-generation beta-lactams	Erythromycins
Third-generation beta-lactams	Clindamycin
Aminoglycosides	Vancomycin
	Metronidazole
	Nitrofurantoin
	Fusidic acid
	Rifampin
	Bacitracin, polymyxins

The reason for this arbitrary classification will become apparent in the subsequent text.

GENERAL-PURPOSE ANTIBIOTICS

Beta-Lactam Antibiotics

With the introduction of newer beta-lactam antibiotics (Table 5.3) (especially the cephalosporins), the status of the penicillins as a distinct group has been diminished and they are now best merged within the entire class of beta-lactam antibiotics. The cephalosporins share the many advantages of the penicillins, making beta-lactams the drugs of first choice for a wide variety of infections due to gram-positive and gram-negative cocci and bacilli. Collectively, their wide spectrum of activity covers the most common clinical infections and as a group these antibiotics share high selective toxicity, bactericidal action, pharmacologic properties that convey good tissue distribution, and a low frequency of adverse effects.

The original natural penicillins remain as useful today as when they were first introduced for the majority of their prime indications. The emergence of infections caused by penicillin-resistant pyogenic cocci and gram-negative bacilli limited the full potential of these antibiotics. Semisynthetic beta-lactams, many only recently introduced, have in large part surmounted the problem of bacterial resistance so that selected agents are now commonly prescribed for severe staphylococcal sepsis, nosocomially resistant gram-negative bacil-

TABLE 5.3. The Beta-lactam Antibiotics

	Penicillins	Cephalosporins
First-generation		
Natural	Penicillin G* and V Procaine and benzathine penicillin G	
Semisynthetic	Oxacillin, cloxacillin, dicloxacillin, flucloxacillin Nafcillin, methicillin Ampicillin, amoxicillin Carbenicillin	Cephalothin, cephazolin, cephalexin, cephradine, cefadroxil, cefaclor
Second-generation	Ticarcillin	Cefamandole Cefoxitin†
Third-generation	Piperacillin Mezlocillin Azlocillin	Moxalactam‡ Cefotaxime Cefoperazone

*Also known as benzyl penicillin or crystalline penicillin G.
†Actually a cephamycin and not a cephalosporin.
‡Actually an oxalactam and not a cephalosporin.

lary sepsis (including *P. aeruginosa*), gonorrhea and syphilis, anaerobic sepsis (including *Bacteroides fragilis*), and infections with *H. influenzae*.

Mechanisms of Action and Resistance

Beta-lactam antibiotics inhibit bacterial cell division with loss of cell viability and cell lysis. They are all bactericidal and have absolute selective toxicity. They interfere exclusively with synthesis and control of the peptidoglycan component of bacterial cell walls. Peptidoglycan synthesis provides the cell wall structure its shape and resilience. A structural defect of completed peptidoglycan is the first step toward penicillin-induced cell lysis. Penicillins bind to a series of proteins (referred to as penicillin-binding proteins or PBPs) contained within the cytoplasmic membrane of both gram-positive and gram-negative bacteria. Each protein may possess one or more enzymatic functions including D,D-carboxypeptidase, transpeptidase, and endopeptidase activities. For example, in *E. coli* K12, six PBPs exist: PBP 1A and 1B for peptidoglycan cross-linking (transpeptidase), which if inhibited cause cell elongation and lysis; PBP 2 for maintenance of rod cell shape, which if inhibited (principally by a unique beta-lactam, mecillinam), causes large ovoid cells that are osmotically stable; PBP 3 for cell septum formation, which if inhibited prevents cell division and results in filament formation; PBP 4 for both D,D-carboxypeptidase and endopeptidase activities; and PBPs 5 and 6 also for carboxypeptidase activities. The PBPs 1B and 3 seem particularly important for the action of most penicillins and cephalosporins. Beta-lactam antibiotics cause filamentous shapes to form when gram-negative bacteria are exposed to low concentrations. If the concentrations are raised, bulging of the cell envelope appears at points of cell division, and eventually cell lysis occurs. Efficacy of beta-lactam antibiotics depends on their relative affinities for the PBPs, their beta-lactamase stability, and their ability to penetrate through the outer membrane of the bacterial cell wall.

The beta-lactam ring interacts with the active site of the penicillin-sensitive enzymes. The ring's beta-lactam bond has been proposed to be a structural analog of the D-alanyl-alanine dipeptide, the cross-linking peptide bond in the final transpeptidation step of cell wall synthesis. This results in poor cross-linking, which in effect prevents cell growth.

Cell lysis (irreversibility of penicillin action) is postulated to result from activation of autolytic activity by major peptidoglycan hydrolases (autolysins). These hydrolyze covalent bonds of peptidoglycan to then expose the cytoplasmic membrane which results in osmotic lysis of the cell. Support for this hypothesis is described by the study of so-called beta-lactam tolerance in several types of bacteria, including *S. aureus*, *S. pneumoniae*, group B streptococci, *E. coli*, *Streptococcus mutans*, and *Streptococcus sanguis*. Tolerant strains resist lysis by penicillins probably because of reduced autolysin activity. Tolerance can be demonstrated *in vitro* when the MBC:MIC ratio of any of the beta-lactam antibiotics exceeds 32 to the organism in question. The other theoretical model for lysis is explained by the presumed continued growth of cytoplasmic mass, with cell disruption occuring at sites of weakened peptidoglycan structure.

Beta-lactamases are enzymes capable of hydrolyzing the beta-lactam ring of this important group of antibiotics. One of the most important examples explains the mechanism of resistance to beta-lactams among staphylococci. This involves inducible beta-lactamases released as extracellular enzymes that hydrolyze penicillins and cephalosporins to unstable and inactive penicilloic acid and cephalosporic acid metabolites respectively. In *S. aureus* this is mediated by an inducible R-plasmid gene. Thus penicillinases of gram-positive bacteria cause resistance by hydrolysis of the extracellular beta-lactam by the accumulation of beta-lactamase within the whole population of bacterial cells. Inducible beta-lactamases activate an antirepressor protein that combines with and then inactivates the repressor protein, thereby allowing synthesis of penicillinase.

The semisynthetic penicillins methicillin and nafcillin, isoxazolyl penicillins such as cloxacillin, and all cephalosporins are chemically modifed such that their beta-lactam nucleus has a very low affinity for staphylococcal beta-lactamase and are therefore resistant to enzymatic hydrolysis. These are key antibiotics for the treatment of beta-lactamase–producing *S. aureus* infections.

Beta-lactamases are widespread in bacteria and those of gram-negative bacteria are particularly important causes of antibiotic resistance. Beta-lactamases of gram-negative bacteria are either chromosomally or R-plasmid–mediated, and are either inducible or constitutive. Chromosomal beta-lactamases are widespread among gram-negative bacteria and are capable of producing resistance to cephalosporins and penicillins. Newer second- and third-generation beta-lactams, especially those with a 7-alpha-methoxy group on the beta-lactam ring (e.g., cefoxitin and moxalactam), are intrinsically resistant to hydrolysis by chromosomal beta-lactamase. These are useful for treating sepsis caused by resistant gram-negative bacilli. There are currently 11 types of R-plasmid–specified beta-lactamases (based on isoelectric focusing). TEM1, whose genes are transposon-borne, is the most widely distributed of the enzymes, accounting for approximately 75% of all R-plasmid beta-lactamases. It is the one type capable of hydrolyzing those penicillins (but not cephalosporins) usually otherwise active against gram-negative bacilli. It is also important to note the homology of TEM-type beta-lactamases among *H. influenzae* and *Neisseria gonorrhoeae* that mediate beta-lactamase production and result in the worldwide problem of penicillin resistance among these pathogens.

Resistance of a beta-lactam to hydrolysis by a beta-lactamase does not necessarily imply that that drug will effectively inhibit that particular bacterium. Permeability refers to the rate of penetration of the beta-lactam through the organism's cell envelope or, in the case of gram-negative bacteria, the outer membrane of the gram-negative cell wall. Outer membrane diffusion is influenced by molecular size, hydrophobicity, and electrical charge of the antibiotic. Permeability competes directly with beta-lactamase affinity before definitive binding to PBPs mediates drug susceptibility. Lowered permeability accounts for differential susceptibility among various beta-lactams and is a favored explanation of low-level resistance to beta-lactam antibiotics. This is a highly effective mechanism of beta-lactam resistance whereby retarded entry of the drug to the periplasmic space allows periplasmic antibiotic detoxification preventing bacterial inhibition. The corollary is illustrated by the situation in which the permeability rate of the antibiotic is such that hydrolysis of periplasmic beta-lactamase is insufficient to detoxify the antibiotic, resulting in PBP binding and cell lysis. The combination of improved permeability and beta-lactamase resistance explains why some second- and all third-generation beta-lactams have an extended spectrum of activity to otherwise beta-lactam–resistant nosocomial gram-negative bacilli.

Decreased affinity for binding to penicillin binding proteins accounts for selected examples of beta-lactam resistance and is best illustrated by the penicillin resistance of very occasional clinical isolates of *S. pneumoniae* and of methicillin resistance of *S. aureus*. These effects are probably the result of several mutations whereby one or more of the PBPs are altered so that beta-lactam binding is reduced. For both examples, clinical occurrence is infrequent and is only a problem in selected outbreaks, especially that of methicillin-resistant *S. aureus* where hospital cross-infection is occasionally reported.

The final mechanism of beta-lactam resistance is tolerance, and has been described for *S. aureus* and *Streptococcus viridans* group (example, *S. sanguis*). Tolerance is defined by the situation whereby the MBC (defined as that concentration necessary for 99.9% cidal activity) exceeds by far the MIC for that organism — an MBC:MIC ratio of at least 32. Such clinically tolerant isolates are deficient in autolytic activity, resulting in bacterial inhibition but not lysis at clinically achievable tissue and blood concentrations.

Microbiologic and Pharmacologic Considerations

Although penicillins and cephalosporins are widely distributed throughout the body, advantage is taken of the fact that these antibiotics can be administered safely in extremely high doses so that bactericidal levels are achieved at most tissue sites of infection. Furthermore, in meningitis, inflammation of the meninges is an essential component to augment antibiotic distribution to the CSF.

Approximately half of the beta-lactams now available are not absorbed from the upper gastrointestinal tract upon oral administration. This is best explained by the relative instability of the beta-lactam ring to gastric acidity. Only acid stable beta-lactams reach the duodenum for absorption. This is certainly the advantage of phenoxymethyl penicillin (penicillin V), which is orally absorbed better than penicillin G. Oral bioavailability is still only a fraction of the dose administered, thus limiting the serum concentration of free drug available for distribution. The parenteral route of administration is frequently selected so that larger doses can be more readily administered.

Most beta-lactams have a short serum half-life (approximately 30 minutes for penicillin G and 60 minutes for most semisynthetic penicillins and cephalosporins) as they are rapidly cleared by the kidneys and excreted in the urine in active form. Frequent oral (four times daily) or intravenous (every four hours) administration is therefore generally recommended. The exceptions to this are cefazolin, moxalactam, and cefoperazone, which have longer half-lives and require less frequent administration. Two cephalosporins, cephalothin and cefotaxime, are metabolized by the liver and their less active metabolites are then excreted in the urine.

To prolong the duration of antibacterial effect, certain pharmaceutical modifications to penicillin G are now classic first-generation penicillins. Procaine penicillin G contains an equimolar mixture of penicillin G and procaine that after intramuscular administration provides the patient with penicillin G serum levels that remain elevated for 18 to 24 hours. It is primarily indicated for treatment of acute genitourinary gonorrhea. Benzathine penicillin is an ammonium salt of benzyl penicillin that maintains low serum concentrations of penicillin G for at least 18 and as long as 28 days. This advantage provides for the single-dose treatment of syphilis and once-monthly prophylaxis for acute beta-hemolytic *S. pyogenes* pharyngitis for the prevention of recurrent rheumatic fever. Both benzathine and procaine penicillins are reserved strictly for intramuscular administration.

Probenecid is an inhibitor of renal tubular organic acid secretion (the mechanism that accounts for 90% of the renal excretion of beta-lactams). It is used as an adjunct to beta-lactams to increase their antibiotic serum concentrations and to prolong their serum half-lives. Probenecid is regularly prescribed with procaine penicillin G, ampicillin, or amoxicillin to take advantage of these two properties in the usual management of acute genitourinary gonorrhea.

Simply stated, there are only a few reasons for not selecting a beta-lactam antibiotic: (1) if the organism is resistant to the penicillin or cephalosporin of choice or if resistance is likely to emerge, and (2) if the host is allergic to the drug. With respect to the former, bacterial resistance has been the principal indication to select a semisynthetic beta-lactam, and for this reason a plethora of new first-, second-, and third-generation beta-lactams have been marketed over approximately the past two decades. These can be further classified as either staphylococcal penicillinase-resistant semisynthetic penicillins and cephalosporins or as extended-spectrum beta-lactams.

The semisynthetic penicillinase-resistant penicillins are methicillin, oxacillin, cloxacillin, and nafcillin (all for parenteral use) and oxacillin, cloxacillin, dicloxacillin, and flucloxacillin (all available as oral preparations). As a group they have specific activity against penicillin-resistant beta-lactamase positive *S. aureus* and much lower (compared to penicillin G) antibacterial activity to the other pyogenic cocci. The first-generation cephalosporins are also staphylococcal beta-lactamase–resistant and act as substitutes for the penicillins for therapy of staphylococcal infections. Less than 5% of infections with *S. aureus,* whether attributed to in-hospital or out-of-hospital sources, are sensitive to penicillin G, and therefore a semisynthetic penicillinase-resistant beta-lactam must initially be prescribed whenever staphylococcal sepsis is suspected.

The extended spectrum of first-generation penicillins — ampicillin and carbenicillin and their two closely related second-generation counterparts, amoxicillin and ticarcillin respectively — were introduced as broad-spectrum agents with activity to common gram-negative bacilli. Ampicillin is particularly active against *E. coli* and *Proteus mirabilis*, the two common etiologic bacilli of acute urinary tract infections. Ampicillin is also important to consider in the therapy of infections with *Salmonella* and *Shigella* species and *H. influenzae*. Unfortunately, beta-lactamase–mediated resistance restricts the use of ampicillin for these conditions. Oral amoxicillin is more completely absorbed than ampicillin and for similar doses, peak blood levels are twice those of ampicillin. Amoxicillin's antibacterial spectrum is identical to that of ampicillin and they share common resistance mechanisms.

Carbenicillin and ticarcillin, on the other hand, have slightly extended spectra. They are active against some strains of *P. aeruginosa*, indole-positive *Proteus* species, *Enterobacter*, and *B. fragilis*. For *Pseudomonas* infections advantage is taken of the fact that carbenicillin and ticarcillin can be safely administered at maximal doses twice that for ampicillin, and when combined with an antipseudomonal aminoglycoside (such as tobramycin), a synergistic antibacterial effect results toward this highly resistant nosocomial pathogen. The mechanism of this synergy is that the penicillins individually augment the aminoglycoside's permeability through the outer membrane of *Pseudomonas*, thereby increasing the bacterial uptake of the aminoglycoside for improved bactericidal activity. Ticarcillin is two to four times more potent an inhibitor of *P. aeruginosa* than carbenicillin and is the preferred antipseudomonal, semisynthetic, beta-lactam for initial therapy of *Pseudomonas* infections. Piperacillin, mezlocillin, and azlocillin are even more active than ticarcillin, and after future reporting of clinical experience, one of these may supercede ticarcillin as the drug of first choice.

First-generation cephalosporins were originally introduced as alternatives to the extended-spectrum and antistaphylococcal semisynthetic penicillins. Their spectrum of activity against Enterobacteriaceae is very similar to that of ampicillin (with the one exception that the cephalosporins are generally more active against *Klebsiella* species).

One reason that cephalosporins gained rapid clinical acceptance was that they can be safely administered to penicillin-allergic patients, at least to those with no history of immediate-onset type of allergic reaction. There is only a 10% to 15% occurrence of cross-hypersensitivity where a penicillin-allergic patient may also be cephalosporin allergic. There are, however, several situations in which a cephalosporin is not the preferred alternative to a penicillin in a penicillin-allergic patient. These are as follows:

1. The first- and second-generation cephalosporins do not cross the blood-CSF barrier as efficiently as penicillins even when the meninges are inflamed, and so they are not drugs of choice for primary bacterial meningitis. This is not the case with third-generation cephalosporins that do cross the blood-CSF barrier and are now first-choice antibiotics for gram-negative bacillary meningitis.
2. The first- and second-generation cephalosporins do not share with ampicillin any activity against *H. influenzae*. Again the exceptions to this are cefaclor, cefamandole, and the third-generation cephalosporins that do indeed have inhibitory activity to *Hemophilus* sp. Both moxalactam and cefotaxime are active against beta-lactamase–producing strains of *H. influenzae*.
3. The cephalosporins are not ideal for penicillin sensitive *T. pallidum* and they should not be prescribed to penicillin-allergic patients who have syphilis. Other antibiotics are better alternatives.
4. The cephalosporins do not act synergistically with aminoglycosides against *S. faecalis*. Vancomycin would be the second choice antibiotic in penicillin-allergic patients.
5. Methicillin-resistant staphylococci (especially *S. epidermidis*) are occasionally recorded as sensitive to cephalosporins *in vitro*. Because the mechanism of methicillin resistance is probably shared to some extent with the cephalosporins, these infections are best managed with vancomycin or possibly fusidic acid.

Second-generation cephalosporins were introduced with an extended spectrum to gram-negative bacilli. Cefoxitin, the prototype cephamycin, with a 7-alpha-methoxy group on the beta-lactam ring, is resistant to beta-lactamases, which explains its extended spectrum. Cefamandole has improved permeability characteristics to sensitive gram-negative bacilli that provide rapid cell inhibition before sufficient beta-lactamase degradation can occur.

The antibacterial advantages of improved permeability and beta-lactamase stability are shared by the third-generation cephalosporins. Nosocomial enteric gram-negative bacilli and *Pseudomonas* are still predominantly resistant to first-generation penicillins and first- and second-generation cephalosporins. Since the introduction of third-generation drugs, we have a potentially effective substitute for the more toxic aminoglycosides in treating these infections. The principal indications for prescribing a third-generation beta-lactam antibiotic are as follows:

1. Parenteral antibiotic therapy of hospitalized patients infected with nosocomially resistant gram-negative bacilli either because the infecting organism is aminoglycoside resistant or, as in the case of *P. aeruginosa,* the organism is more susceptible to the combination of tobramycin plus a newer third-generation antipseudomonal beta-lactam such as piperacillin or cefoperazone.
2. To substitute for an aminoglycoside antibiotic in situations where aminoglycoside treatment is either less preferable or potentially more toxic. A patient with progressive renal dysfunction will frequently benefit from a third-generation beta-lactam to avoid not only aminoglycoside toxicity but the situation of prescribing aminoglycosides at lower doses or at excessively long dose intervals.
3. To take advantages of the fact that third-generation beta-lactams have particular antibacterial potency to *H. influenzae, B. fragilis,* and *N. gonorrhoeae,* providing effective beta-lactam therapy to these relatively resistant pathogens.
4. For gram-negative bacillary meningitis by virtue of the ease with which most of the third-generation beta-lactam antibiotics cross the inflamed meninges. The higher CSF concentrations achieved in combination with the significantly lower MICs to these antibiotics give them the advantage over first- and second-generation penicillins and cephalosporins in the treatment of this relatively unusual form of meningitis. It is hoped that future clinical trials will justify also using these third-generation beta-lactams in neonatal gram-negative and *H. influenzae* meningitis.

Third-generation beta-lactams must not be selected for prophylactic indications or as general antibiotics for blind therapy of presumed gram-negative sepsis unless hospital susceptibility profiles of nosocomial gram-negative isolates show widespread aminoglycoside and beta-lactam resistance. Patterns of use for individual hospitals must take into consideration the higher cost of these newest beta-lactams and the real risk of promoting the development of low-level permeability type beta-lactam resistance.

Adverse Effects

The adverse effects of the beta-lactams are listed below:

1. Hypersensitivity
   Immediate-onset allergic reactions: anaphylaxis, angioneurotic edema, urticaria
   Late-onset allergic reactions: urticaria, other skin rashes (maculopapular rashes), drug-induced fever, serum sickness
2. Dose-related toxicities
   CNS
   Electrolyte disturbances
   Bleeding diathesis
3. Interstitial nephritis

Allergic reactions, which account for the majority of side effects, are estimated to occur in 3% to 5% of the population and as many as 10% of patients who have previously received a beta-lactam antibiotic. Anaphylaxis, the most serious immediate-onset allergic reaction, begins 10 to 30 minutes after administration and is recognized as respiratory stridor (secondary to bronchospasm and laryngeal edema) followed by hypotension and collapse of the patient. Subcutaneous and, if necessary, intravenous epinephrine, 0.3 to 0.5 ml of a 1:1000 solution, is the antidote to administer immediately, although aminophylline, corticosteroids, respiratory intubation, or tracheostomy and oxygen may also be necessary. The unpredictable nature of such severe allergy is only best prevented by never prescribing any beta-lactam antibiotic to patients with a history of immediate-onset allergic reactions to penicillins or cephalosporins. Although one can perform skin tests for penicillin allergy with penicilloyl polylysine (PPL), which is commercially available, most physicians do not have the minor determinant mixture (MDM) available. Thus the absolute confidence of the test is thwarted for those potentially allergic patients who are hypersensitive to minor haptenic determinants of penicillins and cephalosporins. In those rare clinical situations where a penicillin or a cephalosporin must be prescribed despite the history of immediate-onset allergy to beta-lactams, desensitization can be tried. Incrementally increasing subcutaneous doses of the antibiotic of choice, under physician supervision and with careful precautions and readiness to treat any immediate-onset reaction, will induce blocking antibodies that frequently allow a full course of beta-lactam therapy without allergic side effects.

An unusual delayed hypersensitivity reaction common to methicillin but occasionally also seen with ampicillin and cloxacillin is interstitial nephritis. Patients develop progressive renal failure with fever, eosinophilia, microscopic hematuria, proteinuria, and pyuria. Renal biopsies reveal tubular damage and interstitial inflammatory changes.

Fortunately, in most clinical situations where a penicillin allergy history is discussed, either the allergy history is of a minor nature so that a cephalosporin can be substituted, or an entirely different antibiotic can be selected.

Maximal-dose penicillin G therapy, especially in patients with renal failure, can cause hallucinations, convulsions, and coma; interference with platelet aggregation resulting in a bleeding diathesis; and electrolyte disturbances, either hyperkalemia from excess potassium salt administration, hypernatremia for a similar reason, or hypokalemic alkalosis from competition for reabsorbable anions at the distal convoluted tubule. It is also prudent to observe for such electrolyte disturbances in patients with congestive failure who may or may not be taking digitalis glycosides.

Moxalactam is singled out as having a more adverse effect than all of the other beta-lactams, at least one that is expressed more frequently with moxalactam alone. Hypoprothrombinemia occurs with regularity and can be associated with an increased risk of hemorrhage. To counteract this, physicians generally administer vitamin K each time they prescribe full-dose moxalactam.

Aminoglycosides

The aminoglycosides in clinical use are neomycin, streptomycin, kanamycin, gentamicin, tobramycin, amikacin, and netilmicin. Neomycin is now used exclusively as a topical preparation. Streptomycin is only prescribed for the treatment of tuberculosis and some more unusual infections such as tularemia, plague, and brucellosis. Kanamycin has essentially been replaced by the newer aminoglycosides, each with an improved spectrum of activity against gram-negative bacilli. Therefore the choice of an aminoglycoside rests among the last four drugs. The selection depends primarily on the differences of potencies and specific activities to gram-negative bacillary pathogens; significant differences of their pharmacologic toxicities are probably of less importance.

Mechanisms of Action and Resistance

Aminoglycosides inhibit the initiation of bacterial protein synthesis and cause misreading of mRNA. The effect of the latter is to produce phenotypic suppression at sublethal concentrations. Their interaction with the 30S ribosomal subunit involves the S12 ribosomal protein component that controls whether or not binding occurs; the exact binding site is unknown. The subsequent change in configuration of the ribosome causes inhibition of dissociation of free ribosomes, decreased stability of initiation complexes, distortions of both the A and P sites, inhibition of ribosome release from mRNA after peptide release, inhibition of peptide termination mediated by peptide release factor, and a possible effect on translocation.

Although these effects on protein synthesis may be adequate to inhibit cell growth, lethality is probably due to the effect of aminoglycosides on cytoplasmic membrane permeability as evidenced by enhanced potassium leakage followed by leakage of high-molecular-weight materials from the cell. Loss of permeability control involves the initial interaction of the positively charged aminoglycoside and the anionic outer surface charge of the outer membrane of gram-negative bacteria, the cytoplasmic membrane-dependent active transfer of the antibiotic across the cell's inner (cytoplasmic) membrane, and the binding to ribosomes involved in a ribosomal cycle.

Resistance to aminoglycosides may be caused by ribosomal mutation of the target site of action, cell membrane impermeability, and lack of transport or enzymatic modification, the last two being the most common mechanisms among clinical isolates of gram-negative bacilli.

Among the Enterobacteriaceae, the most frequent form of resistance is R-factor — mediated enzymatic modification of the antibiotic (*N*-acetylation, *O*-phosphorylation, or *O*-nucleotidylation). Enzymatic resistance depends on the relative rates of inactivation and cell membrane transport. Only a small fraction of the total aminoglycoside in the medium surrounding the organism is taken up by the bacterial cell and the transported drug is then subsequently modified so that it no longer binds to its ribosomal target. It is difficult to predict cross-resistance among the aminoglycosides (i.e., resistance to more than just a single aminoglycoside). Generally, however, amikacin and netilmicin tend to be more resistant antibiotics to the enzymatic modification of some gram-negative bacilli. Permeability rates depend on cell energy, concentration of transport antagonists (especially divalent cations), pH, and periplasmic drug concentrations normally achieved in gram-negative bacilli.

Aminoglycoside-resistant *P. aeruginosa,* which is representative of nosocomially resistant gram-negative bacteria, may show resistance to all tested aminoglycosides including those that are resistant to inactivating enzymes. This common mechanism of resistance is entirely due to their relative impermeability to aminoglycosides. This low-level permeability resistance of *P. aeruginosa* can be overcome by the concomitant use of an antipseudomonal beta-lactam antibiotic such as ticarcillin or piperacillin (and soon to be released, newer third-generation beta-lactams with improved antipseudomonal activity to those third-generation drugs already available). Physiologic factors that reduce aminoglycoside bioactivity include ionized divalent cations such as magnesium and calcium that reduce permeability of the drug through the gram-negative cell's outer membrane, polyanions such as DNA in purulent secretions that bind the drug and thus reduce its bioavailability to the infected tissue site, and the low-pH anaerobic milieu of abscesses that again inhibit those cellular energy processes necessary for efficient drug uptake.

Microbiologic and Pharmacologic Considerations

Aminoglycosides are generally prescribed for their extended spectrum to Enterobacteriaceae that are for the most part sensitive to all aminoglycosides, and to *Pseudomonas* organisms and other nosocomial pathogens that may be gentamicin resistant but sensitive to tobramycin, amikacin, or netilmicin. Selection is based on knowledge of the susceptibility profile of the infecting gram-negative pathogen or, until this is available, the local hospital pattern of susceptibilities. In most instances, gentamicin remains the selection of choice for blind initial therapy of serious gram-negative sepsis. Tobramycin is less active than gentamicin to the common infecting Enterobacteriaceae, yet is of real value for infections with *P. aeruginosa* where it has a twofold to fourfold advantage, by virtue of its improved permeability characteristics. Amikacin is also an alternative to gentamicin for empirical therapy of gram-negative sepsis, especially in areas where gentamicin-resistant bacilli are frequently isolated. Amikacin's major pharmacologic advantage is its resistance to aminoglycoside-inactivating enzymes. Netilmicin's spectrum of activity is very similar to that of gentamicin.

Aminoglycosides are not absorbed orally, and parenteral systemic administration is now generally confined to intravenous delivery as intermittent infusions. Intramuscular injections are limited by the volume necessary for each dose and the patient's reduced compliance to injections compared to infusions.

Aminoglycosides are not bound to serum proteins and therefore have a large volume of distribution. Although diffusion to synovial, pleural, and pericardial tissues is high, effective concentrations are not achieved in the brain, CSF, vitreous and aqueous humors of the eye, and the prostate. Achievable pulmonary tissue concentrations are low, and this plus the physiologic resistance factors make maximal-dose therapy mandatory, with careful monitoring of peak and trough serum levels.

Because of the relatively low susceptibility of Enterobacteriaceae and *Pseudomonas* species, the physician must not only select the microbiologically most active drug but must prescribe that drug in pharmacologically effective dosages that will not cause adverse effects.

Aminoglycosides are eliminated exclusively by the kidneys and are concentrated in the urine. Accumulation occurs in the renal cortex as a manifestation of the exceedingly prolonged true elimination half-life from the body. Impaired renal function further delays drug excretion, and major dosage modifications are therefore necessary to avoid toxic accumulation. Either an increase in dosage interval or a decrease in the amount of drug will reduce the risk of toxic accumulation. Nomograms and mnemonics are available to facilitate safe estimation of the required amount and dosage interval in patients with reduced renal function.

Adverse Effects

Aminoglycoside therapy is limited by the risk of toxicity, especially nephrotoxicity and ototoxicity (vestibular and auditory). The frequency with which these conditions develop depends on the aminoglycoside prescribed. For example, nephrotoxicity is more common than ototoxicity with gentamicin and the reverse is true for tobramycin. Tobramycin and amikacin are less nephrotoxic than gentamicin, and netilmicin exhibits

TABLE 5.4. Pharmacologic Administration of Aminoglycosides

	Recommended Therapeutic Serum Levels (μg/ml)		*Recommended Individual Doses on the Basis of*		
Agent	*Peak**	*Trough†*	*Weight (mg/kg)*	*Surface Area (mg/m²)*	*Usual Dosage Interval (hrs)*
Gentamicin	8±2	1.0±0.5	1.5–2.0	50–60	8
Tobramycin	8±2	1.0±0.5	1.5–2.0	50–60	8
Netilmicin	8±2	1.0±0.5	1.5–2.0	50–60	8
Amikacin	15–25	1–5	7.5	300	12

*Peak serum level is defined as the serum concentration taken 15 minutes after the end of a 15- to 30-minute intravenous drug infusion. Higher peak levels may be acceptable in patients with normal renal function with gram-negative bacillary infections of low susceptibility to aminoglycosides.

†Trough level is that serum concentration just before the next dose is administered.

fewer adverse effects on the eighth cranial nerve.

To avoid these reactions, it is important to prevent toxic accumulation of these drugs in the body. This requires specific dose and dosage interval selection based on the patient's body weight or surface area, renal function, and age, as well as close monitoring of peak and trough blood levels throughout therapy.

To achieve therapeutic serum levels it is important to prescribe an aminoglycoside dosage sufficient to produce peak serum concentrations in excess of the organism's aminoglycoside MIC without exceeding the toxic upper limit for safe drug administration. The dosage interval is then adjusted to bring the trough level to a detectable yet low serum concentration. The most frequent doses, intervals, and peak and trough serum levels for these four aminoglycosides are summarized in Table 5.4.

Patients with renal failure eliminate aminoglycosides relatively gradually and risk toxic accumulation unless the dosage and/or the interval are adjusted to compensate for the degree of reduced renal function. The combined use of aminoglycosides and cephalosporins is also recognized to enhance aminoglycoside nephrotoxicity. Patients who are prescribed both aminoglycosides and loop diuretics have an increased risk of ototoxicity.

A rare adverse effect of aminoglycosides is enhancement of the neuromuscular blockade of curariform drugs during general anesthesia.

SPECIFIC-USE ANTIBIOTICS

Sulfonamides and Trimethoprim

Sulfonamides are the oldest systemic antibiotics still in regular use. Their renewed popularity has been partly due to the introduction of trimethoprim/sulfamethoxazole (cotrimoxazole or TMP/SMZ). Both the sulfonamides and trimethoprim are broad-spectrum bacteriostatic antibiotics and presently available individually or in a fixed-drug combination (80 mg trimethoprim and 400 mg sulfamethoxazole).

Sulfonamides alone are only prescribed systemically for urinary tract infections caused by susceptible Enterobacteriaceae or topically as sulfacetamide eye drops for bacterial conjunctivitis and silver sulfadiazine and sulfamylon both for burn wound sepsis. Similarly, trimethoprim alone is best indicated for the treatment of acute urinary tract infections and acute and chronic bacterial prostatitis, and as prophylaxis for chronic recurrent lower urinary tract infections.

The combination of TMP/SMZ has significantly extended these indications to include also *Salmonella* enteric fevers, *Shigella* enteritis, infantile diarrhea caused by enteropathogenic *E. coli,* prophylaxis for traveler's diarrhea, otitis media (including that caused by ampicillin-resistant *H. influenzae*), prophylaxis of acute infectious exacerbations of chronic bronchitis, *Pneumocystis carinii* pneumonia, nocardiosis, and a variety of sexually transmitted diseases including gonorrhea, lymphogranuloma venereum, and chancroid. It is also prescribed for chemoprophylaxis of bacterial infections in immunocompromised hosts with cancer or patients who are undergoing bone marrow transplantation.

Sulfonamides are prescribed in combination with pyrimethamine for malaria chemoprophylaxis (pyrimethamine plus sulfadoxine), for treatment of uncomplicated attacks of chloroquine-resistant *Plasmodium falciparum* malaria (pyrimethamine plus sulfadiazine), and treatment of toxoplasmosis (pyrimethamine plus triple sulfonamides).

Mechanisms of Action and Resistance

The mechanisms of action of both sulfonamides and trimethoprim have been reviewed (see under Selective Toxicity). Acquired resistance to sulfonamides is relatively common and mainly plasmid mediated. An altered dihydropteroate synthetase is produced that differs from the chromosomal enzyme in that it has reduced affinity for sulfonamides but not *p*-aminobenzoic acid. This represents a mechanism of resistance whereby the new enzyme allows the site of sulfonamide inhibition to be bypassed with synthesis of dihydropteroic acid. Resistance is carried by several transposable elements.

Trimethoprim resistance has a similar bypass mechanism to that for sulfonamides. Plasmid-derived and transposable dihydrofolate reductases have a lowered affinity for trimethoprim with several thousandfold increases in the drug concentration required for 50% enzyme inhibition. This allows for full bacterial synthesis of tetrahydrofolate.

Resistance to both sulfonamide and trimethoprim can also be explained in part by reduced drug permeability.

Microbiologic and Pharmacologic Considerations

The pharmacology of trimethoprim is straightforward compared to that of the sulfonamides. Trimethoprim is orally well absorbed and it is distributed widely in most body tissues. Thirty percent of the drug is metabolized and the remainder is excreted unchanged in the urine. When renal function is normal, trimethoprim achieves high urinary concentrations for inhibition of most common bacterial urinary tract pathogens. Its elimination half-life is 10 to 12 hours and significantly longer in patients with renal dysfunction. Trimethoprim concentrates in prostatic acinar tissues, making it the drug of choice for bacterial prostatitis. It also concentrates in saliva, inflamed lung tissues, and bile.

Sulfonamides are also well absorbed orally (with the exception of some rarely used nonabsorbable preparations) and equally well distributed within the body. In the circulation, sulfonamides are bound to albumin, which can significantly interfere with other albumin-bound drugs and compounds (especially bilirubin; see under Adverse Effects). Sulfonamides are acetylated by the liver and these inactive metabolites are then excreted in the urine. Sulfonamides and their conjugated metabolites are generally insoluble in urine, resulting in their precipitation as crystals in the urine filtrate. Crystalluria blocks renal tubules and can cause renal failure. Although the problem can be partially prevented by forced-fluid diuresis to maintain a high urine flow through the renal tubules, or by alkalinization of the urine, which improves sulfonamide solubilities, crystalluria has limited the popular use of many older sulfonamides that were most likely to cause this adverse effect. An example of an older but popular systemic sulfonamide preparation was triple sulfonamides (trisulfapyrimidines), which was a combination of sulfadiazine, sulfamerazine, and sulfathiazole. In this mixture, the three sulfonamides each retained their individual urine solubilities, and by limiting the dose of each, the risk of crystalluria was significantly reduced.

The sulfonamides prescribed today are specifically selected, as they are very unlikely to cause crystalluria. Sulfasoxizole is an example of this in that it is a short-acting sulfonamide that is not only excreted rapidly but is highly soluble in urine and therefore safely prescribed. These last pharmacologic properties have promoted this popularly prescribed sulfonamide to be used almost exclusively in the treatment of acute urinary tract infections. Adequate tissue levels are not achieved using sulfasoxizole.

Another approach to circumvent the problem of crystalluria was to prescribe medium- and long-acting sulfonamides that are slowly excreted. The long-acting sulfonamides have been discontinued from clinical use as they were recognized frequently to cause the Stevens-Johnson syndrome (see under Adverse Effects). Sulfamethoxazole is a medium-acting preparation that has been retained in popular clinical use as the sulfonamide component of TMP/SMZ.

The optimal ratio of serum concentrations of TMP to SMZ for maximal synergistic effect to most susceptible bacteria is approximately 1:20. The fixed oral and intravenous preparations are a combination of TMP and SMZ in a 1:5 ratio that will achieve the approximate synergistic levels in serum. Both antibiotics are variably absorbed when prescribed orally and therefore intravenous administration is more predictable. Tissue concentrations of sulfamethoxazole are generally less than those for trimethoprim when expressed as a percentage of serum concentrations.

Adverse Effects

Sulfonamide-induced crystalluria causing renal damage is now a rare clinical occurrence. The major adverse effects of sulfonamides are hypersensitivity reactions manifesting as drug fevers, eosinophilia, urticaria, maculopapular rashes, serum sickness, and the Stevens-Johnson syndrome, a subset of erythema multiforme. Sulfonamides also cause bone marrow depression of leukopoiesis, which occasionally causes symptoms of agranulocytosis. Hemolytic anemia is also described in patients with inherited glucose-6-phosphate dehydrogenase deficiency.

Sulfonamides are contraindicated in the newborn and during the last trimester of pregnancy (principally because they readily diffuse across the placenta) because they compete with bilirubin for albumin-binding sites. Fetal albumin more easily displaces free bilirubin, resulting in kernicterus. Sulfonamides are also contraindicated in premature infants, who are unable to conjugate them before elimination can occur.

Trimethoprim is generally well tolerated with only a low frequency of gastrointestinal upset. Folate deficiency and hematologic side effects are unusual. Folate-depleted patients who take high doses of trimethoprim for prolonged courses of treatment can be given folinic acid without diminishing trimethoprim's antibacterial activity.

Chloramphenicol

The indications for prescribing chloramphenicol are few and limited principally because of its well-described bone marrow toxicities. Chloramphenicol is usually considered the drug of choice for the following infections, although in many instances suitable substitutes are now available:

1. Typhoid fever and enteric fevers caused by nontyphoidal *Salmonella* species.
2. Anaerobic infections caused by *B. fragilis*, especially if systemically severe or associated with brain abscess.
3. Pneumococcal, meningococcal, and *H. influenzae* meningitis in penicillin-allergic patients.
4. *H. influenzae* meningitis due to ampicillin-resistant (beta-lactamase–positive) strains. In pediatric meningitis, chloramphenicol is always considered a first choice antibiotic until *H. influenzae* is excluded or until the etiologic strain of the organism is proved susceptible to ampicillin.

Although these infections usually respond well to chloramphenicol, it is now recognized that occasional isolates of *Salmonella typhi* and *H. influenzae* are chloramphenicol resistant. Thus proving *in vitro* susceptibility is still important before fully relying on this antibiotic as the first choice for therapy. In addition, several alternatives to chloramphenicol for anaerobic infections with *B. fragilis* are available and one in particular, metronidazole, is a suitable substitute in the management of anaerobic suppurative brain abscess. Moxalactam and possibly other new third-generation beta-lactams may, in the future, replace chloramphenicol for the treatment of beta-lactamase–positive *H. influenzae* meningitis.

Mechanisms of Action and Resistance

The mechanisms of action of chloramphenicol have been reviewed above (see under Selective Toxicity). The common explanation for acquired chloramphenicol resistance is a plasmid-mediated and transposable chloramphenicol acetyl transferase that causes enzymatic acetylation of chloramphenicol. Acetylated chloramphenicol is inactive as an antibiotic, accounting for the bacterial resistance. Some gram-negative bacteria that do not possess R factors have their low-level chloramphenicol resistance explained on the basis of reduced outer membrane permeability.

Microbiologic and Pharmacologic Considerations

Chloramphenicol is a lipid-soluble, broad-spectrum, bacteriostatic antibiotic with some distinct pharmacologic advantages. Namely, it is well absorbed and diffuses readily into most tissues including both the brain and CSF. The risk of aplastic anemia restricts its use, however, and for infections in general, with susceptible gram-positive and gram-negative organisms, chloramphenicol is generally contraindicated.

Chloramphenicol is metabolized in the liver by conjugation with glucuronic acid to inactive metabolites. Ninety percent of the drug and its metabolites are excreted by the kidneys. The immaturity of the enzyme glucuronyl transferase in neonates accounts for the severe dosage limitations of chloramphenicol to newborns. To prevent the development of the gray-baby syndrome, the daily dosage of chloramphenicol to newborns should not exceed 25 mg per kg, and both peak and trough blood levels should be closely monitored to prevent toxic accumulation of drug in the body.

Adverse Effects

The bone marrow toxicities of chloramphenicol occur in two forms: a dose-related condition probably due to chloramphenicol's inhibition of mitochondrial protein synthesis (chloramphenicol also inhibits the uptake of iron by normoblasts) and an idiosyncratic reaction of unknown etiology. Both toxicities cause similar clinical manifestations such as onset of anemia, leukopenia, or thrombocytopenia, or combinations of these. Dose-related toxicity is quite common and if one examines for reticulocytopenia or an increased serum iron concentration, all patients receiving usual dosages of chloramphenicol for long periods of time or patients prescribed amounts in excess of 4 to 6 gm per day will manifest this toxicity. Serious dose-related bone marrow suppression is unusual if chloramphenicol is promptly discontinued whenever the white blood cell counts decrease to less than 4.0×10^9 per liter, or if the percentage of polymorphonuclear cells decreases to less than 40%. The dose-related toxicity is promptly reversed once the antibiotic has been eliminated from the body.

Examination of bone marrow smears easily distinguishes dose-related toxicities from idiosyncratic pancytopenias. The former is characterized by a hypercellular marrow with unique vacuolization of the erythroid and myeloid cells, while the latter appears as a hypocellular marrow with depression of all cell type precursors.

Aplastic anemia secondary to chloramphenicol is rare — the approximate incidence is 1 patient in 40,000 courses of therapy. Aplastic anemia is more likely to occur in patients given chloramphenicol by the oral route of administration (although cases have occurred in patients given intravenous chloramphenicol only) or if the patient is prescribed chloramphenicol on numerous occasions or for prolonged periods of time. This most unfortunate adverse reaction is well described to occur after chloramphenicol therapy has been discontinued, and in such cases the mortality increases if the interval between the drug and the toxicity exceeds two months.

Chloramphenicol's other adverse effects include the following:

1. The gray-baby syndrome is manifest as an ashen skin discoloration, hypothermia, abdominal distention, failure to suck, flaccidity, and death in 40% of patients. It is due to the failure of the neonate's liver to metabolize chloramphenicol. The drug is therefore relatively contraindicated in newborns, at least until their glucuronyl transferase enzyme systems mature in the first few weeks of life. Careful dosage selection and monitoring of serum levels are mandatory whenever it is prescribed under these circumstances.
2. Inhibition of hepatic microsomal enzymatic metabolism of other agents such as oral anticoagulants, phenytoin, and oral hypoglycemic drugs, increases their serum half-lives and contributes to adverse interactions.
3. Antibiotic-associated pseudomembranous colitis.
4. In rare circumstances (described principally in patients with cystic fibrosis) chloramphenicol has also been blamed for optic neuritis.

Tetracyclines

The tetracyclines are bacteriostatic broad-spectrum antibiotics of relatively low selective toxicity. They are prescribed for urinary tract infections, *Chlamydia trachomatis* genitourinary and pelvic infections, as second-line drugs for gonorrhea and syphilis in penicillin-allergic patients, for acute management of *Mycoplasma pneumoniae* pneumonia, for intermittent suppressive management of lower respiratory tract infections in patients with chronic obstructive pulmonary disease or bronchiectasis, as prophylaxis for traveler's diarrhea due to enterotoxigenic *E. coli,* and for a variety of miscellaneous infections including brucellosis, actinomycosis, rickettsial infections, nocardiosis, and tularemia. There are several tetracyclines, such as oxytetracycline, chlortetracycline, and rolitetracycline, that are essentially indistinguishable from generic tetracyline hydrochloride. Doxycycline and minocycline are somewhat different, as is discussed below.

Mechanisms of Action and Resistance

The mechanisms of action of tetracyclines have been reviewed above (see under Selective Toxicity). The mechanism of tetracycline resistance remains unknown, but evidence suggests that in most bacteria, it is under the control of a plasmid-derived repressor protein. This is associated with inducible resistance and reduction in the rate of tetracycline accumulation. It isn't clear if reduced accumulation is due to lowered influx or enhanced efflux but recent evidence favors the latter. It is also possible that intracellular tetracycline interacts less effectively with the 30S ribosomal subunit.

Microbiologic and Pharmacologic Considerations

In addition to the disadvantages of the low selective toxicity of tetracyclines, there are several microbiologic and pharmacologic reasons to limit their application as antibiotic drugs except for the above indications. Microbiologically they are contraindicated in the management of common gram-positive pyogenic coccal infections because of the prevalence of resistant strains, which could expose patients to treatment failure. *Streptococcus pneumoniae* is commonly tetracycline resistant. Tetracycline often fails to eradicate *S. pyogenes* in the treatment of group A beta-hemolytic streptococcal pharyngitis. Tetracycline is not a satisfactory antistaphylococcal antibiotic and should not be prescribed as an alternative to the beta-lactams in allergic patients when treating infections caused by *S. aureus*.

From a pharmacologic perspective, tetracyclines are further disadvantaged because they are contraindicated in children, pregnant women, or patients with any degree of renal insufficiency. Tetracycline complexes with calcium in the hydroxyapatite of teeth and bones, and if administered prior to permanent tooth eruption (ages 8 to 12 years) they cause permanent brown discoloration of the tooth enamel with resultant increased dental caries. If administered during pregnancy, tetracycline may retard fetal bone growth and will also affect the fetal development of normal teeth. Tetracyclines (with the exception of doxycycline) accumulate if administered to patients with renal failure and this results in increased azotemia and associated catabolic effects of the inhibited protein synthesis by the liver.

Tetracyclines are active *in vitro* against common gram-negative bacillary urinary tract pathogens and are prescribed for uncomplicated acute upper and lower tract infections in adults. They are also drugs of choice for *C. trachomatis* infections and for acute gonorrhea and syphilis in penicillin-allergic patients. Tetracyclines are active against *M. pneumoniae* and are agents of choice second to erythromycin for treatment of that organism. Tetracycline has broad-spectrum activity to gram-positive and gram-negative cocci and bacilli of the normal respiratory flora, including most upper respiratory isolates of *H. influenzae* and some Enterobacteriaceae. This group of organisms frequently cause lower respiratory tract infections in patients with chronic pulmonary diseases, and tetracycline remains among the few popular antibiotics to treat the relapsing bronchopneumonia of such patients with chronic bronchitis or bronchiectasis.

Doxycycline is a long-acting tetracycline (half-life 18 to 22 hours) that can be prescribed twice daily for improved patient compliance. It is also of confirmed benefit for antibiotic prophylaxis of traveler's diarrhea due to enterotoxigenic *E. coli*. Minocycline shares similar properties of complete absorption and a long half-life but has the distinct disadvantage of causing tinnitus and severe vestibular toxicities. Minocycline is therefore only prescribed for the occasional patient with nocardiosis or as a third-line drug for eradication of asymptomatic meningococcal pharyngeal colonization.

Tetracyclines in low daily doses are effective treatment for acne probably by both inhibiting *Propionibacterium* acne and preventing lipolytic activity within sebum.

Tetracycline hydrochloride is incompletely absorbed, partially metabolized by the liver, and excreted in the bile. It is primarily excreted by the kidneys and when administered to patients with renal failure toxic accumulation will therefore occur. Doxycycline, however, is completely absorbed, also metabolized, and principally excreted in the feces by back diffusion across the intestinal wall into its lumen. It therefore does not accumulate in renal failure and is safe to use whenever a tetracycline is indicated.

The absorption of all tetracyclines is impaired if they are coadministered with cations such as calcium or magnesium that chelate the drug. Tetracyclines should not be given with milk or antacids.

Adverse Effects

In addition to causing tooth discoloration and dental caries, retarded fetal bone maturation, and azotemia and catabolic side effects in renal failure (all mentioned above), tetracyclines also cause hepatotoxicity (only if intravenously administered to pregnant women), photosensitivity dermatitis, and candidal suprainfections (especially oral thrush and candidal vaginitis). Gastrointestinal irritation is quite common and antibiotic-associated diarrhea or pseudomembranous colitis is also well documented. These toxicities combined with the contraindications of tetracycline to children, pregnant women, and patients with renal failure significantly limit the popularity of tetracycline as a regular antibiotic choice for common bacterial infections.

Erythromycin

Erythromycin is a popularly prescribed antibiotic with the following general indications. It is a substitute for beta-lactams in the oral outpatient therapy of common infections such as streptococcal pharyngitis, otitis media, gonorrhea and syphilis (restricted to the treatment of these infections in penicillin-allergic pregnant women in place of tetracycline), minor superficial staphylococcal infections, prophylaxis for dental procedures in penicillin-allergic patients with valvular heart diseases, and prophylaxis for recurrent *S. pyogenes* infections in penicillin-allergic patients with rheumatic fever. For these indications alone, erythromycin has gained justifiable popularity.

Erythromycin is also the first choice treatment of both *Mycoplasma* and *Legionella* pneumonias and the first choice treatment of *Campylobacter jejuni* enterocolitis. These further extend erythromycin's application to include septically ill hospitalized patients.

Mechanisms of Action and Resistance

Erythromycins are macrolide antibiotics (a macrocyclic lactone ring with a neutral and an amino-deoxy sugar in glycosidic linkage) that bind to the 50S ribosomal subunit to interfere with positioning of peptidyl-tRNA and to inhibit translocation. Maximal activity may depend on lipid solubility (maximal at pH 8.6) in the bacterial cytoplasmic membrane and declines with acid pH. Erythromycin binds more avidly to the larger ribosomal subunit than clindamycin and may displace the latter, although the binding sites are not identified.

Resistance to erythromycin and clindamycin, particularly of *S. aureus, S. pyogenes,* and *S. faecalis,* normally results from an inducible and plasmid-borne enzyme that causes methylation of the two adenine residues in the 23S segment of ribosomal RNA. Methylated rRNA results in reduced ribosomal binding affinity for erythromycin and clindamycin.

Microbiologic and Pharmacologic Considerations

Erythromycin is not complex from either the microbiologic or pharmacologic points of view. It is well absorbed orally, distributes readily to most infected tissue sites (it is not prescribed for meningitis), and is primarily excreted in the bile. The estolate formulation of erythromycin has the pharmacologic advantage of improved bioavailability but the disadvantage that it can cause allergic cholestatic hepatitis, which essentially detracts from its popularity.

Adverse Effects

The only significant adverse effect of erythromycin itself is gastrointestinal intolerance. Nausea, indigestion, and mild diarrhea restrict its use, especially in adults, to low doses and short durations. Cholestatic hepatitis with erythromycin estolate causes upper abdominal pain, fever, hepatic enlargement, hyperbilirubinemia, and eosinophilia, and is only seen occasionally with the estolate form and usually only after 14 or more continuous days of treatment. The intravenous formulations of erythromycin are generally venoirritative and high doses must be infused slowly.

Clindamycin

Clindamycin was originally introduced as a substitute for penicillins and erythromycin in the management of minor upper respiratory tract infections and superficial staphylococcal sepsis. It was soon apparent that it was an effective bacteriostatic antibiotic for severe systemic anaerobic sepsis with most anaerobic organisms including *B. fragilis*. Because clindamycin is a frequent cause of antibiotic-associated diarrhea and pseudomembranous colitis, it is now mainly reserved as one of the prime antibiotic choices for anaerobic sepsis due to *B. fragilis*.

Mechanisms of Action and Resistance

Clindamycin binds to the 50S ribosomal subunit by weak hydrophobic interactions with a protein involved in the ribosomal A site, and this primarily interferes with aminoacyl-tRNA binding to prevent peptide synthesis. The mechanism of resistance is similar to that for erythromycin described above.

Microbiologic and Pharmacologic Considerations

Clindamycin is well absorbed orally and distributes well to most tissues. The notable exception is that it does not cross the blood-brain barrier and is therefore not to be prescribed for treatment of anaerobic brain abscesses. Clindamycin is metabolized by the liver and is safe to use in patients with renal failure.

Adverse Effects

Diarrhea due to toxigenic *Clostridium difficile* overgrowth in the colon is the only important adverse effect of clindamycin. Diarrhea occurs more frequently with clindamycin than other antibiotics and will develop whether the drug is prescribed orally or parenterally. Clindamycin-associated diarrhea frequently occurs days after the antibiotic has been discontinued. As a rule of thumb, one in every four or five patients with diarrhea caused by any antibiotic will subsequently develop pseudomembranous colitis — a much more serious problem than diarrhea alone.

Antibiotic-associated pseudomembranous colitis is recognized by its clinical association with antibiotic therapy, its localization to the colon only, the presence of pseudomembranes on sigmoidoscopic or colonoscopic examinations (superficial luminal plaques attached to the colonic or rectal mucosa at sites of ulceration), and the typical histologic mucosal changes on rectal mucosal biopsy (focal areas of swelling, inflammation, and ulceration with necrotic cells and inflammatory debris enmeshed in a fibrin membrane). Patients with pseudomembranous colitis experience sudden onset of severe abdominal pain, fever, and a rapid intestinal exudation of fluid and protein resulting in dehydration, circulatory collapse, and metabolic acidosis, bacteremia, and shock. Prompt discontinuation of antibiotic immediately followed by aggressive fluid and electrolyte replacement is as important as the prescription of oral vancomycin or metronidazole to inhibit *C. difficile* overgrowth. Because clindamycin frequently causes diarrhea, the frequency with which it causes pseudomembranous colitis is higher, and this alone justifies restricting the drug to clinical situations in which it is specifically indicated.

Vancomycin

Vancomycin is a narrow-spectrum bactericidal antibiotic prescribed to patients who are allergic to penicillins and cephalosporins, who have severe staphylococcal infections or with *S. faecalis* endocarditis (enterococcal endocarditis). It is also the drug of choice in treating infections caused by methicillin-resistant staphylococci (both *S. aureus* and *S. epidermidis*) and is prescribed for the treatment of antibiotic-associated pseudomembranous colitis caused by toxigenic *C. difficile*. Vancomycin has a narrow therapeutic range, and toxicity limits its popularity as a potent systemic antibiotic for other gram-positive streptococcal and staphylococcal infections.

Mechanisms of Action and Resistance

Vancomycin inhibits the synthesis of peptidoglycan in gram-positive cell walls. It is a high-molecular-weight glycopolypeptide whose chemical structure (only recently described) prevents permeation through the outer membrane of gram-negative bacilli, thus the narrow spectrum to gram-positive cocci and bacilli only. At the level of the cytoplasmic membrane of susceptible organisms, vancomycin blocks the transfer of peptidoglycan subunits to the growing point of peptidoglycan. It is also an inhibitor of glycopeptide synthetase. Resistance to vancomycin is uncommon.

Microbiologic and Pharmacologic Considerations

Vancomycin is an effective bactericidal antibiotic for infections caused by *S. aureus, S. epidermidis,* and *Corynebacterium* species (aerobic diphtheroids, an occasional etiology of endocarditis). Group D streptococci and *S. viridans,* however, may occasionally be inhibited but not lysed at serum concentrations achieved by therapeutic doses, implying that vancomycin should be prescribed in combination with an aminoglycoside, especially when treating endocarditis caused by these organisms. The MBC and serum cidal titers are important *in vitro* aids to monitor the bactericidal efficacy of vancomycin.

Vancomycin is not absorbed following oral administration and is therefore the first choice antibiotic to treat the intestinal overgrowth of *C. difficile* that causes antibiotic-associated pseudomembranous colitis. In this situation it is usually prescribed in oral dosages of 500 mg four times daily. It is not recommended for intramuscular administration and thus intravenous vancomycin is the route of administration selected for treatment of systemic infections. The drug distributes well within most body tissue sites including the CSF, provided that the meninges are inflamed.

Vancomycin is excreted by the kidneys. Although its elimination half-life is approximately 6 hours in patients with normal renal function (the usual dose for adults is 1 gm every 12 hours or 25 to 40 mg/kg/day for children), the dosage interval must be increased for administration to patients with any degree of renal insufficiency (a major dosage modification). Vancomycin is not removed by hemodialysis or peritoneal dialysis and must not be prescribed more often than once per week to patients with anuric renal failure.

After a 1-gm intravenous dose, vancomycin peak serum levels are 25 to 40 μg per ml, and at the end of a 12-hour dose the interval trough serum levels average 5 to 10 μg per ml. Safe maintenance of these serum levels in patients with renal dysfunction is only feasible if a vancomycin assay is available.

Adverse Effects

Vancomycin has a low margin of safety, and toxic serum levels are easily exceeded if doses are not monitored carefully. The most important clinical adverse effect is directed to the eighth cranial nerve, manifesting almost exclusively as auditory toxicity. Regular audiometric evaluation is recommended and the drug should be promptly discontinued if toxicity is recorded. Vestibulotoxicity and nephrotoxicity are unusual if they occur at all. The only other frequently encountered problem is venoirritation with phlebitis upon intravenous administration.

Metronidazole

Metronidazole is a 5-nitroimidazole antibiotic with bactericidal activity to a restricted range of infecting microorganisms. It is selectively toxic to anaerobic organisms, both gram-positive and -negative cocci and rods, with the specific inclusion of *B. fragilis*. It is also an effective drug for the treatment of infections caused by anaerobic protozoans such as *Entamoeba histolytica*, *Giardia lamblia*, and *Trichomonas vaginalis*. The only worrisome resistance patterns are seen in gram-positive, anaerobic, nonspore-forming bacilli.

Mechanisms of Action and Resistance

Metronidazole's selective toxicity to microbial cells that have anaerobic metabolic pathways is based on the cell possessing electron transfer components of sufficiently low redox potential (as is the case with ferredoxin) to reduce the drug's nitro group. The transiently produced nitro-group reduction products of metronidazole bind to DNA, causing destabilization of the DNA helix, a lowering of the molecular weight range of DNA, and an increase of the molecular weight of DNA, all due to the formation of single- and double-strand breaks of DNA. Metronidazole-resistant anaerobic bacteria fail to efficiently reduce metronidazole's nitro group to these nitroradical anions by reduction of either drug transport or supply of electron donors (i.e., ferredoxin), the latter possibly by the mutational absence of pyruvate dehydrogenase activity. Resistance among obligate anaerobic bacteria (especially *B. fragilis*) is uncommon.

Microbiologic and Pharmacologic Considerations

Metronidazole is absorbed from the upper gastrointestinal tract with 100% bioavailability. It distributes well to all tissues including the CSF and brain. The drug is excreted by the kidneys, although some 20% to 40% is metabolized to active water-soluble hydroxy and acid metabolites.

Metronidazole is the only cidal antibiotic active against *B. fragilis* and therefore plays an important role in the management of *B. fragilis* endocarditis and suppurative anaerobic brain abscesses. In addition to its excellent pharmacologic properties and bactericidal action, it is comparatively free of the bone marrow suppressive toxicities of chloramphenicol and the risk of pseudomembranous colitis of clindamycin. Thus it is a preferred antibiotic to prescribe in combination with aminoglycosides in the management of mixed aerobic and anaerobic intraabdominal and pelvic sepsis.

The antibiotic is also prescribed for vaginitis with *T. vaginalis* or *Gardnerella vaginalis*, dysenteric and extraintestinal amebiasis, giardiasis, necrotizing gingivitis, and toxigenic *C. difficile* pseudomembranous colitis.

Adverse Effects

Dose-related nausea and vomiting are the only clinically evident adverse effects. Much attention has been placed on the fact that metronidazole is mutagenic (as tested by the Ames's method of mutation response in *Salmonella typhimurium*) as well as being carcinogenic in some small animal models of tumor production. It is on this basis that there is a relative contraindication to prescribing metronidazole during pregnancy. There is no clinical evidence of increased tumor risk to patients in 25 years of its active clinical use. Nevertheless, *in vitro* mutagenicity test results suggest that the antibiotic should only be prescribed for absolute clinical and microbiologic indications and then as specific doses for defined durations of treatment.

Nitrofurantoin

Nitrofurantoin is the principal member of the nitrofuran group of antibiotics. They are bactericidal agents that are effective primarily against gram-negative bacillary urinary tract pathogens.

Mechanisms of Action and Resistance
Nitrofurans act in a manner similar to that of nitroimidazoles. Both share the common feature of nitro-group reduction before biologic activity is assumed. The major difference is that the nitrofurans have a more positive redox potential and they are reduced by nicotinamide adenine dinucleotide- (NADH) and nicotinamide adenine dinucleotide phosphate- (NADPH) linked bacterial nitroreductases. Bacterial mutants resistant to nitrofurans lack the oxygen-insensitive NADPH-linked nitroreductase, resulting in absent reduction of nitrofurantoin to its active intermediates. Acquired clinical resistance is not common.

Microbiologic and Pharmacologic Considerations
Nitrofurantoin is available as a macrocrystalline formulation that is readily absorbed without excessive nausea. Its rapid absorption and renal elimination result in low serum levels and negligible tissue concentrations, thus confining nitrofurantoin to use in acute and chronic upper and lower urinary tract infections.

The rapid and complete intestinal absorption also affords nitrofurantoin one other clinical advantage in the long-term suppressive or prophylactic treatment of urinary tract infections. Because it is completely absorbed, the drug has a negligible influence on the normal gut flora, thus preventing suppression of normally sensitive bacteria with resultant overgrowth of resistant strains. Therefore patients treated with nitrofurantoin are unlikely to become colonized with nitrofurantoin-resistant bacilli that could subsequently reinfect the lower genitourinary tract.

Adverse Effects
There are three adverse effects of nitrofurantoin, each quite different in its clinical features. Digestive tract irritation is the most common, and causes limited patient compliance. The macrocrystalline formulation has reduced the frequency of this effect. Nitrofurantoin also causes a well-documented drug-induced hypersensitivity pneumonitis with resultant pulmonary fibrosis. This must be recognized early to prevent significant lung damage. Finally, nitrofurantoin is known to cause a mixed motor and sensory peripheral neuropathy. This is most frequently described in patients with renal failure in whom elimination of the drug is delayed. For this reason nitrofurantoin is absolutely contraindicated in patients in renal failure.

Fusidic Acid

Sodium fusidate is a nontoxic relatively narrow-spectrum bacteriostatic antibiotic that is inhibitory to *S. aureus*. This organism is generally sensitive regardless of its sensitivities to other antibiotics and whether or not it produces a beta-lactamase. *In vitro* resistance to fusidic acid emerges rapidly, however, and when clinically prescribed to patients with staphylococcal infections, treatment failures are known to occur.

Mechanisms of Action and Resistance
Fusidic acid is a selective inhibitor of elongation factor G in bacteria by stabilizing the ribosome-factor G guanosine diphosphate complex, thereby inhibiting factor G-mediated GTP hydrolysis. It also inhibits binding of aminoacyl-tRNA to ribosomes. Both effects result in inhibition of protein synthesis. Clinical isolates of *S. aureus* that are resistant to fusidic acid may be due to mutational or plasmid-associated mechanisms. Mutational resistance is due to modification of elongation factor G, causing reduced affinity for fusidic acid. Plasmid-mediated resistance results from modifications of cell membrane lipids that reduce fusidic acid's permeability and thus its intracellular concentrations.

Microbiologic and Pharmacologic Considerations
Fusidic acid is well absorbed following oral administration. An intravenous preparation is also available. Distribution is excellent to most tissue sites with the notable exception that it does not cross the blood-CSF or the blood-brain barrier (even when inflammation is present). Inhibitory concentrations are achieved in infected bone tissue and joint fluid. Fusidic acid is conjugated and excreted in the bile. No renal excretion occurs and no dosage modification in renal failure is therefore necessary.

Fusidic acid has been successfully used to treat staphylococcal infections often after other antibiotics have been tried and have failed. Particular benefit is claimed for its use in the management of acute and chronic staphylococcal bone and joint infections. The major disadvantage of fusidic acid is its propensity to cause resistance during clinical therapy. It is generally recommended therefore that fusidic acid not be used alone but always in combination with an antistaphylococcal beta-lactam to prevent the emergence of fusidic acid-resistant organisms. This presents the problem of antagonism between fusidic acid and the selected beta-lactam whereby the infecting strain of *S. aureus* fails to be inhibited and lysed. This is easily demonstrated *in vitro* and the possibility of such antagonism *in vivo* must be kept in mind.

An important pharmacologic factor to consider when using fusidic acid plus an antistaphylococcal beta-lactam is that the fusidic acid is widely distributed in the body, whereas the beta-lactam may not closely follow this pattern of distribution. In this regard, possible other alternatives to the beta-lactams could be tried. Fusidic acid plus erythromycin or clindamycin has been reported to be effective in the treatment of osteomycelitis.

There has been too little clinical experience in treating severe staphylococcal sepsis to judge the true clinical efficacy of fusidic acid alone or in combination with other antibiotics. Widespread experience, especially in North America, using fusidic acid for osteomyelitis is not available and, although some reports support its use, the physician must certainly decide only to use this agent with careful clinical monitoring for resistance and treatment failure.

Adverse Effects

Oral fusidic acid is generally safely prescribed, with only mild gastrointestinal disturbances and occasional skin rashes reported. No other significant local or systemic side effects have been reported. Intravenous fusidic acid may be associated with hyperbilirubinemia.

Rifampin

Rifampin (also known as rifampicin) is a potent antituberculous drug with excellent antistaphylococcal antibacterial properties. Alone or in combination with other antistaphylococcal antibiotics (such as erythromycin) it is an effective third-line choice for some occasional clinical infections. Rifampin is also indicated as a first choice in the treatment of meningococcal carriers and the chemoprophylaxis of close household contacts (i.e., children under the age of 4 years) of persons with *H. influenzae* meningitis.

Mechanisms of Action and Resistance

Rifampin binds to the beta subunit of bacterial RNA polymerase causing inhibition of RNA synthesis. The large size of the rifampin molecule prevents penetration through the outer membrane of gram-negative bacilli, and thus the drug is mainly active against gram-positive and -negative pyogenic cocci and mycobacteria. Although clinically acquired resistance is uncommon, mutational changes in the RNA polymerase do account for the laboratory demonstration of *in vitro* resistance, and has been the basis of resistance seen with prophylactic use of this drug.

Microbiologic and Pharmacologic Considerations

Rifampin is well absorbed orally and distributes to most tissues of the body, with therapeutic concentrations in the lung, bronchial and salivary secretions, pleural fluid, CSF, liver, bile, and urine. It is deacetylated in the liver and both the free drug and its metabolite are excreted in the urine.

Adverse Effects

Rifampin can cause several adverse effects. One that all patients should be alerted to is the orange-pink color it produces in the urine, saliva, sweat, and tears. Abnormalities of liver function are common, although careful observation of these is important as rifampin also causes hepatotoxicity with significant elevation of levels of serum alkaline phosphatase and bilirubin.

Intermittent or interrupted therapy is unusual in that when restarting therapy with rifampin, patients can develop autoimmune hemolytic anemia, thrombocytopenia, fever, arthralgia, acute renal failure, and a hepatorenal syndrome.

Rifampin induces liver microsomal oxidoreductases with resultant drug interactions to effectively reduce serum levels of oral birth control pills, warfarin anticoagulants, oral hypoglycemic drugs, and other agents so metabolized by these liver enzymes.

ADDITIONAL CONSIDERATIONS

Combination Antibiotic Therapy

There are many instances in which combined antibiotics are appropriately indicated:

1. To achieve a synergistic effect. Two examples of this are the combination of tobramycin and one of the antipseudomonal beta-lactams (ticarcillin or piperacillin) for synergistic inhibition of *P. aeruginosa*; and the combination of a penicillin (usually either penicillin G or ampicillin) and an aminoglycoside (either gentamicin or tobramycin) in the

management of group D streptococcal (enterococcal) endocarditis.

2. Whenever infections are polymicrobial in etiology.
3. Blind therapy and/or broad-spectrum antimicrobial coverage are indications for combination therapy. The initial choice of antibiotics to cover gram-positive pyogenic organisms including *S. aureus* and gram-negative bacilli, as in patients with septicemia, often includes a penicillin, an antistaphylococcal beta-lactam, and an aminoglycoside until the etiologic organism is identified.
4. To prevent the emergence of resistant organisms, which is best exemplified by the combination antibiotic therapy used in the treatment of active tuberculosis. Drugs prescribed on an individual basis are likely to induce resistance, whereas combinations of antituberculous medications prevent this.
5. To permit a reduced dosage of a potentially toxic drug. Synergistic combinations of tobramycin and antipseudomonal beta-lactams provide effective antipseudomonal therapy without single high-dose and potentially toxic tobramycin therapy.

Combination antibiotic therapy has adverse effects that include antagonism between prescribed antibiotics, antibiotic incompatibilities, and an increased risk of additive toxicity.

Antibiotics in Renal Failure

Pharmacologically, the aim of antibiotic therapy is to establish and maintain therapeutic and nontoxic tissue levels of drugs. Because the kidney is the major route of excretion for many antibiotics, careful consideration must be given to the effect of renal impairment on drug selection and administration. When renal function is impaired, any drug normally excreted by the kidneys will be retained and will accumulate in the body. Retention of some drugs, especially those antibiotics with a low margin of safety, has the potential for the development of serious toxicity. For this purpose, antibiotics in renal failure can be classified into four categories:

1. Those that are absolutely contraindicated in the presence of renal failure, as specific and unavoidable toxicity will occur with even the slightest accumulation of drug in the body.
2. Those that have the potential for serious toxicity, but with a major dosage modification they can still be prescribed to achieve safe therapeutic concentrations without toxic accumulation.
3. Some with toxicities that only occur in the presence of significant drug accumulation, as would be the case in patients with advanced renal failure. For these drugs only a minor dosage modification is required.
4. Some that are safe to use in the presence of renal failure.

The agents in each of these categories are summarized below:

1. Antibiotics contraindicated in patients with renal failure: tetracycline, nitrofurantoin
2. Antibiotics requiring major dosage modification in renal failure: all aminoglycosides, vancomycin, most cephalosporins, moxalactam, carbenicillin, ticarcillin, piperacillin, trimethoprim, TMP/SMZ, sulfonamides
3. Antibiotics requiring minor dosage modification in renal failure: most penicillins, cephalothin, cefotaxime
4. Antibiotics not requiring dosage modification in renal failure: chloramphenicol, clindamycin, doxycycline, erythromycin, fusidic acid, metronidazole

A major modification is a strictly defined reduction in dosage or increase in dosage interval that must be made in the presence of any degree of renal impairment. Major modification usually implies the use of nomograms to establish safe dosage selections, and where feasible, these antibiotics should be monitored by serum antimicrobial assays. A minor modification is a reduction in dosage only, and is only required in a patient with advanced renal dysfunction. It usually means a halving the dose in the presence of significant renal impairment.

For reasons already reviewed, tetracycline and nitrofurantoin are the only two antibiotics absolutely contraindicated in the presence of renal failure. The syndrome of toxic effects that occurs when tetracyclines accumulate in the body includes exaggerated antianabolic action resulting in negative nitrogen balance and increased azotemia, and pronounced anorexia associated with weight loss, nausea, vomiting, and dehydration. Hyperphosphatemia and acidosis are possible with more serious toxic accumulation. The patient with renal failure who takes nitrofurantoin may develop neurotoxicity, which is usually manifested as a mixed motor and sensory disturbance with severe pains, depressed reflexes, and muscle atrophy. This neurotoxicity is not related to the megaloblastic anemia sometimes seen with nitrofurantoin or the folate deficiency anemia of chronic renal failure. The other two major side effects of the nitrofurantoins, hemolysis and hypersensitivity pneumonitis, are not more frequently seen in renal failure. For both tetracycline and nitrofurantoin, these toxicities are usually reversible if recognized early and if medication is promptly discontinued.

Aminoglycosides, vancomycin, most cephalosporins, moxalactam, and cefoperazone all require major dosage modifications to achieve satisfactory safe serum levels without toxic accumulation. The aminoglycosides and vancomycin have narrow therapeutic dosage ranges and can cause major dose-related toxicities if permitted to accumulate to toxic tissue concentrations.

The toxicity potential of most first- and second-generation cephalosporins, moxalactam, and cefoperazone is not as critical as that of the aminoglycosides. Nevertheless, accumulation does occur in renal failure and because of the potential for nephrotoxicity, major dosage modifications are recommended.

The antipseudomonal penicillins, carbenicillin, ticarcillin and piperacillin, and trimethoprim or TMP/SMZ are all included in the major dosage modification category not because they have narrow therapeutic dosage ranges, but because if allowed to accumulate, they will cause hematologic disturbances and a bleeding diathesis. Interference with adenosine diphosphate-induced platelet aggregation and prolongation of bleeding time is the explanation for the purpura induced by carbenicillin (and probably also ticarcillin and piperacillin) when administered in high doses to patients with renal dysfunctions. Accumulation of trimethoprim in the presence of renal insufficiency may be associated with an increased risk of megaloblastic bone marrow toxicities. Dosage modifications for trimethoprim have not been clearly established and its use in these situations is best determined by clinical necessity.

The many antibiotics that require a minor dosage modification are relatively safer to administer in the presence of renal failure as these drugs have alternate routes of excretion (i.e., liver metabolism or general degradation in peripheral tissues). Their wider therapeutic range and less serious toxicities usually require only a reduction in dosage while maintaining the usual dosage intervals, and these modifications are only necessary in patients with severe renal impairment.

The principle of a major dosage modification is to begin therapy with the administration of a single usual recommended dose that will achieve an initial desirable serum antibiotic level. Then the physician has a choice of either a variable-dosage regimen or a variable-frequency regimen. The principle of the former is to lower the dosage and maintain the usual interval. For this the physician requires a published nomogram or a memorized mnemonic as a guide to dosage selection. The variable-frequency regimen involves administering the usual dosage but at an increased interval (again with the use of nomograms or mnemonics). Wherever possible, serum levels should be closely monitored. It is important to be assured of both therapeutic peak and safe trough serum concentrations. Most hospital microbiology laboratories are now able to provide an assay procedure for at least some of these more toxic antibiotics, especially the aminoglycosides.

Antibiotic therapy to patients receiving dialysis is also best tailored by closely monitoring peak and trough serum levels as well as predialysis and postdialysis serum levels. In such situations it is preferable either to prescribe antibiotics that are safe to administer in renal failure or to select only those antibiotics that are easily monitored and for which there is an available serum assay.

For the patient who has renal failure one can now compensate for the increased risk of toxicities by administering antibiotic therapy according to guidelines and principles, and in this manner all but a very few antibiotics can be safely prescribed with excellent therapeutic efficacy.

ANTIFUNGAL ANTIBIOTICS

In contrast to the large number of antibacterial antibiotics that have been developed, there is a dearth of clinically applicable antifungal agents. The major reason for this is a similarity between mammalian and fungal cells (both are eukaryotic) making it very difficult to develop drugs that exploit the difference between these cells with good therapeutic indices.

Table 5.5 summarizes various classes of antifungal drugs.

Polyene Antibiotics

The most important polyenes used clinically are amphotericin B and nystatin.

Mechanisms of Action and Resistance

These antibiotics are composed of a macrolide ring with hydroxyl group substitution and a conjugated dou-

TABLE 5.5. Antifungal Agents, Mode of Administration, Dose, and Specific Therapeutic Indications

Class	*Drug*	*Mode of Administration*	*Dose*	*Therapeutic Indications*
Polyenes	Nystatin	topical	100,000 units q8h	Oral, vaginal, cutaneous candidiasis
	Nystatin	p.o.	500,000 units q6h	Esophageal, intestinal candidiasis
	Amphotericin B	i.v.	5–50 mg q24h*	Systemic candidiasis, histoplasmosis, coccidioidomycosis, cryptococcosis, blastomycosis, aspergillosis, mucormycosis, systemic sporotrichosis
Imidazoles	Ketoconazole	p.o.	200–1200 mg q24h	Chronic mucocutaneous candidiasis, acute mucocutaneous candidiasis, histoplasmosis†, coccidioidomycosis†, cryptococcosis†, blastomycosis†, dermatophytosis†
	Miconazole	i.v.	400–1200 mg q8h	Coccidioidomycosis, cryptococcosis
	Miconazole	topical	Cream/suppository	Vaginal, cutaneous candidiasis, dermatophytosis
	Clotrimazole	topical	Cream/suppository	Vaginal, cutaneous candidiasis, dermatophytosis
	Econazole	topical	Suppository	Vaginal candidiasis
Antimetabolite	Flucytosine	p.o.	25–35mg/kg q6h	Cryptococcosis, urinary candidiasis, systemic candidiasis
Penicillium derived	Griseofulvin	p.o.	330 mg q24h (ultramicrosize) 250 mg q12h (microsize)	Dermatophytosis
Chemical	Potassium iodide (1gm/ml)	p.o.	1–4 gm q8h	Lymphocutaneous sporotrichosis

*Usual dose is 0.6 mg/kg/24 hr, but occasionally may use up to 1 mg/kg in severe overwhelming infection.
†Use of ketoconazole in deep mycosis has not been well established.

ble bond system. They combine with sterols, principally ergosterol in the fungal cell membrane, and cause membrane leakage of cellular constituents and cell death. The major constituent of mammalian cell membranes, in contrast, is cholesterol, for which the polyenes have less affinity and therefore cause less toxicity.

Nystatin and amphotericin B produce a static effect at low concentrations but a fungicidal effect at high concentrations. An interesting and possibly therapeutic feature of amphotericin B is its apparent immunoadjuvant effect on both cell mediated and humoral immunity in the host.

Microbiologic and Pharmacologic Considerations

The chemical configuration of the polyenes results in water insolubility and virtually no absorption through the gut. As a result of this property, nystatin, and less often amphotericin B are used orally in the treatment of mucosal (oral, esophageal), and intestinal candidiasis.

The pharmacokinetics of amphotericin B following intravenous infusion are very complex, reflecting distribution into at least several peripheral compartments. The complexity of distribution is reflected in the two phases of elimination of the drug, an early one with a half-life of approximately 24 hours but a later one with

TABLE 5.6. Pharmacokinetic Profiles of Selected Systemic Anti-fungal Agents

Drug	*Dose*	*Peak Serum Level (μg/ml)*	*Serum Half-life*	*Urine Excretion (Unmetabolized Drug)*	*CSF Levels*
Amphotericin B*	1 mg/kg i.v.	0.5–3.5	24–48h (early) 15 days (late)	<10%	Low
Miconazole	500 mg i.v.	5–10	24h	<10%	Low
Ketoconazole	200 mg p.o.	3	8h	<1%	30% serum levels
Flucytosine**	100 mg/kg	10–30	3–8h	>80%	>50% serum levels
Griseofulvin	500 mg	<1	10–24h	<1%	—

*Doses of 0.5–1mg/kg i.v. depending on severity of infection.
**Usual dose is 100–150 mg/kg/day in 4 divided doses at intervals of 6 hours.

a half-life of approximately 15 days. A simplistic model of the distribution of amphotericin B might be to consider the cell membranes of the host as a sponge to which amphotericin B binds. Specific pharmacokinetic variables are summarized in Table 5.6.

How tissue or serum concentrations are related to the fungicidal effect of amphotericin B is ill-defined and further complicated by the fact that the determination of fungal susceptibility in vitro has not been standardized.

Dose and clinical indications are summarized in Tables 5.5 and 5.7.

The dose of amphotericin B is usually increased by increments of 5 mg per day to a total dose of 50 mg per day. In very ill patients, this may be accelerated at the rate of 0.3 mg/kg per day. Generally one doesn't give more than 50 mg per day but in some cases of severe or longstanding infection up to 1 mg/kg can be given. In such cases alternate-day therapy is usually used.

The duration of dosing of amphotericin B is empirical and has to be individualized in each clinical situation. In Table 5.7, suggested guidelines for total doses of amphotericin B for selected fungal infections are outlined.

Because of the variable penetration into the cerebrospinal fluid, amphotericin B must be given intrathecally for coccidioidal meningitis and for cases of cryptococcal meningitis that do not respond to the combination of amphotericin B and flucytosine. Because of the irritative effect of amphotericin B on the meninges, very small doses are given intrathecally initially (i.e., 0.025 mg) with the dose gradually increased over two weeks to a maximum dose of 0.5 mg. The intrathecal dose is usually given twice weekly after the maximum dose has been reached. The drug may be administered intrathecally in the lumbar area, intracisternally, or intraventricularly via an ommaya reservoir.

TABLE 5.7. Guidelines for Determining the Total Dose of Systemic Amphotericin B in Various Fungal Infections*

Infection	*Total Dose*
Candidemia	
'Line' associated†	0–250 mg
Non 'line' associated	1–2/gm
Candidiasis	
Oesophageal	250 mg
Urinary (pyelonephritis)	500 mg–1gm
Disseminated	1–2gm
Histoplasmosis	1.5–2.5gm
Coccidioidomycosis	1–2gm
Blastomycosis	2gm
Cryptococcosis	1–2gm‡
Aspergillosis	1–2gm

*Clinical and laboratory responses must be used in conjunction with these guidelines.
†Removal of central line essential for treatment.
‡Amphotericin B used in combination with flucytosine.

Adverse Effects

The toxicity of topical nystatin is minimal and local because of the lack of systemic absorption. The side effects with oral nystatin include mild diarrhea, nausea, and vomiting.

Intravenous amphotericin B has many toxic effects, some of which can be very serious. Acutely, amphotericin B can produce an endotoxin-like effect with chills, rigors, fever, hypotension, tachycardia (and arrhythmias), headache, nausea and vomiting, arthralgias and myalgias. In addition, another common and early complication is severe phlebitis at the site of peripheral intravenous infusion. Usually with repetitive dosing, the acute side effects lessen to some extent. More chronically, nephrotoxicity with prolonged dosing invariably occurs, although often the degree of renal impairment reaches a plateau after there is a rise of serum creatinine to approximately three times normal. No dosage alteration is necessary in renal failure. However for continued therapy amphotericin B can be administered on an alternate day basis. Also, a potassium losing nephropathy can occur and potassium supplementation may be required. The nephrotoxicity is usually reversible within several months, although permanent damage can occur with prolonged therapy, especially in cases where the serum creatinine rises to greater than 3 to 4 times normal.

Hepatic and bone marrow toxicity as well as skin rash are seen less commonly.

Because of its toxicity, administration of amphotericin is more complicated than that for most other drugs. A test dose of 1 mg over approximately 2 hours is usually given to determine the patient's immediate response. If the patient experiences a severe reaction, as noted above, the necessity for the drug should be carefully reconsidered. If it is definitely required, pre-medicating the patient with 25 to 100 mg of hydrocortisone succinate intravenously will reduce the endotoxin-like effects, and adding 1000 units of heparin to the amphotericin B infusion can reduce the incidence of phlebitis. Patients can also be given acetinominophen plus diphenhydramine 1 hour before infusion and every 4 hours during infusion to reduce fever and chills. Oral meperidine may also help. The daily dose should be infused over a long interval (i.e., 6 hours), the slower infusion rate usually associated with fewer adverse reactions.

Very recent evidence suggests that maintaining a high salt load may reduce the nephrotoxicity of amphotericin B.

Imidazole Antibiotics

The most important imidazoles used clinically are miconazole, ketoconazole, clotrimazole, and econazole.

Mechanisms of Action and Resistance

The basic structure of the imidazoles is a five-membered ring consisting of two nitrogen atoms and two double bonds. Various substituents have been attached to this nucleus which give the compounds different antifungal activities and pharmacokinetic properties. These drugs are fungistatic and appear to inhibit ergosterol synthesis in the fungal cell membrane with the accumulation of toxic methyl sterols which cause permeability abnormalities in the fungal membrane and inhibition of growth. Other biochemical effects have been noted with specific imidazoles including a disproportionate increase in saturated fatty acids in the cell membrane which may inhibit certain membrane bound enzymes and lead to the accumulation of toxic concentrations of hydrogen peroxide.

Microbiology and Pharmacologic Considerations

Ketoconazole and miconazole are the only drugs that have proved clinically useful when given systematically, the former orally, and the latter intravenously. The pharmacokinetics of these two drugs are summarized in Table 5.6. Clotrimazole and econazole are used topically.

Dose and clinical indications are summarized in Table 5.5.

Adverse Effects

Parenteral miconazole is associated with side effects similar to those of amphotericin B infusion but which are much milder. These include fever, chills and rigors, pruritus (often severe and prolonged), nausea, and tachycardia. Hyponatremia (in contrast to hypokalemia caused by amphotericin B) and pancytopenia can also occur. Like amphotericin B, phlebitis is also a common problem with prolonged treatment. A test dose of 200 mg is recommended.

Compared with miconazole and amphotericin B, ketoconazole is associated with relatively few side effects and has the advantage of oral administration. However, with increasing use of the drug, severe hepatotoxicity has been demonstrated in approximately 1 per 15,000 treated patients. Up to 10% of patients, however, may demonstrate abnormalities in liver enzymes. Patients treated with ketoconazole, therefore, should be alerted to the symptoms of hepatitis and also monitored monthly with biochemical determinations if they are on long-term therapy. Additional minor side effects of ketoconazole include nausea and vomiting, abdominal pain, and diarrhea. Pruritus and rash occur in less than 1% of patients.

Antimetabolite Antibiotic

Flucytosine is the only clinically important antifungal which is an antimetabolite.

Mechanisms of Action and Resistance
Flucytosine is a fluorinated pyrimidine which is converted enzymatically in yeast to 5-fluoruracil. This compound inhibits RNA synthesis and also likely DNA synthesis. Natural resistance to flucytosine exists in about 10% of *Candida albicans* isolates and less than 2% of *Cryptococcus neoformans* strains. Resistance has also been shown, however, to develop at a high frequency when flucytosine is used alone in the treatment of fungal infections. When it is used clinically, apart from the treatment of urinary tract infections, flucytosine should be combined with amphotericin B.

Microbiology and Pharmacologic Considerations
These are summarized in Table 5.6. Its major advantages include oral dosing, excellent penetration into the cerebrospinal fluid (especially useful in the treatment of cryptococcal meningitis in combination with amphotericin B), and high urinary excretion rate (useful in the treatment of Candida urinary tract infections).

Dose and clinical indications are summarized in Table 5.5.

When flucytosine is used in combination with amphotericin B, the dose of flucytosine must be monitored carefully. Serum levels above 100 ug/ml are considered toxic. Because amphotericin B is associated with impairment of renal function, the dose of flucytosine is reduced with increasing duration of amphotericin B treatment. The necessity to reduce the dose, if levels are not monitored in the serum, is usually heralded by bone marrow depression and diarrhea.

Adverse Effects
Because the drug is an antimetabolite, its major toxicity is associated with bone marrow depression. Diarrhea, hepatotoxicity, and rarely, bowel perforation, are also reported.

Penicillium-Derived Drugs

The only clinically important antifungal agent in this category is griseofulvin.

Mechanism of Action and Resistance
Griseofulvin consists of two six-membered and one five-membered ring with chlorine, methoxy, methyl, and oxygen substituents. Griseofulvin is fungistatic and appears to inhibit microtubules which results in inhibition of nucleic acid synthesis and chitin synthesis in the fungal cell wall.

Microbiologic and Pharmacologic Considerations
Dose and clinical indications are summarized in Table 5.5.

Adverse Effects
Griseofulvin is a relatively non-toxic drug, although initial treatment may be associated with the development of headaches which, however, usually disappear without discontinuing treatment. Rash and gastrointestinal upset can also occur and rarely, leukopenia has been reported. Griseofulvin can induce hepatic enzymes and therefore a modification in dosage of other drugs, if they are metabolized by the liver, may be necessary.

Chemical Antifungal Agents

Potassium iodide is the only commonly used chemical antifungal agent which is used parenterally. It is effective in the treatment of lymphocutaneous sporotrichosis.

Mechanisms of Action and Resistance
A saturated solution of potassium iodide (1 gm/ml) is effective against *Sporothrix schenkii* when given for several months. The duration of therapy is empirical but if the drug is given for at least one month after resolution of the lesion, relapses are unusual. The mechanism of action is obscure. The effect of the iodide may not be on the fungus itself but in improving the host response by stimulating neutrophil chemotaxis or intracellular killing of the fungus.

Microbiologic and Pharmacologic Considerations
Dose and clinical indications are summarized in Table 5.5.

Toxicity and Side Effects
Evidence of iodine toxicity include excessive lacrimation, parotid swelling, acne, and gastrointestinal upset. The dose used in the treatment of the infection is titrated against these adverse effects to a maximum of 12 gm per day.

ANNOTATED BIBLIOGRAPHY

Atkinson AJ, Bennett JE. Amphotericin B pharmacokinetics in humans. Antimicrob Agents Chemother 1978;13:271–276.
Development of pharmacokinetic model and determination of kinetic parameters for amphotericin B.

Bennett WM, Muther RS, Parker RA, et al. Drug therapy in renal failure: dosing guidelines for adults. Part I. Antimicrobial agents, analgesics. Ann Intern Med 1980;93:62–89.
This provides specific dosage recommendations for prescribing antibiotics to patients with renal dysfunction.

Bryan LE. Bacterial resistance and susceptibility to chemotherapeutic agents. Cambridge, New York, Melbourne: Cambridge University Press, 1982.
A very readable, comprehensive review of the basic microbiology and pharmacology of antibiotic mechanisms of action and resistance.

Geddes AM, ed. Good antimicrobial prescribing. Lancet 1983;2:82, 83–88, 140–143, 197–199, 252–255, 311–315, 370–373, 425–429, 478–480, 532–537, 537–539.
An excellent general and up-to-date reference on current antibiotics.

Hermans PE, ed. Symposium on antimicrobial agents. Mayo Clin Proc 1983;58:3–32, 79–102, 147–168, 217–231.
Another excellent general and up-to-date reference on current antibiotics.

Hoeprich PD, ed. Infectious diseases. A modern treatise of infectious processes, 2nd edition. Hagerstown, Maryland: Harper and Row, 1977.
Detailed therapeutic approach to superficial and deep mycosis.

Levine HB, ed. Ketoconazole in the management of fungal disease. New York: ADIS Press, 1982.
Review of all antifungal agents, structure, mode of action, pharmacokinetics, spectrum of activity with special reference to ketoconazole.

McCracken GH, Nelson JD. Antimicrobial therapy for newborns. New York: Grune & Stratton, 1983.
This is an excellent reference source for the guidelines to safe antimicrobial therapy of infections in newborns.

Medoff G, Kobayashi GS. Strategies in the treatment of systemic fungal infections. N Engl J Med 1980;302:145–155.
Well referenced, practical approach to antifungal therapy.

6 ANTIVIRAL CHEMOTHERAPY

M. John Gill and D. Lorne J. Tyrrell

Until recently, little has been known about the molecular biology of viral infections. The control of viral disease was achieved first by prevention in the form of vaccination, and then by case isolation as determined by known epidemiology. Effective chemotherapy remained elusive despite the considerable effort made to develop antiviral drugs after the discovery of antibiotics. Most investigators believed that once a virus penetrated a target cell, it used host cell enzymes to replicate, making selective targeting of antiviral agents almost impossible. A few agents with antiviral activity were found, but it is only in recent years that the pace of these discoveries has accelerated. This expansion resulted from the discovery that some antineoplastic agents such as idoxuridine (IDU) inhibited certain DNA viruses. Furthermore, it was recognized that a number of viruses specified distinct enzymes for replication. These enzymes have become the targets or the specific activators of new antiviral chemotherapeutic agents which have acceptable therapeutic indexes.

Accompanying this development of antiviral agents, there has been a significant improvement in the ability to diagnose viral infections rapidly and accurately using techniques such as electron microscopy, immunofluorescence, radioimmunoassays, and enzyme-linked immunosorbent assays. These advances have further stimulated the development of antiviral agents.

Antiviral therapy can be directed at a number of sites involved with viral replication:

1. Viral binding to cell
2. Penetration of virus into cell
3. Uncoating of viral particle
4. Viral nucleic acid synthesis
5. Viral protein synthesis
6. Viral assembly
7. Budding from the cell

The exact mode of action of some antiviral agents is still poorly understood. Below are listed the agents for which there is fairly strong evidence pointing to a site of action.

1. Virus penetration or uncoating
   - Amantadine and rimantadine
   - Arildone
2. Viral nucleic acid synthesis
   - Idoxuridine
   - Trifluorothymidine
   - Adenine arabinoside
   - Acyclovir
   - Phosphonoformic acid
   - Bromovinyldeoxyuridine
   - Ribavirin
   - Enviroxine
3. Viral protein synthesis
   - Interferon
   - Methisazone

This chapter reviews current knowledge regarding the mode of action, clinical indications, pharmacology, and side effects of antiviral agents that are licensed or are likely to be licensed in the near future.

NUCLEOSIDE ANALOGS

Most of the new and effective antiviral agents are classified as nucleoside analogs. Many of these agents have proven efficacy in the treatment of herpetic infections. They have not been shown to be effective in infections caused by RNA viruses or other DNA viruses.

Adenine Arabinoside

Adenine arabinoside (ara-A, vidarabine) was developed in the late 1950s as an antineoplastic agent. By 1973 it had been demonstrated to be a potent antiherpetic agent when given either systemically or topically

TABLE 6.1. Therapy for HSV-1 Infections

Infection	*Drug*	*Regimen*
Keratitis	Idoxuridine, 0.5%	Topical 5 × daily
	Adenine arabinoside, 3%	
	Trifluorothymidine, 2%	
	Acyclovir, 3%	
	Interferon	
Herpes encephalitis	Adenine arabinoside	15 mg/kg/d IV over 12 h × 10 d
	Acyclovir*	500 mg/m² IV q8h × 10 d
Mucocutaneous herpes (immunocompromised host)	Acyclovir, prophylaxis or therapy	250 mg/m² IV q8h
Herpes labialis	None	

* = promising agent not yet proved effective.

(ophthalmic). Activity is limited to the herpes group, in particular, herpes simplex 1 (HSV-1) (Table 6.1), herpes simplex 2 (HSV-2) (Table 6.2), and varicella zoster (VZ) (Table 6.3). Ara-A appears to work by binding preferentially to the virally specified DNA polymerase, thus inhibiting viral DNA replication.

Ara-A is not effective orally and is usually used topically or intravenously. It is poorly soluble and a therapeutic dose usually entails administering over 2 liters of fluid intravenously per day. It has a half-life of less than 15 minutes and is rapidly deaminated to hypoxanthine arabinoside (ara-H), which has some antiviral activity and may be responsible for some of the observed side effects of ara-A. Ara-H is excreted in the urine with a half-life of about four hours; therefore dosage modification is required in patients with renal impairment. A dose reduction of 25% to 75% is recommended according to the degree of renal insufficiency.

Ara-A administered topically as a 3% solution has been shown to be effective in treating herpetic keratitis; however, it has no effect on labial herpes (cold sore), genital herpes, or VZ infections. In immunocompromised patients with VZ infections, ara-A given intravenously at a dosage of 10 mg per kg per day for 5 days will accelerate healing and reduce complications if started within 72 hours of onset. In biopsy-proven HSV-1 encephalitis, intravenous ara-A, 15 mg per kg per day for 10 days, reduced the mortality and morbidity significantly, particularly in patients under 30 years of age who were not comatose at the start of therapy. Herpes neonatorum (HSV-1 and HSV-2) also responds favorably to intravenous ara-A at the same dosage. The mortality rate is significantly reduced, as is the rate of moderate and severe neurologic sequelae in the survivors. The drug is licensed for the treatment of HSV encephalitis and herpes neonatorum.

Documented side effects include nausea, vomiting, and diarrhea, which occur infrequently. Bone marrow suppression, central nervous system (CNS) agitation, and muscle pain have been reported and may necessitate dosage modification.

Acyclovir

Acyclovir (Zovirax, acycloguanosine 9-(2-hydroxyethoxymethyl)-guanine) is a purine analog that was first described in 1977 and since then has become recognized as the first of a new class of potent, highly specific, antiherpetic agents.

The specificity of acyclovir is derived from the fact that cells infected with HSV-1, HSV-2, and VZ contain both cellular and virally specified thymidine kinase (TK) and cellular and virally specified DNA polymerase. The virally specified enzymes have similar but not identical substrate specificities to the host's enzymes. This difference in specificity can be used to inhibit viral but not host cell DNA replication.

Acyclovir is relatively inert as it is not recognized by host cell enzymes. However, it is recognized by the virally specified TK in herpes infected cells. The viral TK phosphorylates acyclovir. After further phosphory-

TABLE 6.2. Therapy for HSV-2 Infections

Infection	*Drug*	*Regimen*
Herpes genitalis*		
Initial	Acyclovir, 5% ointment	5× daily
	Acyclovir, oral	200 mg po 5× daily × 10 d
	Acyclovir, intravenous	250 mg/m²/q8h × 10 d
Recurrent	Acyclovir, oral, initiated by patient	200 mg po 5 × daily × 10 d
Prophylaxis	Acyclovir oral	200 mg po 2× daily
Herpes neonatorum*	Adenine arabinoside	15 mg/kg/d IV over 12 hrs × 10 d
	Acyclovir†	500 mg/m² IV q8h × 10 d

*These infections are predominantly HSV-2, but HSV-1 may occur.
†Promising agent not yet proved effective.

TABLE 6.3. Therapy for Other Viral Infections

Infection	*Drug*	*Regimen*
Varicella zoster (immunocompromised host)	Adenine arabinoside	10 mg/kg/d IV over 12h × 5 d
	Interferon	2–5 × 10^5 IU/kg/d IM or sc × 5–7 d
	Acyclovir*	500 mg/m² IV q8h × 7 d
Influenza A prophylaxis	Amantadine	100 mg po bid
	Rimantadine	100 mg po bid

* = promising agent not yet proved effective.

lation by host cell enzymes to acyclovir-triphosphate it interacts with the virally specified DNA polymerase and inhibits DNA replication. It has only minimal inhibition of the host cell DNA polymerase. As acyclovir interacts mainly with virally specified enzymes, it has only minimal toxicity.

Clinical Uses

Acyclovir is an effective antiherpetic agent. It appears to have only minor activity against Epstein-Barr virus and questionable activity against human cytomegalovirus infections, but is very potent against HSV-1, HSV-2, and VZ infections.

Topical Acyclovir

Topical acyclovir administered as a 3% ointment appears effective in promoting healing of (herpetic) corneal ulcers. It appears to be equal or superior to IDU, trifluorothymidine (TFT), and ara-A in the treatment of these ulcers.

In the primary episode of genital herpes, topical administration of acyclovir, 5% ointment, four times a day for 1 week has been shown to reduce the period of virus shedding from 7 to 4.1 days and accelerate crusting of the lesions from 10.5 to 7.1 days. The drug does not prevent viral latency or decrease the risk of further recurrences. In recurrent genital herpes, acyclovir does not have such a dramatic effect, although it may slightly decrease the duration of virus shedding.

Acyclovir has been used in topical therapy of mucocutaneous herpes infections in the immunocompromised patient. Although application of 5% ointment four times a day for 10 days failed to improve healing, it did reduce pain and the period of virus shedding significantly.

Oral Acyclovir

Acyclovir is well absorbed and appears to reach and maintain significant antiviral plasma levels. Its role in several herpes infections is still under evaluation.

In primary genital herpes, oral acyclovir, 200 mg five times daily for 10 days, has been shown to reduce the duration of viral shedding, itching, pain, and time to crusting and healing. In recurrent infections, the agent also appears to speed healing and reduce the period of infectivity. Recently it has been shown that continuous oral acyclovir at the above dosage is effective in suppressing recurrences, although cessation of treatment is followed by a return of infection. It has been found that initiation of treatment with oral acyclovir at the first symptom of a recurrence of genital herpes may abort the recurrence.

No trials have been published evaluating oral acyclovir in the therapy of early VZ infection; however, the intravenous drug, as discussed in the next section of this chapter, has a beneficial effect in both healthy and immunosuppressed patients. Since the inhibitory $dose_{50}$ (ID_{50}) for VZ is higher than the ID_{50} for HSV types 1 or 2, and since oral absorption is variable, clinical trials comparing oral acyclovir to placebo are required before this form of therapy can be routinely recommended.

Intravenous Acyclovir

In a double-blind, placebo-controlled trial, intravenous acyclovir in dosage of 5 mg per kg every eight hours for five days significantly accelerated healing and diminished both new lesion formation and duration of vesicles in primary genital herpes. In animal studies, initiation of this agent within hours of the primary infection reduced viral latency. Unfortunately, this effect has not been demonstrated in clinical trials since most patients begin therapy outside the time frame when acyclovir could affect latency.

Mucocutaneous herpes infections may cause considerable morbidity, particularly in immunosuppressed patients in whom mucosal damage may have been caused by irradiation and/or chemotherapy. Intravenous acyclovir has been demonstrated to alleviate pain and accelerate healing. In some cases it has been effective in cases where ara-A was not.

Varicella zoster infections may be severe and life threatening, particularly in immunocompromised patients. Acyclovir has in vitro activity against VZ virus. In a preliminary trial, intravenous drug, 500 mg per m^2 per day every eight hours, in immunocompromised patients with VZ infections decreased postherpetic neuralgia, accelerated healing, and restricted dissemination.

In healthy adults with shingles, acyclovir significantly reduces pain, reduces virus shedding, and accelerates healing when used intravenously at 500 mg per m^2 every eight hours. Intravenous acyclovir has been shown to be ineffective in reducing the prevalence of postherpetic neuralgia in patients with shingles. This finding has been disappointing, as this is a major complication of shingles.

In animal studies acyclovir has been shown to reduce significantly the mortality of herpes encephalitis. It has considerable promise for the treatment of this condition in humans.

Side Effects

In clinical studies, the mild inflammation at the injection site and transient rises in creatinine and blood urea nitrogen levels are the only side effects noted so far. Neither the toxic nor the therapeutic levels for acyclovir have been completely established. In significant renal failure, a modification of either the dosage or dosage interval appears prudent. For intravenous acyclovir the suggested modifications in dosage interval are: creatinine clearance (Cl_{Cr})greater than 50 ml per min, every 8 hours; Cl_{Cr} 25 to 50 ml per min, every 12 hours; Cl_{Cr} 10 to 25 ml per min, every 24 hours; and Cl_{Cr} 0 to 10 ml per min, one-half of the recommended dose every 24 hours. Since oral acyclovir is not completely absorbed, no modification is recommended (200 mg five times/day) unless Cl_{Cr} is below 10 ml per min, when the dosage should be decreased to 200 mg twice daily.

Bromovinyldeoxyuridine

Bromovinyldeoxyuridine (BVDU) is a new antiviral agent under clinical investigation that is extremely potent in vitro against HSV-1 and VZ. This activity has been documented in animal studies in which BVDU appears effective in treatment of HSV-1 keratitis, HSV-1 cutaneous infections, and herpes encephalitis. The drug is less effective against HSV-2 infections. It appears to be a promising agent with little toxicity.

Idoxuridine

Idoxuridine (5-iodo-2′-deoxyuridine, IDU) was shown in 1961 to have in vitro activity against the herpes viruses. The following year this antiviral activity was demonstrated in an animal model of herpetic keratitis, and soon IDU became the accepted treatment for the human disease. Several attempts were made to use IDU as a systemic agent for severe herpes infections such as HSV encephalitis. Unfortunately, its lack of specificity for viral replication caused considerable host toxicity, thereby precluding its systemic use. Topical use in herpetic keratitis has become increasingly restricted by the identification of resistant infections and allergic keratoconjunctivitis. As newer antiviral agents become licensed, the role of IDU will diminish.

Although commonly used, IDU has no proven efficacy in the treatment of herpes labialis. Other nucleoside analogs have been tried for that condition, but none is effective without the benefit of dimethylsulfoxide (DMSO) as a solute carrier. Without DMSO, these drugs do not penetrate keratinized skin.

Trifluorothymidine

Trifluorothymidine (5-trifluoromethyl-2′-deoxyuridine, TFT) was originally derived as an antineoplastic agent due to its ability to inhibit DNA polymerase. Soon it was found to inhibit in vitro DNA virus replication of the herpes and vaccinia viruses. Unfortunately, its toxicity to the host precludes TFT's systemic use. However, it is effective topically in the treatment of herpatic keratitis. It appears to be significantly superior to IDU in herpetic keratitis, with fewer treatment failures and fewer local side effects.

INTERFERONS

In 1957 Isaacs and Lindenman described a naturally occurring substance that interfered with viral replication. This stimulated the study of interferon and interferon inducers as agents to treat human viral infections. Interferons have a broad spectrum of activity and are active against both RNA and DNA viruses. Despite their early promise, limited supply at a high cost and unexpected toxicity with systemic administration have resulted in restricted use of these agents as antiviral therapy. With the advent of genetic engineering and DNA cloning, however, highly purified interferons of various types and reasonable quantities are becoming commercially available, warranting a new look at them as antiviral agents.

Although there appear to be many molecular species of interferons, three broad types can be defined: interferon-α (HuIFN-α; at least eight species) produced from human leucocytes is the most widely tested interferon; interferon-β (HuIFN-β; at least two species) is produced from human fibroblasts; and interferon-γ (HuIFN-γ; many species) is induced in lymphoid cells by mitogens to which the cell has been sensitized.

The majority of interferon used in clinical trials has been provided by the Finnish Red Cross Service. The activity of these preparations has been approximately 10^4 to 10^6 units per milligram of protein. Pure interferon contains between 10^8 and 10^9 units per milligram of protein. Trials using the highly purified interferons are continuing in anticipation of increased efficacy and fewer side effects.

The interferons are glycoproteins with molecular weights of approximately 15,000 to 20,000. They are not effective orally and are administered topically or systemically to treat viral infections of mucous membranes, and intravenously or intramuscularly to treat systemic viral illnesses. They do not cross the blood-brain barrier and have been tried intrathecally without success as treatment of viral CNS infections.

The mechanisms by which interferons inhibit viral replication are still incompletely understood. Interferons bind to the surface of the infected cell, triggering a series of events leading to the antiviral state. This is achieved by the indirect induction of a specific ribonuclease, which cleaves single-stranded RNA and another enzyme that inhibits protein synthesis. These effects of interferon on target cells are reversible.

Until their clinical role is defined, interferon use in viral infections should be limited to therapeutic trials. Topical interferon is effective in the treatment of herpes keratitis, but has no advantage over the less expensive antiviral compounds.

Intranasal interferon is ineffective in treating influenza or rhinovirus infection. In most studies, the intranasal form had to be administered prior to viral challenge to show even minimal benefit, thereby limiting its potential value in clinical practice.

Systemic interferon may be of value in several viral illnesses. Cytomegalovirus (CMV) shed in the urine of congenitally infected infants and renal transplant recipients can be decreased by systemic interferon, but no clinical benefit is gained. Interferon at 6.4×10^5 units per kg per day has had little effect on CMV pneumonia after bone marrow transplantation.

Attempts to alter the course of chronic hepatitis B virus infection with systemic interferon, either alone or in combination with adenine arabinoside, have shown early promise. Considerable host toxicity was encountered, however, and the role of this treatment remains unresolved.

Intramuscular interferon has been used in the treatment of varicella zoster infections in immunocompromised patients. At doses of 1 to 3×10^6 units per day, it decreased pain and led to earlier crusting, and limited dissemination. Similarly, systemic interferon decreased the complication rate of varicella infection in immunocompromised children.

Several side effects have been reported with the systemic use of interferons. Hematologic problems include pancytopenia and thrombocytopenia. Fever is dose related and almost invariably present. Malaise and fatigue are similarly dose related and are more common with prolonged interferon use. All these problems disappear when the drug is stopped. Despite early hopes, cloned interferon of high purity produces similar side effects.

Twenty-five years after the discovery, the role of interferon as therapy for viral infections remains unclear. On the one hand, the prospects of obtaining highly purifed, cloned interferon at an affordable price is exciting. On the other hand, difficulties in appropriate timing of therapy, the significant side effects, and the biologic and pharmacologic differences of the many species of interferon await clarification and will delay their routine use.

AMANTADINE AND RIMANTADINE

Amantadine (Symmetrel) was discovered in 1964 and is one of the oldest antiviral compounds. It is currently licensed for prophylaxis against all strains of influenza A. Recently, a derivative, rimantadine, has been shown to be equally effective with less toxicity.

In tissue cultures, amantadine inhibits many RNA viruses, including the myxoviruses, paramyxoviruses, and togaviruses. It appears to interfere with virus penetration and then uncoating of the virus, and has a 50% to 70% efficacy rate compared to placebo when used prophylactically in high-risk individuals during influenza A epidemics. High-risk individuals include unvaccinated children and adults with underlying pulmonary, cardiovascular, metabolic, and neuromuscular disease or immunologic deficiencies; and selected unvaccinated contacts of index cases, for example, household contacts, hospital personnel, and persons in institutions during nosocomial outbreaks.

It is effective against all of the influenza A strains, but is ineffective against influenza B. Amantadine given orally has not been shown convincingly to be effective in treating influenza pneumonia. One study has demonstrated that aerosolized amantadine, 1 gm per 100 ml distilled water, three times a day for four days, significantly improved the resolution of symptoms and signs of influenza A pneumonia with only minor side effects. The value of amantadine as a therapeutic agent in established influenza A pneumonia remains controversial and must be evaluated further.

The usual adult dosage is 200 mg once a day or 100 mg twice a day, of which 90% is absorbed. The amount must be reduced in those with renal impairment. Up to 5% of patients who take amantadine may complain of poor concentration, agitation, and insomnia.

OTHER AGENTS

Many agents other than those named above are being evaluated for their antiviral activity.

Ribavirin

In 1969 a nucleoside antibiotic pyrazomycin was discovered to have considerable antiviral activity, but it was toxic. In 1972 a derivative ribavirin was found that induced less host toxicity yet still had the ability to inhibit viral replication with a broad spectrum of antiviral activity. Since then, in vitro activity has been demonstrated against both DNA viruses (including HSV-1, HSV-2, adenovirus, and human CMV) and RNA viruses (including influenza A, B, measles, and respiratory syncytial virus). Ribavirin is virustatic. Its main mechanism of action appears to be inhibition of RNA polymerase.

Clinical trials on the efficacy of oral ribavirin in influenza have provided conflicting results. Some have shown clinical improvement with decreased viral shedding when treatment was initiated early in the infection. At least one large multicenter trial failed to confirm these findings. Oral ribavirin has been tried in the treatment of several other viral illnesses including measles, viral hepatitis, and herpes genitalis. The results in most of these studies have been less than convincing.

In 1981 administration of ribavirin by small-particle aerosol was used successfully to treat 14 patients with influenza. Further trials using this route of administration have also shown a beneficial effect in the treatment of both respiratory syncytial virus and influenza B infection. These results are encouraging but they all must be confirmed in large-scale, placebo-controlled, double-blind studies. At present ribavirin is not licensed for use.

Arildone

Arildone belongs to a group of acyclic diketones. In tissue culture it and its derivatives have been shown to inhibit viral uncoating. In vitro it is most effective against herpes simplex viruses and varicella zoster, and also has activity against CMV, picornaviruses, and rhinoviruses. It is still undergoing evaluation.

Enviroxine

Enviroxine has been found to have antiviral activity against rhinoviruses, echovirus, and coxsackieviruses in tissue culture. It is not virucidal, but diminishes both viral RNA and protein synthesis. In the open studies it appears to have promise both as a prophylactic and therapeutic agent for rhinovirus infections.

Phosphonoformic Acid

In 1978 trisodium phosphonoformic acid (PFA), an organophosphorus compound, was found to have significant antiviral activity. Since then PFA has been demonstrated to be active against HSV-1, HSV-2, and influenza A in vitro. In animal studies it appears promising in HSV infections, but clinical trials still must confirm its efficacy.

Methisazone

In 1950 the thiosemicarbazone group was shown to be active against poxvirus infections in mice by inhibiting translation of late viral mRNA. In humans it has been effective prophylactically against smallpox but ineffective as therapy of established infection. The main reported side effect is vomiting when given as 200 mg per kg loading dose and 50 mg per kg every six hours for eight doses. With the eradication of smallpox, the interest in methisazone is mainly historical.

UNPROVEN AGENTS

Many other agents and treatments have been claimed to be effective against viral infections. Numerous vaccines including smallpox, polio, BCG, and influenza have been tried, as non specific immunostimulators against viral infection, but in controlled studies they have failed to prevent recurrences of herpes simplex. These vaccines all have certain risks and should be used only when the benefits clearly outweigh risks. Other therapeutic modalities ranging from herbal preparations and immune stimulants to chemicals and ultraviolet irradiation have also failed to show any definite benefit. They include flavinoids, L-lysine, 2′deoxy-D-glucose, lithium or zinc creams, ether, and butylated-hydroxy-toluene (BHT, a food preservative).

The value of these agents as antiviral therapy or for palliation is unproved and their potential side effects are unknown. Reports of their effectiveness are anecdotal and they must be properly tested in double-blind, controlled trials before they can be recommended to a public only too willing to purchase cures and remedies for viral infections.

CONCLUSION

Vaccination and good public health measures including case isolation remain the most important measures in controlling viral infections; however, significant advances in the understanding of the molecular biology of viruses have enabled scientists to develop new agents to inhibit these pathogens selectively. The newer agents are becoming increasingly important both as prophylactic and therapeutic agents in given clinical situations. As with antibiotics, there is some concern that resistance to antiviral agents will become common; some resistant mutants have been produced in laboratory strains of HSV and several resistant clinical isolates have also been reported. This would suggest that care should be taken to prescribe antivirals responsibly.

ANNOTATED BIBLIOGRAPHY

Chang TW, and Heel RC. Ribavirin and inosiplex: a review of their present status in viral diseases. Drugs 1981; 22:111–128.

Dolin R, Reichman RC, Madore HP, et al. A controlled trial of amantadine and rimantadine in the prophylaxis of influenza A infection. N Engl J. Med 1982; 307:580–584.

A well-designed clinical trial demonstrates the beneficial effects of prophylaxis for influenza A epidemics.

Hirsch MS, Schooley RT. Treatment of herpesvirus infections. N Engl J Med 1983; 309:963–970; 1034–1039.

A comprehensive, well-referenced review covers both the antiviral agents for herpes virus infections and their appropriate use.

Lengyel P. Biochemistry of interferons and their action. Ann Rev Biochem 1982; 51:251–282.
A good review explaining some of the basic biochemistry of the action of interferon.

King DH, Gallasso G, eds. Acyclovir symposium. Am J Med 1982; (July): 1–391.
Proceedings of a conference in which the biochemistry, pharmacology, and clinical uses of acyclovir were fully discussed.

Pollard RB. Interferon and interferon inducers: development of clinical usefulness and therapeutic promise. Drugs 1982: 23:37–55.
The clinical promise and problems of interferon use are discussed.

U.S. Department of Health and Human Services. Georgia. Ineffective therapies for genital herpes infections. Pamphlet 00-3728. Atlanta: Centers for Disease Control,
A brief summary, designed for the patient, discusses ineffective treatments of genital herpes infections.

7 CHEMOPROPHYLAXIS OF INFECTIONS

Lindsay E. Nicolle

Chemoprophylaxis is the use of antimicrobial agents to prevent infections from occurring rather than to treat those that are already established. Optimal prophylaxis requires that the appropriate agent be present in the appropriate concentration at the potential site of infection when the individual is exposed to the infecting agent. Chemoprophylaxis can be medical or surgical. It may be given on a short-term basis to cover a specific risk situation, as in perioperative surgical prophylaxis, or for a more extended period targeted against either a single organism, such as penicillin given to prevent group A streptococcal infections, or a number of potential pathogens, as with prophylaxis for urinary tract infection or granulocytopenia.

The prophylactic use of antimicrobials is associated with several undesirable features. These include adverse drug effects and expense, but of major concern is the modification of endogenous host microbial flora, potentiating the emergence of resistant organisms. Such organisms may then not only produce infection in the individual receiving prophylaxis, but contribute to the spread of resistance factors among organisms in an institution or geographic area. Thus chemoprophylaxis should be used only in situations where there is acceptable proof of efficacy, with care being taken that the dosage and duration of therapy are appropriate. Ideally, the efficacy of a prophylactic regimen for a given situation should have been demonstrated in prospective, randomized, controlled studies. Many recently introduced indications for prophylaxis, such as the use of rifampin for *Hemophilus influenzae* meningitis, have met this criteria. Other accepted uses of prophylaxis, however, such as periprocedure antimicrobials to prevent bacterial endocarditis, have never had their efficacy documented in acceptable clinical trials, and their continued recommendation is based upon past medical practice and an assessment of the risk of the infection.

MEDICAL CHEMOPROPHYLAXIS

Medical prophylaxis is given for infection caused by agents exogenous to the host, such as malaria prophylaxis for travelers, or against infection by agents that may be part of the endogenous flora. This distinction between exogenous and endogenous organisms may be somewhat arbitrary. For example, in bacterial meningitis, prophylaxis is considered to be against an exogenous organism, but that organism must colonize the nasopharynx, thus becoming endogenous before it causes disease. The distinction is useful conceptually, however, and is maintained in this discussion.

Infection Caused by Exogenous Agents

Rheumatic Fever

Prophylactic antibiotics should be given to any person who experiences one or more episodes of rheumatic fever. The goal is to prevent streptococcal pharyngitis and thus second attacks of rheumatic fever. This is considered secondary prevention of rheumatic fever, as compared with primary prevention of initial episodes by treating all streptococcal pharyngitis. The most effective regimen (Table 7.1) in the prevention of second attacks of rheumatic fever is intramuscular benzathine penicillin, at least partially because it obviates many of the problems of compliance intrinsic in courses of oral medication. The duration of prophylaxis remains controversial. Some practitioners favor continuing medi-

TABLE 7.1. Medical Chemoprophylaxis: Exogenous Organisms

Disease	*Organism*	*Chemoprophylaxis*	
		Agent	*Dose and Duration*
Rheumatic fever	*S. pyogenes* (Group A streptococcus)	Penicillin V	125–250 mg po bid
		or Benzathine penicillin	1.2 MU IM every 4 wks
		or Sulfadiazine	1 gm po od (0.5 gm if <25 kg)
		or Erythromycin	250 mg po bid
Bacterial meningitis	*N. meningitidis*	Sulfadiazine*	1 gm bid × 2 d
		Rifampin	600 mg (<1 mo, 5 mg/kg; >1 mo, 10 mg/kg) bid × 2 d
		Minocycline	200 mg then 100 mg q12h for 5 additional doses
	H. influenzae	Rifampin†	20 mg/kg (max. 600 mg) daily × 4 d
Ophthalmia neonatorum	*N. gonorrhoeae* *C. trachomatis*	Silver nitrate, 1 or 2%‡ Erythromycin, 0.5% or ophthalmic ointment Tetracycline, 1% ophthalmic ointment	Applied to both eyes, topically, immediately after birth
Influenza	Influenza A	Amantadine	100 mg po bid
Pneumocystis	*P. carinii*	TMP/SMZ**	5 mg TMP, 25 mg SMZ/kg/d, in two doses
Tuberculosis	*M. tuberculosis*	Isoniazid	5 mg/kg (max. 300 mg) daily for 1 yr
Leprosy	*M. leprae*	Dapsone	<6 mo 6 mg; 6–23 mo 12 mg; 2–5 yrs 25 mg: twice a week 6–12 yrs 25 mg; >12 yrs 50 mg: daily for 3 yrs
Plague	*Y. pestis*	Tetracycline	15–20 mg/kg/24 hr, (1.2 gm max.) in 4 doses × 7 d
		Sulfonamide	40 mg/kg/d po × 7 d
Pertussis§	*B. pertussis*	Erythromycin	40–50 mg/kg/24 hrs in 4 doses × 14 d
Diphtheria§	*C. diphtheriae*	Erythromycin	40–50 mg/kg/24 hrs in 4 doses × 7 d
		or Benzathine penicillin	1.2 MU (600,000 U if <5 yrs) IM one dose

*Sulfadiazine should be used for prophylaxis for *N. meningitidis* only if the disease-producing strain is known to be susceptible to this agent.

†Rifampin is indicated for day-care center contacts and all family members if there is an unaffected sibling under 4 years of age.

‡Silver nitrate is not effective in preventing *C. trachomatis* ophthalmia neonatorum.

§Indicated for nonimmune close contacts.

**Trimethoprim-sulfamethoxazole

cation for a lifetime, while others would discontinue it at age 20 in individuals who have not had carditis and who experienced their last attack at least five years earlier. Prophylaxis should be continued for the lifetime of persons who have experienced rheumatic carditis, and also for any adult with frequent exposure to young children.

Bacterial Meningitis

Chemoprophylaxis is effective in preventing secondary cases of bacterial meningitis in close contacts of patients with meningitis or other invasive disease due to *Neisseria meningitidis* or *H. influenzae*. These organisms colonize the nasopharynx, and effective prophylaxis to eradicate the carrier state requires adequate levels of antimicrobials in the saliva. Agents such as penicillin, ampicillin, and chloramphenicol, which are used successfully in the therapy of bacterial meningitis, are not effective prophylactically to eradicate carriage, and their inefficacy probably reflects the low levels these agents attain in saliva. Sulfadiazine was widely used for prophylaxis of *N. meningitidis* in the 1950s, and is clearly effective in terminating outbreaks in closed populations. The emergence of sulfonamide-resistant organisms, perhaps partially due to indiscriminate large-scale use of sulfas, necessitated the development of alternative prophylactic agents. Thus while sulfonamides are useful against *N. meningitidis* infection because of their documented efficacy and relative inexpensiveness, they should only be used if the disease-producing strain is known to be sulfonamide-sensitive. Rifampin is the alternative agent of choice. Minocycline is also effective, but as it is a tetracycline, it must be avoided in pregnant women and young children, and in civilian populations its prophylactic use has been associated with an unacceptably high incidence of vestibular side effects.

Only rifampin has been shown to be effective in the chemoprophylaxis of invasive disease, including meningitis, due to *H. influenzae* type b. It does not however, eradicate *H. influenzae* if given in the dose recommended as prophylaxis for *N. meningitidis*, however; a single daily dose over a longer period of time — four days — is required.

Prophylaxis for sporadic *N. meningitidis* disease should be given to the patient's household or day-care contacts. Contacts of individuals residing in closed populations, such as college dormitories or military camps, should receive medication in an epidemic, but indications for prophylaxis for contacts of sporadically affected persons in such populations are not clear. Such cases should be dealt with individually, based on exposure. Health care workers in contact with a patient do not require prophylaxis unless prolonged, intimate exposure to nasopharyngeal secretions (e.g., mouth-to-mouth resuscitation) has occurred. Prophylaxis for *H. influenzae* meningitis is controversial but is currently recommended for all household contacts if there is a second, noninfected sibling under 4 years of age, and for day-care center contacts. Patients with disease due to *H. influenzae* should also receive prophylactic therapy, as treatment will not necessarily eradicate the infecting organism from the nasopharynx.

Ophthalmia Neonatorum

The routine instillation of silver nitrate in newborn infants' eyes has decreased the incidence of ophthalmia neonatorum due to *N. gonorrhoeae*. Currently, most infectious ophthalmia neonatorum is caused by *Chlamydia trachomatis*, and silver nitrate is not effective in preventing disease due to this agent. Both erythromycin and tetracycline ophthalmic ointments will prevent the disease caused by *C. trachomatis*, and are also effective for *N. gonorrhoeae*. Thus they appear to be more rational prophylaxis for the newborn, although their use may be associated with sensitization.

Influenza

Amantadine prophylaxis has been shown to be 75% to 90% effective in the prevention of influenza A during an epidemic. It is currently recommended for selected high-risk populations such as those for whom vaccination is recommended (persons over 65 years or those with significant chronic cardiac, respiratory, renal, or endocrine disease) but contraindicated (those with allergies to eggs). Persons at risk who were vaccinated immediately prior to or during an influenza epidemic should receive amantadine prophylaxis for two weeks after vaccination, until a protective antibody response from vaccination has developed. Other suggested recommendations include household contacts of an individual with influenza, and unvaccinated staff and patients in hospitals or institutions during an epidemic. Prophylaxis in these situations has not been well studied, however, and is not currently widely used.

Pneumocystis carinii

Trimethoprim/sulfamethoxazole (TMP/SMZ) prevents the development of *Pneumocystis carinii* pneumonia in children receiving chemotherapy for leukemia. Continuous prophylaxis without significant adverse effects has been given for up to two years. The risk of acquisition of *P. carinii* infection in such children appears to vary among institutions, and a decision whether or not to give the drug must consider the local experience. The prophylactic efficacy of TMP/SMZ in adults has not been documented. Its prophylactic and therapeutic use in patients with the acquired immunodeficiency syndrome has been associated with a high rate of cutaneous reactions, and its efficacy, if any, remains unknown.

Tuberculosis

Isoniazid therapy is recommended for Mantoux-negative household contacts of persons with active tuberculosis, and is true prophylactic therapy in this instance. Those contacts who have Mantoux conversion at 8 to 12 weeks after exposure and are assumed to have been infected should continue isoniazid for one full year, but therapy can be discontinued in those who remain Mantoux negative at repeat testing. Other commonly accepted recommendations for isoniazid, as developed by the American Thoracic Society, are more appropriately considered therapeutic rather than prophylactic, as medication is given to individuals with infection with tuberculosis, albeit without active disease. Suggested indications include persons of any age who have not received adequate therapy for tuberculosis and have an abnormal chest x-ray, those with recent (less than two years) documented conversion of the tuberculin test, and a Mantoux-positive individual of any age with underlying illness such as diabetes, silicosis, gastric resection, or malignancy, or who is undergoing immunosuppressive therapy. Isoniazid is also recommended for individuals under 35 years of age with a positive skin test alone and no other risk factors. Some authors feel that this recommendation is overly inclusive and suggest isoniazid therapy only for skin test-positive children (under 20 years) or for older individuals only with one of the other risk factors. With isoniazid prophylaxis, transient increases in levels of liver enzymes are common, but do not usually require discontinuation of the drug. Any clinical evidence of hepatitis necessitates discontinuation of the drug. The risk of significant hepatotoxicity from isoniazid increases with increasing age, and is greater in individuals with significant underlying hepatic disease.

Leprosy

Dapsone therapy should be given to household contacts under 25 years of age of persons with lepromatous or dimorphous leprosy, and continued for three years. This decreases the subsequent occurrence of leprosy in these contacts by approximately 50%. Dapsone is an oxidant drug, however, and may produce hemolysis in persons with glucose-6-phosphate dehydrogenase deficiency who receive it for prophylaxis.

Plague

Chemoprophylaxis with tetracycline or a sulfonamide is recommended for household contacts, hospital staff, or other persons who are close contacts of an individual with suspected or confirmed primary or secondary plague pneumonia. In addition, household contacts of an individual with flea-borne plague have an increased risk of developing that disease, and should also receive prophylaxis.

Pertussis and Diphtheria

Unimmunized children under 5 years of age who are contacts of patients with pertussis and unimmunized persons of any age who are contacts of individuals with diphtheria should receive chemoprophylaxis to prevent infection. The efficacy of prophylaxis in these situations is unproved, but the morbidity of infection and the risk of infection after exposure are felt to be high enough to warrant this use of antibiotics.

Prophylaxis for Travelers

Malaria

Travelers from nonmalarious areas of the world are at high risk for acquisition of malaria when they travel to endemic areas. Effective preventive chemotherapy requires knowledge of geographic areas of the world where malaria is endemic, and in which of these areas chloroquine-resistant *Plasmodium falciparum* is prevalent (Table 7.2). Chloroquine-resistant organisms are currently found in certain areas of South and Central America, the Indian subcontinent, Southeast Asia, the Indonesian archipelago, and East Africa. The geography of malaria and of chloroquine-resistant *P. falciparum* may vary from year to year, and physicians can consult current updates from various sources including the Centers for Disease Control, Atlanta, Georgia, in making a decision as to whether a traveler to a certain area requires prophylaxis and if so, what type.

Travelers to malarious areas where the organism is chloroquine-sensitive should take chloroquine phosphate starting one to two weeks before departure, then weekly while in the endemic area, and for six weeks

TABLE 7.2. Medical Chemoprophylaxis for Travelers: Exogenous Organisms

Disease	*Organism*	*Agent*	*Dose and Duration*
Malaria	*P. vivax* *P. ovale* *P. malariae* *P. falciparum* (chloroquine-sensitive)	Chloroquine phosphate	300 mg base (500 mg salt) (5 mg base/kg for children) initiated 2 wks before entering an endemic area and taken weekly while residing in and for 6 wks after leaving endemic area
	P. falciparum (chloroquine-resistant)	Pyrimethamine/sulfadoxine (Fansidar)	25 mg/500 mg (1 tablet) (0.5 mg/kg and 10 mg/kg for children) once weekly during and for × 6 wks after exposure in endemic area
Traveler's diarrhea	Enterotoxigenic *E. coli* Other	Doxycycline or	100 mg po daily
		TMP/SMZ†	160/800 mg (1 double-strength tablet) bid, in two doses
		or Bismuth subsalicylate*	57 gm qid daily

*Not recommended for persons younger than 12 years.
†Trimethoprim-sulfamethoxazole

after leaving. For those going to geographic areas of the world where acquisition of chloroquine-resistant *P. falciparum* is a risk, pyrimethamine/sulfadoxine (Fansidar) should be taken *in addition to* chloroquine. The pyrimethamine/sulfadoxine combination is effective prophylaxis for chloroquine-resistant *P. falciparum,* but is not reliable prophylaxis for *P. vivax,* and its efficacy for *P. ovale* and *P. malariae* is currently unknown. Pregnant women, infants under 2 years of age, and persons with a history of allergy to sulfa should not receive pyrimethamine/sulfadoxine. In some parts of Southeast Asia, chloroquine- and pyrimethamine/sulfadoxine-resistant malaria have been identified, but effective prophylaxis for these strains has not yet been defined. Malarial prophylaxis is not 100% effective, and all individuals returning from malarious regions who have taken prophylaxis should be advised to seek medical assistance for any febrile illness after their return, and to advise the medical personnel consulted at that time of any recent travel history.

Traveler's Diarrhea

From 25% to 50% of travelers to developing countries develop diarrheal illness. The major pathogen responsible for the condition is enterotoxigenic *Escherichia coli,* with *Shigella* sp., *Salmonella* sp., and protozoa also contributing. Recommendations for chemoprophylaxis to prevent traveler's diarrhea remain controversial, but several agents (Table 7.2) have been shown in prospective, controlled, randomized studies to prevent this disease. Doxycycline and TMP/SMZ are approximately 90% effective, while bismuth subsalicylate (Pepto-Bismol) has been shown to be about 60% effective. Despite this proven efficacy, antimicrobial prophylaxis for travelers at risk of acquiring diarrheal illness is not generally recommended due to concern that the widespread use of these drugs will promote the emergence and dissemination of antibiotic-resistant toxigenic strains. Clearly, the prophylactic use of these agents also carries with it the risk of adverse effects, including photosensitivity with doxycycline. An alternative effective approach is early treatment should symptoms develop, which should minimize associated adverse effects and antimicrobial resistance. Effective early treatment regimens include trimethoprim/sulfamethoxazole, one regular strength tablet twice a day for five days; trimethoprim alone, 200 mg twice a day for five days; or bismuth subsalicylate, 30 to 60 ml every half-hour for eight doses. Bismuth subsalicylate should not be used in children, as it may cause salicylate intoxication.

Chemoprophylaxis to Prevent Bacterial Endocarditis

Bacterial endocarditis is one condition for which prophylaxis is given to prevent infection with endogenous organisms. Optimal management for the prevention of bacterial endocarditis has three components. First, the individual with a cardiac lesion that places him or her at risk for developing endocarditis must be identified. Second, specific procedures associated with a frequency and degree of bacteremia sufficient to warrant periprocedure prophylaxis must be recognized. Finally, the individual must receive the appropriate prophylactic regimen with respect to agent, dose, and route and timing of administration.

In general, any individual with known heart disease, particularly a condition involving the valves, should be considered a candidate for prophylaxis. This includes persons with congenital heart disease (excluding uncomplicated secundum atrial septal defects or ligated and divided patent ductus arteriosus), acquired valvular lesions, prolapsing mitral valve, idiopathic hypertrophic subaortic stenosis, calcified mitral annulus, or intracardiac prostheses. Any person who has previously experienced an episode of infective endocarditis should also receive prophylaxis. Currently, prophylaxis is not felt to be indicated for individuals with permanent transvenous pacemakers.

Factors important in determining which procedures warrant prophylaxis include the concentration of organisms at the site at which the procedure is performed and the amount of associated trauma, both of which correlate with the extent of bacteremia. Specific indications include dental procedures accompanied by bleeding, such as extraction, deep scaling, and operations for periodontal infections; surgery involving the upper respiratory tract, including bronchoscopy with a rigid scope; operation or instrumentation of the gastrointestinal or genitourinary tract; cardiac surgery involving extracorporeal circulation; and surgical procedures in which infected or contaminated tissues or abscesses are invaded. Generally, endoscopy with fiberoptic devices, including bronchoscopy, gastroscopy, and colonoscopy, does not require prophylactic therapy; nor does insertion or removal of intrauterine devices and uncomplicated delivery. Despite the low risk of bacteremia in these instances, however, some authors recommend prophylaxis for any patient with a prosthetic valve. There is insufficient evidence to allow formulation of definite recommendations.

The efficacy of prophylaxis in preventing bacterial endocarditis is unknown, as it has never been tested in any randomized clinical studies. Many features are controversial, including whether or not prophylaxis is effective, which agents or combination of agents should be used, by what route they should be given, and for what duration. For logistic and cost reasons, it is unlikely that studies will be carried out to resolve these controversies. The American Heart Association guidelines for prophylaxis (Table 7.3) are based upon current knowledge and estimates of risk of endocarditis in humans as well as data from animal studies. It seems reasonable, in the absence of definitive studies and until further information becomes available, to follow these guidelines.

Prophylaxis is targeted against gram-positive organisms, such as viridans streptococci, enterococci, other streptococci, and staphylococci, which are the etiologic agents in over 90% of endocarditis. Recommended regimens have been chosen to ensure bactericidal activity against these potential pathogens. Thus the addition of an aminoglycoside to penicillin or vancomycin for gastrointestinal and genitourinary procedures is for synergistic activity against *S. faecalis*. Prophylaxis should not be initiated until immediately before the procedure, as prolonged preprocedure therapy may facilitate the emergence of flora resistant to the chemotherapeutic agent and render it ineffective. For individuals receiving penicillin prophylaxis for the secondary prevention of rheumatic fever, a nonpenicillin should be given for perioperative prophylaxis against bacterial endocarditis, as the flora of these persons is likely to indicate penicillin-resistant organisms. Alternately, parenteral regimens with higher doses of penicillin and an aminoglycoside may be used. The duration of prophylaxis may be modified depending on the duration of the procedure. For brief procedures, lasting only a few minutes, a single preprocedure dose may well suffice, while prolonged operations or procedures may necessitate administration of several additional doses.

Prophylaxis for Other Infections Caused by Endogenous Organisms

Urinary Tract Infection

Approximately 10% of women experience recurrent, symptomatic, lower urinary tract infection. Infection is usually caused by organisms resident in the fecal flora

TABLE 7.3. Prophylaxis Against Bacterial Endocarditis

Procedure	*For Patients with Native Valves*	*For Patients with Prosthetic Valves*
Any dental procedure associated with bleeding, or respiratory tract instrumentation	Aqueous crystalline penicillin G, 1 MU, (30,000 U/kg for children), with procaine penicillin G, 600,000 U IM 30–60 min preprocedure; then penicillin V, 500 mg (250 mg for children <30 kg) po q6h × 8 doses or Penicillin V, 2.0 gm (1.0 gm for <30 kg) po 30–60 min before and 500 mg (250 mg for <30 kg), po q6h × 8 doses or Erythromycin, 1.0 gm (20 mg/kg for children) po 1–2 hrs before; then 500 mg (10 mg/kg for children) q6h × 8 doses* or Either regimen recommended for patients with prosthetic valves	Aqueous crystalline penicillin G, 1 MU (30,000 U/kg for children), with procaine penicillin G, 600,000 U IM *plus* gentamicin, 1.5 mg/kg IM 30–60 min before; then penicillin V, 500 mg (250 mg for children <30 kg), po q6h for 8 doses or Vancomycin 0.5–1.0 gm (20 mg/kg for children) infused slowly over 1 hr starting 30–60 min before procedure; then erythromycin, 500 mg (10 mg/kg for children) q6h × 8 doses*
	All Patients	
Gastrointestinal or genitourinary surgery or Abscess drainage or incision of infected tissues	Aqueous crystalline penicillin G, 2 MU (30,000 U/kg for children) or Ampicillin, 1.0 gm (50 mg/kg for children) IM or IV before procedure plus Gentamicin, 1.5 mg/kg IM or IV Repeat both drugs for 2 additional doses q8h or *Vancomycin, 0.5–1.0 gm (20 mg/kg for children) IV infused slowly over 1 hr plus Gentamicin, 1.5 mg/kg IM or IV Repeat both drugs once 12 hrs later	

*Regimens recommended for penicillin-allergic patients.

and is preceded by periurethral colonization by these organisms. For women who have experienced two or more symptomatic infections in a six-month period, low-dose antimicrobial prophylaxis, which will virtually eliminate symptomatic infection, is recommended. Prophylaxis is not indicated for women with recurrent relapse of infection from upper tract disease or with associated genitourinary abnormalities such as renal stones, as these infections require suppressive, not prophylactic, therapy. The pattern of recurrence, reinfection or relapse, should be established for each patient before prophylaxis is initiated.

Regimens of documented efficacy are shown in Table 7.4. The prophylactic antimicrobial should be taken at bedtime to maximize the time the agent remains in the urinary bladder. The three regimens listed are all equally efficacious, and the choice will usually be determined by patient tolerance. Prophylaxis for recurrent cystitis is generally prescribed for a six-month period. For patients who continue to have recurrent symptomatic infections, continuous prophylaxis with trimethoprim/sulfamethoxazole for up to two years has been reported not to cause adverse effects and to maintain therapeutic efficacy.

TABLE 7.4. Medical Chemoprophylaxis: Endogenous Organisms

		Chemoprophylaxis	
Disease	*Organism*	*Agent*	*Dose*
Recurrent symptomatic lower urinary tract infection	*E. coli* *S. saprophyticus*	TMP/SMZ*	40/200 mg (one-half of a regular-strength tablet) daily or 3 times/wk
		Trimethoprim	50 mg daily
		Nitrofurantoin	50 mg daily
		Nitrofurantoin macrocrystals	100 mg daily
Prolonged (>7 days) granulocytopenia	Gram-negative, aerobic, enteric flora	TMP/SMZ*	160/800 mg (2 regular-strength tablets or 1 double-strength) po q8h or q12h
		Nalidixic acid	2 gm po q6h
Otitis media	*S. pneumoniae* *H. influenzae* *B. catarrhalis* *S. pyogenes*	Ampicillin or Sulfisoxazole	125 mg (<2½ yrs) or 250 mg (>2½ yrs) po daily 500 mg bid daily

*Trimethoprim-sulfamethoxazole.

Granulocytopenia

Individuals with granulocytopenia, usually defined as an absolute polymorphonuclear leukocyte count of fewer than 1000, are at risk of developing infection. The degree of risk is inversely proportional to the level of absolute granulocyte count. The source of sepsis is frequently endogenous flora colonizing the upper airway or gastrointestinal tract. Antimicrobial prophylaxis decreases the incidence of infection in patients with profound granulocytopenia anticipated to be of limited duration, such as leukemic patients undergoing induction chemotherapy. Currently, prophylaxis is recommended for any such patient anticipated to have granulocytopenia for seven days or longer.

Trimethoprim/sulfamethoxazole, started when the granulocyte count first falls below 1000, has been most widely used. One study comparing TMP/SMZ and nalidixic acid suggests the former is superior in preventing infections due to gram-negative organisms, but may prolong granulocytopenia and be associated with increased systemic fungal disease. Numerous other regimens of oral nonabsorbable antibiotics, including gentamicin alone, gentamicin plus vancomycin, vancomycin plus polymixin and kanamycin, and neomycin and polymixin B, have also been shown to be effective prophylactically, but have been associated with patient intolerance due to gastrointestinal side effects and emergence of aminoglycoside-resistant organisms. Thus they cannot currently be recommended. Many prophylactic regimens have included an antifungal agent, such as nystatin, 1 million units every four or six hours, or amphotericin B, but evidence that such therapy prevents colonization or infection with yeast or fungi is not convincing. Prophylaxis, once initiated, should be continued until the granulocyte count has returned to over 1000.

Otitis Media

Organisms isolated from the middle ear in acute otitis media are usually resident colonizers of the nasopharynx. Otitis media is thought to occur when these organisms gain access to the inner ear, usually from the eustachian tube, in the presence of secretory otitis media, or obstruction to drainage. In young children, this infection is common and has a tendency to recur. Two randomized, controlled, prospective studies have demonstrated the efficacy of prophylaxis in the prevention of recurrent otitis media in high-risk populations, one of Alaskan Eskimos, the other of children with frequent reinfections seen in urban pediatric practice. Prophylaxis, although not widely used, could be considered as an option for the management of children under 6 years of age who have experienced at least three episodes of acute otitis media in the preceding 18 months. The efficacy of this therapy compared with surgical procedures such as ear drainage tubes has not been studied.

SURGICAL CHEMOPROPHYLAXIS

Infection is a complication of approximately 5% of all surgical wounds. It results in delayed healing and prolonged hospitalization, and may require antimicrobial therapy or further surgery. Thus prevention is important to reduce patient morbidity and prolonged hospitalization. Good surgical technique remains the most important preventive method, including avoiding preoperative shaving of the operative site, minimizing tissue trauma and bleeding at surgery, avoiding the placement of foreign material in the wound, eliminating dead space, adequately debriding devitalized tissue, and maintaining as short an operative time as technically feasible. In addition to these considerations, antimicrobial prophylaxis can reduce the frequency of postoperative wound infection for selected procedures.

Surgical prophylaxis is responsible for 25% to 50% of antibiotic use in most general hospitals. Several reviews have reported that a large proportion of this usage is inappropriate and can lead to unnecessary expense, adverse drug effects, and modification in the susceptibility of hospital flora, resulting in the emergence and persistence of resistant organisms. With this potential for significant harm, it is important that antimicrobial prophylaxis used in surgery adhere to accepted guidelines based on data derived from well-controlled studies. Such studies, performed largely during the last decade, have permitted the development of some general principles (Table 7.5).

Types of Surgery

Prophylaxis should only be given for specific, selected types of surgery, principally, in certain clean-contaminated procedures; that is, those in which the respiratory, genitourinary, or alimentary tract is entered under controlled conditions and without unusual contamination, and where prophylaxis has been documented by suitable prospective trials to be efficacious. Specific operations include surgery on the oral cavity, some types of gastroduodenal surgery, hepatobiliary surgery in patients likely to have bactibilia (including persons over 70 years, those with obstructive jaundice, a common duct stone with or without jaundice, acute cholecystitis, or previous hepatobiliary surgery), colorectal surgery, including appendectomy, and procedures involving the female genital tract.

For most clean surgical procedures, that is, where wounds are nontraumatic and uninfected, where inflammation is not encountered, there is no break in technique, and mucous membranes are not entered, the rate of postoperative infection is so low, usually less than 2%, that little benefit is gained from prophylaxis and it is not indicated. For clean procedures in which a prosthetic device is implanted, such as cardiac valves or hip replacement, the morbidity and mortality of prosthetic infection is considered of such magnitude that prophylaxis is recommended, despite the lack of data to document its efficacy. The low infection rates inherent in this type of surgery would require a large number of patients to document prophylactic efficacy, and again, due to the expense and difficulty of performing such large-scale studies, the value of prophylaxis may never be adequately tested.

While antimicrobial therapy is usually given for contaminated and dirty wounds, the antimicrobial agents used in these circumstances are therapeutic rather than prophylactic and are not discussed further. For genitourinary surgery, prophylaxis is not currently recommended if the urine is uninfected. In the presence of infected urine, antimicrobial therapy is indicated, but is prescribed not as prophylaxis but as treatment of the urinary tract infection.

Timing of Prophylaxis

For prophylaxis to be effective, the antibiotic should have reached a satisfactory tissue level at the site of surgery when the incision is made. Antimicrobials started after the incision are less effective, and if given over three hours after incision, will not alter postoperative infections. Thus the initial dose must be given preoperatively, usually on call to the OR or at the time of anesthetic induction. One exception to preoperative timing is in cesarean sections, where antimicrobial prophylaxis is given when the cord is clamped, thus avoiding transplacental transfer of the drug to the newborn infant.

The duration of antimicrobial therapy should be strictly perioperative. Extended therapy does not increase prophylactic efficacy and is associated with in-

TABLE 7.5. Surgical Prophylaxis

Type of Surgery	*Recommended Prophylaxis*
Clean-contaminated	
Oropharyngeal	Cefazolin, 1 gm IV or IM on call to the operating room, repeat q4h during operation
Gastroduodenal	
Gastric tumor, gastric ulcer, GI bleeding, pyloric obstruction, perforated duodenal ulcer	
Biliary tract	
Patients >70 years, with jaundice, common duct stone, acute cholecystitis, previous biliary surgery	
Hysterectomy	
Vaginal or abdominal	
Cesarean section, emergency	Cefazolin, 1 gm IV immediately after cord clamped
Appendectomy	Cefoxitin, 1 gm IM or IV on call to the operating room, repeat q4h during surgery
Colorectal	Oral: erythromycin base, 1 gm and neomycin sulfate, 1 gm at 1:00 P.M., 11:00 P.M., and 2:00 A.M. on day before surgery
All surgery	Parenteral: cefoxitin, 1 gm IM or IV on call to the operating room, repeat q4h during surgery
Clean	
Cardiac surgery	Cefazolin, 1 gm IM or IV on call to the operating room, repeat q4h during operative procedure or Cloxacillin, 1 or 2 gm IV on call to the operating room, repeat q4h during operative procedure
Prosthetic valve insertion, coronary artery bypass, grafts	
Peripheral vascular surgery	
Graft insertion for abdominal aorta or lower leg bypass	
Artificial joint insertion	
Hip fracture for pinning	
Trauma and burns	
Open fractures	Cefazolin, 1 gm IV q8h started within 3 hrs of injury and continued 3–7 d
Burn wounds (second and third degree)	Topical: 0.5% silver nitrate solution 10% mafenide acetate cream 1% silver sulfadiazine

creased adverse drug effects, cost, and alterations in microbial flora to a more resistant pattern. While some authors recommend continued prophylaxis for 24 to 48 hours following the surgery, even this is probably excessive, as several reports have shown that a single preoperative dose is as effective as extended therapy. Brief procedures undoubtedly require only a single preoperative dose. For more prolonged surgery, the antibiotic should be repeated every four hours during the procedure to ensure adequate tissue levels are maintained throughout the procedure. Prophylaxis for clean and clean-contaminated procedures should, based on current knowledge, never be extended for longer than 48 hours postsurgery.

Choice of Agent

The ideal prophylactic agent is targeted against organisms that are anticipated to cause infection for a given procedure. For oropharyngeal surgery this is oral streptococci and anaerobes. Gastroduodenal and biliary procedures require enteric gram-negative coverage as well, and colonic procedures require *Bacteroides fragilis* to be covered adequately. For clean procedures with prosthetic insertions, gram-positive cocci, particularly coagulase-negative staphylococci and *S. aureus,* are the most important pathogens.

In practice, one of the broad-spectrum antimicrobial agents that is effective against many types of organisms, usually a first-generation cephalosporin, has been used, and considerable experience concerning their efficacy has been reported. For most clean and for clean-contaminated surgical procedures not involving the colon, studies suggest the first-, second-, and third-generation cephalosporins are equally effective. As the first-generation cephalosporins are considerably cheaper, they seem to be preferable. Cefazolin, with a prolonged half-life, higher serum levels, capability of being given intramuscularly, and relative low cost, is perhaps the most attractive among these. It has documented efficacy for a number of different surgical procedures and it is widely recommended (Table 7.5). Other first-generation cephalosporins could also be used, depending on cost considerations, although they may not be well tolerated on intramuscular administration.

These drugs provide wide coverage, including gram-positive aerobes, some gram-negative aerobes, and some anaerobes, but are not adequate prophylaxis for infections where *Bacteroides fragilis* is a significant pathogen, such as in colorectal surgery. For these procedures, several regimens with better anaerobic coverage may be used; recommended oral and parenteral regimens are shown in Table 7.5. Prophylaxis for colorectal surgery should be either oral or parenteral, but not both, as the two forms combined have not been shown to be superior to either alone.

While the cephalosporins have been the class of antibiotics most widely used and evaluated for prophylaxis, other agents or regimens may be equally efficacious, and any with demonstrated efficacy in controlled clinical trials would be suitable for prophylaxis. Regimens with documented efficacy include: for biliary tract surgery, gentamicin, trimethoprim/sulfamethoxazole, and tobramycin plus vancomycin; carbenicillin and metronidazole for abdominal hysterectomy; penicillin G, carbenicillin, metronidazole, and trimethoprim/sulfamethoxazole for vaginal hysterectomy; a combination of ampicillin and cloxacillin for otolaryngologic surgery. For colonic surgery, oral regimens including tetracycline or metronidazole with neomycin, metronidazole and kanamycin, and doxycycline alone, and parenteral regimens including clindamycin or metronidazole with gentamicin, and erythromycin or metronidazole with tobramycin have all been shown to be effective. It seems preferable, however, to adopt one or two standard regimens for prophylaxis and use these routinely, as thorough experience with one regimen is likely to minimize errors in usage.

PROPHYLAXIS FOR TRAUMA AND BURN WOUNDS

Antibiotic therapy is indicated for patients with open fractures, although controversy still exists over the terminology of this as prophylactic or therapeutic. While some authors feel that it is therapy for a contaminated wound, others argue that, if given within three hours of trauma, it may be considered prophylaxis in preventing infection. As *S. aureus* is the most common infecting pathogen, first-generation cephalosporins are appropriate and have been demonstrated to be superior to placebo or penicillin plus aminoglycoside in at least one study. The current recommended duration of therapy is five days, although future studies may show that shorter courses would be equally efficacious.

Penicillin G is widely prescribed to prevent pneumococcal meningitis for head injuries with cerebrospinal fluid leaks. The efficacy of such therapy is untested and questionable, and it cannot be recommended as routine practice. Similarly, penicillin G has been widely prescribed in the immediate postburn period to prevent early group A streptococcal infection. Recent studies suggest that this organism is now an infrequent cause of burn wound sepsis, and such prophylaxis is no longer indicated. Topical therapy of burn wounds can, however, prevent colonization and decrease wound sepsis due to *S. aureus* and gram-negative organisms, and is indicated for all second- and third-degree burns (see Chapter 24).

ANNOTATED BIBLIOGRAPHY

Gorbach SL. Traveler's diarrhea. N Engl J Med 1982;307:881–882.

An editorial examining options for prophylaxis and treatment of traveler's diarrhea.

Hirschmann JV. Rational antibiotic prophylaxis. Hosp Pract 1981;November:105–123.

A complete general review of the use of prophylactic antimicrobials.

Hurley DL, Howard P, Hahn HH. Perioperative prophylactic antibiotics in abdominal surgery: a review of recent progress. Surg Clin North Am 1979;59:919–933.

A complete review of current rationale and clinical studies of surgical prophylaxis.

Jackson GG. Considerations of antibiotic prophylaxis in non-surgical high-risk patients. Am J Med 1981;70:467–473.

A review of the problems inherent in the use of antibiotics for non-surgical prophylaxis, especially as relates to nosocomial infections.

Jacoby I, Mandell LA, Weinstein L. The chemoprophylaxis of infection: a brief review of recent studies. Med Clin North Am 1978;62:1083–1098.

A general review of use of antimicrobial prophylaxis with emphasis on usage validated by properly performed clinical studies.

Kaplan EL, Anthony BF, Bisno A, et al. AHA committee report: prevention of bacterial endocarditis. Circulation 1977;56:139A–143A.

Statement of the American Heart Association's recommendations for antibiotic prophylaxis for bacterial endocarditis.

8 IMMUNIZATION

Ronald Gold

Immunization against the common childhood infections — diphtheria, tetanus, pertussis, poliomyelitis, measles, mumps, and rubella — has been the single most effective action of modern medicine in reducing overall morbidity and mortality rates. The success of immunization programs provides the most clear-cut demonstration of the advantages of prevention over treatment and rehabilitation. Recent changes in immunization policy in the United States, which combine emphasis on public education to obtain high levels of voluntary participation with laws requiring proof of immunization at school entry, have resulted in the almost complete elimination of indigenous measles and rubella.

TYPES OF IMMUNIZATIONS

Active immunization refers to the administration of an antigen to induce humoral and/or cellular immunity. Passive immunization refers to the provision of specific preformed antibody.

The characteristics of an ideal vaccine include: (1) ability to induce long-lasting protection, (2) lack of adverse effects, (3) stability during distribution and storage, and (4) effectiveness after a single dose. No presently available vaccine meets all of these criteria. The degree of departure from the ideal will become apparent in the discussion of each agent.

Vaccines can be divided into two types: (1) inactivated or purified fractions of microbes and (2) live, attenuated microbes. Live vacccines have the advantage of requiring a small dose since the microbe multiplies in the recipient, producing long-lasting immunity. They have the disadvantage of requiring special handling during distribution and storage prior to use in order to prevent inadvertent inactivation. They can cause disease if administered to immunosuppressed patients.

Passive immunizing agents should (1) be of human origin so as to minimize reaction, (2) be free of hepatitis B virus and other infectious agents, (3) have high, specific antibody titers, (4) be inexpensive, and (5) be readily available.

ACTIVE IMMUNIZATION

General Precautions and Contraindications

1. When administering any immunizing agent, the possibility of anaphylaxis must be considered and epinephrine should always be at hand.
2. Minor infections such as the common cold and most other respiratory tract infections are not a contraindication to immunization. An illness with fever is a reason to postpone immunization.
3. If a severe reaction (convulsion, collapse, marked lethargy, prolonged screaming for more than three hours, or fever over 40.5°C) follows administration of pertussis vaccine (as in DPT or DPT-polio), further doses of this vaccine should be avoided. There is no evidence that fractional doses of vaccines are either efficacious or less likely to cause severe reactions.
4. Interruption of the immunization schedule for any reason does not require starting the series over again, regardless of the interval.
5. Live, attenuated, viral vaccines (measles, mumps, rubella, oral polio, yellow fever) must never be given to individuals known to have impaired immunity resulting from

a. Immunodeficiency diseases (agammaglobulinemia, severe combined immunodeficiency)
b. Leukemia, lymphoma, or generalized malignancy
c. Immunosuppressive therapy with corticosteroids, cytotoxic drugs, or irradiation.

6. Anaphylaxis or other systemic allergic reactions after eating eggs is a contraindication to the use of live viral vaccines prepared in chicken or duck embryo tissue cultures (measles and mumps) and of killed viral vaccine produced in embryonated eggs (influenza).
7. Atopic diseases such as eczema, asthma, etc., are not a contraindication to immunization.
8. Pregnancy is generally a contraindication to immunization, especially with live viral vaccines such as rubella and measles, because of the risk of viremia and transplacental exposure of the fetus. Yellow fever and polio vaccines can be given if exposure is likely; toxoids and killed vaccines may also be given to pregnant women when indicated.
9. In children with neurologic disorders, the advantages of protection induced by the vaccine generally outweigh the risks of accentuating the neurologic problem (see under Pertussis Vaccine).
10. The following combinations of vaccines have been shown to be effective and have no increase in adverse reactions when given simultaneously at different sites:
    a. DPT and oral polio vaccine (OPV)
    b. Measles, mumps, and/or rubella vaccines (MMR, MR), etc.
    c. MMR and OPV
    d. DPT and MMR

TABLE 8.1. Routine Immunization Schedule for Infants and Children

Age	*Vaccines*	
2 mo	DPT*	Polio†[(a)]
4 mo	DPT	Polio
6 mo	DPT	Polio
12 mo	MMR‡	
18 mo	DPT	Polio
4–6 yr	DPT	Polio
14–16 yr	Td§	Polio†[(b)]

*DPT — diphtheria toxoid, pertussis vaccine, tetanus toxoid, alum-adsorbed.

†Polio — either live (oral) poliovirus vaccine or inactivated poliovirus vaccine combined with DPT.
(a) Optional if live (oral) poliovirus vaccine is used.
(b) Not necessary if live (oral) poliovirus vaccine is used. The need for subsequent boosters of inactivated poliovirus vaccine is not established.

‡MMR — measles, mumps, rubella virus vaccines. Because slightly higher rates of seroconversion are achieved by immunization at 15 instead of 12 months of age, 15 months is the recommended age in the United States.

§Td — diphtheria toxoid, tetanus toxoid, alum-adsorbed, for use in persons over 7 years of age. Contains a smaller amount of diphtheria toxoid than that used for younger children in order to reduce reaction rates. Should be administered every 10 years throughout life after completion of the basic series.

Immunization Schedules for Infants and Children

The schedules given in Tables 8.1 and 8.2 reflect the recommendations of the National Advisory Committee on Immunization of Canada, the American Academy of Pediatrics, and the United States Public Health Service.

Changes in the recommended immunizing agents and schedules occur as a result of medical advances. Thus alum-adsorbed DPT has recently been introduced into Canada. Because the adsorbed vaccines are significantly more immunogenic with respect to both diphtheria and tetanus toxoids and pertussis vaccine, their use is recommended over fluid vaccines.

Active Immunizing Agents

BCG Vaccine

Bacille Calmette-Guérin vaccine (BCG) is a lyophilized preparation of a live attenuated strain of *Mycobacterium bovis*. It should be administered by the intradermal route in accordance with the manufacturer's instructions. The scarification method is no longer recommended. This vaccine varies widely throughout the world in immunogenicity, efficacy, and reactogenicity. Considerable controversy exists concerning the efficacy and hence the use of BCG in preventing clinical tuberculosis.

TABLE 8.2. Immunization Schedule for Children or Adults Not Immunized in Early Infancy

	Age	
Timing	*1–6 Years*	*Over 6 Years*
First visit	DPT*-polio†	Td-polio
Interval after first visit		
1 mo	MMR‡	MMR
2 mo	DPT-polio†[(a)]	Td-polio
4 mo	DPT-polio	—
10–16 mo	DPT-polio	Td-polio
14–16 yrs	Td§-polio†[(b)]	Td-polio

*DPT — diphtheria toxoid, pertussis vaccine, tetanus toxoid, alum-adsorbed.

†Polio — either live (oral) poliovirus vaccine or inactivated poliovirus vaccine combined with DPT.
(a) Optional if live (oral) poliovirus vaccine is used.
(b) Not necessary if live (oral) poliovirus vaccine is used. The need for subsequent boosters of inactivated poliovirus vaccine is not established.

‡MMR — measles, mumps, rubella virus vaccines. Because slightly higher rates of seroconversion are achieved by immunization at 15 instead of 12 months of age, 15 months is the recommended age in the United States.

§Td — diphtheria toxoid, tetanus toxoid, alum-adsorbed, for use in persons over 7 years of age. Contains a smaller amount of diphtheria toxoid than that used for younger children in order to reduce reaction rates. Should be administered every 10 years throughout life after completion of the basic series.

Recommended usage. BCG vaccine should be used only in groups at high risk of developing tuberculosis, including

1. Individuals repeatedly exposed to untreated, active tuberculosis.
2. Communities with high rates of infection.
3. Health workers who handle tubercle bacilli or who are at high risk of exposure to undiagnosed pulmonary tuberculosis.
4. Newborn infants whose mothers have infectious tuberculosis at the time of delivery, only if mother and infant are separated until conversion to positive tuberculin reactivity is demonstrated. If separation is not possible or desirable, the infant should receive isoniazid for three months after mother is no longer infectious, at which time isoniazid can be discontinued if results of the tuberculin test and chest x-ray are both negative.

Adverse reactions. Up to 5% of recipients develop persistent or spreading skin ulcers, inflamed regional lymph nodes, or keloid formation. Suppurative lymphadenitis occurs at a rate of 0.1%, and is usually responsive to isoniazid therapy. Severe osteitis and generalized BCG infection are very rare.

Contraindications. Positive tuberculin test, impaired immunity, extensive skin disease, pregnancy, and measles or mumps vaccine in preceding four weeks.

Cholera Vaccine

Cholera vaccine is a killed, phenol-preserved suspension of both the Inaba and Ogawa serotypes of *Vibrio cholerae*. The vaccine is thought to prevent cholera in 50% of recipients for three to six months.

Recommended usage. Travelers to areas where cholera is endemic or epidemic should be vaccinated. The vaccine does not prevent acquisition of asymptomatic carrier state of *V. cholerae* and should not be used to control disease transmission. Primary immunization consists of two to three doses administered four weeks apart. Boosters are required every six months if the risk of exposure continues.

Adverse Reactions. Local reactions, fever, and malaise lasting one to two days are common.

Contraindications. Serious reaction to previous cholera vaccination. Safety in pregnancy is unknown, so that use must be based on individual need.

Diphtheria Toxoid

Diphtheria toxoid is prepared by formalin inactivation of diphtheria toxin. Immunity is directed only against the toxin but does not prevent carriage of *Corynebacterium diphtheriae*. Alum-adsorbed toxoid is significantly more immunogenic than fluid preparations. Diphtheria toxoid is rarely used alone; it is usually combined with tetanus toxoid and pertussis vaccine (DPT) or with tetanus toxide (dt, DT).

Recommended usage. See schedules in Tables 8.1 and 8.2. Since immunity to clinical diphtheria depends on adequate levels of antitoxin antibody, routine immunization is recommended for everyone.

Adverse reactions. Several local reactions with fever may occur in older children and adults. Reaction rates increase in frequency with age, quantity of toxoid used, and number of doses given. Adult-type diphtheria toxoid should be used in children over 6 years of age or adults.

Contraindications. Serious reaction to previous dose of diphtheria toxoid.

Influenza Vaccine

Influenza vaccine consists of two or more strains of inactivated virus partially purified by centrifugation. The virus strains are chosen so as to include antigens of the most recently isolated strains of influenza A and B. Vaccines may contain whole virus particles or disrupted virus. The latter are used only in children. Influenza vaccine provides approximately 70% protection for about one year against clinical influenza.

Recommended usage. The vaccine is recommended primarily for those at risk of suffering severe illness or death from influenza:

1. Persons over 65 years of age
2. Persons with
   a. Heart disease associated with pulmonary congestion
   b. Chronic pulmonary disease
   c. Chronic renal disease
   d. Diabetes mellitus
   e. Sickle cell disease
   f. Immunodeficiency

Immunization should be performed annually in high-risk persons, preferably before the start of the influenza season (December-March).

Adverse reactions. Fever, myalgia, and malaise lasting one to two days are not infrequent, especially after administration of whole-virus vaccine. An increased incidence of Guillain-Barré syndrome was seen after use of the swine influenza vaccine in 1976, but has not been observed with subsequent influenza vaccines.

Contraindications. Egg hypersensitivity is a contraindication to the use of the vaccine because of the risk of severe allergic reaction to the trace amounts of egg protein in the vaccine.

Measles Vaccine

Measles vaccine consists of a live, attenuated virus that can be used alone or in combination with rubella and/or mumps vaccine. The vaccine is 90% to 95% effective in preventing disease. Failures occur most often because of improper handling and refrigeration of the vaccine during distribution or storage.

Recommended usage. All children should receive measles vaccine at 12 months of age or as soon as practicable thereafter. The vaccine should not be given before the first birthday because of an increased frequency of vaccine failure as a consequence of persisting transplacental antibody. When epidemics occur, however, measles vaccine should be given at 6 months of age, followed by reimmunization at 12 to 15 months of age. The following children should also be reimmunized:

1. Those originally immunized prior to 12 months of age
2. Those given immune serum globulin together with measles vaccine
3. Those previously immunized with killed measles vaccine (not used after 1970)

Adverse reactions. About 15% of recipients develop mild fever, with or without rash, 5 to 12 days after immunization. The incidence of encephalitis after measles vaccine may be 1 per million. The risk of subacute sclerosing paraencephalitis (SSPE) appears to be at least 10-fold lower after measles vaccine than after natural measles.

Contraindications

1. Anaphylaxis or systemic allergic reactions after eating eggs are contraindications to the use of live measles vaccine (and MME).
2. Immunodeficiency or immunosuppression.
3. Pregnancy.
4. There is no evidence that measles vaccine exacerbates clinical tuberculosis, although it does transiently suppress positive tuberculin tests. Tuberculin skin testing is not required before measles immunization.

Meningococcal Polysaccharide Vaccines

Vaccines composed of purified capsular polysaccharides from group A and group C meningococci are available. Vaccines against groups Y, W135, and 29E are under investigation. The group A and C vaccines provide at least 90% protection in children and adults against homotypic meningococcal disease for at least two years. The group A vaccine is effective in infants as young as 3 months, but no protection of infants under 18 to 24 months has been observed with the group C vaccine.

Recommended usage. The vaccine is administered for epidemic control, to travelers to areas of the world where epidemics are occurring, and to household contacts of affected persons.

Adverse reactions. Local erytherma and pain may occur.

Contraindications. Serious reaction to previous dose of meningococcal vaccine.

Mumps Vaccine

Mumps vaccine consists of live attenuated virus grown in cell cultures of chick embryos. The seroconversion rate is over 95% in susceptible recipients. Antibodies persist for at least 12 years after immunization. Boosters are not necessary.

Recommended usage. Mumps vaccine is recommended for all children at or soon after their first birthday, and is usually combined with measles and rubella vaccines. Mumps vaccine should also be given to children nearing puberty and adults, especially males, who have had neither mumps nor prior mumps vaccine.

Adverse reactions. Rare.

Contraindications. The vaccine should not be given to pregnant women or to immunodeficient or immunosuppressed patients. Anaphylaxis or systemic allergic reactions after eating eggs are contraindications to the use of mumps vaccine.

Pertussis Vaccine

Pertussis vaccine is a suspension of killed *Bordetella pertussis*. The alum-adsorbed preparations are significantly more immunogenic than plain or fluid vaccines. Pertussis vaccine is almost always given in combination with diphtheria and tetanus toxoids (DPT), and a combination of DPT plus inactivated poliovirus vaccine (DPT-polio) is also available. Adsorbed pertussis vaccine is 70% to 90% effective in preventing clinical pertussis. Severe disease is rare in children who are fully immunized with adsorbed vaccine.

Recommended usage. All infants and children under age 6 years should be immunized against pertussis using the schedules in Tables 8.1 and 8.2. The adsorbed vaccines containing aluminum salts must be given intramuscularly. Because adverse reactions are very common in older children and adults, pertussis vaccine is not recommended for persons over 6 years of age.

Adverse reactions. Minor reactions (fever <40°, local redness, swelling, pain, tenderness at the injection site, increased irritability, and crying) are very common, occurring in up to 50% of infants. Moderate reactions, such as sterile abscess, occur with a rate of 0.1 per 1000 immunizations. The most common cause of a sterile abscess is subcutaneous rather than intramuscular injection of alum-adsorbed DPT. Severe reactions have been reported to occur as follows: persistent screaming for more than three hours (1:1000), seizures (1:2000), and marked lethargy and pallor (1:2000). Encephalopathy with permanent brain damage was estimated to occur with a rate of 1 per 300,000 immunizations. The frequency of seizures, encephalopathy, brain damage, and death is significantly higher after pertussis than after pertussis vaccine.

Contraindications. The vaccine should be withheld in the presence of an evolving or progressive neurologic disorder and in those demonstrating a severe reaction to a previous dose of pertussis vaccine (as above). A family history of epilepsy or other neurologic disease is *not* a contraindication to pertussis vaccine. There are no data demonstrating a correlation between such a family history and an increased risk of adverse reaction.

There are no data indicating the safety or efficacy of fractional doses of pertussis vaccine. If severe reactions occur, the vaccine should not be administered again.

Plague Vaccine

Plague vaccine is a formalin-killed, phenol-preserved suspension of *Yersinia pestis*.

Recommended usage. Persons having contact with wild rodents in any area where plague is enzootic (western United States) and laboratory personnel working with plague.

Adverse reactions. Mild local reactions, fever, headache, and malaise are common.

Contraindications. A serious reaction to previous dose of plague vaccine.

Pneumococcal Polysaccharide Vaccine

Pneumococcal vaccine is composed of purified capsular polysaccharides from each of the 23 most common serotypes of *Streptococcus pneumoniae*. These 23 serotypes (1, 2, 3, 4, 6A, 6B, 7F, 8, 9N, 9V, 10A, 11A, 12F, 14, 15B, 17F, 18C, 19A, 19F, 20, 22F, 23F, 25F, and 33F) cause 85–90% of pneumococcal bacteremia and meningitis. High seroconversion rates and protection against disease caused by vaccine strains has been observed in healthy young adults. Protection has not yet been demonstrated in infants less than 2 or in the elderly over 65 years of age, the two age groups at greatest risk of fatal pneumococcal disease. Moreover, the efficacy in immunocompromised persons and those with absent or deficient splenic function is uncertain.

Recommended usage. Routine immunization of persons of any age is not recommended. Vaccine may be of benefit to persons over 2 years of age who are at increased risk of severe pneumococcal disease, including persons with the following conditions:

1. Asplenia, splenic dysfunction, or sickle cell disease
2. Chronic renal disease, cirrhosis, chronic alcoholism, chronic pulmonary disease
3. Hodgkin's disease (vaccine should be given as soon as diagnosis is made, prior to chemotherapy or splenectomy)

Adverse reactions. Local soreness and erythema are common. After repeated doses of vaccine, severe local reactions frequently occur. Boosters are not recommended.

Contraindications. Serious reaction to previous dose of pneumococcal vaccine. Safety in pregnancy in not known.

Poliovirus Vaccines

Two kinds of poliovirus vaccines are available: inactivated and live, attenuated. Inactivated vaccine (Salk) contains types 1, 2, and 3 poliovirus grown in monkey tissue culture and inactivated with formalin. It is available alone or combined with DPT. The seroconversion rate after the full course of inactivated vaccine is over 90%. The vaccine is highly effective in preventing paralytic disease; however, it induces little local immunity in the intestinal tract and does not prevent infection and subsequent excretion of poliovirus in the feces.

The live oral poliovirus vaccine (Sabin) consists of attenuated strains of serotypes 1, 2, and 3 poliovirus grown in monkey cell or human diploid cell cultures. Both humoral and local intestinal immunity are induced by the live vaccine. The vaccine strains infect the intestinal tract and are excreted in the feces, frequently resulting in infection of susceptible, close contacts.

Recommended usage. Immunization against poliomyelitis can be achieved with either inactivated or live poliovirus vaccine, using the recommended schedules in Table 8.1 or 8.2. Breast-feeding does not interfere with the effectiveness of the live oral vaccine in infants. Routine immunization of adults living in North America is not recommended. Poliovirus vaccination for adults should be considered as follows:

1. Those who travel to areas where poliomyelitis is endemic or epidemic
2. Laboratory workers working with poliovirus
3. Nonvaccinated parents of infants who are to be given oral live poliovirus vaccine

Unvaccinated adults should be immunized with inactivated poliovirus vaccine (see Table 8.2). Unvaccinated parents of infants who are to receive live oral vaccine should either be immunized with inactivated vaccine prior to immunization of the child or receive oral live vaccine at the same time as the child. Previously immunized adults who are in an at-risk category should be given a single dose of inactivated poliovaccine if more than 10 years have elapsed since the last dose. In case of an epidemic of poliomyelitis, oral poliovirus vaccine should be given to all persons over 6 weeks of age who are at risk and who are not fully immunized. Inactivated vaccine is not recommended to control outbreaks.

Adverse reactions. The inactivated vaccine has not been reported to produce any adverse effects. Oral live poliovirus vaccine has rarely been associated with paralytic disease in recipients or in close contacts of recipients. The incidence of vaccine-associated paralytic disease in recipients is 1 per 4 to 8 million doses distributed and in contacts is 1 per 2 to 4 million doses distributed.

Contraindications. Immunodeficiency or immunosuppression

Rabies Vaccine

Rabies is established in skunks, foxes, bats, and raccoons in North America. If unimmunized, dogs and cats can also transmit the disease. Human rabies has never been documented to occur after bites by mice, squirrels, voles, hamsters, gerbils, rabbits, chipmunks, or other rodents.

Several types of rabies vaccines have been used: (1) Semple type, 14% suspension of rabbit brain containing phenol-inactivated rabies virus; (2) duck embryo vaccine, rabies virus grown in embryonated duck eggs and inactivated with beta-propiolactone; (3) hamster tissue culture vaccine; and (4) human diploid cell vaccine (HDCV), inactivated rabies virus grown in human tissue culture. Both the Semple and duck embryo vaccines have been associated with severe and occasionally fatal reactions. Neither is currently being manufactured or recommended for use in North America. The HDCV is recommended for both preexposure and postexposure prophylaxis. It is highly immunogenic, is very effective in preventing rabies after bites by rabid animals, and is very safe.

Recommended usage. Preexposure prophylaxis should be considered for the following high-risk groups: veterinarians, animal handlers, certain laboratory workers, spelunkers, and others at risk of exposure to rabid animals. Human diploid cell vaccine induces protective levels of antibody when given by the intradermal route. The schedule is 0.1 ml intradermally on days 0, 7, and 21, followed by intradermal boosters every two years. Serologic testing is recommended when the intradermal route is used.

For postexposure prophylaxis (Table 8.3) HDCV should be given on days 0, 3, 7, 14, and 28. Serologic testing of antibody response is not necessary when using HDCV. Rabies immune globulin (RIG) is preferable to equine rabies antiserum and should be used in a dose of 20 IU per kg, one-half infiltrated around the wound, if possible, and one-half given intramuscularly. The combination of vaccine plus RIG should always be used for postexposure prophylaxis, as fatal rabies has occurred after the use of HDCV alone.

TABLE 8.3. Postexposure Prophylaxis for Rabies

Animal Species	*Condition of Animal*	*Treatment*
Dog, cat	Healthy and available for observation for 10 days	Local wound care. HDCV* + RIG† at first sign of rabies in dog or cat, which should be killed and examined
	Rabid or suspected rabid	HDCV + RIG
	Escaped and cannot be found	HDCV + RIG if rabies suspected
Wild animals: skunk, fox, raccoon, coyote, bat, other carnivores	Regard as rabid; if available, kill and test animal	HDCV + RIG

*HDCV; five 1-ml doses IM on days 0, 3, 7, 14, and 28.
†RIG; 20 U/kg, half infiltrated around wound and half IM. If RIG is unavailable, use antirabies serum (equine), 40 U/kg.

Adverse reaction. Occasionally, patients experience local tenderness at the injection site. Serum sickness and anaphylactoid reactions are rare.

Contraindications. Known previous hypersensitivity to the vaccine.

Rubella Vaccine

Rubella vaccine currently available in North America is an attenuated live virus strain grown in human diploid cell culture. The seroconversion rate with this vaccine is over 95%, and long-term protection against clinical disease is expected since antibody persists at least 10 years. Transmission of the vaccine strain from vaccinees to susceptible contracts has not been observed. The purpose of rubella immunization is to prevent occurrence of the congenital rubella syndrome. Two strategies have been proposed to achieve this goal: (1) immunization of all children at 1 year of age in order to interrupt transmission of rubella or (2) selective immunization of all girls at 10 to 12 years of age to ensure that all women of child-bearing age are immune to rubella. Either policy should work if the immunization program is effective in reaching the entire target population; however, the first has substantial cost benefits over the second.

Recommended usage. All children should be immunized with rubella vaccine combined with measles and mumps vaccines (MMR) at 12 to 15 months of age. In addition, rubella vaccine should be given to all adolescent girls and women of child-bearing age who lack a documented history of rubella immunization or who lack rubella antibodies. Serologic testing is not necessary prior to rubella immunization. The rate of adverse reactions appears to be less in immune than in susceptible women receiving the vaccine.

Adverse reactions. Transient arthralgias occur in 15% to 20% of adult women and frequency increases with age. Arthritis is much less common. Recurrent or chronic arthritis is very rare.

Contraindications. The vaccine strain has been demonstrated to cross the placenta and infect the fetus; however, congenital malformations have not been observed in infants born to susceptible mothers who receive rubella vaccine in the first trimester. It should not be given to immunosuppressed or immunodeficient persons. Allergy to eggs is not a contraindication to the use of rubella vaccine (see measles and mumps vaccines).

Smallpox Vaccine

Worldwide eradication of smallpox was declared by the World Health Organization in May 1980. There are now no indications for the use of smallpox vaccine in civilian populations and the vaccine is no longer required for travel to any country. It should never be used in the treatment of recurrent herpes simplex, warts, or any other disease.

Tetanus Toxoid

Tetanus toxoid is prepared by treatment of tetanus toxin with formalin. The toxoid is highly immunogenic and highly effective. Tetanus has rarely if ever occurred in a fully immunized person.

TABLE 8.4. Tetanus Prophylaxis in Wounds

Immunization History (doses)	*Clean, Minor Wounds*		*All Other Wounds*	
	Toxoid	*TIG**	*Toxoid*	*TIG*
Uncertain	Yes	No	Yes	Yes
0–1	Yes	No	Yes	Yes
2	Yes	No	Yes	No§
3 or more	No†	No	No‡	No

*Tetanus immune globulin, human (250 units).
†Unless more than 10 years since last booster.
‡Unless more than 5 years since last booster.
§Unless wound more than 24 hours old.

Recommended usage. Tetanus toxoid may be used alone or in combination with diphtheria toxoid and pertussis vaccine (DPT), with diphtheria toxoid (dT), or with DPT and inactivated polio. The immunizing schedules are given in Tables 8.1 and 8.2. Adsorbed toxoid is preferred to fluid toxoid. Boosters should be given every 10 years.

Tetanus prophylaxis in wounds. Prompt, complete cleaning and debridement of wounds is the most important aspect of tetanus prophylaxis. The indications for administration of toxoid and tetanus immune globulin (TIG) are given in Table 8.4.

Adverse reactions. Local and systemic reactions correlate directly with preexisting antitoxin levels. High levels that may result in severe local reactions are usually the result of too frequent administration. Except under unusual circumstances, tetanus toxoid should not be given to any person who has received a booster within five years.

Contraindications. Severe systemic reaction to previous dose of tetanus toxoid. Persons experiencing a severe local reaction should not be given further boosters more frequently than every 10 years.

Typhoid Vaccine

Two kinds of typhoid vaccine are available: a heat-phenol inactivated vaccine and an acetone-dried vaccine. The latter is significantly more effective.

Recommended usage. Routine immuniation is not recommended. It should be administered in the event of exposure to chronic carrier of *Salmonella typhi* and for those planning to travel to areas where typhoid fever is endemic.

Adverse reactions. Local reactions, headache, fever, and malaise are common. Severe reactions are rare.

Contraindications. Severe reaction to previous typhoid immunization.

Yellow Fever Vaccine
Yellow fever vaccine is a live attenuated vaccine grown in chick embryos. It is recommended for persons living or traveling in areas where yellow fever is endemic. It is also required of persons going from endemic areas to certain other countries where the disease is not present but could be introduced. Yellow fever vaccine is available only at centers approved by the World Health Organization. Immunity lasts for more than 10 years. No serious adverse reactions have been reported, even in persons allergic to eggs.

Passive Immunizing Agents

Passive immunization refers to conferring protection against an infection by administering preformed, specific antibodies. As a general rule, passive immunization is used when no active immunizing agent is available, or when immediate protection is required following exposure. Two types of agents are available: standard human immune serum globulin, which is also called immune globulin or gamma globulin, and special preparations of human or animal sera containing high titers of specific antibodies to a particular microbe or toxin. Human preparations are preferable to those of animal origin because of the higher frequency of allergic reactions with the latter and the longer duration of protection with the former.

Immune Serum Globulin
Immune serum globulin is a gamma globulin fraction (mainly IgG with only traces of IgA and IgM) prepared from pooled human plasma. It is free of hepatitis viruses. It is most often administered intramuscularly but an intravenous preparation has recently become available.

Recommended usage. When administered in a dose of 0.25 ml per kg within 72 hours of exposure, immune serum globulin is highly effective in preventing measles. It should be used for household and other close contacts of measles, especially infants, who have no history of natural measles or measles vaccination. Immunocompromised patients should receive 0.5 ml per kg (maximum dose 15 ml).

Immune globulin will prevent or modify hepatitis A infection when given before exposure or within two weeks after exposure. Postexposure prophylaxis, 0.02 to 0.04 ml per kg, is recommended for all household contacts and for inmates and staff of institutions experiencing an outbreak of hepatitis A. It is not indicated for hospital personnel in contact with a case, or for school exposures. Preexposure prophylaxis is recommended for travelers to developing countries (0.02 ml/kg) and to persons residing or working in developing countries (0.05 ml/kg, repeated once in four to six months).

Adverse reactions. Local pain and tenderness.

Contraindications. Bleeding diasthesis; use intravenous preparation.

Botulism Antitoxin, Equine
For use in persons exposed to botulinum toxin or ill with botulism.

Adverse reactions. Serum sickness

Contraindications. Anaphylaxis to horse serum.

Diphtheria Antitoxin, Equine
For use in prevention of diphtheria in unimmunized exposed persons and in treatment of the disease. Unimmunized, asymptomatic household members or close contacts of a patient with diphtheria should receive antitoxin (1000 units) in addition to antibiotic prophylaxis if they cannot be observed daily for seven days. Antitoxin should be given as therapy when diphtheria is suspected on clinical grounds, without waiting for bacteriologic confirmation. Dose (20,000 to 120,000 units) and route of administration vary with age, severity, and duration of illness. Details are given in the manufacturer's package insert.

Adverse effects. Serum sickness.

TABLE 8.5. Postexposure Prophylaxis of HBV

Status of Donor	*HBs Testing*	*Management*
HBsAg-positive		HBIG immediately, 0.06 ml/kg, and 1 mo later
HBsAg status unknown		
High-risk source*	Yes†	ISG, 0.06 ml/kg immediately and *if test positive,* HBIG immediately and 1 mo later. If test negative, nothing.
Low-risk source	No	Nothing
Source unknown	No	Nothing or ISG

*High-risk: Those with acute hepatitis; institutionalized with Down's syndrome, hemodialysis recipients, persons of Asian origin, male homosexuals, illicit drug users.

†Test if results can be known within seven days of exposure.

Contraindications. Anaphylaxis to horse serum.

Hepatitis B Immune Globulin

Immune serum globulin prepared from human plasma pools contains variable amounts of antibody to hepatitis B surface antigen (anti-HBs). Hepatitis B immune globulin (HBIG) contains an anti-HBs titer of at least 1:100,000 and is effective in preventing hepatitis B infection after needle stick exposure to blood containing HBsAg. Because immune serum globulin contains anti-HBs with a titer of at least 1:100, however, it is also somewhat effective, and is an alternative to HBIG if the latter is unavailable. Table 8.5 summarizes the use of HBIG following percutaneous (needle stick) or mucosal exposure to blood.

Infants born to HBsAg-positive mothers are at high risk of developing hepatitis B infection or chronic liver disease, or becoming chronic carriers. Such risk can be reduced by at least 75% by the use of HBIG. A dose of 0.5 ml should be given to the infant immediately after birth. Hepatitis B vaccine should be given within the first week of life followed by injections at 1 and 6 months of age.

The vaccine is discussed as part of the chapter dealing with hepatitis (Chapter 15).

Tables 8.6 and 8.7 are summaries of currently available active and passive immunizing agents.

Rabies Immune Globulin, Human, and Rabies Antiserum, Equine

Both are used in postexposure prophylaxis of rabies (see Rabies Vaccine). The former is the agent of choice.

Tetanus Immune Globulin, Human

Recommendations for use of tetanus immune globulin (TIG) are given in Table 8.4. For prophylaxis in wounds, TIG is used in non-immunized persons with tetanus-prone wounds. The dose is 250 units. It is also used in the treatment of tetanus to try to neutralize toxin in body fluids. The dose is 10,000 units.

Varicella Zoster Immune Globulin, Human

This vaccine is prepared from pooled human plasma containing high titers of varicella zoster antibody.

Recommended usage. After exposure to chickenpox, VZIG should be given to susceptible children with leukemia, lymphoma, immunodeficiency, or immunosuppressive therapy; and to newborn infants whose mothers develop chickenpox from four days before to 2 days after delivery.

The vaccine should be given within 96 hours of intimate exposure to prevent or modify disease. It is not effective in treating chickenpox or zoster. It should not be used in children or adults with a past history of chickenpox except in patients who have received a bone marrow transplantation. The duration of protection with VZIG is not known. If a high-risk child is exposed for a second time, a second dose should be given if the exposure occurs more than 21 to 28 days after the first dose.

Adverse reactions for RIG, TIG, and VZIG. Local pain and tenderness.

Contraindications. Bleeding diathesis.

The following preparations are of no proven value and are not recommended for prophylaxis or treatment:

1. Gas gangrene antitoxin, equine
2. Mumps immune globulin, human
3. Pertussis immune globulin, human

ANNOTATED BIBLIOGRAPHY

American Academy of Pediatrics. Report of the Committee on Infectious Diseases, 19th edition. Evanston, Ill: American Academy of Pediatrics, 1982.

The "red book" contains the official recommenda-

TABLE 8.6. Summary of Currently Available Active Immunizing Agents

Vaccine	*Type*	*Routine Use* *Children*	*Adults*	*Special Circumstances*	*Efficacy*
BCG	Live, bacterial	No	No	Yes	?
Cholera	Killed, bacterial	No	No	Yes	50%
Diphtheria	Toxoid	Yes	Yes	—	Very high
Hepatitis B	Purified antigen	No	No	Yes	Very high
Influenza	Killed, viral	No	No	Yes	65–75%
Measles	Live, viral	Yes	Yes*	—	90–95%
Meningococcal	Purified antigen	No	No	Yes	90–95%
Mumps	Live, viral	Yes	Yes*	—	90%
Pertussis	Killed, bacterial	Yes	No	—	70–90%
Plague	Killed, bacterial	No	No	Yes	?
Pneumococcal	Purified antigen	No	No	Yes	?
Polio	Killed, viral	Yes	Yes*	Yes	Very high
Polio	Live, viral	Yes	No	Yes	Very high
Rabies	Killed, viral	No	No	Yes	Very high
Rubella	Live, viral	Yes	Yes*	—	95%
Smallpox	Live, viral	No	No	No	—
Tetanus	Toxoid	Yes	Yes	—	100%
Typhoid	Killed, bacterial	No	No	Yes	?
Yellow fever	Live, viral	No	No	Yes	Very high

*Should be given only if recipient is susceptible to the disease.

TABLE 8.7. Current Available Passive Immunizing Agents

Agent	*Abbreviation*	*Source*	*Uses*
Immune globulin	IG	Human	Measles, hepatitis A & B
Botulism antitoxin	—	Horse	Botulism
Diphtheria antitoxin	—	Horse	Diphtheria
Hepatitis B immune globulin	HBIG	Human	Hepatitis B
Rabies immune globulin	RIG	Human	Rabies
Rabies antiserum	RAS	Horse	Rabies
Tetanus immune globulin	TIG	Human	Tetanus
Varicella zoster immune globulin	VZIG	Human	Chickenpox/zoster

tions of the American Academy of Pediatrics on immunization policies and practices. It is also a superb summary of the entire field of infectious diseases.

Benenson AS. Control of communicable diseases in man, 12th edition. New York: American Public Health Association, 1980.

Recommendations of the American Public Health Association.

Centers for Disease Control. Immunization against disease 1980. Atlanta, Ga.: U.S. Public Health Service, 1980.

This monograph reviews the current worldwide epidemiology of each infection for which immunization is available and then presents the official recommendations of the Advisory Committee on Immunization Practices of the U.S. Public Health Services. Updated and new recommendations are published in Morbidity and Mortality Weekly Reports, a free publication available from the Centers for Disease Control, U.S. Public Health Service, Atlanta, Georgia, 30333.

National Advisory Committee on Immunization. A guide to immunization for Canadians. Ottawa: Health and Welfare Canada, 1979.

Official recommendations on immunization of the National Advisory Committee on Immunization (NACI). A new edition of the "green book" is in preparation. Updated and new information is published in Canada Diseases Weekly Report, available free from Bureau of Epidemiology, Laboratory Center for Disease Control, Tunney's Pasture, Ottawa, Ontario K1A OL2.

II ORGAN SYSTEM INFECTIONS

9 INFECTIONS OF THE CENTRAL NERVOUS SYSTEM

Thomas W. Austin

Infections of the central nervous system can represent a real test of the diagnostic and therapeutic acumen of the attending physician. These infections are a fascinating group of disease entities that primarily affect the leptomeninges or the brain parenchyma itself.

Their etiology, manifestation, treatment, and outcome vary, but it must always be kept in mind that these infections can result in serious disease with occasionally devastating sequelae and even death. They must never be underestimated and particularly in the case of acute bacterial meningitis and encephalitis, must be regarded as medical emergencies. To deal with these infections in a rational manner, a clear understanding of the etiology, epidemiology, and pathogenetic mechanisms is essential.

ACUTE MENINGITIS

Acute meningitis can be caused by a number of different microbiological agents and can also be due to noninfectious causes. It is easiest to consider the acute meningitis syndrome as either bacterial or aseptic. The latter category can be further subdivided into infections that do and do not require antimicrobial therapy.

Etiology

Bacterial meningitis. The agents that cause bacterial meningitis vary in importance based upon the patient's age as well as any underlying diseases that may be present. In the neonatal period, group B streptococci and enteric gram-negative rods, in particular *Escherichia coli,* are of major importance. Less often, other gram-negative organisms and the gram-positive bacillus *Listeria monocytogenes* may cause disease. Beyond the first few months of life and up to the sixth year, *Hemophilus influenzae* accounts for many of the cases of meningeal infection, but *Neisseria meningitidis, Streptoccus pneumoniae, and Streptococcus* sp. must always be considered and ruled out. *Neisseria meningitidis* is important as a cause of epidemic meningitis as well as sporadic disease in young adults, while *S. pneumoniae* is a frequent cause of infection in the middle-aged and elderly population. Common causes of meningitis after head trauma, head surgery, or in association with cerebrospinal fluid shunts are staphylococci, both coagulase-positive and -negative. Less often, enteric gram-negative rods and *S. pneumoniae* (basal skull fractures) are seen in this group (Table 9.1).

Aseptic meningitis. The syndrome of aseptic meningitis can be thought of as a symptom complex that may be produced by a number of infectious or noninfectious agents. Most infectious causes are viral, and those most frequently encountered are the enteroviruses (usually varying serotypes of echo and coxsackieviruses), mumps viruses, and arboviruses. The last derived their name from the fact that they are *ar*thropod-*bor*ne.

Other viruses that have been associated with meningitis include the herpesviruses (herpes simplex types I and II, herpes zoster, cytomegalovirus, and Epstein-Barr), hepatitis, measles, adenoviruses, and lymphocytic choriomeningitis virus.

Bacteria may create a picture of aseptic meningitis if the process has been partially treated. This is typically seen, for example, in a patient who is feeling unwell and takes some antibiotics such as ampicillin, possibly left over in the medicine cabinet, prescribed for a previous illness. The patient may take enough antibiotics to suppress growth of organisms so that results of lumbar

TABLE 9.1. Bacterial Meningitis: Etiologic Organisms and Epidemiology

Age Group	*Agent*	*Epidemiologic Setting*	*Clinical Associations*
Newborn	Lancefield group B streptococci; enteric gram-negative rods; *Listeria monocytogenes*	Maternal transmission; prolonged labor; premature rupture of membranes; low birth weight	Temperature, respiratory, or cardiovascular instability; failure to nurse; concomitant bacteremia
Preschooler	*H. influenzae, N. meningitidis, S. pneumoniae,* and streptococci sp.; also potential pathogens	Sporadic disease; increased risk of disease in case of contacts in same age group	Upper respiratory tract infection
Young adult	*N. meningitidis*	Sporadic disease in open communities; epidemic disease in closed communities	Concomitant bacteremia; hemorrhagic skin lesions
Adult	*S. pneumoniae*	Sporadic disease	May have concomitant pneumonia and bacteremia
Variable	*S. aureus* and coagulase-negative staphylococci; enteric gram-negative rods; *S. pneumoniae*	Sporadic disease	Head trauma, head surgery, intracranial shunts

puncture indicate aseptic disease, but not enough to cure the infection. Partially treated meningitis therefore is potentially lethal since it may lull the physician into thinking that perhaps the lack of organisms on Gram's stain or culture means that the patient has a viral meningitis.

A similar pattern in the cerebrospinal fluid (CSF) can be seen with a parameningeal focus of infection such as a brain abscess. This is discussed more fully later in this chapter.

Primary amebic meningoencephalitis (PAME) is an acute aseptic form caused by the ameba *Naegleria fowleri*.

A number of organisms typically cause chronic meningitis but may occasionally cause disease that appears to be an acute meningitis. These are discussed in greater detail later in this chapter and are only mentioned briefly here. Fungi such as *Candida* and *Cryptococcus* sp. and *Coccidioides immitis* may cause acute disease, particularly in patients who are immunosuppressed. The same can be said of tuberculous meningitis. Other diseases that infrequently lead to acute meningitis include leptospirosis and syphilis. In its acute form, syphilis is probably the result of spread of the organism to the central nervous system during the secondary stage of disease.

Involvement of the meninges with resultant inflammation can be due to a number of noninfectious causes as well. These include tumors, chemicals (e.g., contrast material), material released from dermoid or epidermoid cysts, and disease entities such as sarcoidosis, Behçet's syndrome, systemic lupus erythematosus, and Mollaret's meningitis.

Epidemiology

The unique susceptibility of the neonate to group B streptococci relates to a lack of protective opsonic antibodies combined with acquisition of the organism, either perinatally from the birth canal or postnatally from colonized contacts. *Listeria* species and the enteric gram-negative rods are generally acquired perinatally. Infants developing meningitis are frequently of low birth weight, products of prolonged labor, and are born after premature rupture of the membranes. Immunoglobulin M (IgM) plays a major role in bacteriolysis of many gram-negative organisms and does not cross the placenta. This may explain the increased susceptibility of newborns to the enteric groups of bacteria.

After the decay of maternally derived immunoglobulins, children lack protective antibodies against *Hemophilus influenzae*. Such antibodies directed against the capsular polysaccharide are of the immunoglobulin G (IgG) class and usually appear by the third to fourth year of life. This presumably reflects exposure of the host to the organism or antigenically similar bacteria. The lack of antibodies fits well with the age-incidence pattern of *Hemophilus* infections. *Hemophilus influenzae* group B infections have increased in frequency in the recent past. In some cases, this may reflect chronic pulmonary sepsis, CSF-upper respiratory tract communication, or a dysproteinemia state. In otherwise normal adults, it may simply reflect an absence of preceding immunologic challenge with the infecting organism. Some authorities attribute this phenomenon to the indiscriminate use of antibiotics in the treatment of upper respiratory tract infections.

Asplenic hosts or individuals deficient in the terminal components of complement appear uniquely susceptible to systemic meningococcal disease. Most individuals with meningococcal meningitis have no apparent preceding humoral or cellular immune defect, however. In the epidemic situation, onset of disease can be co-related with increased frequency of meningoccoccal carriage in the upper airway of healthy individuals. In such populations, it appears the carrier does not develop disease, rather the disease, when it occurs, closely follows acquisition of the organism. Thus the carrier is believed important in transmission of the infectious agent to susceptible persons. The same may apply in the sporadic case; however, this is less well defined.

Infections that occur after cranial trauma or surgery generally arise from contamination of the CSF by organisms present on the adjacent skin or mucous membrane.

As mentioned above, several viral agents can cause aseptic meningitis, but those most frequently encountered in North America are the enteroviruses and mumps viruses. Infections with the former have a peak frequency in the late summer and early fall; those with mumps virus as a cause of meningitis peak in the late winter and spring.

Pathophysiology

Meningitis can develop in one of several ways. Usually the organisms gain access to the central nervous system (CNS) through hematogenous spread. Occasionally, infection may arise secondary to a parameningeal focus that seeds the meninges, or as a result of direct inoculation of organisms into the CSF after trauma or surgery. In some cases of viral meningitis, the infecting pathogen may reach the CNS by neural pathways or the olfactory tract.

When spread is hematogenous, both viruses and bacteria may reach the meninges and/or brain. Viruses gain access to the body through portals of entry that vary with different viral agents, for example, the skin with arboviruses and pharynx with mumps. Viral replication then occurs in adjacent sites, followed by a primary viremia with involvement of organs outside the CNS. Further viral replication and a secondary viremia then occur, with passage of the virus into the meninges and/or brain.

Bacteria may gain access to the circulatory system from sites of infection or colonization and then, by a mechanism not yet completely understood, ultimately enter the CNS through the choroid plexuses of the cerebral ventricles. If local clearance mechanisms are not sufficient to clear the organisms, enough bacteria may eventually be present to cause infection. Once this occurs, as the infectious process progresses, a combination of inflammation, tissue necrosis, and vasculitis results in hypoxia, edema, and impairment of CSF flow. These factors can cause impairment of neurologic function as well as increased intracranial pressure that may at times be severe enough to result in herniation and death. In some cases, particularly with meningococcal infections, the course can be a fulminant one, resulting in death within several hours as a result of bilateral adrenal hemorrhage. This is possibly due to disseminated intravascular coagulation.

Tuberculous meningitis may occur either as a result of a subependymal tubercle rupturing (a form of contiguous focus) or during the course of miliary tuberculosis.

Focal meningitis probably occurs as a result of hematogenous spread. Primary amebic meningoencephalitis is contracted during swimming in infected water. The portals of entry for the free-living organisms are the nasal mucosa and the olfactory nerve.

Clinical Manifestations

Findings associated with acute meningitis are due to infections of the CNS and complications of the infections, such as increased intracranial pressure and hypoxia.

With the initial stages of infection, the patient experiences chills and fever and a severe headache. In addition, there may be signs and symptoms relating to the original site of infection such as pneumonia, sinusitis, or otitis media. In the case of viral meningitis, the symptoms are similar to those seen with bacterial meningitis but tend not to be as severe.

As described in the previous section, as the infection progresses, several events take place, resulting in hypoxia and increased intracranial pressure. Once this happens, the headache obviously will persist but vomiting may begin and evidence of neurologic dysfunction may become obvious. The changes in neurologic function may be global as seen, for example, with alterations in mental status ranging from mild confusion to coma, or they may be localized. Focal findings are usually the result of cerebritis or vascular occlusion secondary to vasculitis or thrombosis.

Significant meningeal irritation can be elicited by attempting to flex the neck passively (Brudzinski's sign) or extend the knees with the hips flexed (Kernig's sign). Both these maneuvers will be resisted and cause pain in the neck and lower back, and hamstring muscles respectively.

Photophobia is quite common but if papilledema is noted, additional complications or alternative diagnoses such as brain abscess, subdural effusion, or herniation should be considered.

Skin lesions can be seen in up to 60% of meningococcal infection and can also be found with certain echoviral infections and pneumococcal meningitis in asplenic patients.

In the neonatal population, the usual signs of meningitis may be lacking. The diagnosis therefore must be considered in any infant showing temperature instability, respiratory difficulties or problems with feeding. Bulging of the fontanelle is a late sign of infection in newborns.

Diagnosis

Whenever dealing with a case of meningitis, the physician must bear in mind that the patient has a potentially lethal disease. Obviously if the patient is stuporous or comatose, it is not possible to obtain a history from the patient, but if family members or close friends are available, every attempt should be made to learn the pattern of signs and symptoms of the present illness and any associated or concurrent illnesses or injuries. It is also important to know whether the patient was taking antibiotics or other medications, whether there was any recent travel history, and whether the patient was in close contact with anyone with any known illnesses, particularly those that might affect the central nervous system. These are only a few of the pieces of information that may help to shed some light on the current illness.

On physical examination, one must look for any evidence of generalized and/or focal neurologic dysfunction, and neck stiffness. Any skin lesions or rashes should be noted as well as clues that might point to a potential source for the infection, such as sinusitis, otitis media, or possibly evidence of congenital heart disease with right-to-left shunting.

The diagnosis of meningitis can be strongly suspected on the basis of the history and physical examination (Figure 9.1). To be absolutely certain and in the absence of contraindications such as bleeding disorders or mass lesions involving the CNS, a lumbar puncture should be done so that the CSF can be examined (Table 9.2).

As mentioned earlier, meningitis can be thought of as either bacterial or aseptic. Aseptic meningitis, usually due to viral infection, classically produces a mononuclear and lymphocytic pleocytosis. During the first 24 to 48 hours, however, the cells can be primarily polymorphonuclear neutrophils (PMN). This should always be kept in mind since physicians tend to associate PMNs with bacterial meningitis only. The total cell count with viral meningitis is usually less than 1000. The CSF protein is generally elevated but the glucose concentration is at least 50% of blood glucose levels drawn at the same time. Some notable exceptions, however, are meningitis due to mumps and lymphocytic choriomeningitis virus, which can occasionally result in low CSF glucose values. Such low values are classically seen with bacterial meningitis and, along with the higher cell count and predominance of neutrophils, are the findings that typically distinguish bacterial from aseptic meningitis. The low glucose is not due to ingestion by the bacteria as was once thought, but to impaired transport of the glucose across the inflamed choroid plexus and increased use of the glucose by host tissues. If viral meningitis is suspected, attempts should be made to culture the virus from stool, throat, and CSF if possible. Sera should also be sent for serologic studies (acute and convalescent samples).

Cases of aseptic meningitis felt to be due to partially treated bacterial meningitis may be diagnosed by trying to detect bacterial antigens using a technique such as counterimmunoelectrophoresis. The organisms most likely to be detected by this technique include *H. influenzae*, pneumococci, and meningococci groups A and C.

The CSF in bacterial meningitis is typically turbid in appearance and under increased pressure. The CSF protein is increased as are the white cells, which are

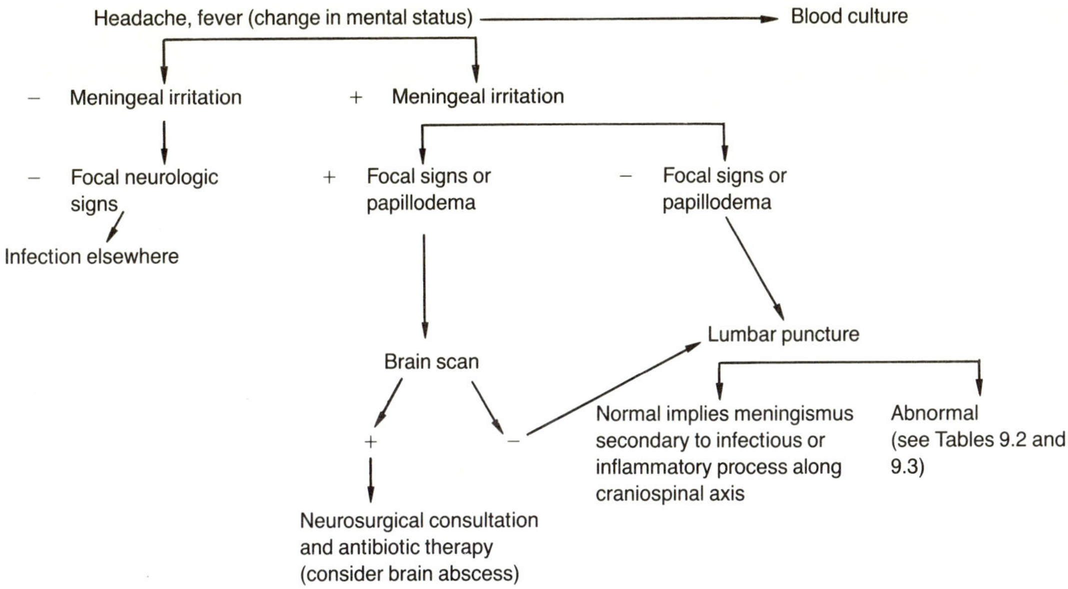

FIGURE 9.1. Flow chart for the investigation of suspected meningitis.

TABLE 9.2. Cerebrospinal Fluid Findings in Central Nervous System Inflammation

	Acute Bacterial Meningitis (Septic)	*Aseptic Meningitis*	*Chronic Meningitis*	*Encephalitis*	*Parameningeal Focus (brain abscess, subdural empyema, epidural abscess)*
Pressure	↑	Normal or ↑	↑	Normal, ↑	↑
White cell count ($\times 10^9$/L)	Generally >1000	Generally <1000	Generally <1000	Generally <1000	Generally <200
Predominant cell type	>90% polymorphonuclear leukocytes	Mononuclear*	Mononuclear	Mononuclear†	Mononuclear
Glucose concentration‡	↓	Normal	↓	Normal or ↓	Normal or ↓
Protein concentration	↑	↑	↑, often markedly	↑	Normal, ↑
Red blood cell count	<100	<100	<100	>100§	<100

Normal values: Pressure (recumbent position) <140 mm H_2O; total white count <5 cells × 10^9/L; glucose >2.2 mmol/L or >50% concomitant blood glucose; protein <500 mg/L; RBC absent.

*In early phase of viral meningitis, can have predominantly polymorphonuclear leukocytes.

†In early phase of viral encephalitis, can have predominantly polymorphonuclear leukocytes.

‡CSF glucose levels are low in bacterial infections and tend also to be reduced in certain viral infections (mumps, lymphocytic choriomeningitis) and in fungal, tuberculous, and amebic infections.

§In certain cases (herpes, *Naegleria* sp., postinfections).

predominantly polymorphonuclear leukocytes. Glucose is reduced in most cases to less than 40 mg per dl, or less than 50% of the simultaneous peripheral blood glucose level. A Gram's stain examination of unspun and spun CSF (cytocentrifuge, if available) should be done immediately in all suspected cases. In approximately 75% of patients with meningitis the organism is visualized on smear. The fluid should also be cultured for both aerobic and anaerobic bacteria, and if clinically indicated, should be examined using India ink for cryptococcus, and cultured for fungi. Finally, where indicated, a search for acid-fast bacilli by smear and culture should be done. The limulus assay has been used with some success in documenting gram-negative rod meningitis, while a serologic assay may detect the cryptococcal antigen in the CSF of a patient with culture-negative cryptococcosis. Some workers have found the CSF lactate and the lactase dehydrogenase (LDH) level a help in distinguishing between bacterial meningitis and infections due to viruses. In general, these substances are higher in the CSF of patients with bacterial infection.

In addition to CSF examination, blood cultures should be obtained in all cases since many patients have a concomitant bacteremia. X-ray examination of the chest and sinuses may help in documenting the initial source of infection.

If a *Hemophilus* infection occurs in an adult or if the patient has recurrent meningococcal meningitis, the possibility of a dysgammaglobulinemic state or an abnormality of the complement system should be considered and immunoglobulin and complement levels (C3, C4, CH50) determined. If there is a history of recurrent pneumococcal meningitis or of previous head trauma, the possibility of a CSF-mucous membrane communication should be considered and skull films, including tomograms and isotope cisternogram, should be done.

Treatment

Therapy of acute meningitis can be divided into specific and supportive measures. Specific forms involve the use of antimicrobial drugs to deal with infecting organisms. Supportive measures are also extremely important and must not be overlooked.

Specific therapy. Before elaborating on the use of specific drugs, certain principles must be recorded. First, if a bacterial meningitis is strongly suspected, therapy based on the likeliest etiologic organisms must be started within one-half hour of seeing the patient. It is not enough simply to choose a drug to which the organism(s) may be sensitive. The drug must also cross the blood-brain barrier or it is useless, and it must be given in an appropriate dose and by the correct route (usually intravenously).

In cases of bacterial meningitis where the Gram's stain is positive, therapy can be initiated as outlined in Table 9.3. Obviously, once culture and sensitivity data are available, any changes felt necessary can be made by the attending clinician. If the Gram's stain of the CSF is negative but a bacterial meningitis is still suspected, one should choose an antibiotic regimen aimed at the likeliest pathogens given the age of the patient and other pertinent epidemiologic or diagnostic data.

In the neonatal period and up to 2 months of age, the most common pathogens are group B streptococci and enteric gram-negative rods. The drugs currently recommended by the American Pediatric Association are ampicillin, 200 to 400 mg per kg per day intravenously; and gentamicin, 2.5 mg per kg per day every 12 hours intravenously if less than 1 week old, otherwise every eight hours. The aminoglycosides do not cross the blood-brain barrier well, so gentamicin is really not particularly effective if gram-negative rods are in fact the pathogens. Third-generation cephalosporins such as moxalactam have excellent activity against nonpseudomonal aerobic gram-negative bacilli, cross the blood-brain barrier, and have potentially less toxicity than aminoglycosides or chloramphenicol. In one study involving the neonatal population, however, the combination of ampicillin plus moxalactam did no better than the combination of ampicillin plus amikacin, and so most pediatric centers begin therapy at least with ampicillin and gentamicin. If culture results indicate a gram-negative rod that is sensitive to one of these newer agents and particularly if a patient is not doing well, ampicillin and gentamicin are discontinued and moxalactam, 150 to 200 mg per kg per day intravenously, is added. If moxalactam is used, vitamin K should be given as well to avoid potential problems with hypoprothrombinemia.

In the age group from 2 months to 6 years of age, *H. influenzae* is the most common etiologic organism. Although the American Pediatric Association recommendation is still ampicillin, 300 to 400 mg per kg per day intravenously, plus chloramphenicol, 50 to 100 mg per kg per day intravenously, most centers now use a third-generation cephalosporin and then switch to ampicillin if sensitivity testing shows that the organism is very sensitive.

TABLE 9.3. Initial Antibiotic Treatment Based on Gram's Stain Examination of the Cerebrospinal Fluid

Organisms	*Antibiotic, First Choice**	*Alternatives*
Gram-positive cocci		
S. pneumoniae, other streptococci; if shunt present or trauma consider *S. aureus* and coagulase-negative staphylococci	Penicillin G, 240,000 U/kg/day; if staphylococci suspected, use cloxacillin, up to 200 mg/kg/day	For *S. pneumoniae* or nonenterococcal streptococci, chloramphenicol, 25–100 mg/kg/day; for staphylococci vancomycin, 20–40 mg/kg/day
Gram-positive rods		
Listeria monocytogenes, rarely clostridia, *Bacillus* sp., or diphtheroids	Ampicillin, 300 mg/kg/day	Erythromycin, 50 mg/kg/day
Gram-negative cocci		
N. meningitidis, rarely other *Neisseria* sp.	Penicillin G, 240,000 U/kg/day	Chloramphenicol, 25–100 mg/kg/day
Gram-negative rods		
H. influenzae — small pleomorphic; enteric aerobes — large rods	Moxalactam, 150–200 mg/kg/day	Ampicillin plus aminoglycoside or chloramphenicol
If pseudomonas is strongly suspected	Tobramycin, 5–6 mg/kg/day plus 5 mg q12h, lumbar, intrathecal, or intraventricular route, and ticarcillin, 250–300 mg/kg/day	

*All drugs are given by intravenous route; tobramycin is also given by lumbar, intrathecal, or intraventricular route. For intrathecal treatment, aminoglycoside without preservative must be used. With moxalactam, prophylactic vitamin K should be used.

In the older age group (greater than 6 years), the usual pathogens in the absence of trauma, recent neurosurgery, or immunosuppression are meningococci and pneumococci. Therefore penicillin G, 240,000 units per kg per day intravenously, would be an appropriate drug to start with. Chloramphenicol, which is normally bacteriostatic for most organisms, is in fact bactericidal for meningococci and pneumococci as well as *H. influenzae,* and so is an appropriate alternative to penicillin in the penicillin-allergic patient.

Patients who have sustained a head injury or have undergone neurosurgery are at risk of infection from *S. aureus* and *S. epidermidis* as well as aerobic gram-negative rods. Empiric therapy in most centers is with a penicillinase-resistant semisynthetic penicillin such as cloxacillin, 200 mg per kg per day intravenously, or oxacillin, plus a third-generation cephalosporin. Once culture and sensitivity results are available, changes can be made if necessary. In cases where *Pseudomonas* is strongly suspected or proved by culture, an aminoglycoside such as tobramycin, 5 to 6 mg per kg per day intravenously plus 5 mg every 12 hours by lumbar, intrathecal, or intraventricular route, plus an antipseudomonal penicillin such as ticarcillin, 250 to 300 mg per kg per day, should be used. Patients are usually treated for approximately two weeks assuming that no complications ensue.

If a pyogenic or bacterial meningitis is less likely and the chances are that one is dealing with an aseptic meningitis syndrome, it is imperative to rule out possible treatable causes such as partially treated bacterial meningitis, a parameningeal focus, tuberculosis, or fungal meningitis. Once the history has been obtained, the patient examined, and appropriate samples sent off for diagnostic work-up, the clinician must carefully consider the possibilities and if one of the above is likely, initiate appropriate therapy guided by the information at hand. As more data become available, the provisional diagnosis may be supported or other diagnostic possibilities may be suggested. Repeat lumbar punctures may help in the assessment of the situation.

If tuberculous meningitis is suspected, therapy should be started with isoniazid, 5 to 7 mg per kg per day, and rifampin, 12 to 15 mg per kg per day, since these are tuberculocidal drugs. Both drugs are given by mouth as a single daily dose and pyridoxine must be given as well to prevent neurologic side effects from isoniazid. Isoniazid readily crosses the blood-brain barrier and, in the presence of meningeal inflammation, rifampin crosses as well. There may be some synergistic hepatotoxicity when both are used together, however, the potential benefits to be gained from their use outweigh the potential risks. Some clinicians also add a third drug such as ethambutol, 15 to 20 mg per kg per day, but this is not a universal practice. Patients are generally treated for one and a half to two years. Steriods can also be used if there is a marked increase in intracranial pressure or if there is danger of obstructing CSF flow because of the inflammatory process. There is some evidence to suggest that the late sequelae of CNS tuberculosis are reduced in steroid-treated patients.

In cases of fungal meningitis, amphotericin B is the drug of choice. In cases due to *Candida* or *Coccidioides* species, the drug is used alone, usually in doses of 0.5 mg per kg per day. Occasionally, higher doses even up to 1 mg per kg per day may be used depending on the sensitivity of the organism and the response of the patient. With *Coccidioides,* however, the drug may have to be given intraventricularly, usually by means of an Ommaya reservoir.

With cryptococcal meningitis, amphotericin is given together with fluorocytosine, since the combined use of these drugs has been shown to be more efficacious than ampotericin alone in treatment of cryptococcal meningitis. The use of the two drugs allows a reduction in the daily dose of amphotericin from 0.5 to 0.3 mg per kg per day, and has generally shortened the duration of treatment from approximately 10 to 6 weeks. In all cases, however, cultures as well as cryptococcal antigen titers should be followed.

Amphotericin B is also used for cases of amebic meningitis, but results unfortunately are poor.

Supportive therapy. Supportive therapy can be every bit as important as specific antimicrobial treatment since patients may die of associated complications just as readily as they can from the primary infection. One of the major problems that may develop is raised intracranial pressure. If this is suspected and is felt to be severe enough, the pressure should be monitored with the use of a device placed intracranially. Several measures can be instituted to decrease the pressure, including steroids (dexamethasone, 4 mg intravenously every six hours) and osmotic diuresis with agents such as mannitol.

Cerebral herniation is a rare complication of meningitis, occurring in less than 5% of all cases. The diagnosis is suggested mainly by a deterioration in the level of consciousness and pupillary changes secondary to uncal herniation. If with the aid of clinical examination and the pressure-monitoring device the raised intracranial pressure is not brought under control, additional measures can be instituted, including use of forced hyperventilation and inducing a hypothermic state.

If shock develops, standard measures such as fluid replacement and pressor agents (if necessary) can be used. The issue of septic shock is discussed in greater detail in Chapter 25. It goes without saying that the underlying infection must be treated with antimicrobial drugs as discussed above. If there is any evidence of a primary focus of infection such as sinusitis or evidence of metastatic infection with suppurative collections, for example in the pleural space or joints, these should be drained.

If disseminated intravascular coagulation should develop, there are essentially three issues to consider: replacement of clotting factors, prevention of end-organ damage, and the role of heparin. Clotting factors can be replaced by giving cryoprecipitate, fresh-frozen plasma, and platelets. End-organ damage is due to deposition of fibrinogen derivatives and is best handled by aggressive fluid replacement. In cases where cerebral edema and increased intracranial pressure are important considerations, fluid replacement must be carefully monitored. If there is evidence of continuing end-organ damage, heparin can be used.

If seizures develop, intravenous diazepam or phenytoin should be given. Seizures are most often seen in cases of bacterial meningitis in the pediatric population.

Finally, the syndrome of inappropriate antidiuretic hormone (ADH) secretion may develop and may lead to severe hyponatremia. Treatment consists of reducing the intake of water. For acute treatment, particularly in severe cases, administration of 0.9% sodium chloride intravenously with concomitant use of furosemide may be considered.

Prognosis

The prognosis for meningitis varies with the infecting agent, the patient's age, the presence of any underlying disease, as well as the rapidity of diagnosis and institution of specific antibiotic therapy. In the neonatal population, the overall mortality is approximately 40%, but is significantly higher when the infection is due to a gram-negative enteric organism as compared to a gram-positive one. This may be due to a more rapid response to antibiotic therapy with the gram-positive organisms.

Hemophilus meningitis in children normally has a mortality rate of less than 10%; with infection due to *Neisseria meningitidis* the rate is somewhat greater than this, and it is even higher with pneumococcal meningitis. The last may reflect the older population affected, and also appears to relate to more severe neurologic injury with pneumococci. The mortality rate in association with gram-negative rod meningitis historically has been in the 50% range. With the advent of the newer cephalosporin drugs, this figure should improve considerably.

Prophylaxis

Vaccine. A vaccine derived from the capsular components of *N. meningitidis* types A and C is available. Its use should be considered for adults during epidemics of disease secondary to these capsular types. It should also be considered for close contacts of patients with sporadic disease secondary to these capsular types since one-half of secondary infections occur one week or more after the index case is diagnosed. No effective vaccine exists for type B meningococcus.

No studies have specifically addressed the efficacy of the pneumococcal vaccine in preventing pneumococcal meningitis. It might be inferred from its ability in immunocompetent hosts to reduce the risk of pneumonia and bacteremia that such a protective effect would occur.

Capsular antigens from the Lancefield group B streptococci have been isolated and used experimentally to induce antibodies in adults. Since the protective antibodies are of the IgG class, such therapy may offer passive protection to the infant when the vaccine is administered to the mother just prior to or during pregnancy. Clinical trials are currently under way.

Antibiotics. Rifampin is the drug of choice for prophylaxis for individuals susceptible to meningococcal disease. This includes close contacts (immediate family, sexual partners) of the sporadic case as well as persons sharing the same closed environment during episodes of epidemic disease. Dosage is 10 mg per kg (maximum 600 mg) given twice daily for two days. To be effective, it should be given as soon as the index case is documented. If the organism is known to be sulfonamide sensitive, a sulfonamide may be used. Minocycline is also effective prophylaxis, but has a higher frequency of nausea, ataxia, and tinnitus. Antibiotics used in the treatment of meningitis, such as penicillin and chloramphenicol, generally fail to eradicate nasopharyngeal carriage and therefore have no role in prophylaxis against meningococcal disease.

It has been recognized recently that preschool-age contacts of patients with *H. influenzae* B meningitis have a 5% to 6% risk of developing serious associated disease and therefore should be considered for prophylaxis. Rifampin has been shown to eradicate *Hemophilus organisms* from the oropharynx and is at present considered the drug of choice in a dosage of 20 mg/kg (maximum 600 mg) once daily for 4 days.

CHRONIC MENINGITIS

Etiology

Although the majority of meningeal infections are acute and secondary to pyogenic bacteria or viruses, a minority are more insidious in onset and manifest a much slower and less dramatic clinical course than their acute counterparts. In fact, clinical and CSF abnormalities lasting a minimum of four weeks are necessary before one can make the diagnosis of chronic meningitis. Most cases are caused by slowly growing organisms such as mycobacteria, fungi, *Nocardia* species, or spirochetes. Other disease entities that have been implicated as causes of chronic meningitis include leptospirosis, coenurosis, cysticercosis, toxoplasmosis, and brucellosis.

Epidemiology

The epidemiology of chronic meningitis is variable and dependent upon the organism involved. Immunosuppressed patients are especially at risk for cryptococcal meningitis, tuberculosis and atypical mycobacterial infection, and nocardiosis. A history of exposure may also suggest certain diseases, particularly ones such as histoplasmosis, syphilis, tuberculosis, and brucellosis.

Pathophysiology

The pathophysiologic mechansims involved with fungal, mycobacterial, and spirochetal infections are probably essentially the same as those discussed under Acute Meningitis.

From animal studies, it appears that leptospires penetrate tissues mechanically rather than being carried there as the result of local hemorrhage. In fact, in humans, it appears that the organisms are able to gain access to the subarachnoid space, with very little inflammatory response being generated on the part of the host.

Toxoplasma organisms can cause an acute infection of the CNS, resulting in either a focal or diffuse meningoencephalitis, or in a more chronic CNS infection. If food, or cat excrement, contaminated with the cysts of *Toxoplasma* is ingested, the organisms are released from their cysts by human digestive enzymes, and invasion of the intestinal tract begins. Organisms ingested by leukocytes or extracellular organisms can then be transported through the blood or lymphatic system to virtually every organ of the body.

Clinical Manifestations

In contrast with acute meningitis where the onset varies from subacute to acute, the onset of chronic meningitis is typically insidious and the course of the disease is much more protracted than that of acute meningitis. Patients can exhibit personality changes or alteration in the level of consciousness. Headaches may also be described, as well as some meningeal signs, but these are much less severe than one would see in a patient with acute bacterial meningitis. Despite the slower course of chronic meningitis, there can be episodes of sudden deterioration of neurologic function. These are usually related to complicating factors such as hydrocephalus and/or cerebral edema.

As a result of the slower course with headache and possibly nausea, vomiting, and other manifestations suggestive of increased intracranial pressure, one may confuse the picture with a tumor. The personality changes that one may find with chronic meningitis are usually the result of hydrocephalus. This is in marked contradistinction to the acute deteriorations of higher neurologic function seen with acute pyogenic meningitis. In the latter, involvement of the meninges is diffuse, affecting all parts of the brain including the frontal cortex. With chronic meningitis, however, meningeal involvement tends to be basilar. Involvement of the underlying brain and spinal cord can result in entrapment of the cranial and spinal nerves.

Diagnosis

A history of the present illness together with details about past illnesses or possible exposure to diseases such as tuberculosis, syphilis, and the like may help in making the diagnosis. The physical examination is generally not particularly helpful and one must usually rely on results of laboratory studies.

The CSF although usually not diagnostic, is at least suggestive. One typically sees a moderate number of leukocytes that are predominantly mononuclear. The CSF glucose concentration is usually reduced, while protein levels are elevated. Any CSF obtained should obviously be stained and cultured and it is always worthwhile for the clinician to discuss the diagnostic possibilities with the microbiologist so that appropriate stains and media can be used to increase the likelihood of finding an etiologic organism. A cytologic examination of the cells should also be done to rule out the possibility of tumor.

Because of the nature of some of the microbiologic agents that can cause chronic meningitis, serologic examination of serum and CSF is worthwhile, particularly if one is considering syphilis or fungi, especially *Cryptococcus* and *Coccidioides* organisms. One must always be careful, however, in interpreting antibody levels in the CSF since if there is any damage to the blood-brain barrier, antibodies present in serum and directed against an organism totally unrelated to the cause of the chronic meningitis may diffuse into the spinal fluid. The normal ratio of antibody in serum to CSF is usually 200:1, but in the presence of CNS infection this ratio may be lowered because of local antibody production in the CSF.

Obviously, skin testing with appropriate controls (to rule out anergy if the tuberculin test is negative) should be done if tuberculosis is suspected. Serology and skin testing are discussed in detail in Chapter 4.

If there is evidence of organ involvement outside the central nervous system, such as pleural fluid collection or skin or lung lesions, attempts should be made to obtain tissue for appropriate work-up. Generally, biopsies of meningeal tissue are done only if no specific answers have been forthcoming and the patient is starting to deteriorate.

Treatment

Treatment will obviously vary with the infecting agent and only a select few are mentioned here. With syphilis, a recommended regimen includes aqueous crystalline penicillin G, 12 to 24 million units intravenously per day for 10 days, followed by benzathine penicillin G, 2.4 million units intramuscularly weekly for three doses. Treatment of tuberculous and fungal meningitis is discussed earlier in this chapter. Nocardiosis is treated with a sulfonamide (sulfadiazine or triple sulfa) in a dose of up to 12 gm per day. In some cases, a second agent is added, either cycloserine or amikacin. Although niclosamide is effective therapy for intraluminal taenia, it has no effect on the cyst form associated with cysticercosis. Consideration should be given to praziquantel, 25 mg per kg per day for three to four days. Neurosurgical intervention may have to be resorted to as well in such cases.

Prognosis

The prognosis of chronic meningitis depends on a number of factors: how far advanced the disease was before diagnosis was made, the infecting agent, and its susceptibility to chemotherapy. An additional major determinant is the presence of any underlying disease in the infected patient, particularly neoplastic or vasculitic diseases.

Prophylaxis

No specific prophylactic measures are available apart from isoniazid for tuberculosis.

FOCAL SUPPURATIVE LESIONS

Although brain abscess is the most common form of focal suppurative infection occurring within the cranium, two other infectious processes must also be considered: subdural empyemas and epidural abscesses. Since brain abscess is the most common of the three, however, it is dealt with in the greatest detail.

Brain Abscess

Etiology

As most cases of brain abscess are secondary to infection in other parts of the body, the etiologic agents generally reflect the organisms causing the underlying infection. In cases of abscess secondary to chronic sinusitis, anaerobes are often found, usually *B. fragilis* and anaerobic streptococci. Aerobic organisms include *H. influenzae*, *S. aureus*, and *S. pneumoniae*. Cases of abscesses arising from an ear focus are due to anaerobes (e.g., *B. fragilis* and anaerobic streptococci) as well as aerobic organisms such as the Enterobacteriaceae and streptococci.

More distant foci of infection such as lung, heart, and abdomen can lead to brain abscess if spread occurs by the hematogenous route. Bacteria seen with lung infection include various streptococci and *Fusobacterium* species. Occasionally, *Nocardia* or *Actinomyces* organisms may be found as well. Cardiac sources depend to a large extent on whether one is dealing with endocarditis (particularly the acute form) or congenital heart disease. In cases of the former, *S. aureus* is often seen, while with congenital heart problems, various types of streptococci may be responsible, such as viridans group, anaerobic, and microaerophilic organisms.

As expected, anaerobes and Enterobacteriaceae are seen when the primary focus of infection is intraabdominal.

In cases where there is no spread from a primary focus of infection but where abscess is due to direct inoculation, as with compound skull fractures and bullet wounds, *S. aureus* is the most common etiologic agent.

To simplify matters pertaining to the etiology of brain abscesses, consider the following: (1) most brain abscesses are secondary to infection at another site (2) mixed infections are not uncommon, and (3) anaerobes as well as aerobes might be causative.

Epidemiology

The exact epidemiology of brain abscesses is hard to define since the epidemiology reflects in part that of the underlying diseases. In terms of sex and age, however, males are affected more often than females and, despite the fact that in general brain abscesses are most frequently seen in patients under 40 years of age, there are two apparent age peaks — 0 to 20 years and 50 to 70 years. Many of the organisms involved are from the patient's endogenous flora, although in certain cases, particularly those associated with trauma, the organisms may be exogenous.

Pathophysiology

Essentially, there are three pathophysiologic mechanisms by which an abscess can develop in the brain: direct extension, hematogenous spread, and direct inoculation. The first two mechanisms are associated with infection elsewhere in the body so that the brain abscess is in fact a secondary site of infection. Direct inoculation involves introduction of pathogenic organisms such as *S. aureus* after trauma such as motor vehicle accident or neurosurgical procedures.

In most cases, it is likely that some sort of damage has occurred to the brain parenchyma prior to or concurrent with the establishment of infection. Obvious examples of CNS damage include trauma and infarction. Consistent with this hypothesis is the fact that most abscesses occur at the site that is the least well perfused — the junction of the gray and white matter. Infections that occur by direct extension usually arise from sites such as the paranasal sinuses, mastoids, or middle ear, and spread is usually through the emissary veins. Hematogenous spread generally arises from sites such as the lung and a congenitally diseased heart (particularly with right-to-left shunting), although other possible foci include skin and soft tissue, pelvis, and abdomen.

Once the organisms reach the brain, an acute inflammatory response ensues, resulting in a focal cerebritis. Sequestration of the infected site begins to occur near the end of the first week, followed by the gradual formation of a fibrous capsule over the next several weeks. The ultimate result is a space-occupying lesion with surrounding edema.

Clinical Manifestations

Since one in fact is dealing with a mass lesion, the signs and symptoms occur as a result of increased intracranial pressure and/or destruction of parenchymal brain tissue. The raised intracranial pressure can be caused by the mass effect of the abscess itself, but may also be due in large part to the edema surrounding the encapsulated focus. Headache is the most common symptom and can be quite severe at times. The pain may be generalized or localized to the site of the abscess. As the intracranial pressure rises, nausea and vomiting can develop as well as changes in mental status, sometimes ending in coma. Findings occurring as a result of destroyed brain tissue vary depending on the site of the brain involved and are not elaborated on here. Some simple examples illustrating this principle are development of focal seizures with cortical lesions, hemisensory defects with parietal lobe lesions, and nystagmus with cerebellar abscesses. It is important to keep in mind, however, that symptoms relating to increased intracranial pressure usually precede focal neurologic abnormalities by a period of days to weeks.

Systemic findings when present often are due to the underlying infection, such as sinusitis. Fever may or may not be present; it is less likely to occur with chronic, well-encapsulated abscesses. Papilledema is usually seen only in more severe cases of increased intracranial pressure.

Diagnosis

It is imperative to take a detailed history and attempt to identify any possible underlying abnormalities or conditions that may predispose or lead to brain abscess. For example, does the patient have congenital heart disease? Is there anything to suggest middle ear or sinus infection? A detailed account of symptomatology is important, particularly headaches, vomiting, change in mental status, or history of neurologic dysfunction.

A detailed physical examination should be performed with careful attention not only to evaluation of the nervous system but to sites that may be serving as primary sources of infection.

If neck stiffness is found, meningitis or subdural empyema should be considered. In the case where meningitis in fact is diagnosed, it is still possible that an abscess is present and that by rupturing or leaking, it caused meningitis. It would be extremely unusual to have a patient with meningitis that then developed into a brain abscess. Some other entities to be considered in the differential diagnosis of a brain abscess include necrotizing viral encephalitides, fungal infection, epidural abscess, toxoplasmosis, cerebral vessel aneurysm, cerebral infarction as the result of a cerebrovascular accident, cerebral thrombophlebitis, and neoplastic lesions (primary or secondary). In cases where brain abscess is suspected a neurosurgical consultation should be obtained.

Several laboratory and radiologic techniques are available to aid in the diagnosis of brain abscess; but their value is quite variable. Hematology data are of minimal value. One may find leukocytosis with some left shift as well as an elevated sedimentation rate, but these are not at all specific.

If primary sites of infection are found, an attempt should be made to obtain cultures. Blood cultures can also be done, although the yield is usually low. Ideally, some CSF should be obtained; however this presents a problem, since if an abscess is present, a lumbar puncture is potentially dangerous. This is particularly true if papilledema is present. It is our practice not to perform a lumbar puncture if there is obvious evidence of a mass effect implying raised intracranial pressure.

If there is still a question as to the diagnosis, we do a computerized tomographic (CT) scan and if this fails to show a mass effect, we proceed with a lumbar puncture. If cerebrospinal fluid is obtained, the pressure should be checked and the fluid examined grossly. It should then be checked for protein and glucose levels (with simultaneous blood glucose level), cell count, and cell type, and stained and cultured for microorganisms. The findings can be variable and range from essentially normal to quite abnormal (Table 9.2). Typical results show a mild to moderate increase in pressure. Some cells are usually present, generally, mononuclear and polymorphonuclear neutrophils. The CSF protein is usually mildly elevated and the glucose is generally normal but may be reduced. Assuming that the abscess is not communicating with CSF in the subarachnoid space, the stain and culture will be negative.

Routine x-rays of the skull with special views to check the paranasal sinuses and mastoids should be done. These may be helpful since a primary focus of infection may be found and one might even see a shift from the midline if the pineal is calcified.

CT scanning is probably the most useful from a diagnostic point of view. When done with intravenous contrast enhancement, an abscess will appear as a central area of decreased density with a surrounding zone of enhancement due to the contrast material. The scan is useful not only for diagnosis but, since it demonstrates the site and size of the abscess, it facilitates follow-up of these patients. Generally, the CT scan is the most sensitive way of diagnosing a brain abscess except in the early stages before encapsulation when cerebritis alone exists. In such cases, radionuclide imaging with technetium can be done, as it will detect an area of cerebritis that the scan might miss.

These techniques, however, are not as useful when one is dealing with abscesses in the posterior fossa region. In such cases, angiography may have to be performed.

Treatment

As with any abscess, a combined surgical and medical approach must be used. Antibiotics, while certainly necessary, are not sufficient. The major exception to this is the treatment of so-called abscesses while they are still in the cerebritis phase and are not yet abscesses in the true sense of the word. In such cases, intensive treatment with antimicrobial drugs alone can result in cure.

Three kinds of surgical approaches can be used: aspiration, drainage, and excision. The best of these appears to be excision, although if the abscess is situated in a vital area of the brain, it may not be possible.

When considering antimicrobial therapy, the physician must know the potential organisms involved and whether or not the drug used can penetrate into the central nervous system. In the Etiology section of this discussion we noted that certain organisms tend to be associated with particular sites of primary infection such as the paranasal sinuses.

If the primary site is the middle ear, sinuses, mouth, or chest, it is our practice to begin with high-dose potassium penicillin G, 4 million units intravenously every four hours, plus chloramphenicol, 1 gm intravenously every 6 hours. If the primary site is cardiac, we treat according to blood culture results. For cases of abscess after trauma or surgery, we include coverage for *S. aureus* — cloxacillin, 2 gm intravenously every 4 hours — as well as for anaerobes and aerobic gram-negative rods — chloramphenicol, 1 gm intravenously every 6 hours. Some of the newer cephalosporins such as cefotaxime or moxalactam may be ideal as well, but at this point there are insufficient data to support their use in the treatment of brain abscesses. Another drug that is excellent for anaerobic organisms is metronidazole. These agents can be changed according to the microbiology results obtained once the abscess is drained or excised. For example, in the case of a brain abscess after head trauma, if *S. aureus* is isolated, cloxacillin alone would be continued and anaerobic or aerobic gram-negative rod coverage would be discontinued.

Unfortunately, no satisfactory studies exist to tell us how long to treat these patients. Most clinicians, however, treat for approximately six to eight weeks with parenteral drugs. Ideally, the lesion can be monitored by CT scan or alternatively by technetium scan.

Prognosis

Mortality figures have varied in the past ranging from 20% to as high as 50%. Recently, however, with the use of CT scanning, mortality in appropriately treated cases has been as low as 5% to 10%.

The most common long-term problem after brain abscess is focal seizures.

Subdural Empyema

The covering of the brain is composed of three layers of meninges: the pia mater and arachnoid, which together form the leptomeninges, and the outermost layer, the dura mater. Meningitis involves the leptomeninges and is an infection in the subarachnoid space. Subdural empyemas represent a focal suppurative collection between the dura and arachnoid layers. An epidural abscess is a focal collection localized between the dura and the skull.

Etiology

Numerous organisms have been associated with this syndrome, including streptococci (aerobic, anaerobic, and microaerophilic), Enterobacteriaceae, and *B. fragilis; S. aureus* and *S. pneumoniae* may also be found.

Epidemiology

Most cases of subdural empyema are secondary to infection involving the paranasal sinuses, with middle ear and mastoid infections next in terms of frequency. Generally, males are involved more frequently than females, with the peak age being the second and third decades.

Pathophysiology

The pathophysiologic mechanisms are similar to those described for brain abscess, that is, direct extension, hematogenous spread, and direct inoculation. In children, subdural empyemas are most often seen as a complication of meningitis.

Clinical Manifestations

Patients generally have fever as well as headaches. The latter are usually localized at least initially to the area of involvement. Because the infection represents a form of space-occupying lesion, increased intracranial pressure can develop together with vomiting and in some cases papilledema. Seizures as well as focal neurologic dysfunction may develop along with some decrease in mental status and signs of meningeal irritation. As the disease progresses, the neurologic damage can become quite extensive, ultimately involving most of the cerebral hemisphere.

Diagnosis

Attempts at a definitive diagnosis should be made on an emergency basis since this is a potentially lethal infection. A history of sinusitis, particularly with recent onset of fever, headache, and any of the findings mentioned above, should make the physician suspicious of an intracranial suppurative process. Blood cultures should be obtained and routine skull films should be done since they may show evidence of sinusitis if this is the predisposing cause. For a more definitive assessment of intracranial status, however, a CT scan or, in its absence, angiography can be done to help delineate the involved area. A lumbar puncture is potentially dangerous because of the increased intracranial pressure.

Treatment

Treatment is dependent upon surgical evacuation of the empyema as well as antimicrobial drugs. If one does not strongly suspect *S. aureus,* initial treatment can be instituted with penicillin G, 20 million units intravenously over 24 hours, plus chloramphenicol 4 to 6 gm intravenously over 24 hours. If staphylococci are suspected, for example, in cases associated with surgery or trauma, a penicillinase-resistant semisynthetic penicillin such as cloxacillin, 12 gm per 24 hours, can be used. Obviously, intraoperative samples should be obtained for culture and any changes in antibiotic therapy can be made on the basis of the culture and sensitivity results. If the intracranial pressure is elevated, steroids may be used as well.

Epidural Abscess

Aside from their location in relation to the dura compared with subdural empyemas and their frequent association with osteomyelitis in overlying bone, intracranial epidural abscesses are essentially identical to subdural empyemas in terms of etiology, epidemiology, and pathophysiology. In fact, it is quite common for the two to coexist since epidural collections frequently extend to the subdural space.

The clinical findings usually consist initially of localized pain and fever. As the process continues, focal neurologic findings, seizures, and evidence of increased intracranial pressure become obvious.

Diagnosis and treatment are similar to those outlined for subdural empyema.

ENCEPHALITIS

The word *encephalitis* refers to inflammation of the brain parenchyma. It is often not confined solely to the brain itself but may involve the meninges (meningoencephalitis) and/or the spinal cord (encephalomyelitis). Encephalitis may occur as a result of direct infection of the brain by a variety of etiologic agents or may be a demyelinating process, possibly due to a hypersensitivity reaction after infection or vaccination.

Etiology

As mentioned, numerous infectious agents can cause encephalitis. Many of these are viral and include arbo, entero, and herpesviruses as well as mumps and adenoviruses. The herpesviruses are of particular interest since herpes simplex (HSV) type I encephalitis is the most common sporadic form of fatal encephalitis in North America and Western Europe. Demyelinating processes have been described after infection with mumps, measles, rubella, and varicella viruses as well as after vaccination, particularly against rabies or smallpox. The postvaccineal form of encephalitis after rabies vaccine was probably due to a hypersensitivity response to neural tissue contained in the vaccine. With the advent of newer rabies vaccines devoid of CNS tissue, the occurrence of such reactions should be greatly reduced.

Several nonviral infectious agents can also cause encephalitis. These include spirochetes such as T. pallidum, fungi, rickettsiae, *Mycoplasma sp.*, protozoa, helminths, and bacteria such as *Brucella, M. tuberculosis,* and *Listeria*. Noninfectious diseases, particularly certain vasculitides, can cause encephalitis as well. The following is a more detailed list of the causes of encephalitis:

1. Infectious causes

    Viruses: arbovirus, enterovirus, herpes simplex, mumps, adenovirus, measles, rubella, varicella zoster, rabies, "slow" viruses

    Bacteria: species of *Listeria* and *Brucella, M. tuberculosis*

    Mycoplasma and *Chlamydia: M. pneumoniae,* psittacosis

    Spirochetes: syphilis, leptospirosis

    Rickettsia: Rocky Mountain spotted fever; murine, epidemic, and scrub typhus

    Fungi: species of *Candida, Aspergillus, Cryptococcus, Histoplasma*

    Protozoa: Toxoplasma sp., ameba, malaria

    Helminths: cysticercosis, schistosomiasis, trichinosis

2. Noninfectious causes

    Vasculitis

    Neoplasms

    Toxins

    Metabolic diseases

In some cases of encephalitis (up to 50% in some series), no specific etiologic agent can be definitely implicated.

Epidemiology

The viruses that we will focus on from an epidemiologic point of view are those primarily responsible for sporadic and epidemic cases, HSV and the arborviruses respectively. When a herpes simplex virus is causative, it is usually HSV type I, except in neonates, in whom type II is generally seen. Since these viruses are found worldwide, the disease follows a similar distribution. There is no seasonal variation and 90% of cases occur after the first year of life. No differences in susceptibility based on race or sex have been found. Person-to-person spread occurs by contact with infected body secretions.

The reservoir is composed of individuals with latent infection. This contrasts sharply, for example, with the arborvirus, for which an animal reservoir exists and man simply represents a terminal host.

In serologic surveys of human populations it has been found that infections with HSV rise as socioeconomic status decreases. Despite the fact that neural infection is the means by which latency is established, symptomatic infection of the CNS is rare.

Arborviruses are responsible for most cases of epidemic encephalitis. The reservoir is fairly extensive and includes certain birds, fowl, rodents, and small mammals. Arthropods are infected with the virus after biting one of the host animals. Replication of the virus then takes place in the arthropods and once their salivary glands are involved, the virus can be transmitted to humans bitten by the arthropods. The geographic distribution, as well as the severity of any particular outbreak, depend on a number of factors, such as the size of the reservoir, the density and activity of arthropod vectors, and the extent of human exposure to the zoonotic cycle. Some arborviral encephalitides are well known with exotic names such as Venezuelan equine encephalitis, Murray Valley encephalitis, and Japanese B encephalitis. Infections most often encountered in North America are eastern and western equine, St. Louis, and California encephalitis.

Pathophysiology

Encephalitis can be the result of either direct or indirect involvement with infectious agents. In the case of direct infection of the brain tissue, organisms generally gain access to the CNS by hematogenous spread or through peripheral nerves. In the case of hematogenous spread, the agents first enter the body through the respiratory tract, for example, and after local replication are disseminated to other organs, including the brain, by the circulatory system. With other infectious agents such as herpes simplex or rabies, spread along peripheral nerves may result. Once the pathogens have reached brain tissue, the effects may be focal or generalized depending on the type of agent, its virulence, and any tropism it may or may not exhibit. In the case of HSV encephalitis, although the lesions can be very widespread, the areas of brain showing the greatest damage are the inferior and medial aspects of the temporal lobe, the orbital part of the frontal lobe, and the insula. At one time it was thought that the virus reached the brain by traveling along the olfactory nerve, but it is now thought that this is incorrect.

During its latency phase, the HSV remains in sensory neurons of the trigeminal ganglion. Neurons from the same ganglion also supply the basilar structures in the anterior and middle fossae corresponding to the frontal and temporal areas described above. It is thought that HSV encephalitis results from the retrograde spread of the virus from the trigeminal ganglion along neurons to the innervative areas of the frontal and temporal lobes. Occasionally, herpes simplex encephalitis may be due to a primary infection with the virus.

In cases of encephalitis caused indirectly by infectious agents, demyelination is the classic finding. This is typically seen, for example, with or shortly after the exanthem of measles, rubella, chickenpox, or smallpox, and after vaccination. The demyelinating process probably is due to a hypersensitivity reaction of some sort, possibly to the myelin, and is not the result of direct invasion by a pathogenic agent. On microscopic examination, areas of demyelination are seen surrounding small and medium-sized veins, with perivascular infiltration by mononuclear cells. The axons are intact.

Clinical Manifestations

Encephalitis is a syndrome that involves parenchymal brain tissue. There may also be some degree of meningeal involvement; therefore, depending on the nature of the causative agent, the host response to it, and the area of brain involved, signs and symptoms can vary tremendously. Classically, encephalitis is an acute febrile illness that causes headache, fever, and a stiff neck; one often finds some changes in mental status. The spectrum can vary from a mild illness with little more than a mild headache and temperature elevation to an acute devastating illness with rapid progression to coma. Returning to the arbovirus and herpesvirus as examples of epidemic and sporadic forms of encephalitis respectively, we see that their clinical manifestations can differ considerably.

Central nervous system infections with arboviruses are generally subclinical. Those that do develop to be clinically overt vary from mild to severe as discussed above. The observed changes can affect any part of the central nervous system but areas typically affected involve the higher levels of thinking and cognition, motor and reflex function.

In overt infections of the CNS with herpes simplex virus, several patterns can be discerned: meningitis, mild diffuse encephalitis, severe diffuse meningoencephalitis, and focal encephalitis. Herpes simplex meningitis is generally a mild disease without focal findings and with no long-term sequelae of consequence. Patients typically have headache, neck stiffness, and fever plus some nausea, vomiting, and photophobia. Herpes encephalitis is generally a much more lethal disease, although the clinical pattern seen can also vary a great deal as well. The common denominator is usually headache, fever, and change in level of consciousness. Manifestations resulting from focal involvement by the encephalitic process include focal seizures, anosmia, speech defects, and olfactory and gustatory hallucinations. Occasionally, patients with herpes encephalitis experience symptoms that are primarily behavioral and may mislead the attending physician into thinking that it is not an encephalitic process.

Diagnosis

The history and physical examination may provide the clinician with enough clues to suggest encephalitis and in certain cases may even suggest potential etiologic agents. This would be particularly true in cases of epidemic arbovirus encephalitis. To make a definitive diagnosis of encephalitis and of the cause of the syndrome, one must usually rely on various radiologic and laboratory techniques.

The investigations that are most helpful in diagnosing encephalitis are examination of the CSF, CT scanning, electroencephalogram (EEG), and technetium brain scans.

Examination of CSF. A lumbar puncture should be performed to allow examination of the CSF (Table 9.2). The opening pressure can vary from normal to elevated and there is generally an increased cell count. Usually, lymphocytes predominate but in severe cases, particularly of herpes simplex encephalitis where tissue necrosis is part of the pathologic picture, one may see PMNs as well as red blood cells. The protein is increased but glucose levels will vary depending on the etiologic agent. With most viral infections, the glucose level is normal, but can be reduced with lymphocytic choriomeningitis and mumps infections. Obviously, if bacteria are responsible for the encephalitis, the glucose level will usually be decreased.

CT scan. The CT scan is of tremendous value because it not only detects areas of parenchymal involvement but picks up cerebral edema. In conjunction with the findings on history, physical examination, and lumbar puncture, the CT scan allows one to make a fairly definitive diagnosis of encephalitis.

Electroencephalogram. The EEG is of value, particularly early in the course of the disease, since it is easy to do and may detect abnormal activity before other tests are able to. The usual pattern in herpes simplex encephalitis is arrhythmic slow-wave activity with periodic spike and wave complexes over one or both temporal lobes.

Technetium scans. These scans, like the EEG, are positive early in the course of the disease. The increased isotope uptake in the area of involvement is nonspecific, however, and simply indicates that there are local breaches in the blood-brain barrier.

Techniques to determine the etiologic agent include examination of tissue, culture, and serologic investigations. To examine tissue, one must first obtain a biopsy specimen from the involved site and this is generally done by prior localization using CT scanning. Once the tissue is obtained, it can be cultured as well as examined by a variety of methods including standard staining for bacteria or fungi, fluorescent antibody staining, and electron microscopy.

For serologic examination, paired samples (acute and convalescent) of serum as well as CSF can be examined for rises in titer to specific agents.

Treatment

As with meningitis, the treatment of encephalitis can be considered in terms of specific and supportive measures. Specific therapy obviously depends on the nature of the causative agent. If it is a spirochete, fungus, or bacterium, antimicrobial drugs suitable for the pathogen can be instituted. If it is viral, the only virus for which specific therapy is available at present is herpes simplex. To date, the only drug licensed to treat herpes simplex encephalitis is adenine arabinoside. This drug is usually given in a dose of 15 mg per kg body weight per day intravenously as a single 12-hour infusion for approximately 10 to 14 days. A newer drug, acycloquanine (acyclovir) is more selective and appears to be less toxic than adenine arabinoside, and is currently undergoing clinical evaluation for the treatment of herpes encephalitis.

Supportive measures are essentially the same as those described for meningitis.

Prognosis

The prognosis for survival varies with the infecting agent. With mumps it is excellent, with the enteroviruses quite good, and with the arboviruses variable. With herpes simplex encephalitis, despite treatment, prognosis is only fair. Complete recovery is the rule with mumps while partial recovery only may occur following an enteroviral or arboviral infection. Partial recovery only tends to be the rule with herpes simplex encephalitis.

Prophylaxis

Immunization for mumps and influenza prevents infective CNS syndromes caused by these viruses. Very rarely, neurologic complications due to hypersensitivity reactions to the vaccines occur. At the present time, there are no specific prophylactic measures available for enteroviral or herpes simplex infections of the CNS. Knowledge of the zoonotic cycle and avoidance of areas with high levels of arthropod infestation, particularly during peak seasons, should help in decreasing the frequency of arborviral encephalitis.

Chronic Encephalitis

Although most of the time when we think of encephalitis we think of an acute or subacute illness, there are chronic encephalitides due to "slow" virus infections. These infections have two major features in common: a long latency period and inexorable progression once clinical symptoms have appeared. At present, there appear to be two types of chronic infections: Those due to conventional viruses and those due to unconventional agents. In the former group, there are three diseases described in humans: subacute sclerosing panencephalitis (SSPE) due to measles virus, progressive multifocal leukoencephalopathy due to a papovavirus, and progressive rubella encephalitis due to rubella virus.

In the second group, two syndromes have been described — kuru and Jakob-Creutzfeldt disease. These are believed to be due to acellular infectious agents called prions. Prions are much smaller in size than viruses and little is known about them at present.

Why infection with some of the standard viruses or these newer agents causes chronic infection is not completely understood. In the case of measles, rubella, or papovavirus infection, obviously the host response does not eliminate the virus. This may result either because the host responses are not initiated in the first place or they are somehow ineffective. Another possibility is that the virus is protected, possibly by persisting within the infected cell, so that any immune response elicited cannot gain access to the virus. In the case of prions or unconventional agents, it appears that no immune response is elicited.

Just as the host response is blunted or thwarted, the virulence of the virus must also be altered in some way or else the host cells would be destroyed. Ultimately, tissue damage may develop as a result of interactions between the immune response of the host and the virus. The CNS lesions are inflammatory, demyelinating, or spongiform. Spongiform changes are classically seen in kuru and Jakob-Creutzfeldt disease.

The diagnosis can usually be made on clinical grounds although the EEG may be helpful, particularly with SSPE where a suppression burst pattern may be seen, and Jakob-Creutzfeldt disease, where one usually sees generalized slowing with occasional high-voltage complexes. In progressive multifocal leukoencephalopathy, CT scans typically show areas of demyelination.

With SSPE and progressive rubella encephalitis, antibody against measles and rubella virus can be detected in the CSF.

There is no specific treatment available for any of these diseases at present.

INTRACRANIAL SHUNT INFECTIONS

Etiology

Infections associated with an intracranial shunt (ventriculoatrial or ventriculoperitoneal) are usually due to skin organisms, in particular coagulase-negative staphylococci and *S. aureus*.

Epidemiology

Most infections occur early, within days or a few months of insertion of the device, although late infections can occur.

Clinical Manifestations

In addition to the usual symptoms and signs of meningitis, additional findings may be elicited. If the shunt is malfunctioning, the patient may demonstrate signs of increased intracranial pressure. Depending on the location of the lower end of the shunt (atrium or peritoneum), signs of extracranial infection may overshadow the CNS infection (endocarditis, peritonitis). Occasionally fever may be the only finding. The infection may be insidious in onset, although in most cases initial contamination is believed to occur at the time of shunt insertion or revision.

Diagnosis

Infection is documented by CSF examination, by the lumbar puncture if the shunt is functioning, otherwise percutaneously through the shunt reservoir.

Treatment

In only a small percentage of cases can the infection be controlled without total removal of the shunt. In general, surgery plays an integral part of initial management. If possible, the shunt is removed for a period of up to one week and then replaced at a site different from where the infection occurred. If the patient is shunt dependent, the alternatives are immediate replacement under antibiotic coverage or a period of external drainage through a closed system, with or without intrathecal antibiotics. In this situation, the CSF is examined on a daily basis. Once the fluid is demonstrated to be sterile, the shunt is replaced. Again, a site remote from the previous site should be chosen whenever possible.

Antibiotic treatment is based on organism susceptibility and penetration of the blood-CSF barrier by the antibiotic.

Prognosis

Because of the serious problem of obstruction of the shunt with infection and the underlying neurologic disorder, the mortality rate may approach 50%. An interesting complication is that of immune-complex glomerulonephritis secondary to persistent antigenic stimulation due to the bacteremia associated with the infection.

Prophylaxis

Although no studies have been carried out to demonstrate the efficacy of perioperative prophylaxis during shunt insertion, such therapy is often prescribed. One approach is to administer cephalothin, 25 mg per kg to a maximum of 2 gm at the time of shunt insertion, with a similar dose at the completion of surgery.

ANNOTATED BIBLIOGRAPHY

Bacterial Meningitis

Abramowicz A, ed. New drugs for enteric gram-negative bacillary meningitis in adults. Med Newsletter 1981;23:73–74.
Discusses the potential role of the third-generation cephalosporins in this difficult problem.

Bennett JE, Dismukes WE, Duma RJ. A comparison of amphotericin B alone and combined with flucytosine in the treatment of cryptococcal meningitis. N Engl J Med 1979;301:126–131.
Documents the efficacy of combined antifungal treatment for cryptococcal CNS infections.

Ellner JJ, Bennett JE. Chronic meningitis. Medicine (Baltimore) 1976;55:341–369.
An excellent discussion of chronic meningitis, its etiology, diagnosis, and management.

Kocen RS. Meningitis: tuberculous meningitis. Br J Hosp Med 1977;17:439–444.
A good short review of the topic.

Norrby R. A review of the penetration of antibiotics into the CSF and its clinical significance. Scand J Infect Dis 1978;14(suppl):296–309.
Examines the importance of CSF antibiotic levels in the successful treatment of bacterial meningitis.

Nyhan WL, Richardson F. Complications of meningitis. Ann Rev Med 1963;14:243–260.
A thorough review of the sequelae of CNS infection.

Swartz MN, Dodge PR. Bacterial meningitis — a review of selected aspects. N Engl J Med 1965;272:725–731, 779–787, 842–848, 889–902, 954–960, 1102–1010.
A good general overview of meningitis.

Brain Abscess

Coonrod JD, Dans PE, Subdural empyema. Am J Med 1972;53:85–91.
An excellent discussion of this uncommon cause of aseptic meningitis requiring rapid diagnosis and surgical treatment for cure.

Samson DS, Clark K. A current review of brain abscesses. Am J Med 1973;54:201–210.
Review of the clinical features and etiology of a large number of cases of brain abscess.

Shaw MDM, Russell JA. Cerebellar abscess: a review of 47 cases. Neurol Neurosurg Psychiatry 1975;38:429–435.
Examines abscesses of the posterior fossa with emphasis on the mode of infection and clinical findings.

Encephalitis

King DH, Gallasso G, eds. Acyclovir symposium. Am J Med 1982; (Suppl): 73;1–391.
Proceedings of a conference dealing with basic and clinical issues as they relate to acyclovir.

Miller JD, Ross CAC. Encephalitis, a four-year survey. Lancet 1968;1:1121–1126.
An overall review of the problem emphasizing the large number of cases for which no etiologic agent can be found.

Wang D, Bortolussi R. Acute viral infections of the central nervous system in children: an 8-year review. Can Med Assoc J 1981;125:585–589.
Despite newer diagnostic techniques, many CNS viral infections still defy etiologic diagnosis.

Whitley RJ, Soong SJ, Hirsch MS. Herpes simplex encephalitis: vidarabine therapy and diagnostic problems. N Engl J Med 1981;304:313–318.
A critical analysis of the pros and cons of indirect versus direct diagnosis of herpes encephalitis as they relate to therapy.

10 INFECTIONS INVOLVING THE CARDIOVASCULAR SYSTEM

Hillar Vellend, William R. Bowie, and
Stanley E. Read

INFECTIVE ENDOCARDITIS

Infective endocarditis is a life-threatening disease and denotes an infection of the endocardial surface of the heart, usually involving a heart valve but occasionally involving the septal or mural endocardium. In the past, the condition was classified by duration and clinical course into acute and subacute categories. Approximately two-thirds of patients have the subacute form, with symptoms of longer than two weeks' duration. They usually have preexisting rheumatic, congenital, or degenerative valvular heart disease. The remainder of patients have acute endocarditis with symptoms of less than two weeks' duration, and approximately two-thirds of these have no history of prior valvular heart disease.

Etiology

Although virtually all bacterial species as well as fungi and rickettsia *(Coxiella burnetii)* have been implicated in infective endocarditis, streptococci and staphylococci remain the most common microorganisms isolated in bacterial endocarditis, accounting for about 80% of cases from recent series (Table 10.1). This fact gives strong support to the dictum that, in the absence of an appreciable seeding focus, patients with streptococcal or staphylococcal bacteremia should be considered to have endocarditis until proved otherwise.

An apparent source of the bacteremia that led to endocarditis can be identified in only 60% of patients. Viridans streptococci organisms usually arise from the mouth, often following dental procedures, whereas enterococci arise from the bowel and genitourinary tract. It is interesting that *S. bovis* endocarditis has been associated with occult carcinoma of the colon. *Staphylococcus aureus* bacteremia is a common complication of intravenous drug abuse and other foci of infection including osteomyelitis, septic arthritis, and soft tissue infection, as well as the use of indwelling intravascular cannulas in hospitalized patients.

Subacute endocarditis is most often due to viridans streptococci or enterococci, whereas acute endocarditis is generally caused by *S. aureus* or beta-hemolytic streptococci, including Lancefield groups A, B, C, and G. Bacteremia due to certain slow-growing, fastidious, gram-negative rods such as *Actinobacillus actinomycetemcomitans, Haemophilus aphrophilus, Cardiobacterium hominis,* and *H. parainfluenzae* should always alert the physician to the high probability of endocarditis.

Fifteen percent of patients have sufficient diagnostic criteria for a clinical diagnosis of probable endocarditis but still have persistently sterile blood cultures. There are several possible causes for culture-negative endocarditis, the most important being the use of empiric antimicrobial therapy for fever before blood cultures are obtained, chronic infective endocarditis (more than three months' duration), fastidious organisms requiring special blood culture techniques such as anaerobes and nutritionally variant streptococci, and nonbacterial causes such as fungi (especially candida and aspergillus) and *C. burnetii* (the cause of Q fever endocarditis).

Epidemiology

Infective endocarditis is an uncommon infection, in large general hospitals accounting for 0.5 to 1.0 per

TABLE 10.1. Causative Microorganisms in Infective Endocarditis

Microorganisms	*Percentage of cases*		*Acute (%)*	*Subacute (%)*
Streptococci		50		
S. viridans	30		5	95
S. faecalis (enterococci)	10		60	40
Others	10		30	70
Staphylococci		30		
S. aureus	25		90	10
S. epidermidis	5		10	90
Miscellaneous		5	15	85
Culture-negative		15	20	80

1000 admissions. Most recent series have continued to observe male predominance, with a male:female ratio of 1.5–2:1. Endocarditis is increasingly a disease of older patients, with a current mean age of 45 to 50 years.

The most definable group at risk are those with preexisting valvular heart disease, although up to one-third of patients with endocarditis have no known prior valvular pathology. Rheumatic valvular heart disease is declining in frequency and now is a predisposing factor in only 20% to 25% of patients with endocarditis. Congenital heart disease remains an important subgroup (approximately 20%), with those with isolated bicuspid aortic valves and ventricular septal defects at particularly high risk. Mitral valve prolapse has become an increasingly important risk factor, comprising up to 15% of all cases of native valve endocarditis in some series. Smaller numbers of patients have underlying valvular disease due to a calcified mitral annulus, previous infective endocarditis, and myocardial infarction.

Pathophysiology

The development of infective endocarditis requires the sequential interaction of several events. The key elements contributing to the development of a vegetation are summarized in Figure 10.1. The endothelium of the valve surface must first be injured by local factors such as rheumatic valvular disease or hemodynamic turbulence. Exposed collagen fibrils may then activate Hageman factor resulting ultimately in the deposition of fibrin and platelets thereby forming a thrombus, sometimes referred to as nonbacterial thrombotic endocarditis. Certain bacterial species that transiently seed the bloodstream, such as streptococci and staphylococci, have a greater intrinsic tendency to adhere to such a thrombus, eventually resulting in a platelet-fibrin-bacterial mass (vegetation) that constitutes the primary pathology of infective endocarditis. Failure to mount a phagocytic cell response to this localized infection results in continuous bacteremia, and the potential for local intracardiac progression as well as remote extracardiac seeding of the infection by septic emboli.

The constant intravascular antigenic stimulus also results in the development of antibodies and the presence of circulating immune complexes that mediate many immunopathologic responses in various organs that are frequently observed in patients with endocarditis. Mechanical dislodgement of the vegetations and their resulting arterial embolization results in end-organ infarction with or without subsequent local infection and possible abscess formation.

Clinical Manifestations

The clinical features of infective endocarditis are explained by five fundamental mechanisms.

Infectious Process on the Involved Valve(s)

The majority (80%) of patients with infective endocarditis have involvement of the left-sided valves — mitral and aortic valve involvement occur with approximately equal frequency — and about 10% have combined mitral and aortic infection. Right-sided endocarditis is seen in about 15% of cases, the tricuspid valve being involved twice as frequently as the pulmonic. It occurs most often in association with intravenous drug abuse and congenital heart disease with a left-to-right shunt.

The vegetation on the involved valve usually leads to a detectable murmur, particularly that of valvular insufficiency. Therefore the development of a previously unrecognized murmur of valvular insufficiency is especially suggestive of endocarditis. The infectious process that begins on the valve may extend into the adjacent myocardium and result in myocarditis, myocardial abscess, pericarditis, intracardiac fistulas, and arrhythmias. The development of atrioventricular conduction block with aortic valve endocarditis is strongly suggestive of a complicating septal abscess.

Congestive cardiac failure remains the most common cause of mortality in endocarditis. It is usually due

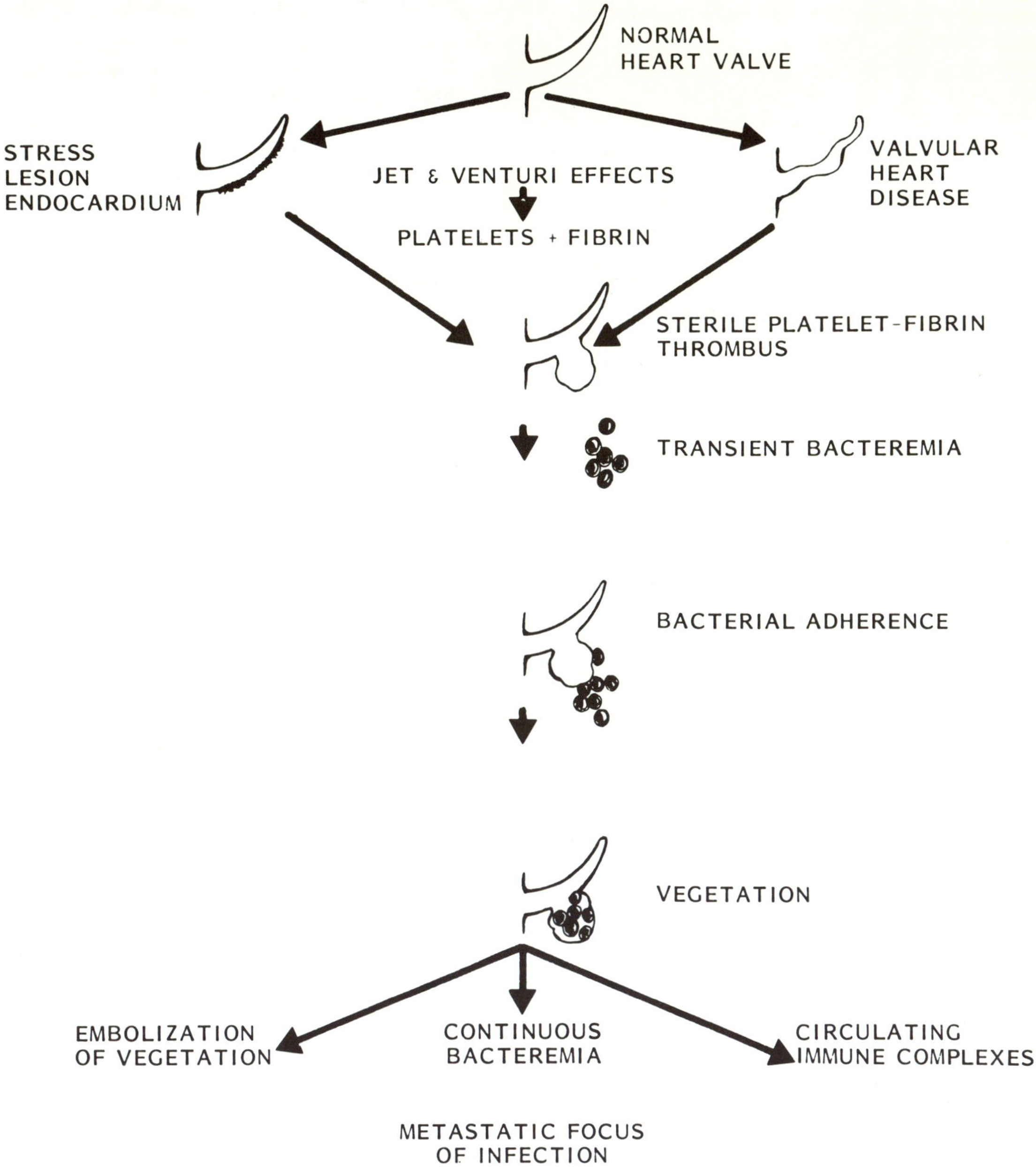

FIGURE 10.1. Pathogenesis of infective endocarditis.

to progressive valvular insufficiency but may be secondary to diffuse myocarditis.

Metastatic Infection

Metastatic (extracardiac) infection occurs in about one-quarter of patients with endocarditis. It may affect any organ but is most commonly seen in the lung in association with right-sided endocarditis. In fact, a septic pulmonary embolus with resulting pneumonia and/or pleurisy may be the principal manifestation of right-sided endocarditis. Another commonly involved site is the brain, with diffuse meningitis/cerebritis predominating before there is any direct evidence of an associated endocarditis. Cases of acute *S. aureus* endocarditis may be initially misdiagnosed clinically as meningococcemia with meningitis because of the associated meningitis, cerebritis, and widespread petechiae in a previously healthy individual.

Mycotic aneurysms usually arise from bacterial invasion of the arterial wall, possibly in association with embolic occlusion of the vasa vasorum. They may be clinically silent but most often declare themselves in the peripheral branches of the cerebral vessels (intracerebral or subarachnoid hemorrhage), splenic and hepatic artery, aorta, or mesenteric arteries.

Immunologically Mediated Phenomena

Immunologically mediated phenomena are seen in up to 75% of patients with infective endocarditis. They are most often manifested as vasculitic cutaneous lesions, such as petechiae, subungual splinter hemorrhages, and maculopapular lesions of the hands and feet (Osler's nodes and Janeway lesions). Ocular findings include subconjunctival hemorrhages and Roth's spots manifested as pale ischemic areas surrounded by a zone of hemorrhage.

Immune complex arthritis has been documented in up to 15% of patients with endocarditis, most often as acute monoarticular synovitis, but occasionally in the polyarticular form. The mechanism of back pain as a primary manifestation of endocarditis is not known.

Arterial Embolization

Arterial embolization can be clinically documented in up to 50% of patients with infective endocarditis. Most often the emboli result in local tissue infarction without secondary bacterial infection. They occur in the cerebral circulation as a so-called stroke syndrome, in the kidney as a renal infarct, and in the spleen as a splenic infarct that is occasionally misdiagnosed as a left lung pulmonary embolus with infarction. Sudden death in endocarditis may be related to coronary emboli.

Nonspecific Systemic Effects of Chronic Infection

Fever is present in 95% of patients with infective endocarditis but there is no characteristic fever pattern. Splenomegaly and clubbing of the extremities are noted in about one-quarter of patients.

Diagnosis

Rigorous application of the diagnostic criteria noted in Table 10.2 should facilitate case definition and result in prompt diagnosis and early institution of effective treatment. Eighty-five percent of patients with infective endocarditis have between four and seven of these clinical signs. Thus the diagnosis of infective endocarditis is *probable* if four or more criteria are present but still *possible* if only three are evident. It is also important to remember that this infection is a dynamic process, and certain manifestations (especially a new regurgitant murmur, immunologically mediated phenomena, an arterial embolus, and echocardiographic imaging of a vegetation) may not even become evident until after treatment is well under way. Definite diagnosis of infective endocarditis requires direct demonstration (at surgery or autopsy) of a vegetation on the endocardium, although it can be made on the basis of constellation of clinical findings supplemented by laboratory tests.

The bacteremia of infective endocarditis is relatively constant and low grade (<100 bacteria/ml blood). Five sets of blood cultures obtained over 12 hours and incubated aerobically and anaerobically will yield the infecting organism in 99% of instances where blood cultures are ultimately positive. Empiric antimicrobial treatment started before endocarditis is suspected may inhibit bacterial growth in blood cultures. The microbiology laboratory should be notified in such instances so that special resins or enzymes (beta-lactamases) may be added to the cultures to inactivate the antibiotics. For some fastidious organisms special media or incubation conditions may be employed. Any metastatic foci of infection should also be cultured if present, and may be positive even when blood cultures are negative. Culturing arterial rather than venous blood usually offers no advantage. Drawing blood specimens at the time of cardiac catheterization rarely increases the yield of positive cultures.

There is usually a leukocytosis in acute endocardi-

TABLE 10.2. Clinical Definition of Infective Endocarditis

Diagnostic Criteria	*Percentage Present*
Fever (≥38°C)	95
Cardiac murmur	95
New regurgitant murmur	60
Positive blood culture (at least 2 separate tubes obtained prior to therapy)	85
Bacteremia (especially due to staphylococci or streptococci) without an apparent feeding focus	65
Arterial embolization	50
Immunologically mediated phenomena	75
Metastatic extracardiac focus of infection	25
Imaging of vegetation by echocardiography	65

tis, although in more chronic disease this may be lacking. Fulminating disease caused, for example by *S. aureus,* may produce disseminated intravascular coagulation. Biochemically, there may be impairment of renal function with elevated levels of serum creatinine and blood urea nitrogen determination secondary to an immune complex glomerulonephritis. A vasomotor nephropathy may result from hypotension in acute sepsis or in endocarditis complicated by congestive heart failure. Nonspecific immunologic tests that may be positive in subacute endocarditis include a positive rheumatoid factor, decreased total hemolytic complement, and the presence of circulating immune complexes.

On chest x-ray there may be evidence of rheumatic valvular or congenital heart disease as well as signs of congestive heart failure. Serologic tests that may be useful include those that detect teichoic acid antibodies in patients suspected of having *S. aureus* endocarditis and antibodies against *C. burnetii* in cases of suspected Q fever endocarditis. Echocardiography, both M-mode (one-dimensional) and two-dimensional have detected vegetations on valves in up to 80% of cases of endocarditis. It has been particularly useful in documenting vegetations in some cases of culture-negative endocarditis. Detection of vegetations by M-mode echocardiography also has some prognostic value since the majority of those patients require surgical intervention. The best yield for detecting vegetations is a combination of both one-dimensional and two-dimensional echocardiography.

Treatment

Antimicrobial Therapy

The principles of antimicrobial therapy of infective endocarditis include: (1) determining in vitro susceptibility of the infecting organism, preferably both the minimum inhibitory concentration (MIC) and the minimum bactericidal concentration (MBC); (2) selecting bactericidal antibiotics in optimal dosage and often in synergistic combinations; (3) using prolonged (minimum of four weeks), uninterrupted therapy with parenteral antibiotics; and (4) in selected cases, laboratory monitoring of efficacy by measuring serum bactericidal titers and maintaining trough levels no lower than 1:8. This is particularly important for infections in which there is a poor therapeutic response, and most cases of gram-negative and fungal endocarditis. The concept of tolerance against cell wall-active antibiotics in *S. aureus* strains in which the MBC is more than 32 times the MIC may be important in selecting appropriate therapy for a bactericidal effect. Adding an aminoglycoside to a beta-lactam antibiotic may be indicated in such cases for more rapid sterilization of the vegetation. Also, treatment of *S. aureus* endocarditis has received considerable attention, with the addition of rifampin or fusidic acid to a beta-lactam antibiotic in poorly responsive cases.

Effective treatment regimens for common microorganisms causing infective endocarditis are summarized in Table 10.3. The dosages recommended for adult patients with normal renal function are as follows:

1. Penicillin G, 4 MU IV q4h
2. Cephalothin, 2 gm IV g4h
3. Vancomycin, 1 gm IV q12h
4. Streptomycin, 15 mg/kg IM q12h
5. Gentamicin, 1–1.5 mg/kg IV q8h
6. Rifampin, 300 mg po q8h

Surgical Therapy

Increasingly aggressive surgical management of patients with complicated endocarditis has greatly influenced the mortality from this infection. The most common indication for surgical therapy is valvular insufficiency resulting in congestive heart failure that is refractory to medical therapy. Other possible indications include: (1) major systemic emboli; (2) failure of optimal antimicrobial drug regimen to sterilize the blood stream and/or vegetation; (3) most cases of prosthetic valve endocarditis; (4) mycotic aneurysms; (5) myocardial abscess and/or intracardiac fistula; (6) pos-

TABLE 10.3. Effective Treatment Regimens for Infective Endocarditis

Infecting Microorganism	*Drug(s) of Choice*	*Effective Alternatives*
S. viridans and β-hemolytic streptococci	Penicillin G ± streptomycin (first 2 wks)	Cephalothin ± streptomycin (first 2 wks) Vancomycin
S. faecalis (enterococcus)	Penicillin G + gentamicin	Vancomycin + gentamicin
S. aureus	Cloxacillin ± rifampin	Cephalothin Vancomycin
S. epidermidis (methicillin-resistant)	Vancomycin plus rifampin ± gentamicin	Cephalothin + rifampin
Culture-negative	Penicillin G + gentamicin	Vancomycin + gentamicin

sibly patients with large vegetations on echocardiography; and (7) fungal endocarditis.

Of those who require surgery (i.e., valve replacement), 75% are cured. The incidence of endocarditis due to the same organism on the prosthetic valve is negligible, irrespective of the timing of the surgery in relation to the duration of prior antibiotic therapy. Surgery in this setting is associated with a higher risk of early mechanical valve dehiscence, however, which may require reoperation.

Prognosis

Untreated endocarditis has a mortality rate approaching 100%, with overall outcome dependent on the development of complications that require surgery. Thus the mortality of medically treated right-sided endocarditis due to *S. aureus* in intravenous drug abusers is small, whereas that with acute aortic valve endocarditis due to *S. faecalis* is 50%. Since most published series come from tertiary referral centers with cardiovascular surgery capability, the outcome of treatment tends to reflect the prognosis of complicated cases. In such centers, approximately 50% of patients are cured medically, an additional 25% require surgical intervention for successful outcome, and 25% die of causes directly related to endocarditis.

Several factors adversely affect outcome: (1) acute endocarditis (40% mortality); (2) endocarditis due to *S. aureus* (33% mortality) and *S. faecalis* (50% mortality); (3) congestive heart failure refractory to medical therapy (45% mortality); and (4) echocardiographically imaged vegetations associated with an increased risk of valve replacement (45% mortality) and major arterial embolization (50% mortality).

Microbiologic relapses within six weeks after apparently adequate initial antibiotic therapy occur in 5% to 10% of patients with infective endocarditis. Forty percent of these patients can be successfully retreated, 40% require additional surgery, and 20% die.

Prophylaxis

There are four key principles in the prevention of infective endocarditis:

1. Systemic antibiotics should be administered to patients with valvular heart disease at the time of procedures associated with a high probability of transient bacteremia.
2. The prophylaxis for dental procedures and upper respiratory tract surgery is directed against viridans streptococci.
3. Prophylaxis for gastrointestinal and genitourinary tract instrumentation and surgery is directed against *S. faecalis*.
4. Antibiotics should be given in such a maanner as to provide effective bactericidal concentrations at the time of the anticipated bacteremia and for no more than 48 hours thereafter.

The efficacy of such prophylaxis has never been proved in humans and these regimens have failed to prevent endocarditis. Prophylaxis, however, has been shown to be effective in animal models.

The drug regimens recommended by the American Heart Association (AHA) Committee on the Prevention of Endocarditis are as follows.

Antibiotic Prophylaxis for Dental Procedures and Surgery of the Upper Respiratory Tract

Adults Without a History of Penicillin Allergy

Regimen A

1. Parenteral-oral combined — aqueous crystalline penicillin G, 1 MU intramuscularly, mixed with procaine penicillin G, 600,000 U intramuscularly followed by penicillin V, 600 mg orally every 6 hours for 8 doses
2. Oral — penicillin V, 2.1 gm orally 1½ to 2 hours prior to procedure, followed by penicillin V, 600 mg orally every 6 hours for 8 doses

Regimen B

1. Penicillin plus streptomycin. Same as regimen A1 (parenteral-oral combined) except that streptomycin, 1.0 gm intramuscularly, is given at the same time as the parenteral penicillin injection

Adults Who Are Allergic to Penicillin

1. Parenteral-oral combined — vancomycin, 1.0 gm intravenously over 30 to 60 minutes. Start initial vancomycin infusion ½ to 1 hour prior to procedure, followed by erythromycin, 500 mg orally every 6 hours for 8 doses
2. Oral — erythromycin, 1.0 gm orally 1½ to 2 hours prior to the procedure, followed by erythromycin, 500 mg orally every 6 hours for 8 doses

Antimicrobial Prophylaxis for Gastrointestinal and Genitourinary Tract Surgery and Instrumentation

Adults Without a History of Penicillin Allergy

Aqueous crystalline penicillin G, 2 MU intramuscularly or intravenously

or

Ampicillin, 1.0 gm intramuscularly or intravenously

plus

Gentamicin, 1.5 mg/kg (not to exceed 80 mg) intramuscularly or intravenously

or

Streptomycin, 1.0 gm intramuscularly

Initial doses given 30 minutes to 1 hour prior to procedure. If gentamicin is used, a similar dose of gentamicin and penicillin (or ampicillin) is given every 8 hours for 2 additional doses. If streptomycin is used a similar dose of streptomycin and penicillin (or ampicillin) is given every 12 hours for two additional doses.

Adults Who Are Allergic to Penicillin

Vancomycin, 1.0 gm intravenously given over 30 to 60 minutes, plus streptomycin, 1.0 gm intramuscularly

A single dose of these antibiotics given 30 to 60 minutes prior to the procedure is probably sufficient, but the same dose may be repeated in 12 hours.

PROSTHETIC VALVE ENDOCARDITIS

Endocarditis is a rare but extremely serious complication of prosthetic valve surgery. It is estimated that the lifetime risk of infection on a prosthetic valve is 1% to 2%, independent of whether a mechanical valve or bioprosthesis is inserted. It is particularly important to employ the recommended prophylactic antibiotics in this population. Although many of the features of prosthetic valve endocarditis (PVE) mimic those of native valve endocarditis, there are some key differences.

Etiology

Staphylococci and streptococci continue to cause over 80% of cases of PVE. In recent years, the single most common cause is *S. epidermidis*. These are often methicillin-resistant. Gram-negative rods, diphtheroids, and fungi (candida, aspergillus) make up the remainder. Culture-negative PVE is very uncommon.

Epidemiology

Although it is traditional to classify PVE into early (occurring within two months of valve implantation) and late forms, this distinction is somewhat arbitrary and does not clearly segregate patients into characteristic groups. The aortic valve is involved almost twice as often as the mitral valve, although this difference has appeared to be less evident in recent years.

Pathophysiology

The infection of a prosthetic valve usually starts in the tissue beneath the site of attachment of the prosthesis to the adjacent valve ring. This infection results in (1) detachment of the valve ring, (2) extension into the adjacent valve ring resulting in a ring abscess, and (3) obstruction by the vegetation.

Clinical Manifestations

The most common clinical features of PVE are fever, early development of a regurgitant murmur due to valve dehiscence, and major systemic emboli, particularly to the cerebral circulation.

Diagnosis

The majority of patients with PVE have positive blood cultures. Sustained bacteremia due to *S. epidermidis, S. aureus,* diphtheroids, or streptococci in a patient with a prosthetic heart valve should lead to treatment for presumptive PVE. Transient bacteremia from an extracardiac feeding focus in the absence of direct evidence of valve involvement should not be considered a reason for treating someone for PVE. Fungal PVE is usually culture negative, and the diagnosis may have to be confirmed by examination of a vegetation that has embolized to a major vessel. Echocardiography is less useful since vegetations are more difficult to image in the presence of a mechanical valve.

Treatment

Antimicrobial Therapy

In the acutely ill patient, once blood cultures have been obtained, treatment should be initiated with vancomycin, 1 gm intravenously every 12 hours, plus an aminoglycoside such as gentamicin or tobramycin, 1.7 mg per kg per dose. This combination provides effective initial therapy for all common causes of PVE except, of course, fungi. Once a specific microbiologic diagnosis has been made, systemic antibiotic therapy should be individualized (see Table 10.3). The duration of parenteral therapy for PVE should be at least six weeks.

Surgical Treatment

Medical cure is uncommon, especially with a mechanical prosthesis, and successful treatment usually requires removal of the infected valve. Prompt surgery is indicated if congestive heart failure occurs, if optimal antibiotic therapy fails to control the systemic or local infection, and when myocardial invasion is suspected on the basis of atrioventricular conduction disturbances and early relapse. Fungal PVE can only be cured by surgery.

Prognosis

Mortality from PVE is high, 60% to 70%. Nonstreptococcal infection, congestive heart failure, new regurgitant murmurs, age, development of renal failure, valvular vegetations on echocardiography, and fungal or staphylococcal infection all constitute risk factors for high mortality. Consideration should be given to earlier surgery in patients with these conditions.

Prophylaxis

Antibiotic prophylaxis for valve replacement is standard practice in all cardiovascular surgery units. Patients with prosthetic valves should receive antibiotic prophylaxis for procedures that are likely to produce transient bacteremia.

MYOCARDITIS AND PERICARDITIS

Inflammation of the myocardium (myocarditis) and/or pericardium (pericarditis) often provides a diagnostic and therapeutic challenge. With many disease processes, both myocardium and pericardium are involved, resulting in myopericarditis; however, either entity may be clinically dominant.

Etiology

The list of organisms that can cause pericarditis or myocarditis includes many viruses, bacteria, fungi, parasites, and rickettsia (Table 10.4). In North American studies, however, approximately 75% of episodes of myopericarditis are due to enteroviruses (coxsackie and echoviruses). The next most common pathogens are pyogenic bacteria and those causing granulomatous diseases (mycobacteria and fungi).

A strong association has been established between myopericarditis and group B coxsackieviruses (types 1 through 6), group A coxsackieviruses (types 4 and 16), and echoviruses (types 9, 11, and 22). In one study, group B coxsackieviruses caused at least 50% of cases of acute myopericarditis and one-third of cases of acute

TABLE 10.4. Selected Examples of Infectious Causes of Myopericarditis

Viruses	*Bacteria*	*Mycobacteria*	*Fungi*	*Parasites*	*Miscellaneous*
Coxsackieviruses A & B	*S. aureus*	*M. tuberculosis*	*Aspergillus* sp.	*E. granulosus*	*M. pneumoniae*
Echoviruses	*S. pyogenes*		*Candida* sp.	*E. histolytica*	*C. psittaci*
	S. pneumoniae		*H. capsulatum*	*T. gondii*	
	Aerobic gram-negative bacilli			*T. spiralis*	

nonbacterial pericarditis. In another study, group A coxsackieviruses caused 23% of acute myopericarditis. The proportion of cases caused by echoviruses is not known.

Bacteria tend to produce only pericarditis, and not myocarditis. At the present time, approximately half the cases of bacterial pericarditis are caused by gram-positive cocci (*S. pneumoniae, S. pyogenes,* and *S. aureus*) and half by gram-negative enteric bacilli. *Staphylococcus aureus* is still the most frequent single bacterial cause (30% to 40%). Bacterial myocarditis is rare but can occur either as a result of direct spread from endocarditis or pericarditis, or embolization from endocarditis. Toxic myocarditis can result from diphtheria and immunologic-mediated myocarditis from acute rheumatic fever.

Granulomatous myocarditis and pericarditis may be caused by *Mycobacterium tuberculosis, M. bovis, Histoplasma capsulatum, Coccidioides immitis,* and *Blastomyces dermatitidis*. Immunocompromised hosts are more susceptible to atypical mycobacteria such as *M. chelonei* and fungi such as *Candida* and *Aspergillus* species. Parasitic infections such as trichinosis, toxoplasmosis, and American trypanosomiasis (Chagas' disease) have a marked predilection for cardiac and skeletal muscles.

Epidemiology

The epidemiology of myopericarditis is diverse and varies depending upon the etiologic agent. Enteroviral infections, spread usually by the fecal-oral route, occur mainly in the summer and fall. Although many of these infections are subclinical, cardiac involvement occurs in about 5% of symptomatic infections and is especially frequent and severe in newborns. The apparent increasing incidence of more severe enteroviral infections in adults may reflect reduced exposure (and hence immunity) to these viruses in childhood as a result of general improvement in sanitation.

Group B coxsackieviruses (types 1, 3, and 4) tend to be endemic, whereas types 2, 5, and 6 usually produce epidemics.

Bacterial pericarditis acquired outside the hospital may result from bacteremia, from contiguous spread from pneumonia, or secondary to chest trauma. Within the hospital setting, it is usually a serious infectious complication of cardiac or thoracic surgery. Tuberculous pericarditis is very uncommon in economically developed countries but should be suspected in high-risk populations, and may result from either a primary or reactivated infection. Fungal pericarditis, also a rare disease, should be suspected in immunocompromised patients.

Each parasitic infection causing myopericarditis has its own particular epidemiology. For example, Chagas' disease is one of the most common causes of heart disease in Central and South America and has its highest frequency in males, 30 to 40 years of age, from rural regions.

Pathophysiology

In the normal heart, there is usually 15 to 20 ml of fluid within the pericardial sac. An inflammatory process that increases or interferes with reabsorption of pericardial fluid can result in cardiac tamponade and mechanical impairment of cardiac function. Myocarditis, in contrast, may result in abnormalities of cardiac rhythm and contractility.

In viral infections, pericarditis is fibrinous, and myocardial inflammation varies from only an interstitial mononuclear infiltrate to marked muscle necrosis. Gross pathologic findings in severe viral myopericarditis include cardiac dilatation and hypertrophy, mural thrombi, and muscle degeneration. Although mild forms may heal without residua, more severe disease often results in scarring and occasionally calcification. Chronic cardiomyopathy may also develop.

Bacterial pericarditis results in a thickened, acutely inflamed pericardium often with increased amounts of purulent pericardial fluid. Direct extension into the myocardium may occur but is unusual. Tuberculous or fungal pericarditis begins as an acute inflammatory reaction that is quickly superceded by a typical granulomatous response that may progress to caseation necrosis, fibrosis, and calcification. Tuberculous and fungal pericarditis may result from either lymphohematogenous spread from a primary focus or direct spread from a hilar or mediastinal lymph node. The pathology of a parasitic myopericarditis depends upon the specific agent.

Clinical Manifestations

Signs and symptoms of bacterial pericarditis are usually more severe than those of viral myopericarditis, but an absolute distinction cannot always be made clinically. With bacterial pericarditis, virtually all patients are acutely ill and in most series, all have fever and rigors, chest pain, muffled heart sounds, and evidence of tamponade. Hepatomegaly, ascites, and peripheral edema also may occur. Systemic symptoms and signs may be attributed initially to an infection at another site that seeded the pericardium. The diagnosis of pericarditis may then only be suspected with the development of cardiac tamponade and shock.

In contrast to bacterial pericarditis, only half of patients with viral myopericarditis are acutely ill; however, the majority have fever, chest pain, and dyspnea. Marked tachycardia (disproportionate to the fever), a faint first heart sound, gallop rhythm, and often arrhythmia may be detected, reflecting myocardial involvement. A history of flulike illness in the patient, close contacts, or in the community is often present.

Pericardial friction rubs can be heard over the precordium in both bacterial and viral pericarditis. The rubs may be transient and variable and usually disappear with an increase in size of the pericardial effusion. Characteristically, rubs are scratchy and are best heard along the left sternal border with the patient in the sitting position and leaning forward. If possible, the patient holds his breath momentarily to minimize obscuring the rub by breath sounds. Rubs may occur during systole or early and late diastole (or during all three phases). A pleural rub may be present concurrently.

Cardiac tamponade, a major complication of bacterial pericarditis in particular, may arise gradually or acutely. Clinically, dyspnea is usually present and the patient may be leaning forward to relieve it. The apical impulse usually is not palpable and the heart sounds are faint or undetectable. A pronounced paradoxical pulse will result in the disappearance of the radial pulse during inspiration. Elevated jugular venous pressure may rise further on inspiration (Kussmaul's sign).

Tuberculosis and other causes of granulomatous pericarditis are usually more chronic and are associated with larger effusions. Specific findings depend upon the activity of the disease elsewhere and the duration of the illness. Often there is only a chronic pericardial effusion, but in later stages calcification may occur, resulting in constrictive pericarditis with markedly elevated jugular venous pressure, hepatomegaly, ascites, and peripheral edema. In healthy hosts, fungal pericarditis with *H. capsulatum, C. immitis,* and *B. dermatitidis* may occur but is usually self-limited. In immunocompromised patients, however, all types of fungal pericarditis may be severe. Parasitic myocarditis and/or pericarditis usually arises as part of a systemic illness with features peculiar to the individual parasitic infection.

Diagnosis

The noninfectious causes of myocarditis and/or pericarditis are as follows:

- Acute myocardial infarction
- Postpericardial injury (Dressler's syndrome)
  - Myocardial infarction
  - Postpericardiotomy
- Uremia
- Collagen-vascular disease
  - Systemic lupus erythematosus, rheumatoid arthritis, scleroderma
  - Drug-induced (procainamide, hydralazine)
- Rheumatic fever
- Familial Mediterranean fever
- Sarcoidosis
- Radiation therapy
- Neoplasms, primary or metastatic
- Myxedema
- Trauma, penetrating or nonpenetrating

The considerations involved in making a diagnosis of myocarditis or pericarditis are outlined in Figure 10.2. It is very important particularly with bacterial

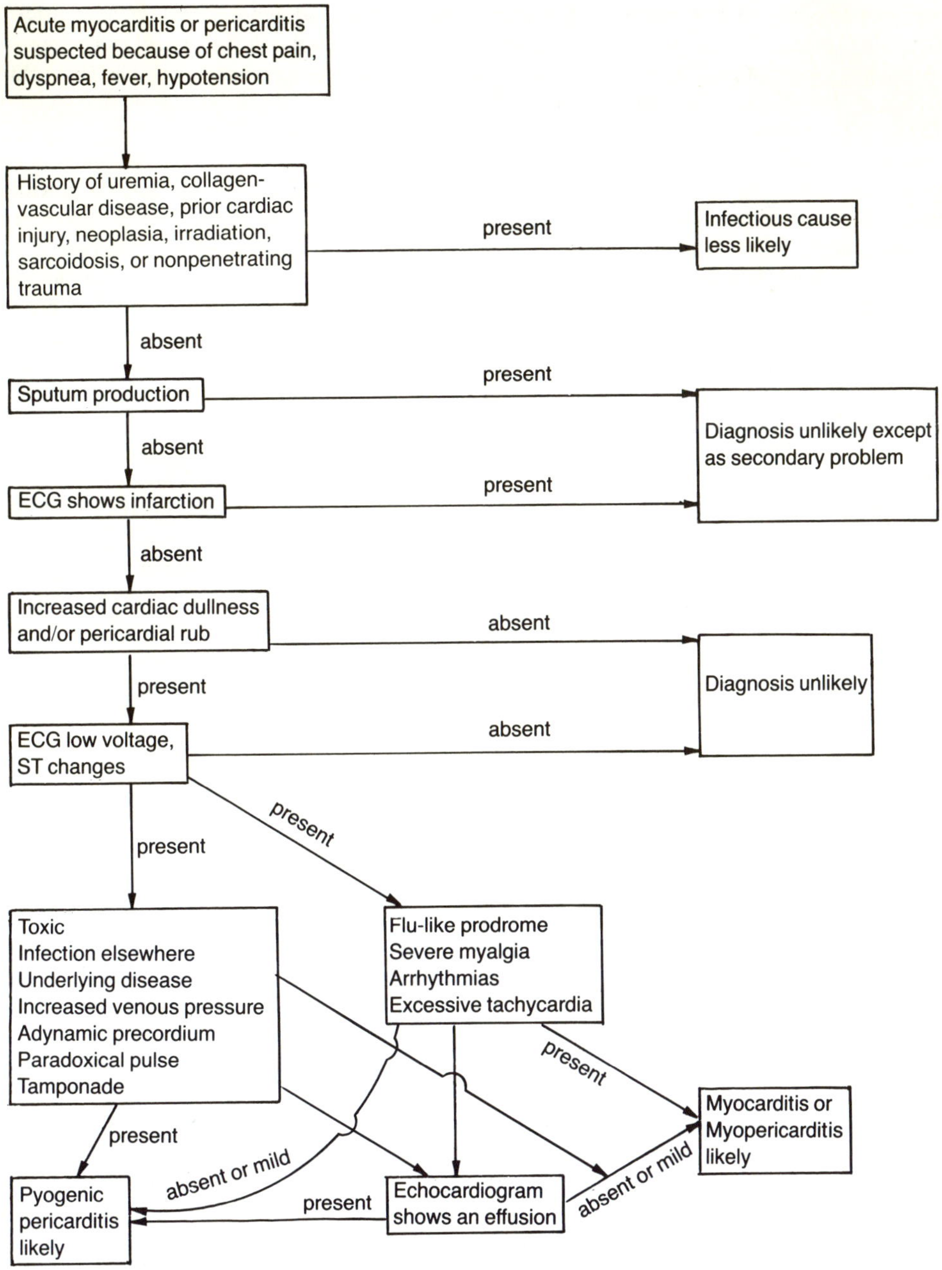

FIGURE 10.2. Considerations involved in diagnosis of myocarditis and pericarditis.

pericarditis, to make the diagnosis early. In numerous series of purulent pericarditis, in a high proportion of cases the diagnosis was not made ante mortem or was made too late in the course of the disease to cure the patient. This may become an increasing problem as more cases are acquired within hospitals (and symptoms and signs are obscured by concomitant illness) or by patients with abnormal host defenses. Another difficulty in recognizing infective pericarditis is that it often develops in patients with preexisting noninfective pericarditis (e.g., uremia or collagen-vascular disease) and may be overlooked.

Apart from clinical manifestations, which are extremely important, various laboratory procedures are helpful in making the diagnosis. Chest x-rays, especially those done serially, may demonstrate a globular cardiac silhouette if there is an associated pericardial effusion, and the epicardial fat line may be seen well inside the lateral margin of the cardiac silhouette. Chest x-rays may also demonstrate another process such as pneumonia, which may have been the initial source for the development of pericarditis. Pleural effusions may also be detected. Electrocardiograms usually show ST and T wave changes, low voltage, and less commonly, arrhythmias, especially in more severe forms of myocarditis. A major distinguishing feature from myocardial infarction is the presence of ST and T wave abnormalities in all leads as opposed to the more localized changes seen in myocardial infarction.

An echocardiogram is a useful noninvasive technique to determine the size of the pericardial effusion and to follow it serially. An isotope scan may also demonstrate an effusion. The most direct means of making a specific diagnosis, however, is by needle aspiration or open surgical drainage to obtain pericardial fluid for examination, and possibly biopsy of pericardial tissue. Myocardial biopsy is usually not indicated except for chronic disease in which cardiomyopathy is suspected. The risk of hemopericardium and cardiac tamponade must be considered, and if direct aspiration is performed it should be done under electrocardiographic monitoring with surgical back-up available. It is important to remember that positive stained smears and/or cultures are diagnostic as opposed to cell counts and biochemical tests of fluid or tissues, which are nonspecific. Depending upon the organisms suspected, the pericardial fluid should have Gram's, acid-fast, and fungal stains; and aerobic, anaerobic, mycobacterial, fungal, and viral cultures. Less specific tests include a differential cell count and determination of protein, sugar, pH, and lactic dehydrogenase (LDH). Any biopsy material should be stained and cultured according to which pathogens are suspected. The yield from pericardial fluid or tissue will vary depending upon the causative pathogen (Table 10.5).

A bloody effusion is usually present in tuberculous or neoplastic pericarditis but may occur with rheumatic fever, uremic pericarditis, and the postmyocardial infarction or postcardiac injury syndrome.

The diagnosis of a specific viral etiology is often difficult. The virus may continue to multiply in the heart after replication in the throat, feces, or urine has ceased, so that cultures from these sites may be negative. Moreover, by the time myopericarditis becomes clinically evident, antibody levels are often already elevated and it may not be possible to demonstrate fourfold increases between acute and convalescent sera. While it is not practical to screen for antibody to all enteroviruses, serologic diagnosis may be facilitated if one is able to isolate a potentially pathogenic virus so that an attempt can be made to detect type-specific IgG or IgM antibody to the isolated virus in the patient's serum. Detection of type-specific IgM antibody is helpful because it is present acutely from a few days to six weeks after onset of infection and is indicative of recent illness. In the absence of a specific viral isolate, serum can be screened for antibody to various group B coxsackieviruses, but a serologic rise in titer may be nonspecific and represent only a heterotypic antibody response. In most cases, viral myopericarditis cannot be specifically proved but can be strongly suspected when clinical and/or laboratory evidence of myopericarditis arises during a nonspecific febrile illness.

Nonenteroviral viral infections can be diagnosed by other findings such as the presence of atypical lymphocytosis and heterophile antibody (Epstein-Barr virus), abnormal hepatic enzymes and serology (hepatitis A or B), isolation of cytomegalovirus from throat or urine, parotitis (mumps), or coexistent influenzal disease.

The specific etiology of bacterial pericarditis, apart from positive stained smears or cultures of pericardial fluid or tissue, can be made by positive blood cultures. Serologic studies are usually not of value; however, in certain laboratories the demonstration of various bacterial antigens (e.g., teichoic acid antibodies for *S. aureus* infections) may be helpful. Diphtheritic myocarditis should be suspected in patients with a history of severe pharyngitis and positive throat cultures or skin cultures for toxigenic *Corynebacterium diphtheriae*. The diagnosis of rheumatic fever depends upon clinical

TABLE 10.5. Yield from Pericardial Fluid or Biopsy

Organism or Class of Organisms	*Microscopic Examination*		*Culture*	
	Fluid	*Tissue*	*Fluid*	*Tissue*
Viruses	–	Fluorescent + +	±	±
Aerobic bacteria	+ + +	+	+ + +	+ + +
Anaerobic bacteria	+ + +	+	+ + +	+ + +
Tuberculosis	+	+ + +	+ +	+ + +
Fungi	Variable	+ + +	+ + +	+ + +
Parasites	Variable	+ + +	Cultures not usually available	

criteria and an antecedent *S. pyogenes* pharyngitis or serologic evidence of streptococcal disease.

The diagnosis of tuberculous pericarditis may be suggested by a less acute course associated with weight loss and a large effusion, a positive skin test (negative skin test, if patient is anergic), a chest x-ray compatible with tuberculosis in approximately 50% of cases, a history of prior tuberculosis, or detection of the infection at other sites. Fungal pericarditis or myocarditis usually is suspected by the presence of a predisposing history or disease at other sites. The serologic diagnosis is discussed in Chapter 4. The diagnosis of parasitic pericarditis or myocarditis depends upon a good epidemiologic history and on other clinical and laboratory findings, including serology. Toxoplasmosis may be congenital or acquired, and may occur in healthy or compromised hosts. Trichinosis should be suspected by clinical findings of myocarditis plus muscle tenderness, periorbital edema, subungual hemorrhages, urticaria, and eosinophilia. Biopsy of peripheral muscle may reveal encysted *Trichinella spiralis* larvae. Acute American trypanosomiasis (Chagas' disease) may result in myocarditis as part of an acute illness with diffuse lymphadenopathy. This may regress but can manifest later as a cardiomyopathy with congestive heart failure, emboli, and cardiac arrhythmias or arteriovenous conduction abnormalities. Amebic pericarditis is a dramatic complication of hepatic amebiasis, which almost always involves the left lobe of the liver.

Treatment

All patients with acute pericarditis must be followed carefully to detect the development of an effusion and tamponade. Treatment requires both specific chemotherapy directed against the infecting organism and adequate drainage of excess pericardial fluid by pericardiocentesis or open surgical drainage, when necessary.

TABLE 10.6. Treatment of Bacterial Pericarditis

Organism	*Antibiotic*
Gram-positive cocci	
S. aureus	Cloxacillin (or other penicillinase-resistant semisynthetic penicillin), 9–12 gm/d IV × 4–6 wks
S. pyogenes	Penicillin G, 20 to 30 MU/d IV × 4–6 wks
S. pneumoniae	Penicillin G, as above
Gram-negative bacilli	
Nonpseudomonas	Moxalactam or cefotaxime, up to 12 gm/d IV × 4–6 wks
P. aeruginosa	Ticarcillin, 18 gm/d IV, plus Tobramycin, 5–6 mg/kg/d IV × 4–6 wks

Organism-specific treatment for bacterial pericarditis is summarized in Table 10.6. High doses of appropriate antimicrobial drugs should be given intravenously for four to six weeks. For the initial therapy of probable acute bacterial pericarditis when the etiology is not known, cefazolin 1 to 2 gm intravenously every eight hours, and tobramycin, 1.5 mg per kg every eight hours, should be started. The treatment of tuberculous and fungal pericarditis follows the precepts for treatment of these organisms as described in Chapter 12. Treatment of parasitic infection depends upon the incriminated pathogen (see Chapter 27). There is no specific antiviral therapy available.

Steroids have been used empirically in viral myopericarditis, especially in cases complicated by persistent pain and cardiac dysfunction on the assumption that chronic myocardial inflammation has an immunologic basis. Prednisone, up to 80 mg daily is given and decreased rapidly over a period of several weeks until the lowest effective dose is reached. Optimal duration of treatment is unknown, and earlier administration of steroids appears to be contraindicated, although pericarditis complicating infectious mononucleosis caused by Epstein-Barr virus may be helped by earlier steroid administration. In tuberculous pericarditis, in addition to specific antituberculous therapy, treatment with steroids in high doses may also reduce the inflammatory response, with reduction in the size of the effusion and subsequent fibrosis and constriction.

Anticoagulation is generally contraindicated in pericarditis because of the risk of hemopericardium.

Rest, with avoidance of strenuous activity for at least a month during convalescence, is probably important for recovery. If there is evidence of severe myocarditis with muscle necrosis, rest should be prolonged, probably for at least three months.

Prognosis

Untreated bacterial pericarditis has a mortality rate of close to 100% but, when treated, mortality decreases to 20% to 40%. If patients survive, there are usually no residua. Similarly, those with tuberculous pericarditis are usually quite ill, but with the use of steroids and prolonged antimicrobial treatment, most survive, although one-third may develop constrictive pericarditis. Fungal pericarditis generally carries a very poor prognosis, usually because severe forms occur in immunocompromised hosts.

In contrast, patients with viral myopericarditis often do not appear very ill initially but may have significant long-term sequelae. In addition, the disease may have a relapsing course in these individuals. In one study of 14 patients followed after group B coxsackievirus myopericarditis, 8 were clinically healthy (4 had abnormal electrocardiograms), 3 had residual chronic congestive heart failure, and 3 had pericardial pain.

Poor prognostic features of myopericarditis include persistent cardiomegaly, congestive heart failure, arrhythmias, and chest pain. All patients, especially those with viral myopericarditis or with these findings, should be carefully followed.

Constrictive pericarditis is an important complication that occurs most frequently with granulomatous diseases like tuberculosis, but is well recognized following bacterial pericarditis, viral or idiopathic pericarditis, and noninfectious causes. Because surgery can be curative for constrictive pericarditis, it is extremely important to differentiate this condition from restrictive cardiomyopathy.

An interesting noninfectious sequela of some cases of infectious pericarditis is a recurrence of findings of pericarditis after a period of partial or total resolution. It appears to be due to a serum sickness-like illness and is often associated with pleuritis, urticaria, arthralgias, or arthritis, and responds to salicylates or steroids. There may be subsequent recurrences, usually of progressively decreasing severity.

Prophylaxis

Routine diphtheria prophylaxis will prevent the subsequent development of diphtheria and diphtheritic myocarditis. Prophylactic antibiotics, usually a cephalosporin or penicillinase-resistant penicillin, are given prior to cardiac surgery to prevent postoperative infections (especially staphylococcal) such as pericarditis. No specific prophylaxis is available to prevent coxsackie or echoviral pericarditis. Preventing various viral communicable diseases such as measles, mumps, rubella, and polio will diminish further the number of rare cases of myopericarditis associated with these illnesses.

RHEUMATIC FEVER

Rheumatic fever is a multisystem disease known to be a sequel to infection with group A streptococci. Although the association between this organism and the disease was made in the 1940s, to date there is no clear explanation for its pathogenesis. In spite of the fact that rheumatic fever is uncommon in the Western world, it remains the leading cause of acquired heart disease worldwide.

Epidemiology

The occurrence of rheumatic fever varies from country to country and is most closely correlated with socioeconomic status, general hygiene, and availability of medical care. Underdeveloped and developing countries have the highest incidence, reaching a maximum of 2% to 5% during outbreaks of streptococcal pharyngitis. The most recent United States information suggests overall incidence of about 15 cases per 100,000 population. There appears to be a limit to the maximum number of cases, which is reached when conditions are optimal for the disease, but it never occurs in epidemic proportions, probably because of genetic predisposition, as is discussed later.

Pathophysiology

The association between pharyngeal infection with group A streptococci and rheumatic fever has been recognized for 40 years, but the actual sequence of events has not yet been elucidated. Onset of disease is usually two to three weeks after pharyngitis and in fact, the streptococci may not be present at the time of onset of the signs and symptoms of rheumatic fever.

It is now generally accepted that the pathogenesis is related to immunologic events. Antibodies to a variety of streptococcal cellular antigens and products including streptolysin O, hyaluronidase, the group-specific carbohydrate, type-specific M protein, as well as cross-reactive heart antigens are generally present in high titers. There is no direct evidence, however, that any of these antibodies is responsible for in vivo damage leading to the classic symptomatology.

For example, the antibody to the cross-reactive antigen present in the streptococcal cell membrane and in human heart sarcolemma can be shown to bind to beating mammalian heart cells in vitro, but it is not cytotoxic. This is probably due to the fact that it does not bind and activate complement, an observation reflected by the lack of complement consumption in vivo during the active disease process.

The most likely mechanism involves lymphocyte sensitization to the cross-reactive antigen. Studies have shown that patients with acute rheumatic fever have lymphocytes that are highly sensitized to group A streptococcal membranes, the site of the cross-reactive antigen(s). This high degree of sensitization persists for several years after the acute attack, even in the absence of intercurrent streptococcal infections.

There is a second cross-reactive antibody present in serum of some patients who have rheumatic fever with chorea. This antibody reacts both to an antigen on the group A streptococcal membrane (distinct from the heart-reactive antigen) and to an antigen in the caudate and subthalamic nuclei of the brain. It is found in about 45% of rheumatics with chorea and the titer rises during periods of increased choreiform activity. As with the heart-reactive antibody, its actual role in the pathogenesis of chorea is unclear.

It is highly unlikely that there is uniform susceptibility to rheumatic fever. Even in conditions most conducive to its development, that is, streptococcal infections, crowded conditions, poor hygiene, and so on, only up to 5% of those with streptococcal pharyngitis develop acute rheumatic fever. This, together with the observation that there is increased familial prevalence of the disease, strongly suggests some form of genetic predisposition. Studies of the HLA-A and B loci in patients with rheumatic fever compared with other family members, persons with nephritis, and controls did not reveal any strong association between the disease and antigens of either of these loci. It has been found, however, that a B-lymphocyte alloantigen, referred to as 883, is present in 75% of persons with rheumatic fever in two groups studied to date, one in Bogota and the other in New York. With a prevalence of only 12% of the general population carrying this marker, the association is one of the highest for any known marker and disease. There is more recent evidence to indicate that most of the remaining 25% of patients with rheumatic fever carry a distinct second marker, now designated 256. Thus it appears that virtually all of these patients can be identified by one of these two genetic markers.

Clinical Manifestations

Rheumatic fever occurs most frequently in children between the ages of 5 and 15 years. Onset is usually not until after the signs and symptoms of pharyngitis have disappeared and varies depending on the major site(s) involved. It is usually abrupt when arthritis is one of the major manifestations, and is accompanied by fever. This is the usual pattern seen in the temperate zones. In tropical and semitropical areas, disease processes without arthritis are more common. Patients in these areas often give a history of one to three weeks of fever, with gradual onset of shortness of breath and chest pain, usually accompanied by arthralgias and weight loss. Chorea is also of insidious onset and often occurs weeks to months after onset of the disease. There are several common clinical manifestations.

1. Fever is almost always present for the first two to three weeks in the untreated patient.
2. Polyarthritis is the most common major manifestation of rheumatic fever in temperate climates. It is classically migratory and usually involves the large joints. The affected joints are red, swollen, and painful. The arthritis of rheumatic fever is extremely responsive to acetylsalicylic acid, showing almost total resolution within a few hours.
3. Carditis is the single aspect of rheumatic fever that can leave the patient with permanent and even eventually fatal damage. The incidence varies from one region to another, but in some tropical and semitropical countries it is the most common major manifestation. The pathogenesis of acute valvular involvement and ultimate fibrosis and scarring may be due in part to inflammation of the endocardium lining the valves. Possibly of even greater importance is involvement of myocardial cells that are present in the proximal one-third of the heart valves.

   Carditis may be sublinical. In clinically recognized cases it may be associated with an organic murmur, a pericardial friction rub, cardiac enlargement on x-ray, prolongation of the PR or QT intervals on electrocardiogram, or congestive heart failure. Of the valves, the mitral is the most commonly affected and a soft mitral regurgitant murmur is the most frequent sign in the acute phase of the disease.
4. Chorea consists of involuntary movements and facial grimaces and may be misdiagnosed as a behavior disorder. The movements are nonrepetitive, rapid, and quasi-purposeful. Chorea may exist without other signs of rheumatic fever, or it may develop before or persist long after other signs of rheumatic activity have disappeared. The prevalence also varies in different countries, for example, in Egypt it occurs in 15% of cases of rheumatic fever.
5. Erythema marginatum is an evanescent rash. It is initially macular and morbilliform with rapid central clearing resulting in red circles that coalesce to form a serpiginous pattern.
6. Subcutaneous nodules usually occur weeks or months after the onset of rheumatic activity. They are nontender, are attached to tendon sheaths or joint capsules, and occur most commonly over bony prominences.

Diagnosis

The diagnosis of acute rheumatic fever is based on the classic major and minor criteria as outlined by Jones:

1. Major manifestations
   - Polyarthritis
   - Carditis
   - Erythema marginatum
   - Subcutaneous nodules
   - Chorea
2. Minor manifestations
   - Fever
   - Arthralgia
   - Previous rheumatic fever
   - Elevated erythrocyte sedimentation rate
   - Positive C-reactive protein
   - Prolonged PR interval on electrocardiogram

Since acute rheumatic fever can cause a variety of symptoms and signs, the modified Jones criteria state that for the physician to make the diagnosis, the patient must have at least two major manifestations or one major and two minor ones, plus evidence of an antecedent streptococcal infection.

The clinical manifestations are the most important, but in addition, two categories of laboratory tests are helpful in the diagnosis: (1) those reflecting acute phase reactants and (2) culture of group A streptococci and/or detection of antibody indicating a recent streptococcal infection:

1. Acute-phase reactants
   a. Erythrocyte sedimentation rate (ESR)
   b. C-reactive protein (CRP)
   c. Complement
2. Streptococcal antibodies
   a. Antistreptolysin O
   b. Anti-group A carbohydrate
   c. Antiheart
   d. Anticaudate nucleus
   e. Anti-DNase B
   f. Antihyaluronidase
   g. Antistreptozyme

In the first category, the most widely used tests are ESR and CRP. Almost without exception, these two tests are elevated during the acute stages of acute rheumatic fever. When chorea is the only manifestation, however, they may be normal. Another acute-phase reactant that is usually elevated in acute disease is complement.

The serologic tests in the second category involve

measuring antibodies to group A streptococci or their products. The most commonly measured antibody is antistreptolysin O. It is elevated in 75% of patients. Other antibodies that can be tested in more specialized laboratories include antihyaluronidase, anti-DNase B, and antibody to the group-specific carbohydrate. A combination of three such tests will result in 95% correlation of streptococcal antibody rise and acute rheumatic fever. Recently, a combined antigen preparation, streptozyme, has been marketed and is capable of detecting more than one antibody.

One of the most reliable antibodies is the antiheart antibody (AHA), which is present in 75% to 80% of patients with acute rheumatic fever. It is not present in significant titers in uncomplicated streptococcal pharyngitis, scarlet fever, or acute poststreptococcal glomerulonephritis. The only other condition with elevated levels of AHA is the postpericardiotomy syndrome, but these antibodies can be differentiated by their lack of cross-reactivity with streptococci.

Differential Diagnosis

Although the diagnosis of rheumatic fever is sometimes difficult, the criteria established by Jones help to limit diagnostic possibilities. The main areas of concern are disease entities that can cause joint swelling, and/or heart murmurs with fever such as rheumatoid arthritis, infectious arthritis, acute osteomyelitis, sickle cell disease, leukemia, postpericardiotomy syndrome, and endocarditis.

Treatment

There are three basic principles involved in the treatment of rheumatic fever: (1) eradicate group A streptococci from the pharynx, (2) minimize or arrest the inflammatory reaction, and (3) prevent recurrence of infection and reactivation of disease.

Antibiotics

The antibiotic of choice for eradication of group A streptococci is penicillin, which can be given either orally or intramuscularly. The oral dose is penicillin G or V, 200,000 to 250,000 units three or four times a day. This must be continued for a full 10-day course. Benzathine penicillin G is given intramuscularly in a dose of 1.2 million units. For children weighing less than 27 kg, the dose is halved. What is often not realized is that even if treatment for streptococcal pharyngitis is initiated up to nine days after onset, it is still effective in preventing the development of rheumatic fever.

Antiinflammatory Agents

Most would agree that antiinflammatory therapy does not affect the final outcome of acute rheumatic fever. The arthritis is extremely responsive to salicylates and it is said that added proof for disease is the dramatic response to these agents. Salicylates are started at 80 mg per kg per day given every four hours and then altered to achieve a serum level of 20 to 40 mg per dl.

In patients who have evidence of carditis, steroids are recommended to attempt to minimize the inflammation and ultimate scarring of the heart valves. Prednisone, 2 mg per kg per day, is given and the response monitored by ESR and CRP. These will return to normal by about two to three weeks and then the steroids are gradually withdrawn. It is important to monitor salicylate levels closely at this time as they are generally lower in the presence of steroids and may rise to toxic levels upon cessation of steroids. The exact explanation of this is not known. It may be due to an increase in salicylate catabolism by steroids.

Some degree of rebound activation frequently occurs with withdrawal of steroids, including mild elevations of C-reactive protein, arthralgias, and occasionally low-grade fevers. These can usually be controlled with salicylates and bedrest.

Prophylaxis

Prevention of the First Attack

Essentially, prevention of the first attack of acute rheumatic fever, or primary prevention, depends upon proper treatment of streptococcal pharyngitis as discussed in the previous section.

With the discovery of genetic markers that are closely linked to the disease (883 and 256 B-cell alloantigens), it should be possible to screen families of known patients to identify susceptible individuals. Until such time as a streptococcal vaccine can be developed that will not sensitize recipients to cross-reactive antigens, these individuals could receive prophylaxis with antibiotics.

Recurrences

Once a patient has had rheumatic fever, susceptibility to recurrences appears to persist throughout life. While the recurrence rate definitely decreases with time after the first attack, there is still a substantial risk of recurrence after five years. With these attacks, the chances of permanent damage to involved heart valves increase.

Prevention of recurrences is equivalent to prevention of reinfection with group A streptococci. Penicillin prophylaxis may take the form of oral preparations, 125 mg twice a day, or monthly injections of benzathine penicillin, 1.2 million units. In penicillin-allergic individuals, sulfadiazine, 0.5 to 1 gm daily, is recommended. If a patient is allergic to both penicillin and sulfas, then either erythromycin or cephalexin may be used. It should be emphasized, however, that there are no long-term studies using either of these antibiotics as prophylactic agents, that as many as 6% to 10% of strains of group A streptococci in some areas may be resistant to erythromycin, and that up to 10% of individuals allergic to penicillins are also allergic to cephalosporins. There is no uniform agreement on duration of prophylaxis. Some recommend continuing to age 20 years, others for life.

Bacterial Endocarditis

Individuals who have damaged rheumatic heart valves must be protected by prophylactic antibiotics to prevent bacterial endocarditis during dental manipulations and certain kinds of surgical intervention. Indications and regimens are outlined in the section of this chapter that discusses endocarditis.

Although a considerable amount of information is known about acute rheumatic fever and the biology of group A streptococci, there are still significant gaps in our understanding of this disease process, particularly regarding the nature of the genetic predisposition and its effect on the immune response to streptococci. Preventing the disease by identifying susceptible individuals and preventing infection with the organism is the only practical approach to solving this major world health problem at the present time.

ANNOTATED BIBLIOGRAPHY

Endocarditis

American Heart Association Committee on Prevention of Bacterial Endocarditis. Prevention of bacterial endocarditis. Circulation 1977;56:139A–143A.
Current recommendations for prophylaxis against endocarditis.

Bisno AL, ed. Treatment of infective endocarditis. New York: Grune & Stratton, 1981.
A multiauthored text providing more detailed descriptions of medical and surgical therapy of patients with infective endocarditis.

Cannady PB Jr, Sanford JP. Negative blood cultures in infective endocarditis: a review. South Med J 1976;69:1420–1424.
Review of culture-negative endocarditis with useful advise about special microbiologic procedures and empiric treatment.

Davis RS, Strom JA, Frishman W, et al. The demonstration of vegetations by echocardiography in bacterial endocarditis. Am J Med 1980;69:57–63.
Thirty patients with endocarditis were studied by echocardiography. Demonstrable vegetations in 57% correlated with a higher incidence of heart failure and need for valve surgery.

Duma RJ, ed. Infections of prosthetic heart valves and vascular grafts: prevention, diagnosis and treatment. Baltimore: University Park Press, 1977.
A detailed account of prevention and treatment of infections of prosthetic heart valves and vascular grafts.

Everett ED, Hirschmann JV. Transient bacteremia and endocarditis prophylaxis: a review. Medicine 1977;56:61–77.
Review of the incidence of transient bacteremia associated with various procedures that may place the patient at risk for endocarditis.

Kaplan EL, Taranta AV, ed. *Infective endocarditis — an American Heart Association symposium*. AHA Monograph no. 52. Dallas: American Heart Association, 1977.
An authoritative monograph reviewing specific aspects of endocarditis in which there is new knowledge.

Phair JP, ed. Recent topics in endocarditis. I. Prog Cardiovasc Dis 1979;22:135–204.
Summary of current state of knowledge of the immunology and surgical treatment of endocarditis as well as review of the problems of prosthetic valve endocarditis and endocarditis in the drug addict.

Weinstein L, Schlesinger JJ. Pathoanatomic, pathophysiologic and clinical correlations in endocarditis. N Engl J Med 1974; 291:832–837, 1122–1126.
Review of the current concepts of the pathophysiology of endocarditis.

Wilson WR, ed. *Symposium on infective endocarditis* Mayo Clin Proc 1982; 57:1–95.
A thorough summary of the Mayo Clinic's extensive experience with this disease.

Myocarditis and Pericarditis

Gould K, Barnett JA, Sanford JP. Purulent pericarditis in the antibiotic era. Arch Intern Med 1974;134:923–927.
A review of 20 cases of purulent pericarditis stressing the importance of aerobic gram-negative rods and anaerobes as causes.

Hirschman SZ, Hammer GS. Coxsackievirus myopericarditis. A microbiological and clinical review. Am J Cardiol 1974;34:224–232.
A description of coxsackieviruses, their epidemiology and clinical manifestations, the difficulty in diagnosis, and a summary of therapy.

Klacsmann PG, Bulkley BH, Hutchins GM. The changed spectrum of purulent pericarditis. An 86-year autopsy experience in 200 patients. Am J Med 1977;63:666–673.
A summary of how the types of patients who develop pericarditis, sources of infection, and relative frequencies of different etiologic agents have changed from the preantimicrobial era to the antimicrobial era.

Montgomerie JZ, Lewis AJ, Fiala M, et al. Pericarditis — teaching conference, University of California, Los Angeles, and Harbor General Hospital, Torrance (specialty conference). West J Med 1975;122:295–309.
A series of presentations on hemodynamic and diagnostic features of pericarditis, viral pericarditis, tuberculous and fungal pericarditis, bacterial pericarditis, and parasitic causes of pericarditis.

Rubin RH, Moellering RC Jr. Clinical, microbiologic and therapeutic aspects of purulent pericarditis. Am J Med 1975;59:68–78.
A review of 26 patients with purulent pericarditis emphasizing the difficulty in making the diagnosis and the importance of host factors in the development of pericarditis.

Sainani GS, Dekate MP, Rao CP. Heart disease caused by coxsackievirus B infection. Br Heart J 1975;37:819–823.
A summary of the features and subsequent course of a group of patients with Coxsackie B virus.

Rheumatic Fever

Agarwal BL. Rheumatic heart disease unabated in developing countries. Lancet 1981;1:910–911.
The prevalence of rheumatic heart disease is discussed in terms of hospital admissions in India as compared with other developing countries as well as the United States and United Kingdom.

Kaplan EL. Prevention of rheumatic fever. Circulation 1977;55:1–4.
The prevention of both primary and recurrent attacks of rheumatic fever is discussed, including antibiotic recommendations for streptococcal upper respiratory infections and for prophylaxis.

Patarroyo ME, Winchester RJ, Vejerano A, et al. Association of a B-cell alloantigen with susceptibility to rheumatic fever. Nature 1979;278:173.
Description of a unique B-lymphocyte alloantigen that is strongly associated with rheumatic fever.

Read SE, Zabriskie JB. Immunologic concepts in rheumatic fever. In: Zabriskie JB, Engle MA, Villarreal Jr. H, eds. Clinical immunology of the heart. New York: John Wiley & Sons, 1981, pp. 51–88.
This chapter reviews the immunologic aspects of rheumatic fever, with emphasis on cross-reactive antigens in the heart and brain and group A streptococcal membrane. Hypothetical immune mechanisms in pathogenesis are discussed, as well as genetic factors that may predispose to these mechanisms.

Stollerman GH. Jones criteria (revised) for guidance in the diagnosis of rheumatic fever. Circulation 1965;32:664–668.
The criteria for the diagnosis of rheumatic fever.

Stollerman GH. Rheumatic fever and streptococcal infections. New York: Grune & Stratton, 1975.
A review of many aspects of rheumatic fever including epidemiology, microbiology, clinical aspects, and management and prevention.

11 INFECTIONS OF THE EAR, NOSE, AND THROAT

Marcoux J. André

Infections of the ears, nose, and throat are the most common illness in children and adolescents. Moreover, adults, and especially the elderly, often compromised in their immunologic defense mechanisms, may display unusual clinical pictures of common upper respiratory tract infectious problems. Relatively few bacterial pathogens and viruses are responsible for most infections at various anatomic sites.

OTITIS MEDIA

Etiology

The common organisms causing acute suppurative or bacterial otitis media are shown in Table 11.1. *Hemophilus influenzae* (non-b type) and *Streptococcus pneumoniae* are responsible for more than 50% of cases in children. The former, although at one time considered restricted to young children, is being isolated more often from older children and teenagers. Group A streptococci *(S. pyogenes)* occur in all age groups but represent less than 15% of isolates. Staphylococci and coliforms are uncommon pathogens in acute otitis media, although they may be isolated in the neonatal period.

Viral causes of acute nonsuppurative or serous otitis media include influenza, parainfluenza, adenovirus, and coxsackievirus. *Mycoplasma pneumoniae* and rarely, *Chlamydia trachomatis* also can cause otitis media. In chronic otitis media, *Staphylococcus aureus,* gram-negative aerobes such as *Escherichia coli, Proteus* organisms, and various anaerobic bacteria predominate.

Epidemiology

Otitis media is the most common infection requiring medical attention and antibiotic therapy in the pediatric age group, with the highest attack rate between 6 and 36 months of age. Disease is more likely to recur when the initial episode occurs during the first year of life. The prevalence of acute otitis media corresponds to that of viral upper respiratory tract infections, which are more common during the winter months. Without adequate treatment, a small percentage of cases of acute otitis media may evolve into a chronic process.

Pathophysiology

For acute suppurative otitis media there is usually a history of preceding viral upper respiratory tract infection. The resultant eustachian tube dysfunction creates increased negative pressure and aspiration of bacterial pathogens from the nasopharynx into the middle ear. Chronic otitis media is usually associated with perforation of the tympanic membrane and mastoiditis.

Clinical Manifestations

Otitis media is characterized by earache, fever, and hearing impairment in most patients. In infants, lethargy, irritability, feeding problems, and diarrhea may dominate the clinical picture. Vertigo, tinnitus, and nystagmus are observed occasionally. Chronic otitis media may be asymptomatic between exacerbations, which resemble acute otitis media and are usually as-

TABLE 11.1. Empiric Antibiotic Treatment Based on Presumptive Clinical Diagnosis of Upper Respiratory Tract Infections

		Antibiotic Treatment		
Clinical Problems	*Probable Etiologies*	*First Choice*	*Alternative*	*Comments*
External otitis	*Pseudomonas aeruginosa,* staphylococci, coliforms	Topical polymyxin B, or gentamicin, hydrocortisone, qid		Swimmer's ear Gentle debridement
Malignant external otitis	*P. aeruginosa*	Tobramycin, IV plus Ticarcillin, IV and topical therapy (above)		Elderly diabetics Bone involvement possible with cranial nerve palsies Surgical debridement as needed Mortality is high
Acute otitis media	*H. influenzae, S. pneumoniae, S. pyogenes, S. aureus*	Amoxicillin	TMP/SMZ or erythromycin plus sulfisoxazole or cefaclor	Tympanocentesis may be necessary; some strains of *H. influenzae* may be resistant to amoxicillin

sociated with ear drainage. Serous otitis media is characterized by less pain and a sensation of fullness in the ear in association with other symptoms of the common cold.

Diagnosis

Because it is such a common infection in children, otitis media should be suspected early in a child with fever. Adequate examination of the tympanic membrane is the key to diagnosis; the ear drum is inflamed, often bulging, with loss of a distinct light reflex, and may have a perforation allowing a purulent exudate to drain. Pneumatic otoscopy, if available, permits assessment of the mobility of the tympanic membrane and the presence of fluid in the middle ear cavity. In otitis media, reduced or lack of movement of the tympanic membrane occurs in contrast to a fluttering movement in a normal ear. The definitive diagnosis is made by tympanocentesis or myringotomy, although this is seldom performed. A Gram's stain and culture of the exudate obtained by this technique or with spontaneous perforation will determine etiology.

In serous otitis media, the tympanic membrane is usually less inflamed, although other signs noted above may be present. Bullous myringitis is classically associated with *Mycoplasma pneumoniae* infection but is uncommon.

Chronic otitis media is diagnosed clinically and etiology determined by aerobic and anaerobic cultures of the discharge through the perforated tympanic membrane or at the time of mastoid surgery.

Treatment

The presumptive antibiotic therapy for acute bacterial otitis media should cover both *H. influenzae* and *S. pneumoniae*. Amoxicillin, 40 mg per kg per day in three equal doses, is the treatment of choice. When penicillin allergy is present, trimethoprim, 8 mg per kg per day, plus sulfamethoxazole, 40 mg per kg per day (TMP/SMZ) in two doses; or a combination of erythromycin, 50 mg per kg per day plus sulfisoxazole, 150 mg per kg per day, in four equal doses may be used. These combinations or cefaclor, an oral cephalosporin, 40 mg per kg per day, in three doses, are also effective against beta-lactamase-producing strains of *H. influenzae*. Local decongestants and antihistamines are of doubtful value.

Treatment of otitis media caused by *M. pneumoniae* is erythromycin in children and erythromycin or tetracycline in adults. Serous otitis media usually is treated symptomatically with decongestants. For chronic otitis media and mastoiditis, surgery is required, with perioperative antimicrobial therapy based on cultures of the discharge.

Prognosis

Most children improve in 24 to 48 hours and therefore reevaluation is necessary at that time for possible changes in antibiotic therapy if no response is noted. Myringotomy or needle aspiration of the middle ear may be necessary to obtain specific microbiologic data in refractory cases.

Prophylaxis

Simple methods such as humidification of the house may help to prevent upper airway infections and secondarily, otitis media, by improving local upper respiratory defense mechanisms. Antibiotic prophylaxis in children with recurrent infections has had some success in high-risk populations (see Chapter 7). Pneumococcal vaccine has been shown to prevent episodes of otitis media due to pneumococcal strains included in the vaccine in children older than 2 years, but is not routinely used for this purpose.

OTITIS EXTERNA

Etiology

Pseudomonas aeruginosa is the most common pathogen isolated in otitis externa. *Staphyloccus aureus,* coagulase-negative staphylococci, diphtheroids, and coliforms may be responsible occasionally. Fungi that cause otitis externa include *Aspergillus fumigatus* and *A. niger.*

Epidemiology

External otitis is a frequent infection in swimmers and patients who insert foreign bodies in their ears (e.g., overuse of cotton swabs to clean the external ear canal).

Pathophysiology

Bacterial and fungal organisms invade locally through macerated epithelium caused by water in the external auditory canal or through superficial erosions of the epithelium caused by trauma. Allergic reactions to hair sprays, high humidity, and heat are other predisposing factors.

Clinical Manifestations

External otitis may be acute or chronic. Acute infection may produce a spectrum of symptoms from pruritus only to excruciating pain. Examination of the canal may be difficult because of severe pain, but usually reveals edema of the wall with partial to complete obstruction and a coating with moist or crusty exudate. In severe cases, marked swelling of the pinna and tender periauricular lymphadenopathy may be present. Systemic symptoms are rare. Chronic otitis externa usually produces less pain but more pruritic symptoms.

Diagnosis

The clinical picture is usually diagnostic. Associated otitis media should be ruled out if possible by proper examination of the tympanic membrane. Careful otoscopy permits visualization of excoriations of skin in the canal, and the exudate confirms the etiology.

Treatment

Topical ear drops containing an antibiotic such as polymyxin B, colistin, or gentamicin to assure adequate coverage against *Pseudomonas* should control the infectious process. A steroid (e.g., hydrocortisone) is usually combined with the antimicrobials to reduce the local inflammatory response. Severe swelling of the external ear canal is first treated with 5% Burow's solution applied to a gauze wick and inserted in the ear, after which the topical antibiotic and steroid may be given.

Systemic antimicrobial agents are necessary when there is clinical evidence of perichondritis or surrounding soft tissue cellulitis and should be chosen based on the organism cultured.

If underlying otitis media cannot be ruled out, systemic antibiotic therapy should also be given.

Prognosis

Acute otitis externa has an excellent prognosis in healthy individuals. Chronic otitis externa, often associated with dermatologic disorders, responds less favorably. Inadequately treated episodes may lead to the chronic form of the disease with stenosis of the ear canal.

Prophylaxis

When the problem is associated with swimming, ear plugs are beneficial. The hazards of foreign bodies placed in the ear canal should be emphasized, especially to children.

MALIGNANT EXTERNAL OTITIS

Etiology

Malignant, or fulminant, external otitis is usually caused by *P. aeruginosa*.

Epidemiology

The entity was described originally in elderly diabetic patients but it can affect children occasionally, especially when acute, localized, external otitis does not respond to topical treatment.

Pathophysiology

The presence of a microangiopathy of the skin overlying the temporal bone leads to poor local vascular perfusion in diabetics. This predisposes localized otitis externa to progress with a necrotizing inflammatory lesion invading surrounding cartilage and producing osteomyelitis of the temporal bone and base of the skull and mastoid. Involvement of several cranial nerves and meningitis can also occur.

Clinical Manifestations

The initial lesion resembles typical external otitis with no systemic involvement. The infection progresses, however, with increasing discomfort and local pain, periauricular cellulitis, and lymphadenopathy, although fever may be minimal. Palsies of facial and other cranial nerves signify deep soft tissue and bony involvement of the skull.

Diagnosis

A diagnostic feature of the disease is the presence of granulation tissue within the external auditory canal at the junction of the bony and cartilaginous portions. Diagnostic clues to suspect malignant external otitis include the presence of severe intractable external otitis, isolation of *P. aeruginosa* from the ear discharge, a history of poorly controlled diabetes mellitus in an elderly patient, and the presence of pain and tenderness around the ear in the mastoid region. It is important to remember that in many cases the early signs and symptoms of the disease do not suggest its potentially lethal nature. Radiologic and radioisotope techniques confirm osteocartilaginous involvement in advanced cases.

Treatment

Effective medical treatment implies early diagnosis and a synergistic antibiotic combination regimen with an aminoglycoside and a semisynthetic penicillin to assure optimal killing of *P. aeruginosa*. Tobramycin (gentamicin), 5 to 7.5 mg per kg per day in three equal doses, adjusted to maintain adequate serum levels, is recommended in combination with ticarcillin, (12 to 18 gm per day, or carbenicillin, 25 to 30 gm per day, in divided doses. Duration of therapy should be prolonged for six to eight weeks. Surgery should be considered early if neurologic complications are present or lateral sinus thrombosis suspected. The complication of pseudo-

TABLE 11.2. Empiric Antibiotic Treatment Based on Presumptive Diagnosis of Upper Respiratory Tract Infections

		Antibiotic Treatment		
Clinical Problems	*Probable Etiologies*	*First Choice*	*Alternatives*	*Comments*
Acute sinusitis	*S. pneumoniae*, *H. influenzae*, *anaerobes*, *S. aureus*, *Streptococcus* sp.	Amoxicillin	TMP/SMZ, cefaclor, dicloxacillin	Surgical drainage may be required
Chronic sinusitis	Anaerobes	Amoxicillin	Penicillin G, IV	Surgery often necessary
Acute mastoiditis	*H. influenzae*, *S. pneumoniae*, *S. pyogenes*, *S. aureus*	Amoxicillin	TMP/SMZ, cefaclor, dicloxacillin	Mastoidectomy if patient remains febrile after 48–72 hrs
Chronic mastoiditis	*S. aureus*, *P. aeruginosa*, coliforms Anaerobes	Cloxacillin plus tobramycin		Mastoidectomy Drainage Tympanoplasty Antibiotic therapy according to microbiologic information

monal meningitis should be treated as outlined in Chapter 9.

Prognosis

A striking increase in mortality (60% and greater) is reported when cranial nerve abnormalities or other deficits of the central nervous system are present. This decreases to less than 20% if no cranial nerve palsies are present. Relapses may occur, usually within one month following treatment. Close follow-up is therefore mandatory.

Prophylaxis

Aggressive treatment of external otitis media in diabetics should be instituted, with early systemic therapy if topical measures are ineffective.

MASTOIDITIS

Etiology

The organisms that cause acute mastoiditis are similar to those causing acute otitis media (Table 11.2).

Epidemiology

Acute mastoiditis was formerly a common complication of acute otitis media. With the introduction and appropriate use of effective antibiotics, it is seen rarely.

Pathophysiology

The natural history of untreated acute middle ear infections almost always includes an extension of the infectious process into the mastoid cells. Erosion and resorption of the bony partitions between mastoid air cells result in a large defect filled with purulent, infected material. Several potentially lethal complications with further extension of the infection can occur, including meningitis, subperiosteal abscess, lateral sinus thrombosis, and brain abscess.

Clinical Manifestations

A throbbing earache, profuse purulent otorrhea, and high fever are present in acute bacterial mastoiditis. There is marked tenderness over the mastoid process, with an erythematous swelling displacing the pinna inferiorly and laterally. Fluctuation may be present when a subperiosteal abscess develops.

Diagnosis

The diagnosis is made clinically. Otoscopy may reveal an intact but inflamed bulging ear drum or more commonly, a perforation through which purulent discharge is observed. Conductive hearing loss may be severe. Radiologic examination may show an increased density of the mastoid, and later a radiolucent abscess may be visualized. Drainage in the external ear canal, if present, may be stained and cultured for a definitive diagnosis.

Treatment

For children with acute mastoiditis secondary to progressive acute otitis media, therapy is directed against *H. influenzae* and *S. pneumoniae* as noted on page 156. For mastoiditis associated with chronic otitis media, broader antibiotic coverage against *S. aureus*, gram-negative enteric rods, and anaerobes may be necessary. A minimum of two weeks of therapy is satisfactory in most cases. When the convalescent stage is reached, simple mastoidectomy should be considered. If patients do not respond to treatment within a few days, especially those with chronic otitis media and mastoiditis, early surgery may be required.

A subperiosteal abscess requires immediate surgical incision and drainage and a complete mastoidectomy. If meningitis is suspected or proved, antibiotic therapy as outlined in Chapter 9 should be employed.

Prognosis

Complete resolution of mastoiditis should occur in two to three weeks in most patients. Those cases complicated by subperiosteal abscess formation, meningitis, or brain abscess have a much poorer prognosis.

Prophylaxis

Early and appropriate therapy of acute otitis media should prevent mastoiditis.

SINUSITIS

Etiology

Streptococcus pneumoniae and *H. influenzae* (non-b type) are the most common causes of sinusitis; staphylococci, *Streptococcus* sp., and gram-negative enteric rods are isolated much less often (Table 11.2). In acute maxillary sinusitis secondary to dental infections, various anaerobic organisms including *Bacteroides* sp., peptostreptococci, and fusobacteria are isolated. In chronic sinusitis, anaerobes are often present in association with gram-negative enteric organisms.

Viral organisms associated with the common cold syndrome also cause acute sinusitis. Fungal causes are very rare but *Candida* and *Aspergillus* sp. may cause sinusitis in immunocompromised hosts and *Rhizopus* sp. can cause sinusitis in diabetics with ketoacidosis.

Epidemiology

Acute sinusitis occurs most frequently during the colder months, usually as a complication of an acute viral upper respiratory tract infection. It is more common in adults than children since the latter do not have fully developed paranasal sinuses.

Chronic sinusitis may result from inadequately treated acute disease and in conditions predisposing to obstruction of the sinus openings (see below).

Pathophysiology

Most cases of acute sinusitis follow an episode of the common cold. Bacterial superinfection occurs as a consequence of impairment of the normal physiology of the mucociliary apparatus caused by the preceding viral infection. An acute inflammatory reaction is produced in the sinus mucosa with further obstruction to sinus drainage. Trauma, dental infections (maxillary sinusitis), nasal polyps, hypertrophied adenoids, congenital abnormalities (e.g., choanae atresia), and cystic fibrosis represent other predisposing conditions. In chronic disease, there is atrophy of the ciliated epithelium and colonization with various bacteria noted above.

Clinical Manifestations

Headache with pain over the involved sinus and nasal congestion with purulent nasal or postnasal discharge are the major features of sinusitis. Anosmia, or a foul taste or smell may also be noted by the patient. Fever is variably present, more commonly in children than adults. In maxillary sinusitis, a dentist is frequently consulted initially because of an aching pain in the front teeth. Inflammatory edema of the eyelids is associated with ethmoidal sinusitis, while swelling of the cheek and forehead represent complications of maxillary and frontal sinusitis, respectively.

Diagnosis

A purulent drainage may be seen below the middle turbinate (frontal, maxillary, or anterior ethmoidal sinuses) or above the middle turbinate (posterior ethmoidal, sphenoidal sinus). Tenderness on palpation over the frontal or maxillary sinuses may be elicited. Complete lack of light transmission through the frontal or maxillary sinuses is also good evidence for infection. The definitive diagnosis is made by x-ray examination, which usually demonstrates a thickened mucosal lining, complete opacification, or the presence of an air-fluid level in the involved sinus. Precise microbiologic diagnosis is usually not necessary; however, if a specific etiology is required, needle aspiration or surgical drainage of the infected sinus is performed and the material is stained and cultured both aerobically and anaerobically. This is indicated in very severe disease with complications or in sinusitis that does not respond to empiric antibiotic treatment.

Treatment

Symptomatic treatment consists of analgesics and nasal decongestants to reduce obstruction of the openings of the sinus and improve drainage. Empiric antibiotic therapy is similar to that for acute bacterial otitis media, with amoxicillin (or ampicillin) as the initial choice, and trimethoprim-sulfamethoxazole in penicillin-allergic patients. Combined sulfisoxazole and erythromycin and a cephalosporin are alternatives.

In chronic disease, where a more diverse group of organisms is possible, treatment should be based on the results of aspiration or surgical drainage. Acute exacerbations of chronic disease usually are caused by *S. pneumoniae* or *H. influenzae* and can be treated as acute sinusitis.

Prognosis

The prognosis is excellent in most cases that are treated appropriately. Chronic sinusitis may develop with inadequate treatment and in cases in which obstruction cannot be relieved. Surgical treatment (e.g., lavage, antrostomy, or the Caldwell-Luc operation) offers better results than medical therapy in the chronic form of the disease.

Prophylaxis

No specific preventive therapy for sinusitis is available.

PARAPHARYNGEAL AND RETROPHARYNGEAL INFECTIONS

Etiology

Anaerobic oropharyngeal flora (e.g., *Bacteroides melaninogenicus, B. oralis, Fusobacterium nucleatum,* peptostreptococci, and peptococci) are the major pathogens in parapharyngeal and retropharyngeal infections. Less commonly, various gram-negative enteric rods, staphylococci, and streptococci are isolated.

Epidemiology

These infections are relatively rare since treatment with antibiotics of predisposing infections is usually effective. Retropharyngeal abscess is seen almost exclusively in infants and young children.

Pathophysiology

Any infection of the pharynx, tonsils, nose, or parotid glands may be complicated by a parapharyngeal infection (peritonsillar abscess, pharyngomaxillary space infection, and masticator space infection). Infections of the nasopharynx or paranasal sinuses, dental infections, or traumatic laceration of the posterior pharyngeal mucosa may progress to a retropharyngeal abscess. The spaces infected by extension are only potential spaces created by the expanding lesion. There is initially an acute inflammatory response that produces a cellulitis that may progress to actual abscess formation with suppuration.

Clinical Manifestations

The patient appears acutely ill, with fever, local pain, trismus (due to irritation of the internal pterygoid muscle), and often bulging of the tonsil or lateral or posterior pharyngeal wall. Cervical swelling may also be present on the side affected with a pharyngomaxillary abscess. Dysphagia with drooling may occur, in addition to airway obstruction in severe cases.

Diagnosis

The diagnosis of a pharyngeal infection is strongly suspected clinically especially after various head and neck infections. X-ray examination, including plain films, and computerized tomographic scan, if available, may confirm the presence of an abscess by demonstrating marked thickening of the prevertebral soft tissues of the cervical region. Blood cultures may also be positive.

Treatment

Adequate surgical drainage must be performed quickly if loculated pus is present. This also provides material for Gram's stain and culture. Initial empiric antibiotic therapy is directed toward the anaerobic oropharyngeal flora. Intravenous doses of aqueous penicillin G, 10 to 20 million units per day, or clindamycin phosphate, 1800 mg per day, in penicillin-allergic patients, is recommended. An aminoglycoside, such as tobramycin or gentamicin, 5 to 7.5 mg per kg per day, and/or an antistaphylococcal drug may be necessary especially in an infection that has developed within a hospital setting. Specific therapy depends on the result of Gram's stain and culture of abscess material.

Prognosis

Early diagnosis is very important for prevention of serious complications. Mortality is increased with airway obstruction, septicemia, hemorrhage, or mediastinitis.

Prophylaxis

Early and appropriate treatment of ear, nose, and throat infections will prevent the development of retropharyngeal and parapharyngeal infections.

LUDWIG'S ANGINA

Etiology

The major pathogens involved in Ludwig's angina include the anaerobic mouth flora — *B. melaninogenicus, B. oralis, F. nucleatum,* peptostreptococci, and peptococci. Staphylococci, streptococci, and gram-negative enteric rods are isolated less commonly.

Epidemiology

Most submandibular space infections are secondary to dental extraction or a periapical abscess of a mandibular molar, especially in the setting of poor dental hygiene. Trauma, fractures of the mandible, foreign bodies, and lacerations of the floor of the mouth may also predispose to this infection.

Pathophysiology

Ludwig's angina is characterized by an acute inflammatory reaction that produces spreading cellulitis, usually without abscess formation, involving the tissue spaces of the floor of the mouth. Dental infection originating from the premolars and first molars usually spreads into the sublingual space, while infection from the second and third mandibular molars usually invades deeper into the submaxillary space. Untreated, the brawny cellulitis will progress to the parapharyngeal or pharyngomaxillary spaces (as described on pages 161–162), with possible extension to the major cervical blood vessels and mediastinum. Lymph nodes and salivary glands are usually not involved.

Clinical Manifestations

A history of lower molar toothache or recent dental extraction is often present. On examination, the patient is febrile and ill-looking, and there is indurated cellulitis of the submandibular area. Within the mouth, usually there is poor dental hygiene and the tongue is elevated and often protrudes. There is pain on palpation of the floor of the mouth, and motion of the neck is restricted. Dysphonia, trismus, and odynophagia with drooling may be present in severe cases, in addition to evidence of progressive airway obstruction with tachypnea, dyspnea, and stridor.

Diagnosis

Diagnosis of the established infection is made from the clinical history and physical examination. Early diagnosis should be suspected in a patient with previous dental problems or instrumentation, who has fever and pain in the submandibular area. If a fluctuant area is felt, direct needle aspiration with Gram's stain and culture of the specimen, both aerobically and anaerobically, will provide the etiology.

Treatment

The patient with Ludwig's angina should be managed in consultation with an otolaryngologist to ensure the maintenance of an adequate airway with frequent monitoring of the respiratory status. High doses of intravenous penicillin G, 10 to 20 million units per day, are begun empirically. A cephalosporin such as cefazolin, 1 gm intravenously every eight hours, or clindamycin phosphate, 600 mg intravenously every eight hours in adults, may be used in penicillin-allergic patients. If an aspiration or surgical specimen is available, a Gram's stain may demonstrate less common organisms such as gram-negative enteric rods or staphylococci, in which cases additional antimicrobial therapy may be added. Results of cultures may also modify subsequent antibiotic therapy.

Early elective tracheostomy is performed if there is progressive airway obstruction to avoid the necessity of emergency tracheostomy. Surgery is necessary if an abscess develops, and some surgeons still believe wide incision of the cellulitis reduces the induration and swelling.

Prognosis

Prior to antibiotic therapy there was a greater than 50% mortality rate for Ludwig's angina, but with appropriate antimicrobial therapy and preservation of the airway there is a good prognosis. An artificial airway is necessary in more than 30% of cases.

Prophylaxis

Proper dental hygiene and early treatment of dental infections should reduce complications of submandibular space infections.

PHARYNGITIS

Etiology

The major cause of bacterial pharyngitis is *S. pyogenes* (group A beta-hemolytic streptococci). Other beta-hemolytic groups, including B, C, and G, may also cause an exudative pharyngitis, although the association is less well defined. *Corynebacterium diphtheriae* is an uncommon cause today but should always be considered. *Neisseria gonorrhoeae* and *N. meningitidis* may also produce a usually mild pharyngitis. A syndrome described as Vincent's angina is caused by oropharyngeal anaerobes, predominantly fusobacteria and spirochetes.

Viral causes of pharyngitis include those producing the common cold syndrome (rhinovirus, coronavirus), adenovirus, enteroviruses (coxsackie and echoviruses), herpesviruses (herpes simplex, cytomegalovirus, Epstein-Barr virus), influenza, and parainfluenza viruses. *Mycoplasma pneumoniae* also commonly causes pharyngitis.

Epidemiology

Most episodes of pharyngitis occur during the colder, damper months and are of viral origin. *Mycoplasma pneumoniae* infections tend to follow the same epidemiologic pattern as viral infections.

Bacterial pharyngitis and tonsillitis occur most often in children and young adults. Particular strains of *S. pyogenes* cause pharyngeal infections with the possible sequela of rheumatic fever. It is not unusual for close contacts of patients with a streptococcal sore throat to be asymptomatic carriers of *S. pyogenes*.

Beta-hemolytic streptococci groups C and G have caused epidemics of pharyngitis similar to those caused by group A, whereas group B disease appears to be sporadic.

Gonococcal pharyngitis or the asymptomatic carrier state is a disease primarily of women and male homosexuals. In disseminated gonococcal infection, pharyngeal infection is often present. Pharyngitis caused by *N. meningitidis* is not necessarily associated with meningitis.

Pharyngitis caused by adenovirus is often accompanied by conjunctivitis and is common in children. The infectious mononucleosis syndrome with pharyngitis is usually caused by Epstein-Barr virus (EBV) and is common in the adolescent and young adult population.

Pathophysiology

Viruses causing the common cold syndrome initially infect the nasal epithelium and subsequently spread to the pharynx. Other viruses, including adenoviruses and enteroviruses, invade pharyngeal tissue directly. The EBV and cytomegalovirus that cause the infectious mononucleosis syndrome not only involve upper respiratory tract tissues but disseminate through other organs in the body.

Streptococcus pyogenes strains causing pharyngitis possess an adherence factor in the surface antigens that is responsible for the affinity of these organisms to human mucous membrane-specific receptors. Resistance to infection in the pharynx, as in other mucosal surfaces, is provided by the resident bacterial flora, an imbalance in which may enable *S. pyogenes* to colonize and multiply.

In diphtheria, the organism rarely invades tissue but produces a toxin that diffuses into surrounding tissues and produces a cytotoxic effect by inhibiting protein synthesis. The local reaction of the toxin causes necrosis of epithelial cells and a collection of fibrin, polymorphonuclear leukocytes, and bacilli that forms a membrane on the tonsil and adjacent pharynx. This may extend down to the larynx. Removal of the membrane leaves a raw, bleeding surface. Other manifestations of diphtheria result from the toxin affecting the heart (myocarditis), nervous system (cranial nerve and peripheral neuropathy), and kidneys.

Clinical Manifestations

Viral pharyngitis usually causes mild to moderately severe pain and erythema of the throat with tender cervical lymphadenopathy and moderate fever. In infectious mononucleosis, the symptoms and signs are often more severe, with a tonsillar exudate and occasionally grossly enlarged tonsils that may cause airway obstruction or dysphagia. In acute streptococcal disease, general symptomatology including high fever, rigors, malaise, headache, nausea, and vomiting is more common than in viral pharyngitis. There is tender cervical lymphadenopathy and marked erythematous swelling of the soft palate and posterior pharynx, with exudate in the tonsillar crypts.

With diphtheritic pharyngitis, the patient may appear extremely ill without a high fever. Marked cervical lymphadenopathy and soft tissue swelling of the neck may produce the so-called "bull" neck. The pharynx and palate in diphtheria are usually covered with a gray, necrotic membrane that may extend downward and cause varying degrees of respiratory impairment. Patients with gonococcal and meningococcal pharyngitis usually have mild symptoms with slight erythema of the pharynx.

Mycoplasma pneumoniae pharyngitis resembles viral pharyngitis clinically.

Diagnosis

The major problem in diagnosis in most cases is differentiating between a treatable bacterial pharyngitis and a viral pharyngitis. Clinical findings alone, although helpful, should be supplemented with throat cultures to establish the diagnosis primarily of group A beta-hemolytic streptococcal disease. Although these organisms can be isolated from asymptomatic carriers, they are usually present only in small numbers in these patients. Therefore in a clinical setting compatible with streptococcal disease, a positive culture is significant.

Early diagnosis of diphtheria is critical. Laboratory personnel should be forewarned of a possible case of diphtheria so that they can examine stained throat swabs for rapid presumptive diagnosis and also inoculate the appropriate media. After isolation of a diphtheria isolate, the toxigenicity of the strain should be confirmed.

Thayer-Martin plates for throat cultures should be used if *N. gonorrhoeae* is suspected.

Viral isolation is not routinely done but should be attempted if facilities are readily available and especially in unusual clinical presentations. Although usually not helpful in the management of specific cases, the culture information will often be useful epidemiologically. Serologic studies may also be used for the diagnosis of adenovirus, cytomegalovirus, EBV, and influenza virus. *Mycoplasma pneumoniae* is usually diagnosed on the basis of complement fixation test, cold agglutinins, and/or culture (although two to three weeks are usually required for culture growth of the organism).

Treatment

Viral pharyngitis requires symptomatic therapy only with analgesics and gargling with warm saline as required. Severe pharyngitis and tonsillitis in infectious mononucleosis are also treated only symptomatically, although high-dose prednisone, 80 mg per day over a few weeks has been used in infection complicated by severe extrapharyngeal disease (hemolytic anemia, thrombocytopenia, or central nervous system involvement).

Bacterial pharyngitis requires specific antimicrobial therapy. For *S. pyogenes,* one intramuscular injection of benzathine penicillin G, 1.2 million units in adults and 600,000 units in children, still offers the best results because of prolonged therapeutic levels of penicillin without the necessity of patient compliance to complete an oral course. The alternative and usual treatment is penicillin V, 500 mg every eight hours in adults, or 20 mg per kg per day in children, for 10 days. A 10-day course results in eradication of the streptococci from the pharynx in almost all patients and prevents relapse and the sequela of rheumatic fever. In penicillin-allergic patients, erythromycin, 2 gm per day in adults, or 30 to 50 mg per kg per day in children, is the best alternative, although an oral cephalosporin may be used if no cross-hypersensitivity exists with penicillin. Initiation of therapy within seven days of the onset of group A beta-hemolytic streptococcal pharyngitis will prevent the development of rheumatic fever.

The treatment of diphtheria requires neutralization of the toxin causing the disease manifestations and eradication of the organism to prevent toxin production and eliminate infectivity. In severe diphtheria, antitoxin, 40,000 to 80,000 units, is given, half the dose by slow (one-hour) infusion intravenously and the remainder intramuscularly. In less severe disease, 40,000 units can be given intramuscularly. Since the antitoxin is derived from horse serum, the patient should be pretested for hypersensitivity by administration of a 1:10 dilution of the antitoxin intradermally and to the conjunctival sac. If the results are positive, the patient must be desensitized by gradually increasing increments of antitoxin under the guidance, preferably, of a clinical allergist. For eradication of the organism, erythromycin 2 gm per day in adults, or 40 mg per kg per day in children, given orally or initially intravenously, is the preferred treatment. An alternative is aqueous procaine penicillin G, 600,000 units intramuscularly every 12 hours, or 1 million units every 4 hours intravenously for two weeks.

Gonococcal pharyngitis is treated effectively with intramuscular procaine penicillin G, 4.8 million units, in combination with probenecid, 1 gm orally, or tetracycline, 500 mg every six hours for five days. Trimethoprim-sulfamethoxazole, nine tablets once daily for five days, is also adequate. Single-dose treatments with ampicillin, amoxicillin, or spectinomycin are inadequate for pharyngitis or asymptomatic pharyngeal carriage. If the patient is infected with a beta-lactamase-producing organism, multiple-dose regimens of intramuscular spectinomycin, cefoxitin, or oral trimethoprim-sulfamethoxazole may be tried.

The treatment of streptococcal pharyngitis caused by other groups (B, C, and G) consists of oral treatment as outlined for group A beta-hemolytic streptococcal strains.

Tetracycline, 500 mg every six hours, or erythromycin, 250 to 500 mg every six hours for seven days, is effective in shortening the duration of *M. pneumoniae* infection.

Prognosis

Viral pharyngitis is usually a transient illness with no complications. It may predispose to bacterial superinfection. Infectious mononucleosis caused by EBV may have severe extrapulmonary complications including thrombocytopenia, hemolytic anemia, diverse neurologic sequelae, hepatitis, and splenic rupture.

In group A beta-hemolytic streptococcal pharyngitis, 10% to 20% of children still have a positive throat culture for *S. pyogenes* after a course of oral therapy. One of the major reasons for this is poor compliance. A culture of the throat after a 10-day course of therapy is therefore recommended. If the cultures are positive, a second course of oral therapy may be given or, preferably, intramuscular benzathine penicillin G. The latter is considered virtually 100% effective. Recurrent streptococcal sore throats in several family members always raise concerns regarding an asymptomatic carrier who is seeding the organism to susceptible members. If such a person is identified and successfully treated, the frequency of infections may be reduced. Other contacts outside the family may also be carriers, however, and in many instances by the time a concerted effort is directed toward identifying such a person, no further infections are experienced. Tonsillectomy does not appear to reduce the number of streptococcal infections, although ones that do occur may be clinically less severe.

Unsuspected diphtheria has a high mortality rate, but even with diagnosis and treatment the mortality rate still approaches 5% because of toxic myocarditis and polyneuritis. These complications are usually secondary to severe pharyngeal diphtheria. Myocarditis tends to occur one or more weeks after the onset of pharyngitis, whereas polyneuritis occurs several weeks after the onset of disease.

After treatment of gonococcal pharyngitis, follow-up cultures must be taken.

Mycoplasma pneumoniae pharyngitis has an excellent prognosis, although extrapharyngeal disease may be associated with a wide variety of potentially serious complications (see Chapter 12).

Prophylaxis

No specific preventive measures exist for viral pharyngitis. For group A streptococcal disease, monthly intramuscular benzathine penicillin, 1.2 million units for adults, and 600,000 units for children, oral daily administration of penicillin V, 250 mg twice daily, or a sulfonamide, 1 gm per day, is recommended for patients to prevent recurrence of rheumatic fever. The duration of such continuous prophylaxis is now considered a matter of judgment depending upon exposure to *S. pyogenes,* the presence or not of rheumatic valvular disease, and the endemicity of rheumatic fever. Generally it is continued for at least five years following rheumatic fever, but beyond this it is difficult to make specific recommendations.

For diphtheria, active immunization with diphtheria toxoid, beginning in childhood, with booster immunizations every 10 years thereafter, is recommended (see Chapter 8).

ACUTE EPIGLOTTITIS

Etiology

Hemophilus influenzae type b causes the majority of cases of acute epiglottitis in children and adults. Very rarely, *H. parainfluenzae, H. aphrophilus, S. pneumoniae,* and *S. aureus* are the causative agents.

Epidemiology

Although primarily a disease of young children (1 to 5 years of age), epiglottitis is being diagnosed more frequently in adults. No seasonal predilection is observed.

Pathophysiology

Epiglottitis is characterized by a rapidly progressive inflammation of any portion of the supraglottic larynx, but especially the epiglottis, which becomes swollen and cherry red. Respiratory obstruction of sudden onset causing death from asphyxia is the main complication. Septicemia is commonly present.

Clinical Manifestations

The prodromal stage is of short duration (often less than 12 hours) and initial symptoms are usually mild. Over a short period of time, however, the patient complains of a severe sore throat and appears anxious and ill, with a high fever. Infants and children are often unable to swallow fluids. A sign of major significance, especially in children, is the onset of respiratory difficulty, which may progress to complete airway obstruction in a very short time if proper treatment is not instituted. Typically, the child is observed sitting up leaning forward with neck extended trying to get air through the swollen epiglottis. Accessory respiratory muscles are used trying to overcome the laryngeal obstruction. "Hot-potato voice" is typical. Adults are usually very anxious and complain of severe dysphagia with drooling. In adults, cervical swelling is reported more frequently than children, and signs of airway obstruction are less commonly noted.

Diagnosis

It is extremely important to suspect acute epiglottitis in any patients, especially children, with upper airway obstruction and acute respiratory difficulties. A presumptive diagnosis is based on the clinical picture and the definitive diagnosis is confirmed by examination of the epiglottis. Inspection of the oropharynx with a tongue blade may permit direct inspection of the supraglottic area, but represents a definite and potentially lethal hazard to an already compromised larynx. Intubation or tracheostomy in suspected cases is a prerequisite before confirmatory inspection or laboratory investigations. A lateral cervical radiograph may show characteristic signs but again, an adequate airway must be assured first. Bacteremia with *H. influenzae* is documented in 70% of cases when blood for cultures is drawn prior to antibiotic administration. Differential diagnoses include diphtheria (a pseudomembrane may be visualized), angioneurotic edema, and foreign body aspiration. Retropharyngeal and peritonsillar abscesses may also compromise the airway.

Treatment

A team approach including a pediatrician or internist, an anesthetist, and an otolaryngologist will assure an optimal result. The primary concern is to provide an adequate airway and administer appropriate antimicrobial therapy. Nasotracheal intubation is generally preferred to tracheostomy by most centers because of the usual rapid response of the underlying disease to antimicrobial agents. Intubation is done, if possible, in the operating room.

Antimicrobial therapy should include a regimen effective against *H. influenzae* strains (including beta-lactamase-producing strains). A combination of intravenous ampicillin, 200 to 400 mg per kg per 24 hours, and chloramphenicol, 100 mg per kg per 24 hours, is the treatment of choice until susceptibilities are known. In penicillin-allergic patients, chloramphenicol alone, or when a staphylococcal infection is suspected, cefamandole, 100 mg per kg per 24 hours, can be used. Therapy is usually continued for seven to ten days because of concomitant bacteremia. Supportive therapy including close nursing care, high-humidity environment, and intravenous fluid administration are essential.

Prognosis

Epiglottitis is a life-threatening disease that if recognized early has a good prognosis. Death by asphyxia will occur when a diagnosis is missed or improper maneuvers are executed that jeopardize the airway.

Prophylaxis

No specific measures to prevent epiglottitis are available.

HERPANGINA

Etiology

Specific serotypes of coxsackievirus A and less commonly coxsackievirus B cause herpangina (Table 11.3).

Epidemiology

Herpangina usually occurs epidemically in children from 3 to 10 years of age during the summer months.

Pathophysiology

The transmission of coxsackievirus is primarily by the fecal-oral route, although spread through respiratory secretions may also occur. Multiplication of viruses occurs in the epithelial cells and lymphoid tissue of the pharynx and intestine, producing viremia with spread of the virus to other tissues. Occasionally, skin and palmar lesions will accompany mouth lesions, a syndrome that is called hand-foot-and-mouth disease.

TABLE 11.3. Infectious Viral Oral Ulcerations

Clinical Entities (Etiology)	*Characteristics*	*Comments*
Acute primary herpetic gingivostomatitis (H. simplex virus type 1)	Mostly in infants; cluster of tiny vesicles → shallow ulcers (≤0.5 cm in diameter) with well demarcated inflammatory margin on gums, lips, buccal mucosa, palate, tongue, floor of the mouth Typical histology	Spontaneous resolution after 1–3 wks, supportive treatment, no steroids
Recurrent intraoral ulcers (H. simplex virus type 1)	Ulcers on fixed mucosa (hard palate, gingival, alveolar ridges) mainly	Same To be differentiated from recurrent aphthous ulcers
Varicella, chickenpox (VZ virus)	Much like herpetic ulcers Typical exanthem	Avoid salicylates (Reye's syndrome in children)
Zoster (VZ virus)	Typical herpetic ulcers, localization depending on ganglia involved (gasserian, geniculate, glossopharyngeal, vagus)	Mainly supportive Vidarabine, IV in selected disseminated forms
Herpangina (coxsackie A-16)	Enanthema on anterior pillar of fauces, tonsils, and soft palate	Healing without sequelae within 1 wk
Hand-foot-and-mouth disease (coxsackie A-16, 5, 10)	Small vesicles and ulcers on soft palate, gingiva, and tongue Identical lesions on the hands and feet	Supportive, complete resolution in 8–10 d

Clinical Manifestations

Herpangina is characterized by an acute febrile illness with lesions present on the anterior pillar of the fauces, tonsils, pharynx, and soft palate. Small 1- to 2-mm vesicles surrounded by an erythematous halo can be visualized in these areas of the mouth, followed by superficial ulcerations after the vesicles break. Dysphagia, headaches, and meningismus may be present. The disease generally lasts from five to seven days.

Diagnosis

The diagnosis is based on clinical findings, depending principally on the appearance of the mouth lesions. For epidemiologic purposes, herpangina can be confirmed by isolation of the virus from the throat or stools in the majority of cases.

Treatment

Symptomatic treatment of herpangina with analgesia and saline gargles can be prescribed.

Prognosis

No serious sequelae occur with herpangina.

Prophylaxis

No prophylactic measures are available.

ACUTE HERPETIC GINGIVOSTOMATITIS

Etiology

Herpes simplex virus type 1 (HSV-1) causes 80% to 90% of cases of herpetic gingivostomatitis, with the remainder caused by HSV-2 (Table 11.3).

Epidemiology

Acute gingivostomatitis usually represents the primary manifestation of invasion with herpes simplex virus in a susceptible host and is seen mainly in children from 6 months to 5 years of age. In the adolescent and young adult population, primary oral herpes infection occurs usually as acute pharyngitis with or without tonsillitis, which may be difficult to distinguish from an acute streptococcal pharyngitis. In most patients, however, primary oropharyngeal herpes is asymptomatic.

Pathophysiology

The source of infection is either a patient with an active herpes infection or an asymptomatic shedder of the virus. The virus invades the epithelial cells at the site of entry and produces a localized primary lesion (cold sore) or several lesions, a gingivostomatitis or pharyngitis. During the initial infection, the virus migrates by way of sensory neurons to the sensory ganglion of the trigeminal nerve where it enters a latent phase. Activation of the virus as a result of precipitating factors, such as fever or psychologic stress, can result in reactivation of the virus with migration to the skin and result in recurrent disease (e.g., herpes labialis). From a primary site, the infection can be spread by direct inoculation to other areas. Pathologically, the lesion is characterized by multinucleated giant cells and intranuclear inclusions in epithelial cells.

Clinical Manifestations

Abrupt onset of fever, general malaise, and irritability precede by one to three days the development of a sore mouth in a child, who often refuses to eat or drink. Typical acute inflammatory changes of the gums are visible on examination. The gingivae are markedly reddened, swollen, and tender, and bleed very easily. Clusters of small vesicles become visible on the gums, lips, buccal mucosa, palate, tongue, and floor of the mouth. The vesicles then progress to tiny shallow ulcerations forming variable-sized, whitish plaques surrounded by erythema. Excessive salivation is frequent in children, and secondary perioral lesions may develop. Halitosis secondary to ulcerations and dehydration often is noted.

Diagnosis

The presumptive diagnosis of gingivostomatitis is based on clinical findings. It can be confirmed by isolation of the virus from the local lesions, by typical pathologic findings of multinucleated giant cells and intranuclear inclusion bodies on Tzanck smear (Giemsa stain) of a scraping of the base of a vesicle, and by serologic tests.

Treatment

Therapy is essentially supportive, relieving pain with analgesics and maintaining adequate hydration and nutrition. Frequent mouthwashes may be soothing and a topical anesthetic solution may facilitate oral hygiene and relieve pain partially. Intravenous fluids may be necessary if the child refuses to drink. Antibiotics are not indicated.

Prognosis

Gingivostomatitis is a self-limited disease of relatively short duration but it may vary considerably in severity. Most patients are free of symptoms after 10 to 14 days. Following the acute episode and after healing of lesions, some patients may continue to shed the virus for several weeks.

Prophylaxis

No specific preventive measures are available.

VINCENT'S SYNDROME

Etiology

The etiology of Vincent's syndrome is probably multifactorial. *Fusobacteria* sp. and oral spirochetes have been implicated as the major pathogens, but other oral bacteria, especially anaerobes, may also be important (Table 11.4).

Epidemiology

This syndrome is seen more commonly in malnourished adolescents and adults in economically underdeveloped countries.

TABLE 11.4. Infectious Bacterial Oral Ulcerations

Clinical Entities (Etiology)	*Characteristics*	*Comments*
Odontogenic infections (oral flora)	Presence of chronic alveolar abscess or odontogenic space abscess Ulcer on alveolar ridge near mucobuccal fold or palate Abnormal x-ray of teeth	Endodontic therapy or extraction
Acute necrotizing ulcerative gingivitis (ANUG) (Anaerobic flora and spirochetes)	Necrotic ulcerations of tips of the interdental papillae; grayish-white pseudomembrane with raw bleeding surface underneath	Oral penicillin Frequent oral rinsing (3% hydrogen peroxide solution) Careful debridement
Acute necrotizing ulcerative mucositis (ANUM) (Anaerobic flora and spirochetes)	More severe than ANUG Debilitated patient	Same as for ANUG Poor prognosis
Syphilis (*T. pallidum*)	Frequently painful, shallow 0.5- to 2-cm ulcer, reddish-brown, with copper-colored halo (lip, tip of tongue, tonsillar region) Tender cervical lymphadenopathy Specific positive serology	Benzathine penicillin G, 2.4×10^6 U IM

Pathophysiology

Poor dental and oral hygiene results in gingival ischemia secondary to capillary stasis, which leads to gingival necrosis. This area then becomes secondarily infected with oral anaerobes, including fusobacteria and spirochetes. In addition to gingivitis, the mucosa of the pharynx and tonsils may be involved (Vincent's angina).

Clinical Manifestations

Various names have been applied to Vincent's syndrome when it involves different parts of the oropharynx. When the gingivae only are affected it is known as trench mouth, Vincent's infection, ulceromembranous gingivitis, or acute necrotizing ulcerative gingivitis (ANUG). When it involves the whole mouth it is known as Vincent's stomatitis or acute necrotizing ulcerative mucositis (ANUM). When it is complicated by involvement of the pharynx or tonsils, it is called Vincent's angina. Vincent's gingivitis (ANUG) causes bleeding and ulcerations of the interdental papillae and gums. Fever and marked halitosis are usually present.

Diagnosis

The clinical diagnosis is based on physical examination. Microscopic examination of a smear from the base of the ulcerative lesions will reveal the typical fusospirochetal flora.

Treatment

Hydrogen peroxide, 3% solution, mouthwashes, and systemic antibiotics for 7 to 10 days are recommended for acute cases. Penicillin V, tetracycline, or metronidazole may be used with satisfactory results. Dental care should be provided after remission to prevent chronic periodontal disease.

Prognosis

The prognosis of Vincent's syndrome is generally good for the acute disease. Rarely, complications such as a severe necrotizing gangrenous lesion of the mouth (noma) may occur.

TABLE 11.5. Infectious Fungal Oral Ulcerations

Clinical Entities (Etiology)	*Characteristics*	*Comments*
Oral moniliasis (*C. albicans*)	Small, soft white plaques resembling milk curds Solitary to diffuse involvement of all mucosal surfaces Raw, bleeding surface underneath	Discontinue broad-spectrum antibiotics as necessary Nystatin, mouthwash or vaginal suppositories Ketoconazole in chronic mucocutaneous disease
Histoplasmosis (*H. capsulatum*)	Large ulceration (≥2 cm) of tongue, palate, epiglottis, and larynx Evidence of disseminated extrapulmonary disease Typical histology Positive specific serology and culture	Amphotericin B

Prophylaxis

Proper nourishment and good oral hygiene will prevent the infection.

ORAL CANDIDIASIS

Etiology

Strains of *Candida albicans* and related species can cause oral candidiasis (Table 11.5).

Epidemiology

Oral candidiasis is a relatively common infection in specific clinical situations: oral candidiasis (thrush) of the newborn of a mother with vaginal candidiasis; patients receiving broad-spectrum antibiotics; the compromised host as a result of underlying disease or immunosuppressive therapy (corticosteroids, cytotoxic drugs); in association with metabolic diseases (diabetes mellitus, hypoparathyroidism, Addison's disease); or in patients with specific cell-mediated immunoincompetence (AIDS).

Pathophysiology

Candida albicans is normally present at a low inoculum in the normal oral flora. As a result of the various epidemiologic factors alluded to above, the organisms may proliferate in the mouth and cause a spectrum of disease ranging from an inflammatory reaction alone with atrophic mucosa to submucosal penetration by ulcers produced in association with other infections such as herpes or certain cytotoxic drugs. Pseudomycelia are usually present in candidiasis and the curdlike white patches seen in many cases consist of the organism, bacterial flora, squamous epithelial cells, and polymorphonuclear leukocytes. The patches may be quite adherent to the underlying mucosa.

Clinical Manifestations

Oral candidiasis (thrush) is characterized by numerous white, elevated patches that resemble coagulated milk on the tongue, throat, palate, and buccal mucosa. When scraped, the mucosa usually bleeds. An acute atrophic form of disease occurs involving the tongue, which is painful and demonstrates inflammation only. Candidae may also cause only a localized inflammation at the corners of the mouth (cheilitis). Esophageal candidiasis is characterized by retrosternal pain and dysphagia.

Diagnosis

The diagnosis is based on clinical findings but can be substantiated by examining a smear of the white patches and noting pseudomycelia and yeast forms.

Culture is not diagnostic because of the presence of *Candida* organisms in normal oral flora. Esophageal candidiasis is diagnosed by characteristic findings on a barium swallow examination, esophagoscopy, and esophageal biopsy.

Treatment

Predisposing factors should be eliminated if possible. Oral nystatin, suspension or vaginal suppositories, is the drug of choice for thrush, 100,000 units four times per day in infants, and 500,000 units four times per day in adults. The suspension can be rinsed in the mouth and then swallowed, and the suppository held in the mouth until it dissolves. Therapy should be continued one week after clinical resolution of the lesions. If this fails, amphotericin B, taken orally, 50 mg in 30 to 60 ml of water three times daily, is usually very effective. It is rinsed in the mouth and then swallowed. Ketoconazole, a new antifungal agent, 200 mg daily, may also be used in cases not responding to topical therapy. For esophageal candidiasis that does not respond to topical therapy, intravenous amphotericin B may be used on a short-term basis (total dose, 250 mg), or ketoconazole, 200 mg once daily.

For chronic mucocutaneous candidiasis, prophylactic ketoconazole, 200 mg once daily, may be necessary.

Prognosis

The prognosis for oral candidiasis is excellent but in susceptible patients, especially immunosuppressed persons, it can progress to esophageal disease and subsequently disseminated disease. Chronic mucocutaneous candidiasis does not result in dissemination but can be painful and cosmetically devastating.

Prophylaxis

In patients who are receiving treatment predisposing to candidiasis, oral nystatin or ketoconazole has been given. On a short-term basis such prophylaxis may be effective, but the tendency to develop resistant candidal strains is significant in long-term prophylaxis.

ANNOTATED BIBLIOGRAPHY

Otitis Media

Bluestone CD. Current concepts in otolaryngology: otitis media in children: to treat or not to treat? N Engl J Med 1982;306(23):1399–1404.
General review with emphasis on etiology, pathogenesis, diagnostic methods of acute otitis media and chronic otitis media with effusion.

Klein JO. Management of acute and chronic otitis media. Curr Clin Topics Infect Dis 1981;2:278–294.
Overview of this common infectious problem, considering pathogenesis, clinical manifestations, microbiology, and management.

Schwartz RH. Bacteriology of otitis media: a review. Otolaryngol Head Neck Surg 1981;89:444–450.
A review of the microbiology of acute otitis media with effusion. Methods of specimen collection are reviewed. The role of *Hemophilus influenzae* in older children is emphasized.

Malignant External Otitis

Chandler JR. Malignant external otitis. Laryngoscope 1968;78:1257–1294.
Original paper by Chandler describes particularly the etiology, pathogenesis, diagnosis, and treatment of this serious infection. Eleven cases are presented.

Dinapoli RP, Thomas JE. Neurologic aspects of malignant external otitis; report of three cases. Mayo Clin Proc 1971;46:339–344.
Fatal neurologic complications are described in detail, as is differential diagnosis.

Mastoiditis

Ginsburg CM, Ruddy R, Nelson JD. Acute mastoiditis in infants and children. Clin Pediatr 1980;19:549–553.
Review of clinical experiences in 57 children with acute mastoiditis (age 2 months to 12 years) in two medical centers in Dallas. Incidence of this infection has decreased but severity of complications is the same. Some form of surgical drainage is necessary in more than 70% of cases in addition to systemic antibiotic therapy.

Sinusitis

Clairmont AA, Per-Lee JH. Complications of acute frontal sinusitis. Am Fam Physician 1975;11(5):80–84.
Anatomic considerations reviewed to explain the physiopathology of the complications of acute frontal sinusitis.

Parapharyngeal and Retropharangeal Infections

Johnson JT, Tucker HM. Recognizing and treating deep neck infection. Postgrad Med 1976;59(6):95–100.
The anatomic relationship of head and neck spaces encourages spread of infection. Emergency hospitalization and management of patient with such a problem is discussed.

Ludwig's Angina

Patterson HC, Kelly JH, Strome M. Ludwig's angina: an update. Laryngoscope 1982;92:370–378.
Historical review, discussion of pathogenesis, and clinical presentation, bacteriology and therapy of this potentially lethal condition are described in 20 cases.

Pharyngitis

Schwartz RH, Wientzen RL Jr, Pedreira F, Feroli EJ, Mella GW, Guandolo VL. Penicillin V for group A streptococcal pharyngotonsillitis — a randomized trial of seven vs ten day's therapy. JAMA 1981;246(16):1790–1795.
Recent therapeutic experiences in treating streptococcal pharyngotonsillitis with oral penicillin during seven days (96 patients) or ten days (95 patients) revealed a greater failure rate (30/96 or 31%) in former group than in latter (17/95 or 18%). In spite of adequate treatment, persistence of streptococci in the throat after adequate therapy may be common.

Epiglottitis

Cherry JD. Acute epiglottitis, laryngitis and croup. Curr Clin Topics Infect Dis 1981;2:1–31.
Comprehensive review of this problem in children and adults including some review of literature. Differential diagnosis well exposed.
Hawkins DB, Miller AH, Sachs GB, Benz RT. Acute epiglottitis in adults. Laryngoscope 1973;83:1211–1220
Clinical review of cases observed at the Los Angeles County/University of Southern California Medical Center during a period of 10 years. An entity more common than generally realized in adults.

Herpangina

Oxman MN. Herpes stomatitis. In Braude AI, Davis CE, Fierer J, eds. Medical microbiology and infectious diseases, vol. 2 of The International Textbook of Medicine. Philadelphia: WB Saunders Co., 1981:860–880.

Vincent's Syndrome

Attebery HR. Vincent's infection. In Braude AI, Davis CE, Fierer J, eds. Medical microbiology and infectious diseases, vol. 2 of The International Textbook of Medicine. Philadelphia: WB Saunders Co., 1981:823–824.

Oral Candidiasis

Armstrong D. Fungal infections in the compromised host. In Rubin RH, Young LS, eds. Clinical approach to infection in the compromised host. New York: Plenum Medical Book Co., 1981:195–228.

12 INFECTIONS OF THE LOWER RESPIRATORY TRACT

Edward D. Ralph

Lower respiratory tract infections are a very common cause of morbidity and mortality in the community and within the hospital setting, and produce a spectrum of disease of mild to life-threatening severity. The different disease entities are as follows: acute tracheobronchitis; chronic bronchitis with or without acute exacerbations; bronchiectasis with or without acute exacerbations; pneumonia, classic bacterial or atypical (bacterial, viral, mycoplasmal, fungal, chlamydial, rickettsial); lung abscess; and empyema. Acute tracheobronchitis and chronic bronchitis are numerically the most common, but usually clinically the least severe.

TRACHEOBRONCHITIS

Etiology

The usual etiologic agents of acute tracheobronchitis (acute bronchitis) in patients without underlying chronic airway disease are as follows:

1. Viral
   - Rhinovirus
   - Coronavirus
   - Influenza
   - Parainfluenza
   - Adenovirus
2. Mycoplasma
   - *Mycoplasma pneumoniae*
3. Bacterial
   - *Bordetella pertussis*

Rhinoviruses and coronaviruses are the principal causes of the common cold syndrome of which tracheobronchitis is one manifestation. Specifically treatable nonviral organisms include *M. pneumoniae* and less commonly *B. pertussis* (whooping cough). Secondary infection of viral tracheobronchitis with bacteria that normally colonize the upper respiratory tract, such as *Streptococcus pneumoniae* and *Hemophilus influenzae,* is unusual. Hospital-acquired pathogens including *Staphylococcus aureus* and a diverse group of gram-negative enteric bacilli may also occasionally cause acute tracheobronchitis.

The condition described above should be distinguished from acute exacerbations in patients with chronic bronchitis, the etiology of which may or may not be infectious.

Epidemiology

Acute tracheobronchitis parallels the occurrence of viral upper respiratory tract and *M. pneumoniae* infections, which occur more frequently during the winter months. *Bordetella pertussis,* in contrast, appears to demonstrate no seasonal variation. The frequency of these illnesses declines with increasing age. Hospital-acquired acute tracheobronchitis usually occurs in debilitated patients, many of whom are intubated and mechanically ventilated.

Pathophysiology

After colonization of the upper respiratory tract, the viruses infect the lining epithelial cells of the tracheobronchial mucosa and cause an acute inflammatory reaction with edema, increased secretions, various degrees of desquamation of the epithelium, and impairment of the mucociliary stream.

Mycoplasma pneumoniae remains extracellularly attached to the respiratory epithelium but can produce similar pathologic changes as viruses. *Bordetella pertussis* also does not usually invade bronchial tissue but multiplies in the mucociliary stream, impairing function and producing inflammation of the bronchial tissues.

Clinical Manifestations

Tracheobronchitis secondary to a viral upper respiratory tract infection is associated with mild fever, cough, and the production of nonpurulent mucoid sputum and usually occurs after upper respiratory tract symptoms begin. A retrosternal burning sensation in the chest, aggravated by coughing, often occurs secondary to mucosal inflammation in the major airways. Severe tracheobronchitis may be associated with minimal hemoptysis, but more serious disease should be considered when a patient produces blood-stained sputum. Superinfection with bacterial pathogens is unusual but is inferred if the sputum becomes copious and purulent, and if there are more severe systemic manifestations but without radiologic evidence of pneumonia. *Mycoplasma pneumoniae* and especially *B. pertussis* infections are usually associated with illness that is more severe and persists longer than the viral syndromes (several weeks as opposed to usually less than a week). Classic pertussis is characterized by bouts of paroxysmal coughing followed by a "whoop" and often vomiting. The disease begins as an upper respiratory tract infection with no fever. In partially immune individuals who have been vaccinated, a short-lived illness with minimal paroxysms of coughing may occur.

Physical examination of a patient with tracheobronchitis may demonstrate upper respiratory tract signs of pharyngitis, cervical lymphadenopathy, and serous otitis. There are no specific pulmonary findings apart from wheezing when there is some degree of lower airway obstruction.

Diagnosis

The majority of cases of tracheobronchitis are diagnosed clinically as part of the common cold syndrome. For epidemiologic purposes, viral cultures of nasal, throat, or sputum specimens and serologic studies may be done to determine or confirm the presence of a specific viral illness in the community. In more severe and prolonged cases, culture and serologic diagnosis of *M. pneumoniae* is warranted (see Chapter 5) as well as nasopharyngeal cultures for *B. pertussis* if the clinical features suggests these diagnoses.

Chest x-ray examination is normal in a patient with no underlying lung disease, although in *B. pertussis* infection there may be accentuation of the bronchial markings in the lower lung zones.

A normal white blood cell count or leukopenia is usually seen in viral infections, mild leukocytosis (less than 15,000 mm^3) in *M. pneumoniae* infections, and marked absolute lymphocytosis in pertussis.

Treatment

Acute viral tracheobronchitis is treated symptomatically with fluids and analgesics as required. If bronchospasm is present, bronchodilators may also be given on a short-term basis.

For suspected or proved *M. pneumoniae* infection, a seven-day course of erythromycin or tetracycline, 1 to 2 gm daily, is usually effective, with response noted in 48 to 72 hours. Relapses can occur following a week's course of antibiotics and an additional two weeks of antibiotic treatment should be prescribed.

For *B. pertussis* infection, a two-week course of erythromycin, 1 to 2 gm daily, is given to reduce the patient's infectivity, although the antibiotics do not appear to affect the clinical course of the disease.

Bacterial infections are usually adequately treated with short courses of antibiotics (amoxicillin, tetracycline, trimethoprim/sulfamethoxazole, or erythromycin). Treatment of hospitalized patients who develop nosocomial gram-negative tracheobronchitis depends upon susceptibility testing, and is similar to that of pneumonia (see Table 12.4).

Prognosis

The prognosis is excellent for tracheobronchitis associated with viral and *M. pneumoniae* infections, and usually the illness resolves within one to two weeks. Progression to bronchopneumonia is unusual and the prognosis then relates to the latter disease. Pertussis is more serious, with greater frequency of complications including pneumonia, atelectasis, bronchiectasis, and cerebral hemorrhage.

Prophylaxis

Prevention of viral respiratory infection is restricted to that of influenza, with yearly administration of vaccine or amantadine to patients at high risk (see Chapter 8). Pertussis vaccine (see Chapter 8) given early in the first year of life to prevent whooping cough loses its efficacy rapidly, resulting in increased susceptibility in the teenage and adult years. Because of this diminished immunity, contacts of patients with pertussis who are proved to be culture-positive in the nasopharynx may be treated prophylactically with 1 to 2 gm of erythromycin per day for a total of 14 days.

CHRONIC BRONCHITIS

Etiology

Chronic bronchitis is an illness characterized by chronic cough and expectoration of sputum for at least three months of the year for more than two successive years. It probably has a multifactorial etiology, the most important causes being cigarette smoking and other air pollutants, with genetic predisposition and infection being of secondary importance. The actual role of microorganisms such as *S. pneumoniae, H. influenzae, H. parainfluenzae, Branhamella catarrhalis,* normal oropharyngeal flora, *M. pneumoniae,* and viruses causing the disease and producing exacerbations is not known.

Epidemiology

Chronic bronchitis is a common disorder in temperate climates with cold, damp winters. It most frequently affects older patients, probably as a result of their prolonged exposure to various air pollutants.

Pathophysiology

After extended exposure, inhaled irritants produce an inflamed mucosa; this is associated with hypertrophy of the mucous glands, with excessive secretions and functional impairment of the mucociliary stream. This results in a reduced ability to clear inhaled particulate matter, including microorganisms. Therefore a larger inoculum of oropharyngeal organisms resides in the tracheobronchial tree of chronic bronchitics, which is in contrast to the relatively sterile tracheobronchial tree of healthy individuals.

It is postulated that the presence of bacteria may produce additional inflammation and aggravate the above pathophysiologic changes. In addition to the chronic effect of microorganisms, acute infections with these may lead to clinical exacerbations of chronic bronchitis with further impairment of respiratory function. It has been difficult to prove, however, that the acute episodes are secondary to infective agents entirely, since (1) the specific organism can be ascertained in fewer than 50% of acute exacerbations and (2) the beneficial effect of antimicrobials, although they are routinely used, is often difficult to prove from clinical trials. The actual role of infection in relationship to other causes of chronic bronchitis, therefore, will probably vary among individuals.

Clinical Manifestations

A wide spectrum of disease is seen in persons with chronic bronchitis from those with a morning cough and no apparent functional respiratory impairment to patients with the syndrome of respiratory failure with chronic cough, copious sputum production, and severe obstructive airway disease. Acute exacerbations of bronchitis are associated with usually mild fever, general malaise, increased production of purulent sputum, and often worsening of respiratory function. The last problem is seen particularly in patients with severe and long-standing airway disease. With recurrent episodes, the patients can usually predict exacerbations quite early, and often note that their sputum increases and has changed from white and mucoid to thick green or yellow.

Physical examination reflects the diversity of clinical disease and ranges from essentially normal to that of a severely incapacitated patient with generalized debilitation, evidence of chronic airway obstruction, and respiratory failure with cyanosis.

Diagnosis

The diagnosis of chronic bronchitis is based on history and the exclusion of other diseases. Chest x-ray may be normal or show evidence of peribronchial thickening, areas of residual fibrosis, and varying degrees of emphysema, both diffuse and localized. During acute exacerbations, there are usually no or minimal changes seen in the chest x-ray but it is very important to compare earlier chest films to exclude pneumonia. Gram's stain of the sputum during acute episodes usually shows polymorphonuclear leukocytes with a mixed bacterial flora or a predominence of one of the more common lower respiratory tract pathogens such as *S. pneumoniae* or *H. influenzae*. Culture of the sputum also may show only a mixed oral flora, or one particular organism may predominate.

The major diagnostic decisions with an acute exacerbation are to determine if it appears to be of bacterial etiology in order to decide on antimicrobial therapy and to exclude more serious diseases such as pneumonia (including tuberculosis), bronchiectasis, lung abscess, or carcinoma (in view of usual history of heavy smoking).

Treatment

Despite the difficulty in proving a direct association between acute infection and the clinical syndrome of ex-

TABLE 12.1. Antimicrobial Treatment of Acute Exacerbations of Chronic Bronchitis and Bronchiectasis

Antibiotic	*Dose*
Amoxicillin	500 mg q8h po
Tetracycline	500 mg q6h po
Trimethoprim/ sulfamethoxazole	160 mg trimethoprim/800 mg with sulfamethoxazole q12h po
Erythromycin	500 mg q6h po

acerbations alluded to above, most patients are treated with antibiotics that would be effective against organisms commonly isolated from the sputum (Table 12-1). The duration of therapy is predicated on systemic response and disappearance of the purulent sputum, and generally continues for seven to ten days. In addition, other therapeutic measures to reduce bronchospasm, if present, can be instituted. Oxygen is used to correct severe hypoxemia while the patient is carefully observed for the retention of carbon dioxide.

Because of the difficulty in many cases in determining a cause-and-effect relationship between acute infection and exacerbations and deterioration in respiratory function, additional studies are required to assess the presence of other infectious agents and the efficacy of antimicrobial agents. Recent studies suggest that symptomatic treatment without antibiotics is as effective.

Prognosis

The effect of acute exacerbations on the prognosis of chronic bronchitis is unknown. Although the patients appear to have acute impairment of respiratory function when they are first seen with an infection, whether or not this in itself impairs respiration chronically has not been proved. Furthermore, the effect of antibiotics in improving the prognosis in these patients is not known.

Prophylaxis

Avoiding air pollutants, especially cigarette smoking, is the main preventive factor in reducing the incidence of chronic bronchitis. In addition, aggressive treatment of lower respiratory tract bacterial infections, especially in children, may reduce the subsequent development of chronic bronchitis in adults who have no smoking history.

To reduce the number of acute exacerbations, several different antibiotic regimens have been tried. Although many studies are inconclusive, it appears that in those bronchitics who have more than one major acute episode per year, long-term antibiotic prophylaxis is beneficial in reducing the total number of exacerbations. Cost, compliance, and patient tolerance affect the agent of choice. Drugs that can be used include ampicillin, amoxicillin, tetracycline, erythromycin, and trimethoprim/sulfamethoxazole (TMP/SMZ). A suggested regimen would be one-half the normal therapeutic dose taken on a daily basis, either year-round or during the winter months when the incidence of acute exacerbations is highest.

Another approach to prophylaxis involves the patient initiating treatment at the earliest onset of symptoms from a home supply of antibiotic. It is theorized that starting early, the disease would be more amenable to treatment. In addition, advantages include reducing both the total amount of antibiotic taken and the emergence of resistant organisms that could develop during continual prophylaxis.

BRONCHIECTASIS

Bronchiectasis is a condition characterized by the irreversible dilatation of bronchi. It may be localized or diffuse in the lungs.

Etiology

Bacterial organisms associated with pneumonia are commonly isolated in patients with bronchiectasis chronically or during acute exacerbations. These include *S. pneumoniae, H. influenzae,* and *S. aureus.* Gram-negative enteric organisms, including *Pseudomonas aeruginosa,* are often found in patients who have more severe bronchiectasis and have undergone numerous courses of antibiotic treatment.

Epidemiology

Bronchiectasis may occur in association with chronic bronchitis or as a complication of asthma, allergic pulmonary aspergillosis, and localized obstructive lesions in the bronchi. There is also a high prevalence of bronchiectasis in patients with chronic sinusitis and in those with systemic diseases, including cystic fibrosis and immunodeficiency complicated by recurrent pneumonias.

Pathophysiology

The major factor predisposing to development of bronchiectasis is the presence of an anatomic or functional obstruction in the bronchi that causes an accumulation of secretions and resultant infection. The inflammatory response results in destruction of the supporting tissue and leads to dilatation of the bronchial walls. The process is self-perpetuating because the dilated bronchi predispose the patient to recurrent infections with further damage.

Clinical Manifestations

Chronic cough with expectoration of large amounts of sputum, usually with hemoptysis, are the cardinal features of bronchiectasis. A continuum of clinical signs and symptoms exists in patients with chronic bronchitis and bronchiectasis, but the presence of persistent hemoptysis and the large volume of sputum reflect more severe destruction of bronchi and erosion into blood vessels. There is also a greater tendency for the development of pneumonia in patients with bronchiectasis, and clubbing of the digits is more common than in chronic bronchitis. With a suppurative focus in the lungs, there is also a possibility of metastatic foci to other parts of the body, including the brain, in patients with bronchiectasis.

Physical examination is always abnormal with bronchiectasis, in contrast to patients with chronic bronchitis, in whom physical findings may be minimal. Areas of bronchiectasis produce coarse crackles and wheezes on auscultation.

Diagnosis

The diagnosis is suspected clinically and usually confirmed by an abnormal chest x-ray that shows localized or diffuse evidence of peribronchial thickening, atelectasis, or on occasion, small cystic lesions in the lungs. The definitive diagnosis is made by bronchography, but unless surgery is contemplated for removal of a specific obstructive lesion or area of localized bronchiectasis, this procedure is usually not indicated.

In acute exacerbations of pneumonia, the patient should be examined as outlined under Bacterial Pneumonia (pages 182–183).

Treatment

Adequate clearance of respiratory secretions from bronchiectatic areas is the mainstay of treatment. This involves the use of postural drainage maneuvers and bronchodilators if a reversible bronchospastic component is also present. Antibiotics are necessary when the complication of pneumonia supervenes, and are usually used when acute exacerbations occur. (Specific treatment regimens are similar to those for pneumonia and are shown in Table 12.4.) Exacerbations not associated with pneumonia are treated in the same way as those of chronic bronchitis (Table 12.1). The presence of more resistant gram-negative rods, such as *P. aeruginosa,* in patients with cystic fibrosis usually requires more aggressive treatment with intravenous antibiotics, including aminoglycosides, cephalosporins, and broad-spectrum penicillins (carbenicillin, ticarcillin, and piperacillin), often in synergistic combinations.

Underlying diseases causing bronchiectasis should be treated, including any local obstructive process that could be excised surgically. Localized areas of bronchiectasis may also be resected, but in general a more conservative surgical approach to bronchiectasis is now being practiced.

Prognosis

Localized bronchiectasis carries a good prognosis, in contrast to diffuse disease, especially that associated with cystic fibrosis and recurrent pneumonias in immunodeficient patients. Complications, including respiratory failure and metastatic foci of infection such as brain abscess, obviously worsen the prognosis.

Prophylaxis

Recognition of underlying diseases that predispose to bronchiectasis is the best form of prophylaxis, including rigorous treatment of childhood bacterial pneumonias and early removal of obstructive lesions. Aggressive treatment of patients with cystic fibrosis may retard subsequent development of bronchiectasis.

Intermittent or continual antimicrobial prophylaxis may be given and is similar to that described for patients with chronic bronchitis (page 178). However, the efficacy of these prophylactic regimens has not been proved and they may result in resistant organisms, which ultimately may cause more severe and difficult-to-treat pneumonias.

PNEUMONIA

Pneumonia is an infection of the terminal airways of the lung involving the respiratory bronchioles, alveolar

TABLE 12.2. Usual Clinical and Laboratory Features of Acute Bacterial and Atypical Pneumonias

Clinical	*Bacterial*	*Atypical*
Setting	Community- or hospital-acquired	Community-acquired
Onset of illness	Acute with rigors	Insidious with chills
Symptoms	Mainly pulmonary and severe	General systemic symptoms (flulike)
Cough	Productive	Dry or minimally productive
Pleuritic pain	Common	Unusual
Laboratory		
Sputum	Purulent Gram's stain and culture positive	Mucoid (if present) Gram's stain and culture negative
Blood	White blood cell count >15,000, positive blood cultures in up to 50% of cases	White blood cell count <15,000, routine blood cultures negative
Chest x-ray	Air-space disease or bronchopneumonia	Interstitial infiltrate
Etiology	Bacterial flora of oropharynx or bacteremia	Acquired, nonindigenous pathogens

ducts and sacs, and alveoli, and is usually visualized radiologically as a parenchymal infiltrate. It can be grouped under the two broad categories of classic bacterial and atypical pneumonia. These are contrasted by clinical and laboratory criteria in Table 12.2. With the initial examination of a patient with pneumonia, it is often possible to categorize a case as one of these major types, which immediately has practical therapeutic implications.

Bacterial Pneumonia

Etiology

The major causes of acute bacterial pneumonia in adults are as follows:

1. Community-acquired
   a. Common organisms
      S. pneumoniae
      H. influenzae
      S. aureus
      Klebsiella pneumoniae
      Oropharyngeal flora, anaerobes and aerobes
   b. Unusual pathogens
      S. pyogenes
      N. meningitidis
      P. multocida
      Salmonella sp.
2. Hospital-acquired
   a. *S. aureus*
   b. Gram-negative enteric rods
      E. coli
      Proteus sp.
      Klebsiella sp.
      Enterobacter sp.
      Actinobacter sp.
      Pseudomonas sp.

The etiology differs depending upon whether the disease is acquired in the community or in hospital. The majority (60% to 70%) of community-acquired bacterial pneumonia is caused by *S. pneumoniae* with the remainder caused by the other organisms shown, including normal oropharyngeal flora composed of anaerobic and aerobic bacteria. Although the organisms listed represent the most common isolates, most clinically important bacteria have been implicated in causing pneumonia.

In children, *S. pneumoniae* and *H. influenzae* are common. In the neonatal period, gram-negative enteric bacilli (e.g., *E. coli*) and group B streptococci predominate.

In contrast to community-acquired disease, pneumonia in the hospital setting is caused primarily by *S. aureus* and gram-negative enteric organisms including *E. coli* and *P. aeruginosa*.

Epidemiology

The epidemiologic setting, whether community or hospital, is very helpful in determining the etiology of pneumonia. Pneumococcal pneumonia, the archetype of bacterial pneumonia, occurs in all age groups but especially in patients suffering from a variety of chronic underlying diseases, and hence is more often found in the elderly population. Although this disease has been studied extensively, the actual percentage of all cases of pneumonia caused by pneumococci is very difficult to determine. In well-documented cases of pneumonia in adults, a rough estimate is 25%; in children this is probably much lower because of the increased frequency of viral pneumonia among young persons.

Certain epidemiologic characteristics are associated with a greater prevalence of specific types of pneumonia. In patients with a preceding influenza pneumonia, *S. pneumoniae* and *S. aureus* are the common superinfecting bacteria. Also, *S. aureus* pneumonia is seen in a high percentage of intravenous-drug abusers who develop bacteremias. *Hemophilus influenzae* pneumonia usually occurs in elderly patients who have a history of chronic airway disease. *Klebsiella pneumoniae* is classically associated with persons with a history of alcohol abuse. *Streptococcus pyogenes* pneumonia, although common in the preantibiotic era, has declined as endemic disease but occurs in isolated epidemics among military recruits, as does *N. meningitidis* pneumonia. *Pasteurella multocida* pneumonia is seen usually in patients with chronic airway disease who have exposure to animals harboring the organism, especially pet cats and dogs.

Hospital-acquired pneumonias occur frequently, especially after surgery. Predisposing factors include debilitating illness, a history of chronic airway disease, and intubation with mechanical ventilation. The epidemiology of nosocomial pneumonia is often characteristic not only for each hospital, but for particular areas of a hospital (for example, intensive and respiratory care units). The flora change periodically under antibiotic selective pressure, and clusters of pneumonia caused by different organisms occur. Debilitated patients have been shown within a few days to acquire hospital flora in their oropharynx, which is the usual source of their pneumonia. Knowing the current bacterial flora in various hospital environments often enables an early etiologic diagnosis before definitive laboratory data are available.

Pathogenesis

Bacterial pneumonia is acquired through four major routes. The most common is aspiration of oropharyngeal contents and this is the usual source of pneumonia caused by *S. pneumoniae, H. influenzae, K. pneumoniae,* and *S. pyogenes*. This "micro" or "occult" aspiration is contrasted with gross aspiration of oropharyngeal and gastric contents in obtunded patients, resulting in so-called aspiration pneumonia. The presence of gastric contents containing food particles and acid acts synergistically with the oropharyngeal flora. Usual sites of aspiration in the lungs are shown in Table 12.3.

TABLE 12.3. Sites of Pneumonia from Aspiration of Oropharyngeal Flora

Position of Patient at Time of Aspiration	*Usual Site of Pneumonia*
Supine	Right and left lower lobes, superior segments
Prone	Right middle lobe and lingula
Right side	Right upper lobe, posterior segment
Left side	Left upper lobe, apical posterior segment
Upright	Lower lobes, basal segments

The second route of infection is through hematogenous spread from a distant infected focus, which is very common with *S. aureus*. The third is through direct spread to the lungs at the time of surgery or trauma, or transdiaphragmatically from intraabdominal sepsis. The fourth route of infection is inhalation through endotracheal tubes, which circumvents certain host defense mechanisms and is a common cause of hospital-acquired pneumonias.

After inoculation and multiplication of bacteria in the peripheral airways, an acute inflammatory reaction is produced, with accumulation of fluid and polymorphonuclear leukocytes in the airways and supporting tissues. As the process evolves, the products of inflammation are ingested by alveolar macrophages. Whether the pneumonia will be localized or widespread depends upon the properties of the infecting bacterium, size of inoculum of the organism, and host response. In classic pneumonia, the alveoli are predominantly involved, with spread among adjacent alveoli resulting in nonsegmental or lobar distribution but patent airways (airspace consolidation). In the other major form, spread may be primarily through the airways and follow segmental patterns, producing more diffuse disease (bronchopneumonia) without patent airways. Numerous focal areas of bronchopneumonia usually result from hematogenously spread infection. The term *consolidation* refers to the solid inflammatory mass within alveoli that is seen both pathologically and radiologically.

The pathologic process may be restricted to the lung parenchyma or spread to the pleural surface (pleurisy, empyema) or other structures adjacent to the lung (pericardium), or disseminate by way of the lymphatics and bloodstream. Resolution of the disease may be complete, as usually occurs in pneumococcal pneumonia, or result in various degrees of necrosis, cavitation, and fibrosis, which is often seen in *S. aureus* and *K. pneumoniae* infections.

Clinical Manifestations

Bacterial pneumonia usually has an acute onset with rigors and high fever, and patients may appear acutely ill to the point of shock. Common symptoms include pleuritic chest pain that causes splinting of the chest wall, cough productive of purulent sputum that is either mixed or streaked with blood, various degrees of respiratory impairment (dyspnea, tachypnea, cyanosis, and ventilatory failure), and cardiovascular responses associated with sepsis. Other physical signs may include those of consolidation with dullness to percussion, increased vocal fremitus, bronchial breathing, and coarse crackles. Decreased breath sounds and/or the presence of crackles alone may be the only finding, however. A pleural rub at the site of pleuritic pain is often heard.

There may be no other clinical symptoms or signs apart from those referable to the respiratory system; however, if present, they may point to a focus of infection that produced a bacteremia and hematogenous seeding of the lung, or an adjacent infection that produced pneumonia by direct spread. A common but nonspecific finding in bacterial pneumonia is the presence of herpes labialis secondary to fever and/or stress of the infection. Although classically associated with pneumococcal pneumonia, it is certainly not diagnostic for this particular bacterial pneumonia.

Diagnosis

In addition to the characteristic clinical features, the diagnosis of bacterial pneumonia is confirmed by sputum examination and culture, blood cultures, and radiologic findings. In many cases, the clinical and laboratory procedures confirm the specific etiologic agent and in others, at least restrict the number of possible etiologies.

Blood for three cultures should be drawn when the patient is seen, and may be done simultaneously or over the course of several hours if the patient does not require immediate antimicrobial treatment. A positive blood culture is unequivocal evidence for the etiology of pneumonia, although very rarely, a polymicrobial infection may exist with only one organism detected in the blood initially.

Blood cultures in gram-positive pneumonias (*S. pneumoniae, S. aureus,* and *S. pyogenes*) are associated with a higher frequency of bacteremia (20% to 50%) than cultures in gram-negative pneumonias (*H. influenzae, K. pneumoniae*) (20%). The presence of a bacteremia usually indicates more severe disease and also suggests the possibility of metastatic foci of infection.

Sputum examination and culture, in contrast, may not only be unrewarding but misleading, and must be interpreted carefully. For sputum examination by Gram's stain, the specimen should be purulent and demonstrate the presence of a large number of polymorphonuclear leukocytes on microscopic examination. The presence of greater than 25 squamous cells in a low-power field (total magnification × 100) indicates excessive contamination with saliva and invalidates interpretation because of the presence of oropharyngeal flora. If a sputum specimen is not initially available, symptomatic treatment with analgesics if pleuritic pain is a major problem, oxygen, and rehydration with fluids often enables the patient to cough up an adequate specimen within a few hours. The presence of a predominant and recognized pathogen on Gram's stain allows a tentative diagnosis of the etiologic agent. Sputum culture often is less reliable than Gram's stain because of overgrowth of flora from the oropharynx. This especially applies in the case of *S. pneumoniae* infection. Therefore failure to grow this organism in sputum should not detract from the diagnosis of pneumococcal pneumonia based on other clinical and laboratory data.

Obtaining a specimen of bronchial secretions or lung tissue for Gram's stain and culture and circumventing the oropharyngeal flora is possible with transtracheal aspiration (TTA) or percutaneous lung biopsy (PLB). Such procedures are necessary especially if an anaerobic infection is suspected and a specific etiology must be determined. The yield of the procedure in terms of modifying therapy must be weighed against possible complications, which include cardiac arrhythmias, hypoxemia, subcutaneous emphysema, hemorrhage, and needle tract infections for TTA, and pneumothorax and hemorrhage for PLB. Because of the complications, suspected anaerobic infections are often treated empirically, and only when a poor response results will these diagnostic procedures be employed.

Results of other laboratory tests in bacterial pneumonia are generally nonspecific and are seen in any type of bacterial sepsis. Usually, there is leukocytosis with a white cell count greater than 15,000 with greater than 5% band cells. Marked leukopenia with thrombocytopenia can occur in overwhelming infection.

The chest x-ray appearance is usually that of air-space disease (nonsegmental, confluent infiltrate with air bronchograms) or bronchopneumonia (segmental, less dense infiltrate without air bronchograms). Each organism can produce either radiologic picture, however, and these findings must be interpreted in the context of other clinical and laboratory data. Certain organisms are more commonly associated with particular radiologic findings and these are summarized below:

Air-space consolidation
- *S. pneumoniae*
- *K. pneumoniae*
- *Proteus* sp.
- Aspiration pneumonia
- *Legionella pneumophila*

Bronchopneumonia
- *H. influenzae*
- *S. aureus*
- *S. pyogenes*
- *N. meningitidis*
- *E. coli*

Interstitial pneumonia
- Viral infection
- *M. pneumoniae*
- *Chlamydia psittaci*
- *Yersinia pestis*
- *Francisella tularensis*
- *Coxiella burnetii*

Effusions, empyema
- *S. aureus*
- *K. pneumoniae*
- *S. pyogenes*
- Aspiration pneumonia

Cavitation
- *S. aureus*
- *K. pneumoniae*
- *P. aeruginosa*
- Aspiration pneumonia

Other diseases that mimic the x-ray picture of acute bacterial pneumonia include pulmonary infarct, pulmonary hemorrhage, atelectasis, carcinoma, and Wegener's granulomatosis.

Treatment

All bacterial pneumonias are potentially life threatening and if facilities are available, patients should be admitted to the hospital at least for initial treatment. Supportive measures include management of fluid balance (many patients are dehydrated), analgesia for pleuritic pain, and oxygen therapy with or without intubation and mechanical ventilation for respiratory failure. In patients with chronic airway disease, oxygen must be given carefully to correct hypoxemia without inducing excessive accumulation of carbon dioxide. Septic shock, if present, is treated as described in Chapter 23.

Specific antimicrobial therapy for community-acquired pneumonia, as shown in Table 12.4, should be instituted after a tentative etiologic diagnosis has been made. Initial therapy should be given parenterally. In the case of pneumococcal infection, this can often be changed to oral therapy several days after defervescence and clinical improvement. Longer courses of parenteral treatment are usually required for the other types of pneumonia. Routine use of broad-spectrum

TABLE 12.4. Parenteral Antimicrobial Treatment of Bacterial Pneumonias

Etiology	*Antibiotic (dosage for 70-kg patient)*
S. pneumoniae	Penicillin G, 1 MU q4h IV or aqueous procaine penicillin G, 600,000 U IM q12h
	Cefazolin, 1 gm q8h IV
	Erythromycin, 500 mg q6h IV
H. influenzae	Ampicillin, 1 gm q4h IV
	Cefamandole 1.5 gm q4h IV
	Choramphenicol, 1 gm q6h IV
	Trimethoprim, 240 mg/sulfamethoxazole, 1200 mg q12h IV
S. aureus	Cloxacillin, 2 gm q6h IV (β-lactamase producing) or penicillin, 2 MU q4h IV (non-β-lactamase producing)
	Cefazolin, 1 gm q8h IV
	Clindamycin, 600 mg q8h IV
	Vancomycin, 1 gm q12h IV
K. pneumoniae	Tobramycin or gentamicin, 1.5 mg/kg q8h IV ± cefazolin, 1.5 gm q8h IV
S. pyogenes	Penicillin G, 1 MU q4h IV
	Cefazolin, 1.0 gm q8h IV
	Erythromycin, 500 mg q6h IV
Oropharyngeal aspiration (Anaerobes, aerobes)	Penicillin G, 2 MU q4h IV
	Clindamycin, 600 mg q8h IV

antibiotic coverage should be avoided if possible. In the extremely ill patient in whom the etiology is not known, however, such therapy is reasonable for most bacterial pathogens but should be modified if and when the specific cause is known. One therapeutic approach for disease in which a reasonably broad spectrum of coverage is wanted, especially for community-acquired pneumonia, is the use of a cephalosporin that covers the majority of these pathogens. Cefamandole, 2 gm intravenously every six hours, or cefuroxime, 750 mg intravenously or intramuscularly every eight hours, both second-generation cephalosporins, are good choices for this initial therapy. They will also cover B-lactamase producing *H. influenzae*. The addition of an aminoglycoside empirically would give additional coverage against gram-negative rods but increase the potential for toxicity.

Combining an aminoglycoside with a penicillinase-resistant penicillin, such as cloxacillin, or a cephalosporin is effective for suspected hospital-acquired pneumonia. The use of a third-generation cephalosporin, such as cefotaxime or moxalactam, may prove to be as effective in this setting. As soon as the specific agent is known, antibiotic therapy, as narrow as possible for the organism, should be selected.

Duration of therapy depends upon the patient's clinical response. Most pneumonias are treated adequately with a total of 10 to 14 days of therapy. More severe pneumonias, for example those associated with abscess formation or empyema, require longer courses of therapy. For the latter complication, surgical drainage or repeated aspiration is necessary.

Prognosis

The prognosis of bacterial pneumonia depends upon the infecting organism, extent of the disease process, and most important, the state of the host defense mechanisms. Pneumococcal pneumonia has a mortality rate of approximately 5%, which increases to 15% if associated with a bacteremia. Higher rates occur in patients with an underlying chronic disease such as coronary artery disease or chronic airway obstruction. *Staphylococcal* and *Klebsiella* pneumonias generally have higher mortality rates (up to 50%) and are associated with more complications.

In general, prompt hospitalization, intensive antibiotic therapy, and early recognition of complications such as lung abscess, empyema, and dissemination of the infection to other organs (e.g., meningitis, endocarditis, and osteomyelitis) reduce the mortality rate.

Prophylaxis

The use of prophylactic antibiotics in preventing bacterial pneumonia in high-risk patients (intubated and ventilated patients in the intensive care unit) is not indicated, and when implemented, usually results in the development of pneumonia with more resistant organisms.

Prophylaxis of *S. pneumoniae* infections is currently available in the form of a vaccine that consists of antigens derived from capsular polysaccharides of 23 strains that cause the majority of pneumococcal disease in the United States. The efficacy of different pneumococcal vaccines has been shown to be as high as 80% in groups where the prevalence of pneumococcal pneumonia is very high. Where this prevalence is low, however, the demonstrated efficacy is marginal. Recommendations for the use of pneumococcal vaccine are discussed in Chapter 8.

Atypical Pneumonia

Atypical pneumonia is a clinical syndrome caused by a diverse group of microorganisms. Although the word "atypical" may be somewhat outdated, it does represent a large group of pneumonias that can be differentiated from classic bacterial pneumonia by several clinical and laboratory features, as noted in Table 12.2. Although these features accentuate the possible differences, there is often overlap between atypical and typical bacterial pneumonias in these areas. Whereas there are relatively few pathogens recognized for the majority of acute bacterial pneumonias, the causes of atypical pneumonias are numerous and represent a wide spectrum of microbiology.

Atypical pneumonias may be further differentiated into acute and chronic, as shown in Table 12.5. This distinction is often useful in diagnosis.

Acute Atypical Pneumonia

Viral Pneumonia

Etiology

Viruses may cause up to 50% of cases of well-documented pneumonias in adults. Those implicated most frequently include influenza A and B, adenovirus, and parainfluenza virus. Less common causes include measles, respiratory syncytial virus, and varicella zoster;

TABLE 12.5. Etiology of Acute and Chronic Atypical Pneumonias

Agents	*Acute Pneumonia*	*Chronic Pneumonia*
Bacteria	*Legionella pneumophila* (legionnaires' disease) *Francisella tularensis* (tularemia) *Yersinia pestis* (plague)	
Mycobacteria	*M. tuberculosis* *M. bovis*	*M. tuberculosis* *M. bovis* *M. Kansasii* *M. avium*-intracellulae complex
Mycoplasma	*M. pneumoniae*	
Chlamydia	*C. psittaci*	
Rickettsia	*Coxiella burnetii*	
Fungi	*Histoplasma capsulatum* (histoplasmosis) *Coccidioides immitis* (coccidioidomycosis)	*Histoplasma capsulatum* (histoplasmosis) *Coccidioides immitis* (coccidioidomycosis) *Blastomyces dermatitidis* (blastomycosis) *Cryptococcus neoformans* (cryptococcosis)
Viruses	Influenza A and B Adenovirus Parainfluenza Measles Respiratory syncytial virus Varicella zoster	
Actinomycetes		*Actinomyces israelii* *Nocardia asteroides*

herpes simplex and cytomegalovirus cause pneumonias primarily in immunosuppressed hosts.

Viral pneumonia is more common in children than in adults. Respiratory syncytial and parainfluenza viruses are especially serious in infants less than 1 year of age.

Epidemiology

Viral pneumonias occur both endemically and epidemically; such epidemics are more widespread than bacterial pneumonias. Influenza A and B infections occur during the late fall and early winter and are the most common viruses producing pneumonia in the civilian population. They tend to occur cyclically in epidemics. The prevalence of influenzal pneumonia is higher in elderly persons, diabetics, and patients with cardiovascular, renal, and chronic lung disease. In contrast, adenovirus causes pneumonia usually in closed populations, such as military recruits. Pneumonia is a frequent complication in adults with varicella, but not in children.

Pathophysiology

Direct inhalation of viral particles in droplets leads to infection of the upper respiratory tract and subsequent spread to the lower airways, causing a tracheobronchitis. The penetration and replication of viruses within the respiratory epithelium impair various cell processes and result in cell death with desquamation. Host defense mechanisms including cell-mediated immune responses, the mucociliary stream to clear secretions, and phagocytic activity may all be compromised by the viral infection. Progression of the infection to the terminal airways and alveoli results in primarily a mononuclear response in the intraalveolar septa and subsequent exudation of fluid into the alveoli.

Because of the impairment of host defense mechanisms, patients with viral pneumonia are at increased risk of a superinfection with acute bacterial pneumonia.

Clinical Manifestations

The onset of viral pneumonia is usually insidious, with other symptoms such as fever, sore throat, earache, and tracheobronchitis preceding the pneumonia by 24 to 48 hours. Thus it is a later manifestation of the underlying viral illness, but once present, the patient can deteriorate clinically very rapidly. Evidence for the presence of pneumonia includes development of tachypnea, dyspnea, cough productive of mucoid sputum or frothy hemoptysis, and in severe cases, cyanosis and progression to respiratory failure. Varicella pneumonia is usually characterized by pleuritic pain because of the presence of vesicular lesions involving the pleura.

Clinical examination of the chest generally understates the degree of lung involvement. Usual ausculatory findings include only the presence of bilateral fine crackles and wheezes. The presence of signs of consolidation supports the diagnosis of a secondary bacterial pneumonia.

Diagnosis

The diagnosis of viral pneumonia is made primarily on clinical and epidemiologic criteria. The latter are especially important, for example, during an influenza outbreak where until the epidemic is recognized, initial cases may be misdiagnosed as other types of atypical pneumonia and occasionally as bacterial pneumonia. Laboratory studies are often not discriminating at the time of first examination since, for example, patients may initially have a polymorphonuclear leukocytosis as seen in bacterial pneumonias, although a normal white blood cell count or relative lymphocytosis is usual in a viral infection. Because cough associated with viral pneumonias is often nonproductive or productive only of mucoid sputum, Gram's stain and culture of the sputum for bacterial pathogens are unrewarding and may be misleading if normal oropharyngeal flora is cultured. Throat and sputum cultures for viral isolation are useful in confirming the diagnosis and defining an epidemic, but practically they do not influence early treatment in the individual case. A diagnosis, apart from culture, is usually confirmed serologically in retrospect (see Chapter 4).

The chest x-ray usually shows an interstitial, unilateral, or bilateral infiltrate. Differential diagnosis of x-ray findings in acute atypical pneumonia includes the following:

1. Hypersensitivity pneumonitis (Löffler's syndrome, farmer's lung, allergic bronchopulmonary aspergillosis)
2. Chemical pneumonitis
3. Collagen-vascular disease (systemic lupus erythematosus)
4. Pulmonary alveolar proteinosis
5. Sarcoidosis
6. Goodpastuer's syndrome

Treatment

Treatment of viral pneumonias is symptomatic. Hospitalization should be strongly considered in most patients so that proper hydration with fluids, analgesia as required, and treatment of respiratory insufficiency and any underlying predisposing disease can be instituted. The routine use of prophylactic antibiotics to prevent bacterial superinfection is not indicated. Instead, this complication should be carefully observed for and treated if the clinical, radiologic, and laboratory criteria indicate a bacterial superinfection.

Bacterial superinfection acquired outside of hospital is usually caused by *S. aureus* or *S. pneumoniae*. Initial treatment, therefore, includes a penicillinase-resistant penicillin, a cephalosporin, erythromycin, or vancomycin. Nosocomial bacterial pneumonia requires broader coverage initially, since gram-negative enteric organisms are common within the hospital setting. Initial coverage therefore should include an aminoglycoside with a penicillinase-resistant penicillin or cephalosporin.

Amantadine, a drug that has been used as a prophylactic agent in the prevention of influenza A, may be helpful in influenza A pneumonia through its ability to reduce peripheral airway resistance and mitigate the signs and symptoms in patients with influenza. Until there is evidence to the contrary, amantadine in a dosage of 200 mg orally daily may be given to patients with influenza pneumonia.

Prognosis

For patients with a viral pneumonia, the prognosis is primarily dependent upon their prior state of health and treatment facilities available including ventilatory support. Because influenza has a higher attack rate in patients with underlying diseases, as opposed to adenovirus and varicella, which may cause pneumonia in young, healthy individuals, influenza pneumonia has a higher case fatality rate than pneumonia caused by other agents. The other important factor adversely affecting prognosis is the development of a secondary bacterial pneumonia.

Prophylaxis

Influenza prophylaxis is the only preventive measure available for viral pneumonia. Influenza vaccine, comprised of inactivated preparations of two or three strains of recent influenza A and B isolates is approximately 80% effective in preventing clinical cases of influenza and is administered yearly to patients who are at high risk of contracting the disease (see Chapter 8).

When vaccination is contraindicated or as an interim measure prior to vaccination, amantadine may be given prophylactically. It has been shown to be as effective as the vaccine in preventing influenza A infection. The recommended dosage of 200 mg per day is similar to that used in treatment. After vaccination, amantadine treatment should continue for two weeks, by which time active immunity to influenza should have developed. Without vaccination, amantadine treatment should continue for the duration of the influenza risk (up to eight weeks). Major drawbacks to this type of prophylaxis are the cost and the neurologic side effects, especially in elderly patients who complain of dizziness, drowsiness, difficulty in concentrating, and insomnia. Side effects may be accentuated in patients with renal impairment and the dosage may have to be reduced.

Bacterial Atypical Pneumonia

Legionnaires' disease, plague, and tularemia are bacterial infections with various systemic manifestations including pneumonia, which may or may not be the dominant finding. These infections contrast with classic bacterial pneumonias in which other systemic manifestations are usually overshadowed by the pulmonary signs and symptoms.

Legionnaire's Disease

Etiology

Legionnaires' disease, a recently described systemic illness with pneumonia as one of its major manifestations, is caused by *Legionella pneumophila,* a pleomorphic gram-negative rod and at least eight related species (e.g., *L. dumoffii, L. micdadei, L. wadsworthii*).

Epidemiology

The organism and disease entity derived their names from the epidemic that occurred at the time of the American Legion convention in Philadelphia in 1976. Subsequent retrospective serologic studies, however, revealed earlier cases of the disease. To date, the majority of patients with legionnaires' disease have been reported from North America and Western Europe. Epidemics are usually associated with specific buildings such as hotels or hospitals, or excavation projects, and appear to be related to environmental contamination with the organism. For example, several epidemics have been traced to contamination of air conditioning systems and water supplies. Immunosuppressed patients and those with underlying debilitating diseases, such as chronic airway obstruction, are predisposed to legionnaires' disease.

Pathophysiology

Inhalation of aerosols contaminated with the organism is the likely mode of spread. No person-to-person transmission has been documented. After it is inhaled, the organism produces an acute inflammatory reaction with both polymorphonuclear and mononuclear cell infiltrates, primarily in the terminal airways. In severe cases, extensive necrosis with cavitation can occur, especially in immunocompromised hosts. The organism has been isolated on rare occasions from the blood.

Clinical Manifestations

Legionnaires' disease has an incubation period of approximately five days and causes a flulike illness. Initially, gastrointestinal symptoms of nausea, vomiting, and diarrhea occur. These are followed by respiratory symptoms, which may be relatively mild or quite progressive in severity, with the development of dyspnea, tachypnea, and in severe cases, respiratory failure requiring ventilation. Pleuritic chest pain can also occur, simulating bacterial pneumonia or a pulmonary embolism. Auscultation usually demonstrates only fine crackles, but signs of consolidation may be present in up to 25% of cases.

Diagnosis

The history of gastrointestinal upset preceding pneumonia, as well as potential epidemiologic exposure, are helpful diagnostic clues clinically. Also, patients who fail to respond to commonly used regimens in bacterial pneumonia, including the penicillins, cephalosporins, and aminoglycosides, should be suspected of having this infection. Confirmation of the diagnosis is usually made serologically using the indirect immunofluorescent technique, in which a fourfold increase in antibody is confirmatory (see Chapter 4). Some cross-reactivity occurs among other lung pathogens that cause atypical pneumonia, including *M. pneumoniae, C. psittaci,* and influenza virus.

The diagnosis may also be confirmed with culture and isolation of the organism from lung tissue, pleural fluid, and rarely, sputum, using special culture media. Direct immunofluorescent staining of sputum or other tissues is a more sensitive and easier technique for diagnosis, although cross-reactivity with other bacteria can occur rarely.

Additional laboratory investigations are nonspecific but may be helpful. Leukocytosis with a marked increase in the number of band forms is often seen, which is unusual for an atypical pneumonia. Also, mild elevations in levels of liver enzymes and serum creatinine and serum urea occur. Additional renal involvement is reflected in hematuria and proteinuria. Hyponatremia and hypophosphatemia are also quite common, the former probably secondary to an inappropriate antidiuretic hormone effect.

Chest x-ray examination differs from most other atypical pneumonias in showing more commonly bronchopneumonia or air-space disease rather than an interstitial pattern only.

Treatment

Although *L. pneumophila* is susceptible in vitro to a large number of antibiotics, studies in animals and treatment responses of patients demonstrate the efficacy of only a few drugs. Most clinical experience has been with erythromycin, 2 to 4 gm intravenously daily initially, which has been shown to lower the case fatality rate significantly. Total duration of therapy is usually 14 days, with the higher dose of 4 gm daily recommended until improvement occurs. The response to treatment is usually fairly dramatic but the diagnosis should not be discarded if a rapid response does not occur. Other antibiotics that are also likely to be efficacious include tetracycline and rifampin, the latter used with erythromycin for synergy in patients who do not respond to the former alone.

Prognosis

The case fatality rate for legionnaires' disease was approximately 15% before the entity became better recognized and the efficacy of erythromycin was known. Treatment with this drug has reduced this rate considerably, although patients who are immunosuppressed or have chronic airway disease still have a poor prognosis.

Prophylaxis

No specific prophylactic measures exist for legionnaires' disease, although when a case is identified, a thorough epidemiologic study should be undertaken looking for a specific environmental source of the organism that could be eradicated by disinfection.

Uncommon Atypical Pneumonias

Pneumonias caused by bacteria (plague, tularemia), chlamydiae (ornithosis), and rickettsiae (Q fever) are summarized in Table 12.6.

Mycoplasma Pneumonia

Etiology

Mycoplasmas are organisms that lack a rigid cell wall but are surrounded by a modified cell membrane. Because of this property, they are resistant to cell wall antibiotics such as the penicillins. They are not related to L-phase variants of bacteria and are able to grow and replicate on cell-free media. *Mycoplasma pneumoniae* is the species that causes pneumonia.

Epidemiology

The source of the illness is human infection. Infections caused by *M. pneumoniae* are endemic but epidemics may occur, especially during the winter months and in closed populations such as military recruits. Approximately 10% of cases of *M. pneumoniae* infection are associated with pneumonia.

Pathophysiology

The organism is transmitted through respiratory secretions. Although it does not penetrate the cell as viruses do, it does adhere to the upper and lower respiratory epithelium by a special terminal organelle. Ciliary activity and metabolic events in the respiratory epithelial cell are inhibited possibly through the production of hydrogen peroxide by the organism. Inflammatory changes with a predominantly mononuclear infiltrate are produced in the tracheobronchial tree and terminal airways, primarily in the alveolar septa.

Dissemination of the organism from the respiratory tract is extremely rare, and manifestations of systemic disease have been attributed to immune complexes or cell-mediated immune reactions.

Clinical Manifestations
Pneumonia is usually preceded by upper respiratory tract symptoms and tracheobronchitis after an incubation period of approximately two to three weeks. As in other atypical pneumonias, cough, while common, is usually nonproductive or productive of only mucoid sputum. On physical examination, the patient may have mild pharyngitis, cervical lymphadenopathy, and fine crackles in the lower lobes with no evidence of consolidation or pleural effusion. Bullous myringitis, often considered a classic finding, is uncommon and nonspecific. Rarely, very severe *M. pneumoniae* infection may mimic an acute bacterial pneumonia.

Diagnosis
The diagnosis should be suspected clinically in a patient with what appears to be a typical viral upper respiratory tract infection that becomes prolonged and associated with tracheobronchitis and signs and symptoms of a mild pneumonia. Chest x-ray examination usually shows a unilateral or bilateral interstitial pneumonia in the lower lobes. A small pleural effusion may be present in up to 25% of cases but is detectable only in the posterior costophrenic angle on lateral x-ray. Very rarely, dense air-space disease may be present.

The white blood cell count is often elevated with polymorphonuclear leukocytosis, but generally less than 15,000 per mm^3. There may be a mild elevation of liver enzymes, although severe hepatitis with jaundice occurs rarely. Nonspecific serologic responses, usually seen in more severe disease, include the presence of cold agglutinins (IgM antibody against I antigen of the red cell). Significant hemolysis as a result of the cold agglutinins is unusual, but can be severe and may occur days to weeks after the onset of the acute illness.

A specific diagnosis is usually made by serology with a complement fixation test (see Chapter 4), but false negative results may occur in up to 50% of cases. The best diagnostic yield uses a combination of tests for cold agglutinins and complement fixation, as well as cultures for *M. pneumoniae* on sputum or throat swabs. The latter may not be available in most laboratories and moreover, may require two to three weeks for growth. It will increase the yield of positive cases, however, and may be important epidemiologically.

Treatment
Erythromycin or tetracycline, 1 to 2 gm orally per day for seven days, is usually effective in shortening the syndrome. After the institution of antibiotic therapy, the organism can often be isolated for up to several weeks despite the absence of symptoms. If a relapse occurs after a week's therapy, an additional two weeks of antibiotic treatment is recommended.

Prognosis
The prognosis for *M. pneumoniae* pneumonia is excellent. Severe complications are rare but obviously worsen the prognosis. These include myocarditis and pericarditis, severe hepatitis, meningoencephalitis, and other neurologic complications involving the brain, spinal cord, and nerve roots, as well as the autoimmune hemolytic anemia alluded to above.

Prophylaxis
No specific prophylactic measures are available.

Actinomycete Pneumonia

Etiology and Epidemiology
The description and epidemiology of pneumonia caused by *Actinomyces israelii* and *Nocardia asteroides* are summarized in Table 12.7.

Pathophysiology
Pulmonary actinomycosis results from aspiration of oropharyngeal secretions. This produces an acute inflammatory reaction followed by marked fibrosis and contiguous spread into adjacent tissues, including the chest wall and mediastinum.

Nocardia infection, in contrast, is acquired by inhalation and often produces multiple abscesses with little or no fibrosis. Spread to other organs is by the hematogenous route.

Clinical Manifestations
Pneumonia caused by *Nocardia* and *Actinomyces* is usually insidious in onset, resembling mycobacterial or fungal infection. Sputum is thick and purulent, often associated with hemoptysis. Metastatic foci of infection, either the result of hematogenous spread (e.g., brain abscesses in nocardiosis) or direct spread (e.g., chest wall sinus tract in actinomycosis) may be the first evidence of clinical disease.

Diagnosis
The diagnosis is confirmed by culture of the organisms from sputum, bronchoscopy, or biopsy of specimens of

TABLE 12.6. Characteristics of Uncommon Acute Atypical Pneumonias

Organism	*Disease*	*Description*	*Epidemiology*	*Reservoir or Vector*	*Pathophysiology*
Bacteria					
Yersinia pestis	Plague	Gram-negative rod (broad, bipolar staining)	Worldwide (esp. Asia, Africa, South America) Incubation period 2–6 days	Fleas, rodents (rats), man	Primary pneumonia acquired from patient by inhalation Secondary pneumonia (rare) from bacteremia with lymphatic disease
Francisella tularensis	Tularemia	Gram-negative rod (small, coccobacilli)	Worldwide (severe forms esp. in North America) Incubation period 1–10 days	Ticks, rabbits, muskrats	Primary pneumonia (rare) acquired from patient by inhalation Secondary pneumonia from bacteremia with glandular forms of disease
Chlamydia					
C. psittaci	Ornithosis (psittacosis)	Obligate intracellular organisms	Worldwide Occupational hazard Incubation period 7–14 days	Birds (wild and domesticated), infected secretions/excretions Man (rare)	Inhalation → primary pneumonia → multiplication in reticuloendothelial system and hematogenous spread with possibly a secondary pneumonia
Rickettsia					
Coxiella burnetii	Q fever	Obligate intracellular coccobacilli	Worldwide Occupational hazard Incubation period 14–21 days	Domesticated animals (sheep, goats, cattle) and their environment Contaminated milk	Inhalation of aerosols or contaminated dust; ingestion of milk Multiplication in vascular endothelium and serosal cells with hematogenous spread to lungs and other organs (granulomatous hepatitis)

* = usual diagnostic test.

Clinical Manifestations	*Diagnosis*	*Treatment*	*Prognosis*	*Prophylaxis*
Mild interstitial pneumonia to severe necrotizing hemorrhagic bronchopneumonia (esp. with primary pneumonias) Presence of regional lymphadenopathy associated with flea or tick bite (ulcer)	Epidemiologic history Culture of lymph node aspirates, sputum, blood (biohazard) Serology*	Strict isolation Streptomycin, 1 gm q8h IM and tetracycline, 1 gm q12h IV (with improvement, 500 mg q6h po) (alternative, chloramphenicol, 1 gm q6h po or IV)	Poor without treatment 10% mortality rate with treatment	Protective clothing Vaccine Antibiotic prophylaxis (tetracycline, 2 gm/day po)
Primary pneumonia, no lymphadenopathy	Epidemiologic history Culture of lymph node aspirates, sputum, blood (biohazard) Serology*	Streptomycin, 1 gm q12h IM (alternative, tetracycline, 500 mg q6h po, chloramphenicol, 1 gm q6h po or IV)	Fair without treatment 5% mortality rate with treatment	Protective clothing Vaccine
Flulike illness with severe headache, sore throat Mild to severe pneumonia with hemorrhage and necrosis	Epidemiologic history Serology* Culture	Tetracycline, 500 mg q6h po (alternative, chloramphenicol, 1 gm q6h po or IV)	Excellent with treatment	Attempted eradication in birds
Flulike illness with headache, myalgias, arthralgias Mild interstitial pneumonia	Epidemiologic history Serology* Culture (biohazard)	Tetracycline, 500 mg q6h po (alternative, chloramphenicol, 1 gm q6h IV or po)	Excellent for pneumonia but poor for endocarditis	Animal management procedures to reduce exposure Pasteurization of milk

TABLE 12.7. Characteristics of Chronic Atypical Pneumonias

Organism	*Disease*	*Description*	*Epidemiology*
Actinomycetes			
A. israelii	Actinomycosis	Gram-positive, branched, anaerobic organisms; non-acid-fast	Worldwide Commensals of mouth and gastrointestinal tract
N. asteroides	Nocardiosis	Gram-positive, branched, aerobic organisms; acid-fast	Worldwide Soil
Fungi			
H. capsulatum	Histoplasmosis	Dimorphic fungus Mycelium-producing spores (infective stage) Yeast form in tissues	Worldwide (North America esp. Mississippi and Ohio River valleys) Soil enriched with starling, pigeon, and bat excreta
C. immitis	Coccidioidomycosis	Dimorphic fungus Mycelium-producing spores (infective stage) Yeast form in tissues (endospores in spherule)	Western hemisphere (North America — southern California to Texas; Mexico) South America and Central America Spores in soil
B. dermatitidis	Blastomycosis (North American)	Dimorphic fungus Mycelium-producing spores (infective stage) Yeast form in tissues	Primarily North America (St. Lawrence, Ohio, Mississippi River valleys) Central America, Africa Probably spores in soil Isolation of organism in dogs
C. neoformans	Cryptococcosis	Yeast form in soil (infective stage) and tissues Large polysaccharide capsule	Worldwide Soil enriched with pigeon excreta

primary or secondary disease. Because the organisms are slow growing, the presence of other bacteria in the sputum may obscure or inhibit their growth. Culture of lung biopsy material or that obtained through transtracheal aspiration uncontaminated by oropharyngeal flora usually eliminates this problem. Gram's stain may be helpful on specimens, with the organisms recognized by being weakly gram-positive with the appearance of beaded, branching filaments. Pathologically, the diagnosis may be made by the presence of so-called sulfur granules, which are clumps of organisms up to a few millimeters in diameter in pus and biopsy specimens. Although more common in actinomycosis, they can also be present in nocardiosis.

Treatment

For pulmonary nocardiosis, sulfonamides remain the treatment of choice. Most clinical experience has been with sulfadiazine, 4 to 8 gm per day orally. This drug may be used alone or combined with either erythromycin, 2 to 4 gm per day orally, or ampicillin, up to 8 gm per day intravenously. A poor response on sulfa drugs alone after two weeks should prompt the addition of either erythromycin or ampicillin. The optimal duration of therapy for nocardiosis is also unknown, but at least six weeks is usually considered necessary.

Pulmonary actinomycosis is usually treated with penicillin G, 10 to 20 million units per day intravenously, for at least two to four weeks after clinical improvement of the infection. Additional treatment orally for up to two months with penicillin V, 2 to 4 gm daily, is also recommended. The duration of therapy is predicated on the clinical response and longer therapy may be required. Several alternative drugs may be given in patients allergic to penicillin or who have had a poor response to penicillin. These include tetracycline or erythromycin, 2 to 3 gm daily orally, and clindamycin, 1.8 to 2.4 gm daily orally or intravenously. Usually medical treatment is curative but if a poor response to medical treatment is noted, surgical excision should be considered.

Prognosis

The prognosis of pulmonary nocardiosis in nonimmunocompromised patients is very good with antibiotic treatment, and the survival rate approaches 90%. Opportunistic infection and dissemination to other tissues adversely affects the survival rate. Uncomplicated pulmonary actinomycosis carries an excellent prognosis despite prolonged therapy. Underlying pulmonary disease and spread to adjacent or distant organs result in a poorer prognosis.

Prophylaxis

No specific chemoprophylaxis or immunoprophylaxis exists. Good oral hygiene including dental and periodontal care will reduce the prevalence of pulmonary actinomycosis.

Mycobacterial Pneumonia

Etiology

Mycobacterium tuberculosis and *M. bovis* (bovine tuberculosis) are the two common strains of mycobacteria that infect humans, the latter being very rare in economically developed countries. The organisms are well adapted pathogens; their major properties that distinguish them from other bacteria are the high lipid content of their cells, which results in marked affinity for certain stains that are resistant to decolorization by acid-alcohol solutions (acid-alcohol-fast); slow generation times; and relative resistance to usual antibiotics and sterilization procedures. They are obligate aerobes and therefore especially pathogenic in tissues with high concentrations of oxygen (e.g., lung apices). Certain atypical mycobacteria are rare causes of pneumonia but are increasing in importance as tuberculosis declines. The most common isolates that produce pneumonia include *M. kansasii* and *M. avium*-intracellulare.

Epidemiology

Tuberculosis is still a very common disease worldwide but has declined markedly in economically developed countries. High-risk groups still exist in these countries, and include recent immigrants from areas where tuberculosis is common, lower socioeconomic populations, predisposed racial groups (Eskimos, native Americans, and Africans), and immunosuppressed patients.

Mycobacterium tuberculosis is acquired from human cases, whereas *M. bovis* is usually contracted through unpasteurized milk. Atypical mycobacterial infection arises from contact with a variety of environmental sources.

Pathophysiology

The primary infection of tuberculosis is acquired by inhalation of droplet nuclei containing the tubercle bacilli from a person with active disease through coughing or sneezing, or through ingestion of unpasteurized milk in the case of bovine tuberculosis. Repeated exposure to the bacillus, such as occurs in a household or closed institutionalized population, or a single large inoculum is usually necessary for infection. After being inhaled, the organisms are carried to a peripheral alveolus, are engulfed by alveolar macrophages, and multiply intracellularly. A mild acute inflammatory reaction is produced. This initial reaction is superceded by typical tubercle or granuloma formation, with the accumulation of lymphocytes and macrophages that differentiate into epitheloid and multinucleated cells (Langhans' giant cells).

With the development of delayed hypersensitivity responses (four to six weeks after the initial infection), the tubercle may undergo caseation necrosis as a result of local ischemic changes in the central part of the lesion. Calcification usually occurs after a period of months to years in areas of caseation.

Early in the course of the illness, at the time of multiplication of bacilli in macrophages, there is lymphatic and hematogenous spread of the organism to regional and distant lymph nodes and various organs of the body. Similar cellular changes in the extrapulmonary organs may then ensue, with tubercle formation.

The initial infection usually resolves spontaneously; however, progressive pulmonary disease or widespread infection involving many different organs in the body (miliary) may occur. Also, although the initial infection may be quiescent for years, a diminution in the immune response can result in reactivation of the infection in the lung or other organs of the body.

A similar series of pathologic events occurs in the gut following ingestion of *M. bovis*. Pulmonary tuberculosis results then from lymphohematogenous spread from the initial focus.

The marker of previous infection to tuberculosis is the tuberculin skin test, which reflects a delayed hypersensitivity response to the tubercle bacillus. Although delayed hypersensitivity is part of the cellular immune response, the two are not necessarily synonymous since the former may be present without evidence of protective immunity.

Clinical Manifestations

A whole spectrum of clinical signs and symptoms is associated with pulmonary tuberculosis. Symptoms of the primary infection are usually self-limited and may go unrecognized or be attributed to a nonspecific flulike illness. Previous exposure to the tubercle bacillus, under these circumstances, is reflected only in a positive tuberculin skin test or in addition, calcified granulomas on chest x-ray. In contrast, the primary infection may be progressive, with tuberculous pneumonia, extrapulmonary organ involvement, or disseminated (miliary).

The usual clinical features in an adult are those of a chronic illness of insidious onset associated with low-grade fever, night sweats, weight loss, and cough productive of mucopurulent sputum. Specific clinical findings relating to complications of pulmonary tuberculosis may also be present. Hemoptysis is quite common but generally is minimal, with streaking of the sputum. Profuse hemoptysis may occur as a result of rupture of aneurysms of the pulmonary arteries caused by adjacent tuberculous infection of the lung parenchyma and lymph nodes. Pleural effusions are common and may be associated with varying degrees of pneumonia. A major complication is the development of a bronchopleural fistula when a large parenchymal lesion erodes into the pleural space and produces an empyema. Cavitation is associated with more extensive disease and greater infectivity. The infection may spread also through the airways to involve not only different parts of the same lung but the opposite lung.

Findings on physical examination cover a whole range from normal to evidence of consolidation, cavitation, pleural effusion, atelectasis, fibrosis, and bronchopleural fistula, and associated with these findings, different degrees of respiratory insufficiency.

Erythema nodosum or erythema multiforme may be present weeks to months after the primary exposure and most likely represent delayed hypersensitivity responses.

Clinical findings for *M. bovis* and atypical mycobacterial pulmonary infection resemble those of *M. tuberculosis*.

Diagnosis

Tuberculosis should be suspected in any patients with chronic atypical pneumonia and especially in those with a high probability of epidemiologic exposure. Clinical features may mimic those of other atypical pneumonias as well as classic bacterial pneumonia, and therefore confirmation of the diagnosis by smear and culture techniques is mandatory. Sputum expectorated spontaneously or after being induced by aerosolized saline inhalations is examined by acid-alcohol-fast stains. If facilities are available, the sputum is usually screened by a fluorochrome technique (auramine-rhodamine) and then confirmed with the Ziehl-Neelsen stain.

Up to five early morning specimens should be stained and cultured for mycobacteria. Culture results are positive in approximately 30% of cases that are negative by smear examination; therefore a positive smear for acid-fast bacilli indicates a moderately severe infection and greater infectivity. Other methods of diagnosis include smear and culture examination of lung tissue specimens or pleura obtained through percutaneous needle or open lung biopsy. Pleural effusions should also be aspirated, stained and cultured for acid-fast bacilli, although the pleural biopsy yields a higher number of positive results. Gastric washings are seldom required for diagnosis from an adult (they may be useful in children), and smears alone of gastric aspirates are often unreliable because of the possibility of nontuberculous acid-fast bacilli in the stomach.

Positive cultures for tuberculosis require two to six weeks of incubation. Positive identification depends upon morphologic characteristics (*M. tuberculosis* and *M. bovis* show cording), as well as certain biochemical criteria.

Chest x-ray examination is often the first diagnostic clue to tuberculosis since the disease may be discovered on a routine examination in a patient with minimal symptoms and signs. The lesion may vary from a small circumscribed area of air-space disease or bronchopneumonia to extensive cavitary disease and fibrosis involving several lobes. Upper lobe involvement predominates, presumably because of the higher oxygen tension in these areas that is favored by the tubercle bacillus. Pleural effusion may or may not be present. A distinctive radiologic finding is that of a diffuse nodular interstitial pattern (miliary) that represents disseminated disease, but which may not be seen for several weeks after severe systemic symptoms ensue. It is important to remember that the radiologic picture of tuberculosis may be extremely variable and the diagnosis cannot be confirmed or excluded by radiologic investigation only.

The tuberculin skin test is a useful epidemiologic marker for tuberculosis and can be used diagnostically in conjunction with other findings in areas where there is low frequency of positivity. A diagnosis of tuberculosis can be made when a recent conversion from a negative to positive test is documented in a patient with an illness consistent with tuberculosis. The tuberculin skin test and its application are described in Chapter 4.

Treatment

Many antimicrobial agents are now available for the treatment of tuberculosis and several common therapeutic regimens are shown in Table 12.8. In the past, treatment usually included two to three drugs for 18 to 24 months. More recently, two drugs, if both are tuberculocidal against intracellular and extracellular bacilli, have been shown to be effective if given for only 9 to 12 months or at least 6 months after conversion of sputum culture to negative.

Using isoniazid (INH) and rifampin in combination as the basic regimen, therapy can be modified for the individual patient. This depends upon (1) the severity of the disease; extensive pneumonia, cavitation, and strongly positive smears suggest severe disease, in which case a third drug, for example, ethambutol or streptomycin, may be added for several months; (2) compliance of the patient (daily or twice-weekly supervised dosing); (3) hypersensitivity or toxicity from treatment drugs; and (4) antimicrobial resistance, which depends upon susceptibility testing of the organisms, which should be done routinely.

The use of tuberculocidal combinations usually eliminates the infectivity of the sputum rapidly and therefore hospitalization may be limited to two weeks. This is dependent upon the patient's understanding of the disease and degree of infectivity, compliance in taking medication, and extent of the disease. If the disease is very severe, longer observation and hospitalization are required. If treated on an outpatient basis, the patient can be seen every two weeks for the first two months, then at monthly visits for six months, and every two to three months for at least one year after cessation of drug therapy. At each visit, in addition to the patient's clinical progress, sputum, if present, should be stained and cultured for tuberculosis, and side effects of the antituberculous drugs must be carefully looked for. Although the agents in general are relatively nontoxic, the duration of treatment and total dose of drug consumed make potential toxicity a significant factor in treatment.

TABLE 12.8. Common Treatment Regimens for Tuberculosis

Regimen	*Drug*	*Dosage*	*Duration (mos)*
Short Course			
Daily	Isoniazid	300 mg po	9–12
	Rifampin	600 mg po	9–12
Twice weekly	Isoniazid	900 mg po	9–12
	Rifampin	600 mg po	9–12
Standard Course			
Daily	Isoniazid	300 mg po	18–24
	Ethambutol	15 mg/kg po	18–24
	Streptomycin	1 gm IM	2

Isoniazid-induced hepatitis is the best-recognized toxic effect of an antituberculous medication. When monitoring for this complication, it is important to inform the patient that if a flulike syndrome should occur he or she must report to the physician for tests of liver function. Although a transient elevation in liver transaminases may occur in asymptomatic persons taking INH, sustained elevation associated with symptoms of hepatitis should result in discontinuing this agent and substituting another. The prevalence of INH toxicity is approximately 2% in persons greater than 50 years of age but is much less in younger age groups. Isoniazid can also induce peripheral neuropathy and anemia secondary to relative pyridoxine deficiency. This usually occurs in elderly, debilitated, or alcoholic patients and is obviated by supplemental pyridoxine, 50 mg daily.

Resistance of tubercle bacilli to usual antituberculous drugs is much higher in patients from areas where the disease is common and in those who have received previous therapy but who have complied poorly with their drug regimens. In treating such individuals, it is important to determine susceptibility of the organisms to the various antituberculous drugs in order to select the best combination. Because a common type of resistance is that to INH, a triple drug regimen consisting of rifampin, ethambutol, and streptomycin may be started. Pyrazinamide or capreomycin may be substituted for any of these drugs. Isoniazid may be included as a fourth drug, if resistance to it is only suspected. Treatment of resistant strains by a triple combination should likely continue for 18–24 months.

Various supportive measures may be superimposed on the basic therapy that has been described. Corticosteroids are rarely necessary but have been employed in patients whose systemic symptoms, including spiking fevers and malaise, fail to resolve after several weeks of appropriate antituberculous therapy. In this setting, doses of prednisone of up to 40 mg daily have been given for short courses to ameliorate these symptoms. Although theoretically corticosteroids could impair cell-mediated immunity, they appear to have no detrimental effect on the clinical course when used on a short-term basis.

The treatment of atypical mycobacterial disease depends upon susceptibility testing of the isolate. This is difficult to predict for many organisms, but in general, they are resistant to usual antituberculous drugs. It is reasonable to start treating a patient with a common regimen initially until the isolate is identified and susceptibility testing is available. When a particularly resistant organism is found, the approach is multiple-drug therapy (often up to six agents) hoping for a synergistic effect, although the organism may be resistant to the individual drugs. Amikacin and ansamycin (a rifampin analogue) may prove efficacious in certain atypical mycobacterial pneumonias.

Prognosis

The prognosis for pulmonary tuberculosis is excellent with proper therapy, and failure of cure should be less than 5% in most cases. Failures are seen in patients with extensive or miliary disease, underlying chest disease, immunoincompetence, previous treatment regimens with poor compliance, and the presence of resistant organisms.

Atypical mycobacterial disease carries a much poorer prognosis because of a deficiency in underlying host defense mechanisms and the relative resistance of many atypical mycobacteria.

Prophylaxis

The prevalence of tuberculosis in many countries has been reduced through improved socioeconomic conditions, treatment, and the use of immunoprophylaxis and chemoprohylaxis. Immunoprophylaxis with bacillus Calmette-Guérin (BCG) is described in Chapter 8.

Chemoprophylaxis with INH has been used extensively, especially in economically developed countries, to protect individuals previously exposed to tuberculosis. The exposure may be recent and based on a recent conversion of the tuberculin skin test to positive, or it may have occurred in the unknown past and be discovered when a tuberculin skin test is positive on routine screening. Prior to the recognition of INH-induced hepatitis as a significant complication, chemoprophylaxis was recommended less selectively. There is still some controversy surrounding the use of INH chemoprophylaxis, but in general it is indicated in the following clinical situations: (1) well-documented recent conversion to tuberculin positivity, (2) children less than 4 years of age after known exposure to a patient with tuberculosis, and (3) positive tuberculin skin test in a patient less than 35 years of age (who has previously not received BCG). The use of INH in patients over age 35 who have a positive tuberculin test of unknown duration must be weighed against the increased likelihood of toxicity. A stronger case for prophylaxis can be made in patients with diseases that impair their immunocompetence, including diabetes mellitus and malignancy, and in those receiving long-term steroid therapy. Even in these situations, however, some physicians prefer to observe the patients for evidence of tuberculosis and withhold prophylaxis. Each patient, therefore, should be carefully assessed regarding the use of chemoprophylaxis.

Fungal Pneumonia

Etiology and Epidemiology

The etiology and epidemiology of common fungal pneumonias are shown in Table 12.7.

Pathophysiology

In histoplasmosis, coccidioidomycosis, and blastomycosis, the organism is inhaled as a spore and transforms into a yeast form in lung tissue. In cryptococcal disease, the infective form is probably the yeast. Multiplication causes an acute inflammatory reaction that is followed by a mononuclear response and granuloma formation (epithelioid and giant cells); necrosis and ultimately, calcification of the lesions occur. Lymphohematogenous spread to various organs in the body occurs early in histoplasmosis. In contrast, coccidioidomycosis disseminates only with progressive pulmonary infection. The time of dissemination of cryptococcosis and blastomycosis is poorly defined. Pyogenic abscesses, in addition to granuloma formation, are often seen in blastomycosis. The large polysaccharide capsule in *C. neoformans* resists phagocytosis, and this organism has a peculiar affinity to cause meningitis, often with minimal or no obvious pulmonary disease.

Clinical Manifestations

The symptoms and signs of fungal pneumonias are similar to those of pulmonary tuberculosis. The initial infections of histoplasmosis, coccidioidomycosis, and cryptococcosus usually produce a flulike syndrome with localized interstitial pneumonia and various degrees of hilar lymphadenopathy. The infection usually goes unrecognized. In contrast, massive exposure to histoplasmosis and coccidioidomycosis may produce a diffuse, severe pneumonia. Skin rashes, including erythema nodosum and erythema multiforme, may be seen several weeks after onset of these infections. Blastomycosis is very rarely an acute infection.

Progressive primary disease is more common with histoplasmosis and coccidioidomycosis and is manifested by symptoms and signs of a severe, acute, atypical pneumonia. Chronic disease occurs subacutely and resembles the usual picture of tuberculosis. The severest form of fungal infection, disseminated disease, may also occur. Histoplasmosis may clinically cause hepatosplenomegaly, generalized lymphadenopathy, ulcerative lesions of the upper respiratory and gastrointestinal tracts, pericarditis, and mediastinitis. Coccidioidomycosis and cryptococcosis often disseminate to the skin, bone, and meninges. Disseminated blastomycosis usually involves the skin, bone, and genitourinary tract.

Diagnosis

Many acute fungal infections are not diagnosed, and a presumed diagnosis is made retrospectively on chest x-ray based on the presence of calcified lesions. If the initial infection is severe pneumonia, which may occur in the case of histoplasmosis and coccidioidomycosis, the diagnosis is made usually on the basis of epidemiologic exposure. Chronic or progressive fungal disease requires precise diagnosis because of important therapeutic implications.

The best method of diagnosis of all fungal infections is by stained smears and cultures of sputum, lung tissue, or other tissues in which specific lesions are found. The bone marrow and liver are other sources of biopsy material. Serology may be helpful in acute and chronic pulmonary disease of histoplasmosis, but it may be negative in severe progressive disease or disseminated disease. In coccidioidomycosis, serology is usually strongly positive in disseminated disease, but only variably positive in nondisseminated disease. In both histoplasmosis and coccidioidomycosis, skin testing is not helpful since it may be negative in patients who are severely ill with progressive or disseminated disease. Serology is difficult to interpret in blastomycosis, and there may be cross-reactivity with histoplasmosis. Cryptococcal antigen may be detected in blood and cerebrospinal fluid and is a precise and sensitive method of diagnosis. Detection of cryptococcal antibody is also sensitive in nondisseminated disease, but is less specific than cryptococcal antigen detection.

The radiologic pictures of the fungal pneumonias resemble those of tuberculosis and can be very diverse, including the presence or absence of a pleural effusion. Cavitary disease appears to be more common with histoplasmosis and coccidioidomycosis; in cryptococcosis, single or multiple nodular bronchopneumonic infiltrates are often seen. No radiologic picture is pathognomonic for any specific fungal pneumonia.

Treatment

No antimicrobial therapy is necessary for the acute, nonprogressive pneumonic form of fungal infection. Patients are usually followed clinically and radiologically to determine the course of the disease. Antimicrobial therapy is indicated if the disease is progressive, nonresolving, or disseminated.

Parenteral amphotericin B is the usual form of treatment for fungal pneumonias. A test dose of 1 mg in 500 ml of 5% dextrose and water solution is infused over four to six hours and side effects are noted. Premedicating the patient with 50 to 100 mg of hydrocortisone succinate tends to ameliorate the chills, rigors, spiking fever, and general malaise that usually accompany amphotericin B infusion. Also, the addition of 1000 units of heparin in the infusion reduces the incidence of phlebitis at the intravenous site. Following the initial 1-mg test dose, if the drug has been tolerated reasonably well, the dosage may be increased by daily increments of 5 mg to a maximum of 50 mg per day. After repetitive doses of amphotericin B the patient generally has fewer uncomfortable side effects such as rigors and fever, but nephrotoxicity assumes a more prominent role. Some degree of nephrotoxicity usually occurs after several weeks of treatment, in which case, giving the drug every two to three days rather than daily usually halts further nephrotoxicity. A common and potentially serious effect is hypokalemia, which is caused by a potassium-losing neuropathy. Potassium supplementation is often required and levels of serum potassium should be watched closely.

The duration of amphotericin B treatment is usually determined by the amount of total drug that is administered. In general, a total dose of 1 to 2 gm is given, which usually requires 6 to 12 weeks of therapy. In cryptococcosis, flucytosine, 150 mg per kg per day in four divided doses, may be given, in which case the dosage of amphotericin B may be reduced to 0.25 mg per kg per day. This reduces the potential toxicity of amphotericin.

Ketoconazole, a new oral antifungal agent, may be useful in patients who fail on amphotericin B or who cannot tolerate the drug because of side effects and toxicity. Optimal dosing schedules with ketoconazole have not been determined and must await further clinical trials; however, a dosage of 200 to 400 mg per day for four to eight months has been effective in the treatment of some fungal pneumonias.

Prognosis

For primary, nonprogressive, fungal pneumonia, the prognosis is excellent without treatment. In patients with primary progressive, chronic cavitary disease and disseminated disease, the prognosis is much less favorable and often the disease continues chronically or relapses despite treatment. The major determining factors in prognosis are the immune competence of the host and the administration of appropriate antifungal therapy, especially amphotericin B, which has improved the prognosis considerably.

Prophylaxis

No chemoprophylactic or immunoprophylactic measures are available for the prevention of fungal pneumonias. Environmental control measures to reduce the number of spores in the soil and the number that are air borne have been attempted for histoplasmosis and coccidioidomycosis on a limited scale. Because the epidemiology of blastomycosis and cryptococcosis is ill-defined, no similar measures have been attempted for these infections.

PYOGENIC LUNG ABSCESS AND EMPYEMA

A lung abscess is a localized collection of necrotic lung debris and an empyema is a purulent, infected, pleural effusion; both are usually complications of necrotizing bacterial pneumonias.

Etiology

Necrotizing pneumonias are caused by aerobic, microaerophilic, and/or anaerobic bacteria, singly or together in polymicrobial infections. With the increasing use of more sensitive anaerobic techniques, anaerobic bacteria arising mainly from the oropharyngeal flora, including *Peptostreptococci, Bacteroides, Fusobacteria,* and *Eubacteria* species, are being isolated more often alone or in association with aerobic organisms from lung abscesses and empyemas. One species, *B. melaninogenicus,* appears to be particularly important. It is likely that the polymicrobial nature of the infections results in a synergistic necrotizing effect on lung tissue.

Staphylococcus aureus, K. pneumoniae, and other gram-negative enteric rods are also common causes of lung abscesses and empyemas.

Epidemiology

Necrotizing pneumonias have been seen classically as a result of aspiration pneumonia in individuals with an altered state of consciousness, including alcohol abusers, accident victims, and those with seizure disorders. Also, *S. aureus* and *K. pneumoniae* pneumonias acquired in the community often result in abscesses and empyema.

Increasing numbers of necrotizing pneumonias caused by a variety of gram-negative enteric bacilli, including *E. coli, Proteus* sp., and *P. aeruginosa* are now acquired within hospitals as a complication of more extensive surgical procedures involving the thorax and abdomen, and the increasing practice of esophageal instrumentation and use of subclavian lines for monitoring.

Pathophysiology

A lung abscess develops with the progression of an acute inflammatory response produced by pneumonia to actual necrosis and formation of a cavity filled with debris consisting of lung tissue, fibrin, and polymorphonuclear leukocytes. In the case of a gross aspiration pneumonia, the additional presence of gastric secretions in combination with organisms contributes to the necrotic reaction.

Empyemas usually develop as a complication of pneumonia through extension of the infection to the pleural space. The inflammatory process at this site is similar to that occurring in the lung parenchyma, and consists of acute inflammation, consolidation, and fibrosis. Empyema may also be caused by direct bacterial seeding of the pleural space at thoractotomy, from ascending infection through chest tubes, transdiaphragmatic spread from an intraabdominal focus, and rarely, through hematogenous spread of infection.

Clinical Manifestations

A lung abscess or empyema may occur either acutely as part of the evolution of a clinically evident necrotizing pneumonia or insidiously after weeks of symptoms, the preceding pneumonia being relatively asymptomatic. There may be systemic symptoms similar to those seen in pneumonia, with pleuritic or dull, steady pain if an empyema is present, or the production of large volumes of purulent sputum with or without hemoptysis if a large, cavitated abscess is present. Particularly foul-smelling sputum or empyema fluid strongly points to anaerobic infection.

For lung abscess, physical examination may be normal, although evidence of a pneumonia surrounding the lesion may be present with crackles and bronchial breathing. The signs of empyema include tracheal deviation away from the side of the lesion, dullness to percussion, and diminished breath sounds over the empyema. An acute empyema may also produce a pleural rub.

Diagnosis

The diagnosis of lung abscess and empyema should be strongly considered in a patient with pneumonia who fails to respond to appropriate antibiotic therapy or who relapses after initial improvement. Other febrile patients with predisposing epidemiologic factors, especially those in an intensive care unit setting, should also be strongly suspected of having empyema and lung abscesses as complications. Confirmation of both lesions is usually obtained by chest x-ray, which demonstrates, in the case of lung abscess, a cavitated lesion with a thick wall and often with an air-fluid level. Certain abscesses may be difficult to see on one x-ray projection and both posteroanterior and lateral views of the chest should be obtained. Rarely, abscesses may not be visualized on chest x-ray and if suspected, isotopic gallium or computerized tomographic (CT) scan of the lung should be done. An empyema will appear as a pleural effusion on chest x-ray (posteroanterior and lateral views). Lack of movement of an effusion with postural changes (lateral decubitus film) indicates a loculated collection. If an empyema is not seen on routine chest x-rays, ultrasound or CT scanning can be performed.

Accurate diagnosis of the infecting organism or organisms may be difficult in a lung abscess if the lesion is due to anaerobes, since sputum specimens will be contaminated with oropharyngeal flora. If it is necessary to determine a specific etiology because, for example, empiric antibiotic therapy is not effective, a percutaneous or transtracheal aspiration may be done. These diagnostic tests are associated with potentially serious side effects and should be carefully considered before being performed. Gram's stain and culture of an adequate sputum specimen (as described on page 182) usually is sufficient for the diagnosis of lung abscesses caused by *S. aureus* or gram-negative enteric organisms. As alluded to above, however, the significance of anaerobic isolates in this situation is difficult to interpret.

As in all cases of suspected bacterial pneumonias, blood for at least three cultures should be drawn and, if positive, the infecting organism(s) confirmed.

All suspected or proved empyemas should be aspirated for diagnosis. Precautions should be taken to ensure that good anaerobic collection, transport, and culture techniques are employed. Gram's stain of the specimen often gives an immediate etiology and determines whether it is caused by a single organism or is polymicrobial, the latter being more indicative of an anaerobic infection. Because of the increased frequency of isolation of *B. melaninogenicus* from empyema fluid and lung abscesses and its relative resistance to the penicillins and other commonly employed drugs, susceptibility testing of anaerobes in addition to aerobic isolates should be routinely undertaken if the specimen has not been contaminated by oropharyngeal flora.

Treatment

The antibiotic treatment of lung abscess and empyema is similar to that of the causative necrotizing pneumonia and is summarized in Table 12.3. All empyemas require drainage, either by repeated aspirations or by chest tubes. In contrast, most lung abscesses resolve without surgical management, although extensive or nonresolving abscesses may require surgical excision. The decision to perform an open thoracotomy with its risks is often difficult, and surgical opinion should be sought early. Percutaneous drainage of an abscess is hazardous because of the potential complications of a bronchopleural fistula with the subsequent development of an empyema. Loculated empyemas may require limited rib resection, breaking down of adhesions, and drainage. Development of a bronchopleural fistula usually requires more extensive surgery.

The duration of antibiotic therapy is longer than in uncomplicated pneumonia and depends upon the time required for adequate drainage of the empyema or resolution of the abscess. After adequate drainage of an empyema, antibiotic treatment should be continued for at least a week after defervescence and the patient's clinical improvement. For lung abscesses, the radiologic picture of cure usually lags behind the systemic response, and actual duration of treatment is difficult to predict. Disappearance of systemic signs and symptoms and lack of sputum production generally indicate resolution of the abscess, but therapy of up to several months' duration may be necessary, especially in anaerobic infections.

Prognosis

The prognosis for lung abscess is dependent upon the extent of the disease (whether a single or multiple abscesses are present, number of lobes involved), and the infecting organism and its susceptibility to antibiotics, and the state of host defense mechanisms. Extensive involvement of the lung with multiple abscesses caused, for example, by *P. aeruginosa* in an immunosuppressed patient obviously carries a very poor prognosis. Another complication with a poor prognosis is gross spillage of an abscess cavity into other parts of the lung, which may be acutely life threatening. Early surgical drainage of large abscesses will prevent this.

The prognosis for empyemas also depends upon the above factors. The presence of a bronchopleural fistula worsens the prognosis and necessitates extensive surgical intervention.

Both lung abscesses and empyema are features of gram-negative and *S. aureus* pneumonias that contribute to the mortality rate of greater than 50% in these types of pneumonia.

Prophylaxis

Early recognition and aggressive treatment of pneumonia reduce the incidence of lung abscess and empyema. Because gross aspiration of oropharyngeal contents is a common cause of necrotizing pneumonia, patients with a decreased level of consciousness should be carefully observed to avoid this possibility and their airway must be protected. Early removal of chest tubes and prophylactic treatment of penetrating chest injuries will reduce the frequency of empyema and lung abscess.

ANNOTATED BIBLIOGRAPHY

Bronchitis

Bates JH. The role of infection during exacerbation of chronic bronchitis. Ann Intern Med 1982;97:130–131.

Tager I, Speizer FE. Role of infection in chronic bronchitis. N Engl J Med 1975;292:563–571.

Critical reviews of data, including antibiotic trials, pertaining to an infectious etiology of chronic bronchitis and acute exacerbations.

Pneumonia

Balows A, Fraser DW, eds. International symposium on legionnaires' disease. Ann Intern Med 1979;90:491–707.

Comprehensive review of etiology, epidemiology, immunology, pathology, and clinical aspects of this disease.

Bartlett JG, Brewer NS, Ryan KJ. Cumitech 7: laboratory diagnosis of lower respiratory tract infections. Washington, DC: American Society for Microbiology, 1978.

Concise review of specimen collection techniques, microscopic examination, and cultural techniques for diagnosis of pneumonia.

Centers for Disease Control. Guidelines for short-course tuberculosis chemotherapy. Morbidity and Mortality Weekly Report 1980;29:97–105.

Glassworth J, Robins AG, Snider DE. Tuberculosis in the 1980s. N Engl J Med 1980;302:1441–1450.

Concise review of the epidemiology, pathogenesis, diagnosis, new therapies, and prophylaxis of tuberculosis, with 121 references.

Johanson WG Jr, Pierce AK, Sandford JP, Thomas GD. Nosocomial respiratory infections with gram-negative bacilli. The significance of colonization of the respiratory tract. Ann Intern Med 1972;77:701–706.

A prospective study of 213 patients admitted to an intensive care unit showed the strong association of colonization of the respiratory tract with gram-negative enteric rods in seriously ill patients and subsequent pneumonia.

Mufson MA, Chang V, Gill V, Wood SC, Romansky MJ, Chanock RM. The role of viruses, mycoplasmas and bacteria in acute pneumonia in civilian adults. Am J Epidemiol 1967;85:526–544.
An epidemiologic study of 427 patients with pneumonia in which the etiology was proved in only one-third of cases, of which 50% were caused by *S. pneumoniae* and the remainder mainly by viruses and rarely mycoplasmas.

Murray HW, Masur H, Senterfit LB, Roberts RB. The protean manifestations of *Mycoplasma pneumoniae* infection in adults. Am J Med 1975;58:229–242
Case presentations of pulmonary and nonpulmonary *M. pneumoniae* disease and review of the literature.

Sullivan RJ, Dowdle WR, Marine WM. Adult pneumonia in a general hospital. Etiology and host risk factors. Arch Intern Med 1972;129:935–942.
A detailed prospective study of 292 patients with pneumonia who were admitted to a city–county hospital. In 57% of the cases, the disease was of proved bacterial etiology and in 25% it was of viral etiology.

Pyogenic Lung Abscess and Empyema

Bartlett JG, Finegold SM. Anaerobic infections of the lung and pleural space. Am Rev Respir Dis 1974;110:56–77.
Comprehensive review of the types of anaerobic respiratory infections, microbiology, clinical features, treatment, and prognoses based on study of 143 patients.

13 INTRAABDOMINAL INFECTIONS

David A. Haase and Godfrey K. M. Harding

Intraabdominal infections are among the most serious life-threatening conditions seen in medical practice. They include infections not only of the abdominal viscera and peritoneal cavity but of the retroperitoneal space. Most result from spread of microorganisms outside of their normal habitat in the gastrointestinal or female genital tracts. Their course may lead to either (1) inflammation of the peritoneum (peritonitis), which may be localized or generalized, or (2) intraabdominal abscess, with collection of purulent material within the intraperitoneal or retroperitoneal space or the intraabdominal viscera. The clinical course is determined by a number of different factors: (1) the nature and site of the primary event; (2) the variety and number of microorganisms involved; (3) the effectiveness of the host defense mechanisms; and (4) the degree and timing of medical and surgical intervention.

ANATOMY

The peritoneal membrane is divided into the visceral peritoneum, which covers the intraperitoneal organs such as the intestines, liver, and spleen, and the parietal peritoneum, which lines the abdominal and pelvic cavities. The retroperitoneal space contains the pancreas, kidneys, ureters, and sections of the duodenum and colon. Also included are major components of the vascular, neurologic, and lymphatic systems, which are directly covered by the peritoneal membrane in some areas. In the female, the uterus and fallopian tubes are almost completely covered by the peritoneal membrane and lie within the peritoneal cavity.

The peritoneal cavity is the potential space between the visceral and parietal peritoneum, and in certain pathologic conditions may contain large quantities of fluid or be totally obliterated by adhesions. It is divided into a number of compartments or spaces by the reflections of the peritoneal membrane that determine the sites and routes of spread of intraperitoneal fluid collections. Major folds of the peritoneal membrane that form the lesser and greater omenta play an important role in limiting the spread of inflammatory processes within the peritoneal cavity. In females, this cavity is not a closed sac, but communicates externally through the open ends of the fallopian tubes.

Insults to the peritoneal membrane causing an inflammatory response can be due to such diverse processes as contamination with bacteria, chemical irritants (blood, bile, gastric acid), or foreign materials (barium, starch, talc). With nonbacterial peritonitis, symptoms and signs may be minimal or they may mimic those of bacterial peritonitis, and the two may be difficult to differentiate. Bacterial peritonitis may be primary or spontaneous without an identifiable intraabdominal source, or secondary with an identifiable intraabdominal source.

PRIMARY BACTERIAL PERITONITIS

Primary bacterial peritonitis, although uncommon, may be seen in all age groups. It may occur in previously healthy persons but is more frequent in those with certain underlying conditions. These include the nephrotic syndrome in children and postnecrotic or alcoholic cirrhosis in adults, especially when ascites is present. It may also be seen in patients with systemic lupus erythematosus. In children, it is more commonly reported in females than in males.

TABLE 13.1. Microorganisms Commonly Isolated in Primary Peritonitis

Age Group	Organisms
Childhood	*Streptococcus pneumoniae,* group A streptococci (gram-negative enteric bacilli, staphylococci, group B streptococci)
Adults	*Escherichia coli, S. pneumoniae,* group A streptococci (anaerobic bacteria)

() = less often isolated.

Etiology

Unlike secondary peritonitis, infection in this group is most often caused by a single microorganism (Table 13.1). In children, *Streptococcus pneumoniae* and group A streptococci are the primary pathogens, although enteric gram-negative organisms and staphylococci have also been isolated. In adults, particularly patients with cirrhosis and ascites, enteric gram-negative organisms are most often involved, however, other pathogens such as *S. pneumoniae* have also been isolated.

Pathophysiology

Microorganisms most likely enter the peritoneal cavity by hematogenous spread from the intestine or from other sites such as the urinary or respiratory tract. Under certain conditions, they may pass directly across the wall of the intestinal tract and in females can also enter through the fallopian tubes. Patients with nephrosis and cirrhosis have defects in host defense mechanisms, with impaired clearance of microorganisms from the blood stream.

Clinical Manifestations

Symptoms and signs may be minimal or totally absent, particularly in the patient with ascites. Usually, however, there is acute onset of fever, abdominal pain and distention, along with systemic upset. Physical examination reveals peritoneal signs of inflammation with involuntary guarding, rebound tenderness, and diminished or absent bowel sounds.

Diagnosis

In patients with the previously mentioned underlying conditions, the diagnosis of primary bacterial peritonitis may be suspected on clinical grounds. Supportive evidence of a continuing inflammatory process, such as leukocytosis in peripheral blood, may be helpful. The diagnosis can be established with certainty by aspirating fluid from the peritoneal cavity, but this is not without risk in some patients.

Biochemical analysis of peritoneal fluid shows features of a transudate (protein, <30 gm/L; lactic dehydrogenase (LDH) <200 IU/L) with an elevated white cell count over 300 per mm^3 with more than 25% polymorphonuclear neutrophils. Gram's stain of the fluid may reveal the infecting organism, and culture should be obtained for aerobes, anaerobes, and fungi. The infecting organism may also be recovered from blood cultures or from another site of infection such as the lung or urinary tract.

Radiographs of the abdomen may be useful in excluding bowel perforation by noting the absence of free air under the diaphragm. Other conditions such as acute pancreatitis, which may mimic primary peritonitis, can be excluded on the basis of the peritoneal fluid analysis (elevated amylase).

Isolation of a single organism favors the diagnosis of primary peritonitis. The final differentiation of primary from secondary bacterial disease may have to be made at exploratory laparotomy. This is seldom necessary in children with gram-positive organisms only, or in patients with end-stage cirrhosis and ascites in whom the likelihood of primary bacterial peritonitis is much higher.

Treatment

Patients with primary bacterial peritonitis generally respond quite promptly to appropriate antimicrobial therapy, often within 48 to 72 hours. Initial therapy should be guided by the clinical situation — age, underlying condition, and Gram's stain of peritoneal fluid if ascites is present. If the stain is negative, therapy should be aimed at the most likely infecting organism for that clinical situation, for example, *E. coli* in adults with cirrhosis, *S. pneumoniae* in children with nephrosis. Single-drug therapy should be adequate in most instances; however, in doubtful cases, broad-spectrum antimicrobial coverage should be used and therapy adjusted when the results of cultures and susceptibility testing of the infecting organism(s) are available (Figure 13.1).

Prognosis

The majority of patients with primary peritonitis due to gram-positive organisms or those who have no under-

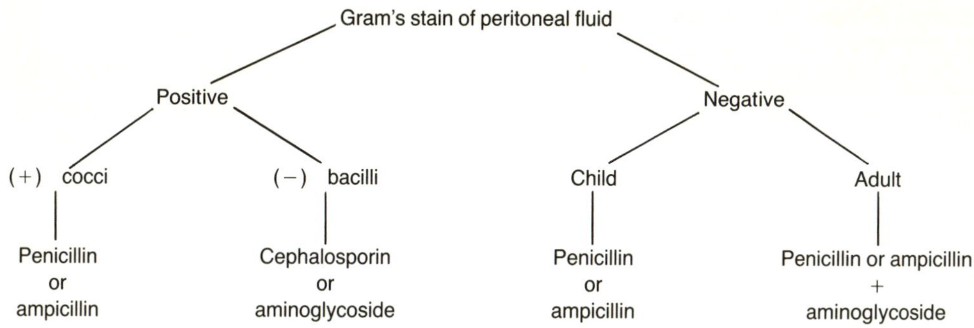

FIGURE 13.1. Suggested initial therapy for primary peritonitis. An antistaphylococcal, semisynthetic penicillin such as cloxacillin may be substituted for penicillin if necessary. A first-generation cephalosporin such as cefazolin may be used alone in most instances.

lying disease recover fully with early diagnosis and therapy. Patients with cirrhosis and ascites often do poorly and have a high mortality rate (80%). This is mostly due to the underlying end-stage liver disease with its associated complications.

TUBERCULOUS PERITONITIS

Tuberculous peritonitis is most often caused by hematogenous spread of *Mycobacterium tuberculosis* to the peritoneum from a primary lung infection. It may only become evident clinically some time after the primary process has healed. Direct spread from lesions in the intestine, lymph nodes, or female genital tract may occur in some cases. Tuberculous infection results in a chronic peritonitis with scattered granulomas over the entire peritoneum, the formation of ascitic fluid, and fibrinous adhesions of the abdominal viscera.

Clinical Manifestations

The onset of symptoms is usually insidious, appearing over weeks or months, but symptoms may be completely absent. Constitutional findings such as anorexia, weakness, weight loss, and night sweats are often present. Fever, abdominal pain and distention may also be prominent. Ascites is often present, with mild abdominal tenderness and a palpable mass. The abdominal wall may have a doughy consistency without rebound tenderness. Symptoms and signs of acute intestinal obstruction may occasionally be the principal features.

Diagnosis

Differential diagnosis includes nontuberculous bacterial peritonitis, starch or foreign body peritonitis, fungal peritonitis, intraabdominal neoplasms, and cirrhosis with ascites. In tuberculous peritonitis the ascitic fluid has the features of an exudate (protein, >30 gm/l; LDH, >200 IU/l) with lymphocytic pleocytosis and may have a decreased glucose concentration below 1.8 mmol per liter. Acid-fast tubercle bacilli are usually not seen on smear, and culture of the ascitic fluid is often negative unless more than 1 liter of fluid is obtained. Definitive diagnosis is based on histology and culture of the peritoneal membrane obtained by percutaneous needle biopsy or at laparoscopy or laparotomy. Granuloma formation is also characteristic of starch or foreign body peritonitis and fungal peritonitis. The tuberculin skin test is generally positive. Evidence of active or healed infection may be present in other organ systems, particularly the lungs.

Treatment

Therapy with isoniazid, 300 mg per day, and rifampin 600 mg per day for 12 to 18 months is usually adequate, but surgical intervention may be necessary to relieve intestinal obstruction.

SECONDARY BACTERIAL PERITONITIS

The secondary form of disease is by far the more common bacterial peritonitis. It is of greater clinical importance and carries a higher morbidity and mortality than

TABLE 13.2. Comparative Features of Primary and Secondary Bacterial Peritonitis

Feature	*Primary Peritonitis*	*Secondary Peritonitis*
Underlying disease	Nephrosis, cirrhosis ± ascites	None except primary intraabdominal disease
Etiology	Often single organism, e.g., *E. coli, S. pneumoniae*	Often several organisms, e.g., *E. coli* and *Bacteroides fragilis*
Route of infection	Hematogenous most common	Direct spread from intraabdominal source
Clinical manifestations	Acute abdomen	Acute abdomen
Antimicrobial agents	Often only single drug necessary	Combined multiple-drug regimen often necessary
Surgery	Rarely required	Always required

TABLE 13.3. Gastrointestinal Microflora

Site	*Organisms*	*Counts/ml or gm of Contents*
Stomach	Viridans streptococci, *Lactobacillus* sp., yeasts	$\leq 10^3$
Small bowel		
Proximal	*Streptococcus* sp., *Lactobacillus* sp. (Enterobacteriaceae, *Bacteroides* sp.)	10^2–10^4
Distal	*Enterobacteriaceae, B. fragilis* group (*Streptococcus* sp., *Lactobacillus* sp.)	10^6–10^7
Large bowel	*B. fragilis* group, *Bifidobacterium, Clostridium* sp., *Eubacterium* sp. (*Enterococci, Enterobacteriaceae*)	10^{11}

() = relatively small numbers.

primary peritonitis. Secondary bacterial peritonitis most often results from perforation of a hollow intraabdominal viscus due to inflammation, obstruction, vascular compromise, or trauma, with subsequent contamination of the peritoneal cavity by endogenous microorganisms. Predisposing conditions are as follows:

1. Trauma
   Blunt or penetrating, with injury to bowel
2. Inflammation
   Intestinal — appendicitis, diverticulitis
   Visceral — cholecystitis, pancreatitis
3. Perforation of the bowel
   Peptic or parasitic ulcers
4. Vascular impairment with ischemia and necrosis of bowel
   Vascular occlusion, arterial or venous
   Mechanical obstruction
5. Rupture of intravisceral abscess
   Renal, hepatic
6. Iatrogenic or postoperative
   Bile peritonitis after liver biopsy
   Intraoperative bowel injury
   Postoperative anastomotic leak
7. Inflammatory conditions of the female genital tract
   Salpingitis, endomyometritis, tubo-ovarian abscess

Rarely, exogenous organisms such as *S. aureus* and *S. epidermidis* from the skin can enter the peritoneal cavity after penetrating trauma, surgical procedures, or infection of intraperitoneal devices and cause peritonitis. Some comparative features of primary and secondary bacterial peritonitis are shown in Table 13.2.

Etiology

The variety and numbers of organisms involved in secondary bacterial peritonitis depend on the site of the primary insult (stomach, small bowel, colon) and on any underlying factors that may alter the normal microflora at that site. The stomach with its low pH normally contains less than 10^3 bacteria per ml (Table 13.3), consisting mainly of oropharyngeal-type organisms. Any condition that increases gastric pH (meals, antacids, cimetidine, ranitidine, blood, achlorhydria) significantly increases the number and type of organisms present.

Bacterial counts rise progressively along the gastrointestinal tract, with higher numbers of gram-negative organisms isolated from the distal small bowel and the colon. The proportion of anaerobic to aerobic organisms also increases along the bowel. In the distal small bowel the anaerobic:aerobic ratio is approximately equal, while in the large bowel it is approximately 1000:1. Gastric achlorhydria or conditions that lead to stasis in the small bowel allow increased growth of microorganisms at these sites. The normal microflora of the intestinal tract may also be significantly altered by antibiotic therapy and immunosuppression, allowing overgrowth of other potential pathogens (*Pseudomonas* sp., *Candida* sp.).

Secondary peritonitis is therefore usually polymicrobial with mixed aerobic and anaerobic organisms. The most commonly isolated aerobes are *E. coli, Proteus* sp., and *Klebsiella* sp. The *Bacteroides fragilis* group, anaerobic cocci, and *Clostridium* sp. are the most common anaerobes. The female genital tract contains numerous organisms as normal flora, anaerobes being the most common. Secondary bacterial peritonitis from this source generally is microbiologically similar to that from intestinal sources.

Pathophysiology

The Wistar rat model of experimental peritonitis has shown the biphasic course of this illness. Aerobic coliform bacteria predominate in the initial acute peritonitis phase, with high mortality; anaerobic bacteria predominate in the secondary, abscess formation, stage. These two groups of organisms, in particular, *E. coli* and *B. fragilis,* have been shown to act synergistically in these mixed infections.

Other factors such as chemical irritants (gastric acid, pancreatic enzymes) or foreign material (barium, blood, bile) may act as adjuvants to increase the virulence of intraperitoneal microorganisms. They may act by direct interference with host defense mechanisms (phagocytosis, intracellular killing) and/or by creating more optimal conditions for bacterial proliferation (tissue injury).

The response of the peritoneal membrane to infection is aimed at limiting the spread of the inflammatory process in the peritoneal cavity and allowing host defense mechanisms, both humoral and cellular, to eliminate the infecting organisms. Initially with local peritoneal inflammation there is exudation of fluid rich in antibodies, complement, neutrophils, and macrophages. These elements of the defense system combine to enhance bacterial phagocytosis and killing. The inflammatory process is further limited by the formation of fibrinous adhesions in the peritoneal cavity, and by the sealing action of the greater omentum. Bacteria and toxins are directly absorbed by the inflamed peritoneum, resulting in bacteremia and endotoxinemia.

The actions of the host defense system may lead to resolution of the inflammatory process or localized abscess formation. If not contained, there is diffuse spread of the inflammatory process, resulting in a generalized peritonitis. Infecting fluid may track into the different spaces of the peritoneal cavity (subhepatic, subphrenic) with resulting abscess formation. Factors that influence this outcome include (1) bacterial virulence, (2) the extent and duration of contamination prior to medical intervention, and (3) the state of the host's defenses.

Many organic systems can also be affected by the consequences of intraabdominal infection. Massive shifts of fluids and electrolytes into the bowel lumen and peritoneal cavity result in decreased circulating blood volume. This is further compounded by fluid loss from fever, vomiting, diarrhea, and nasogastric suction. In addition, endotoxin increases capillary permeability and pooling of fluid in peripheral tissues. Respiratory function may be compromised mechanically by the intraabdominal process with resultant ventilation/perfusion abnormalities and by low-pressure pulmonary edema. The ultimate effects of uncontrolled infection may be septic shock with hypotension, hypoxemia, a hypercatabolic state, metabolic acidosis, renal failure, and death.

Clinical Manifestations

Clinical manifestations depend on the primary underlying cause of infection and the resulting peritoneal response. Past history may reveal a predisposing condition such as peptic ulcer disease, diverticulosis, or pelvic inflammatory disease. Abdominal pain increased by movement or breathing is a frequent complaint. At first it may be felt in a localized area, then later may become generalized. Other possible symptoms include anorexia, nausea, vomiting, fever, chills, decreased urination, obstipation, and abdominal distention.

The clinical signs reflect the continuing infectious process with fever, tachycardia, low pulse pressure, and tachypnea. The patient may appear restless, irritable, or reluctant to move in bed, and later may become lethargic and stuporous. Abdominal distention with generalized tenderness on palpation may be present, or tenderness may be maximal over the affected organ together with involuntary guarding, rigidity, and rebound tenderness. Percussion may detect decreased liver dullness due to free air from intestinal perforation, and bowel sounds may be hypoactive or absent. Rectal examination should be performed, and in the female, pelvic examination may detect a primary process such as a tubo-ovarian abscess or salpingitis. Abdominal signs may be minimal or absent in the very young, the very old, in patients receiving steroid therapy or those in whom the intraabdominal process does not affect the anterior abdominal wall.

Diagnosis

Differential diagnosis of the so-called acute abdomen is quite extensive, and a few of the common causes are listed below:

1. Surgical
   - Inflammatory — acute appendicitis, diverticulitis, pancreatitis
   - Obstructive — acute intestinal obstruction, acute cholecystitis
   - Perforation — peptic or gastric ulcer, inflamed viscera
   - Vascular — ruptured aortic aneurysm, mesenteric vascular occlusion
2. Medical
   - Metabolic — diabetic ketoacidosis, acute porphyria, lead poisoning
   - Hematologic — sickle cell crisis, hemophilia
   - Neurologic — tabes dorsalis, herpes zoster
   - Inflammatory — acute hepatitis, enteric fever, inflammatory bowel disease, pseudomembranous colitis
3. Gynecologic — torsion or rupture of ovarian cyst, acute salpingitis, ruptured ectopic pregnancy, pelvic inflammatory disease

Appropriate laboratory and investigative procedures are necessary for differentiation. Peripheral leukocytosis greater than 15,000 per mm^3 is often present, with a predominance of neutrophils and a shift to immature forms. The hematocrit and blood urea nitrogen are often elevated, reflecting decreased blood volume and there may be evidence of metabolic and respiratory acidosis. Biochemical evaluations such as serum amylase and liver function tests are useful for detecting pancreatic or liver disease. Abnormalities in the results of these studies may be nonspecific, for example, intestinal obstruction in perforated peptic ulcer also causes an elevated serum amylase. Other tests such as blood glucose, electrolytes, urinalysis, and urine culture may assist in diagnosis and patient management. Bacteremia is a frequent occurrence in bacterial peritonitis, and blood cultures are essential.

Needle aspiration of peritoneal fluid is a valuable procedure. Diagnosis is based on gross appearance, biochemical analysis, white cell count, and differential. Gram's stain with culture for aerobes and anaerobes may reveal the infecting organisms; however, a negative tap does not exclude intraabdominal infection.

Radiologic procedures should include plain abdominal films with supine, upright, or lateral decubitus views, and upright chest radiographs. These may show nonspecific changes such as bowel distention due to paralytic ileus, or have features that suggest specific diagnoses. Free air in the peritoneal cavity seen beneath the diaphragm on upright chest x-ray is indicative of bowel perforation. Specialized radiologic procedures may be required to detect the underlying disorder. These include intravenous pyelography, cholangiography, and contrast studies of the bowel (barium is contraindicated in bowel perforation).

Treatment

Treatment of the patient with secondary bacterial peritonitis is supportive, with antimicrobial agents and surgery.

Supportive therapy. It is essential to establish nasogastric suction for gastrointestinal decompression, as well as intravenous lines for administration of fluids, electrolytes, and antimicrobial agents. Respiratory support may also be required. Frequent monitoring of temperature, pulse, blood pressure, respiratory rate, and urine output is necessary. Measurement of central venous pressures or pulmonary venous wedge pressures by central catheters allows for more accurate assessment of hemodynamic status, particularly in the elderly. Biochemical (blood urea nitrogen, creatinine, electrolytes) and hematological values (hematocrit, white blood cell count) plus arterial blood gases should also be monitored. Replacement of fluid and electrolytes guided by the results of monitoring procedures should account for gastric loss and loss into the peritoneal cavity and bowel lumen, plus normal maintenance requirements. Generally, crystalloid solutions such as Ringer's lactate are adequate, but with severe hypovolemia, colloid solutions such as albumin or plasma may be necessary. Nutritional support is also essential in these patients, as metabolic requirements are markedly increased; intravenous hyperalimentation may be necessary.

Antimicrobial therapy. Appropriate antimicrobial therapy is of great importance in the patient with bacterial peritonitis and is adjunctive to surgical therapy.

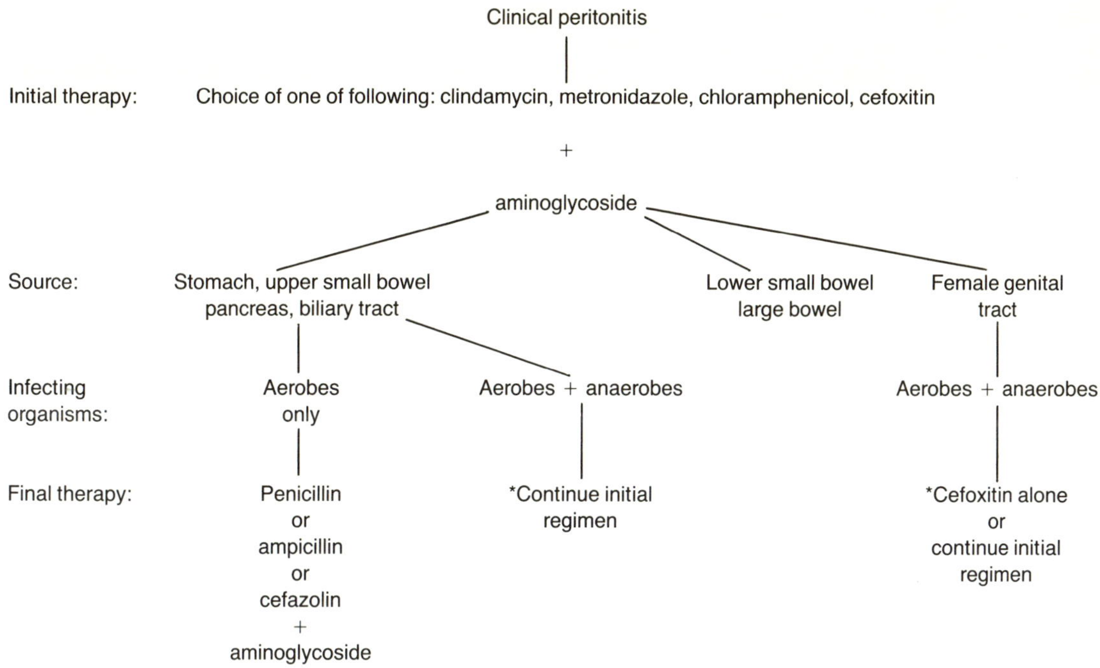

FIGURE 13.2. Suggested approach to antimicrobial therapy in secondary bacterial peritonitis. Final therapy is based on the source of infection and the infecting organisms. Penicillin or ampicillin should be added if enterococcal bacteremia is detected. Penicillin may be added to any regimen if *Clostridium* sp. is thought to be an important pathogen.
*Unless an organism (other than *S. faecalis*) that is resistant to both agents is isolated from the infected exudate.

Medication should be started as soon as the diagnosis is made and appropriate cultures are obtained. Antimicrobial therapy helps to limit the spread of initial infection and reduce the complications of bacteremia, septicemia, and abscess formation. These agents have allowed a significant reduction in mortality. Initial therapy is often empiric, based on knowledge of the source of infection and microorganisms that are potentially responsible for the peritoneal contamination. Therapy must therefore include coverage for aerobic gram-negative organisms such as *E. coli* and anaerobic organisms such as the *B. fragilis* group. This usually requires the use of several agents. With the results of culture and susceptibility testing, therapy may be adjusted, particularly if resistant organisms are isolated (Figure 13.2).

The aminoglycosides gentamicin, tobramycin, netilmicin, and amikacin provide coverage for gram-negative aerobic organisms and should be combined with drugs that cover anaerobic organisms, including the *B. fragilis* group. These include clindamycin, chloramphenicol, cefoxitin, metronidazole, ticarcillin, and carbenicillin. The role of the enterococci in intraabdominal infection is not entirely clear, but if they are isolated from the blood, additional coverage with penicillin or ampicillin is required. Penicillin may be added if *Clostridium* sp. is thought to be an important pathogen.

In cases of infection associated with the stomach, upper small intestine, pancreas, and biliary tract, although anaerobic isolates are infrequent, initial therapy should include aerobic and anaerobic coverage (Figure 13.2). If aerobes only are isolated, the patient can be treated with penicillin or cefazolin plus an aminoglycoside (Figure 13.2). Serum levels of aminoglycoside and renal function should be monitored. One must be cautious, however, particularly with liver abscesses, since in certain instances anaerobes can play a role as discussed later in this chapter. Newer beta-lactam antimicrobial agents such as moxalactam, piperacillin, and ceftizoxime may be potentially useful in intraabdominal infection but are still under investigation. Intravenous steroids may be of benefit in the treatment of patients in septic shock, and recently antiserum to J5 *E. coli* has been shown to be beneficial, but this is still experimental.

Surgical therapy. Surgery is the most important modality in the management of patients with intraabdominal infection and should not be delayed unnecessarily. The aims of exploratory laparotomy are firstly to identify and eliminate the primary source of contamination and secondly to remove infected fluids, foreign material, and necrotic tissue from the peritoneal cavity. Saline irrigation of the peritoneal cavity may be useful in some instances, such as when there is gross fecal contamination. Intraoperative or postoperative irrigation with antibiotic or antiseptic solutions is not generally recommended. Specimens of material from the peritoneal cavity should be submitted for Gram's stain plus aerobic and anaerobic culture.

Prognosis

In recent prospective trials with appropriate antimicrobial agents and surgery the failure rate has been as high as 20% and the mortality rate up to 10%. The two most important factors that influence outcome are age and underlying disease (diabetes, emphysema, malignancy). Death in patients with intraabdominal infection may result from failure of the cardiovascular, respiratory, and renal systems.

SPECIFIC SOURCES OF INTRAABDOMINAL INFECTION

The most common causes of intraabdominal infection are appendicitis, diverticulitis, cholecystitis, and pancreatitis. These conditions may lead to local peritonitis adjacent to the inflamed organ or to perforation of the organ with localized abscess formation or generalized peritonitis and distant abscess formation (subphrenic, pelvic). Bacteremia is common and transportation of organisms by way of portal circulation to the liver may result in liver abscesses. The infecting organisms involved in these conditions are most often mixed and originate in the bowel directly associated with the inflamed organ. When dealing with a patient who has an acute abdomen, it is important to keep in mind that a number of possibilities might explain the clinical picture (see page 208).

Appendicitis

Acute inflammation of the appendix may result from primary infection of the submucosal lymphatic tissue as occurs in *Salmonella* infection. The majority of cases arise secondary to mechanical obstruction of the lumen by fecoliths, enlarged lymphoid tissue, or parasitic worms. The ensuing stasis leads to increased bacterial multiplication and infection, while the increased intraluminal pressure results in vascular obstruction with ischemia and gangrene. Subsequent perforation results in secondary bacterial peritonitis as described. The site of localized peritonitis and periappendiceal abscess formation depends on the anatomic location of the appendix such as retrocecal or pelvic.

Clinical features include colicky epigastric or periumbilical pain that later shifts to the right lower quadrant as the adjacent parietal peritoneum becomes inflamed. Constipation is common but diarrhea may also be a feature. A mass may be palpable through the abdominal wall in patients with a periappendiceal abscess, and rectal examination may elicit tenderness. Plain radiographs assist in excluding other causes of an acute abdomen and may show an air-fluid level, gas in the right lower quadrant, or loss of the psoas shadow. Barium examination may outline an abscess or show displacement of adjacent viscera.

Early appendectomy before perforation occurs is curative, but this may be delayed in the very young and the elderly who may display atypical features. Perioperative antimicrobial therapy is only recommended in the patient with suspected perforation of the appendix. Postoperative wound infection and dehiscence are common. The management of secondary bacterial peritonitis is as previously described.

Diverticulitis

The pathogenesis is similar to that of appendicitis, with obstruction by a fecolith and resulting infection. Complications include perforation with localized peritonitis or abscess formation, generalized peritonitis with its sequelae, and the formation of fistulae in the bladder, vagina, abdominal wall, or perineum. The clinical features are similar to those of other causes of the acute abdomen. Abdominal pain and tenderness may be localized to the left lower quadrant and constipation may be present. Plain radiographs of the abdomen may show the air-fluid level of an abscess, and a contrast enema with a water-soluble agent may outline an abscess or perforated diverticulum. Antimicrobial therapy and surgery where indicated are necessary to cure the patient of the infection.

Cholecystitis

Acute cholecystitis occurs when there is stasis of the gallbladder contents and subsequent colonization with bowel microorganisms, either directly by way of the biliary tree or through the blood stream or lymphatics. In the majority of cases stasis is caused by obstruction with a gallstone; however, in some instances obstruction may be secondary to other causes such as a neoplasm or enlarged lymph node. Occasionally no obstruction is detected (acalculous cholecystitis). The predominant pathogens are *E. coli, Klebsiella* sp., and *S. faecalis*. Anaerobic organisms such as *B. fragilis* and *Clostridium perfringens* are less frequently isolated. Complications include empyema, ischemia with gangrene and perforation, secondary bacterial peritonitis, and abscess formation. Acute cholangitis may also occur, particularly when there is obstruction of the common bile duct.

The clinical features of acute cholecystitis include right upper quadrant pain and tenderness with radiation to the scapula and right shoulder. Palpation may elicit a positive Murphy's sign or detect a tender enlarged gallbladder. Liver function testing may show abnormalities in many patients. It may be necessary to perform preoperative ultrasonography or intravenous cholangiography to demonstrate the presence of cholelithiasis and biliary tract obstruction. The course of acute cholecystitis may lead to resolution, particularly if there is spontaneous relief of biliary tract obstruction. However, complications may arise and surgical intervention may then become necessary. The antimicrobial regimen most often employed is ampicillin in combination with an aminoglycoside such as gentamicin or tobramycin.

Pancreatitis

Inflammation of the pancreas may arise from conditions such as trauma, alcoholism, and biliary tract obstruction. Initially, there is a release of pancreatic enzymes causing chemical peritonitis and tissue injury, but secondary bacterial infection may occur. This is commonly seen in the severe hemorrhagic or necrotizing forms of pancreatitis. The infecting organisms may arise directly from adjacent bowel, by hematogenous spread, or from the infected biliary tree when there is biliary obstruction. Complications include peritonitis, abscess formation, and pseudocyst formation. Major septic complications, although infrequent, have a high mortality rate.

Clinical features include persistent fever with severe epigastric pain and tenderness. Hypotension plus hypocalcemia and tetany may also be present. Plain abdominal radiographs may reveal a sentinel loop of localized duodenal ileus. Spasm of the colon at the splenic flexure (colon cut-off sign) may be demonstrated in the plain radiographs or by a contrast enema. Ultrasonography and computed tomography are useful in the diagnosis of secondary complications such as abscess and pseudocyst formation.

Aggressive supportive management is necessary and surgical therapy is aimed at removing necrotic material and draining pancreatic abscesses. Appropriate antimicrobial therapy and nutritional support are also necessary.

PERITONEAL DIALYSIS AND PERITONITIS

Peritonitis is a major complication associatd with peritoneal dialysis in hospitalized and ambulatory patients. It may occur in one of several ways: (1) perforation of the bowel during placement of a dialysis catheter; (2) passage of organisms directly across the bowel wall; (3) colonization and infection with skin organisms through the dialysis catheter; and (4) contamination of the dialysis fluid with bacteria or endotoxin. The common infecting organisms are *S. aureus, S. epidermidis,* and streptococci; however, gram-negative organisms such as *Pseudomonas* sp. and *Serratia* sp. may be isolated. Yeasts such as *Candida* sp. may also cause infection in these patients.

Clinical symptoms and signs of bacterial peritonitis have already been described. The dialysate drainage is cloudy and a specimen of fluid should be sent for white cell count, Gram's stain, plus culture and susceptibility testing prior to starting antimicrobial therapy. The infecting organisms may be isolated in approximately 75% of patients with clinical infection. Antibiotics are often administered by the intraperitoneal route with or without simultaneous intravenous therapy, and the agent(s) employed can be chosen on the basis of the Gram's stain of the dialysate. If this is unavailable or not helpful, presumptive therapy should include an antistaphylococcal agent such as cloxacillin or cefazolin plus an aminoglycoside. Further adjustment can be made when the results of culture and susceptibility testing are available.

INTRAABDOMINAL ABSCESSES

Localized collections of purulent material in the abdominal cavity are another manifestation of intraabdominal infection. They consist of necrotic debris, bacteria, and white blood cells surrounded by a fairly well-defined wall of fibrinous material. Abscesses may form within the peritoneal cavity, a visceral organ, or in the retroperitoneal space.

Intraperitoneal Abscess

Etiology

The majority of intraperitoneal abscesses occur after secondary bacterial peritonitis caused by conditions such as appendicitis, diverticulitis, cholecystitis, pancreatitis, trauma, and abdominal surgery. They may be single or multiple and form either adjacent to the inflamed organ or in specific anatomic areas of the peritoneal cavity. The peritoneal reflections form channels and potential spaces that allow fluid collections to form, particularly in recumbent patients. These include the subdiaphragmatic or subphrenic spaces, the intermesenteric and paracolic areas, and the pelvic cavity. The location of an abscess depends to a large extent on the site of primary inflammation and the position of the patient at the time of peritoneal contamination.

The microorganisms isolated from intraabdominal abscesses are mixed, with anaerobic organisms such as the *B. fragilis* group being the most common. In addition, aerobic organisms such as *E. coli, Klebsiella* sp., *P. aeruginosa, S. aureus,* and enterococci are frequently isolated. These reflect the endogenous microflora from the site of primary inflammation.

Pathophysiology

The response of the peritoneum to infection is aimed at limiting the spread of the inflammatory process and is initially localized to the area of primary infection. If successful, bacteria, neutrophils, and inflammatory debris are surrounded by a fibrinous wall and form a localized abscess such as a periappendiceal or pericolic abscess. If the infection is not contained, generalized peritonitis occurs with free inflammatory exudate within the peritoneal cavity. This infected fluid subsequently forms abscesses in areas away from the site of primary infection. The abscess creates an ideal environment for proliferation of anaerobic organisms, and the capsule impairs the penetration of phagocytic cells, antibodies, and antimicrobial agents. The net result is an enlarging collection of purulent material with bacteria and inflammatory debris, which may rupture, releasing its contents into the peritoneal cavity, adjacent viscera, or an extraabdominal site such as the pleural cavity. Bacteremia may also occur in the patient with an intraperitoneal abscess.

Clinical Manifestations

The presence of intermittent spiking fever with shaking chills, particularly in the postoperative patient, is a prominent feature of an intraabdominal abscess. Other symptoms and signs vary depending on the location and source of the abscess, and may be difficult to interpret, particularly postoperatively. Abdominal distention, tenderness, and diminished bowel sounds are nonspecific, and a mass may be palpable in some instances through the abdominal wall or on rectal examination. The disease may be acute or patients can have a more chronic course in the presence of continuing antibiotic therapy.

Subphrenic Abscess

Any source of intraabdominal infection may lead to a subphrenic abscess with a collection of purulent material in one or more of the subphrenic spaces located above or below the liver. These abscesses most commonly occur after major abdominal surgery but are frequently seen with other conditions such as a perforated peptic ulcer, ruptured appendix, diverticulitis, and anastomotic leaks. Abscesses in the lesser sac commonly follow primary infection in an adjacent organ such as the stomach, duodenum, colon, or pancreas, or infection of a pancreatic pseudocyst.

The clinical features are often insidious with delay in diagnosis, but may include fever, chills, and tachycardia with other nonspecific systemic symptoms. Jaundice may be present along with upper abdominal pain and tenderness, or patients may have dyspnea, chest pain, or shoulder tip pain. Pleural effusion, atelectasis, and elevation of the diaphragm may be detected.

Pelvic Abscess

Pelvic abscesses may arise from primary inflammation in a pelvic organ or from purulent drainage originating in the upper abdomen. They may form adjacent to or in a pelvic organ, for example, a tubo-ovarian abscess, or in the peritoneal cul-de-sac between the rectum and bladder in males or uterus in females. The bacteriology is similar to that of abscesses in other areas except for isolation of *N. gonorrhoeae* in females. Clinical features of lower abdominal pain and tenderness are nonspecific but a tender mass may be detected on rectal and vaginal examinations.

Diagnosis

The clinical features are of great importance in suspecting a diagnosis of intraperitoneal abscess. Isolation of an anaerobic organism such as a member of the *B. fragilis* group from blood culture is an important diagnostic clue. Other noninvasive diagnostic tests such as plain radiographs, ultrasonography, and isotope scanning may be useful in detecting and localizing the intraabdominal or intrapelvic abscess. Definitive diagnosis can be confirmed by surgical exploration or by percutaneous needle aspiration guided by ultrasonography or computed tomography.

The chest radiograph in subphrenic abscess may show a pleural effusion, elevation of the hemidiaphragm, and other pulmonary abnormalities suggestive of pneumonia, pulmonary embolism, or postoperative atelectasis. Free air under the diaphragm indicates a postoperative anastomotic leak or perforation of a hollow viscus, while an air-fluid level indicates a subphrenic abscess. The plain abdominal radiograph may show evidence of paralytic ileus or intestinal obstruction and occasionally, also characteristic gas collections. Contrast studies are often useful in outlining an abscess or demonstrating displacement of the stomach or intestine by the abscess mass.

The more specialized noninvasive tests may give more accurate localization of the intraabdominal abscess but are time consuming and costly. Therapy should not be unduly delayed while waiting for results of these tests. Ultrasonography can be used to detect abscesses in the abdomen or pelvis and can distinguish solid from cystic structures. More recently it has been used in guiding percutaneous needle aspiration for diagnosis and drainage of intraabdominal abscesses. The overlying abdominal wall must be intact, and the presence of gas- or contrast-filled structures such as stomach or bowel may prevent proper delineation of underlying masses. Radionuclide imaging using technetium 99m (Tc 99) sulfur colloid, gallium 67 citrate (Ga 67), and more recently indium 111 oxine- (In 111) labeled autologous neutrophils has been successful in establishing the diagnosis. Computed tomography of the abdomen with or without contrast material has improved the detection of abscesses and can also be used to guide percutaneous needle sampling of intraabdominal masses for diagnosis and drainage if necessary. Like the ultrasound, it distinguishes solid from cystic masses, but it is more expensive and cumbersome. Various combinations of these techniques may be used in the patient with suspected intraabdominal abscess, and because they essentially rely on different mechanisms for detection of masses, they are often complementary.

Treatment

Optimal treatment includes parenteral administration of antibiotics and early surgical drainage. The initial antibiotic regimen should cover both aerobic and anaerobic organisms with an aminoglycoside plus a drug such as chloramphenicol, clindamycin, metronidazole, or cefoxitin, as discussed in the section on bacterial peritonitis. Therapy may be guided by results of cultures of material aspirated prior to surgery and blood. Penicillin or ampicillin should be added if enterococci or *Clostridium* sp. are isolated from the blood. Adequate drainage of the intraperitoneal abscess is mandatory and may be accomplished at laparotomy. This also allows exploration of the abdomen for the primary source of infection and detection of other abscesses that may be present. More recently, percutaneous needle aspiration guided by ultrasound and computed tomography has been performed. The results have been favorable and this technique may be useful in the critically ill patient who is unable to undergo immediate surgery. The results of culture of material obtained during surgery may be misleading, as antibiotic therapy started preoperatively can suppress growth of pathogenic organisms.

Prognosis

The morbidity and mortality are considerable in the patient with intraperitoneal abscess, particularly after abdominal surgery. Delay in diagnosis and inadequate drainage are two important contributing factors. The mortality rate may range from 30% to 50% in some series and is highest in older patients, those who have had emergency surgery, or persons who have several abscesses.

Intravisceral Abscess

Abscesses developing within abdominal organs such as the liver and spleen are uncommon. They are more frequently caused by hematogenous spread of organisms from a distant site of infection, but may develop from infection in an adjacent site or from penetrating trauma.

Liver Abscess

Etiology and Pathophysiology

Liver abscesses may either be secondary to bacterial infection or a complication of amebic colitis. Bacterial abscesses are far more frequent, particularly in North America, and may arise by (1) hematogenous seeding through either the hepatic artery during systemic infection or the portal vein in cases of intestinal infection; (2) ascending infection from the biliary tract; (3) blunt or penetrating injury; (4) contiguous spread from an adjacent focus such as the gallbladder; or (5) cryptogenically with no obvious source of infection found. Preexisting cysts or tumors may also be secondarily infected. Historically, liver abscesses were more common following intestinal infection but the majority in more recent years have been secondary to trauma, biliary tract infection (cholecystitis, cholangitis), and systemic bacteremia from causes such as endocarditis and pyelonephritis. Many patients with one or more liver abscesses often have chronic debilitating diseases such as diabetes mellitus or cirrhosis.

Multiple liver abscesses are generally due to hematogenous spread of infection and may predominate in one lobe or the other. The presence of a pyogenic liver abscess may induce an inflammatory response in adjacent structures such as overlying peritoneum or diaphragm, with the formation of adhesions and sterile pleural effusions. Liver enlargement due to an abscess may displace adjacent diaphragm and stomach and may even involve the overlying abdominal wall. Subsequent rupture of the abscess may occur either onto the skin or into the chest, peritoneal cavity, or stomach.

Bacterial isolates from pyogenic liver abscesses vary with the underlying disease. Anaerobic organisms such as anaerobic and microaerophilic streptococci, *Fusobacterium* sp., and *Bacteroides* sp., especially the *B. fragilis* group, can cause liver abscesses, particularly when secondary to intraabdominal infection. One-third of these will have concomitant aerobic isolates. In liver abscesses secondary to biliary tract infections, enteric gram-negative organisms such as *E. coli* are often the only organisms isolated. Liver abscess is the most common extraintestinal manifestation of amebiasis. Over 50% of affected patients have no history of diarrhea and negative stools for ova and parasites. Organisms are carried to the liver by way of the portal vein and commonly form a solitary abscess in the right lobe of the liver. Secondary bacterial infection of an amebic abscess may occur.

Clinical Manifestations

Symptoms and signs may be minimal. Patients may have fever of unknown origin; anorexia, malaise, weight loss, fever, right upper abdominal pain, and tender hepatomegaly are generally present. Occasionally, pain may be felt in the left upper quadrant or epigastrium, or diffusely. Respiratory findings may be present with cough, pleuritic chest pain, shoulder tip pain, pleural effusion, and atelectasis. Jaundice may also be present. Laboratory tests show anemia, polymorphonuclear leukocytosis with a left shift, and elevated levels of serum alkaline phosphatase. Other liver function tests may be mildly abnormal and anaerobic bacteremia may be present.

Clinical differentiation of an amebic from a pyogenic liver abscess may be difficult. The history of travel to an area endemic for amebiasis is helpful. Diarrhea, although more common with amebiasis, may also occur in the patient with a pyogenic abscess. Spiking fever is more common in the latter while point tenderness over the liver is more common with the former.

Diagnosis

Plain radiographs of the chest and abdomen may show an elevated hemidiaphragm, pleural effusion, basal atelectasis, or air within the abscess cavity. Radionuclide scans are the most valuable procedures in the diagnosis of liver abscess. The technetium scan shows an area of decreased uptake in both pyogenic and amebic abscesses, and the gallium scan shows an area of increased uptake in the pyogenic abscess and an area of decreased uptake in the amebic abscess. Ultrasound or computed tomography of the abdomen assists in the diagnosis and helps distinguish between a solid mass such as a tumor and a fluid-filled abscess. Angiography reveals distortion of the vasculature by an avascular mass. Needle aspiration of the abscess guided by ultrasound or computed tomography is diagnostic. Purulent material shows bacteria on Gram's stain and culture. Amebic abscesses commonly contain a reddish-brown material and may show trophozoites of *E. histolytica* on microscopic examination or culture. Serologic tests are positive in most patients with amebic liver abscesses (90%) and needle aspiration may not be required.

Treatment

There are three approaches to therapy of a pyogenic liver abscess: (1) open surgical drainage plus antimicrobial therapy, (2) percutaneous needle aspiration and catheter drainage plus antimicrobial therapy, and (3) antimicrobial therapy alone. Initial antimicrobial therapy should be directed against anaerobic organisms such as the *B. fragilis* group and aerobic enteric organisms. The combination of an aminoglycoside (gentamicin, tobramycin) plus clindamycin, chloramphenicol, metronidazole, or cefoxitin is sufficient. Results of culture of material obtained by needle aspiration should be used to modify therapy if necessary. Amebic liver abscesses rarely require needle aspiration or open surgical drainage and can be successfully treated with metronidazole or emetine. During therapy patients should be followed with serial computed tomography scans or ultrasonography to ensure resolution of the abscess.

Prognosis

Multiple pyogenic liver abscesses have a higher mortality rate than solitary abscesses, since complete surgical drainage may not be feasible and there is often infection in other organ systems. Undiagnosed, undrained abscesses have a high mortality and uncomplicated amebic abscesses have a low mortality. With rupture into chest, pericardium, or peritoneum, the mortality rate rises.

Splenic Abscess

Etiology and Pathophysiology

Splenic abscesses are most commonly caused by hematogenous spread of bacteria from a distant focus such as in cases of bacterial endocarditis. Patients with splenic infarcts from hemoglobinopathies such as sickle cell anemia and blunt trauma with hematoma formation are also more susceptible to splenic infection and abscess formation. Streptococci and *S. aureus* are the most common bacterial isolates, particularly when the condition is due to hematogenous spread. Enteric gram-negative organisms have also been isolated, but anaerobic organisms are less frequently seen.

Clinical Manifestations and Diagnosis

Commonly there is left upper quadrant pain, spiking fever, and tender splenomegaly. Pain may also be felt over the lower chest area or at the tip of the left shoulder. Peripheral leukocytosis and bacteremia may be present. A history of trauma may precede clinical symptoms by weeks or months. Plain chest radiographs may show elevation of the left hemidiaphragm, left pleural effusion, or atelectasis. Abdominal films may show a soft tissue mass or an air-fluid level in the left upper abdomen. Contrast studies of the gastrointestinal tract are often helpful, but radionuclide scanning with technetium 99m, gallium 67, or indium 111-labeled neutrophils are of greater assistance in the diagnosis.

Treatment

Since presumptive antimicrobial therapy should cover aerobic gram-positive cocci and gram-negative bacilli as well as anaerobic organisms, the combination of clindamycin or cefoxitin plus an aminoglycoside (gentamicin, tobramycin, or netilmicin) is appropriate. Therapy can be modified when results of culture and susceptibility testing of blood and abscess contents are available. Ideally, splenectomy should be performed when possible, but in certain instances only incision and drainage can be undertaken.

Pancreatic Abscess

Etiology and Pathophysiology

The majority of pancreatic abscesses develop after severe hemorrhagic or necrotizing pancreatitis and after pancreatitis secondary to biliary tract disease. In these conditions bacteria from the adjacent bowel damaged by proteolytic enzymes or from the infected biliary tree have direct access to the inflamed pancreas. In most instances, enteric organisms are isolated, for example *E. coli, Klebsiella* sp., *Enterobacter* sp., enterococci, and viridans streptococci. Occasionally *S. aureus* is also isolated, but anaerobic organisms are less frequently seen. Pancreatic abscesses may cause erosion of the stomach, duodenum, or colon, with perforation and fistula formation. Spread of the infection to, and abscess formation in the retroperitoneal area may occur, along with abscesses in the lesser sac and subphrenic spaces.

Clinical Manifestations and Diagnosis

Patients may experience clinical deterioration after initial resolution of acute pancreatitis. There may be persistent fever with upper abdominal pain and tenderness, and an abdominal mass may be palpable. Leukocytosis and high levels of serum amylase may be present and bacteremia is often detected.

Plain abdominal radiographs may show an air-fluid level or anterior displacement of the gastric air bubble. Ultrasonography and computed tomography are extremely useful in the detection of pancreatic or lesser sac abscesses. Radionuclide scans such as gallium 67 or indium-labeled neutrophils may also be helpful in highlighting a pancreatic abscess, but are less reliable.

Treatment

Antimicrobial therapy should be instituted early in the patient with suspected pancreatic abscess. The combination of clindamycin or cefoxitin plus gentamicin or tobramycin provides adequate coverage. Antimicrobial therapy can be modified when the results of culture and susceptibility testing of blood and surgical material are available. Surgical drainage of the pancreatic abscess or infected pseudocyst is essential. If present, predisposing factors such as cholelithiasis should also be removed. Complications such as a perforated bowel and spread of infection within the retroperitoneal space must also be identified and appropriately managed. Recurrent or persistent abscess formation may necessitate repeat laparotomy. Nutritional support with reduction of pancreatic activity using total parenteral nutrition is also essential.

The mortality rate without surgical drainage of the pancreatic abscess is near 100%, particularly in older patients with underlying disease.

Retroperitoneal Abscess

The potential space between the posterior peritoneal membrane and the transversalis fascia lining the abdominal and pelvic cavities may be the site of abscess formation. The majority of these form in relation to structures that lie within or adjacent to the retroperitoneal space. In the abdomen these include portions of the duodenum and colon, plus the pancreas and appendix anteriorly, and the kidneys, aorta, and vertebral column posteriorly. Most commonly seen is the perinephric abscess arising secondary to pyelonephritis or a renal abscess. Perforation of the bowel, appendicitis, and pancreatitis also frequently cause retroperitoneal abscesses as described above. These are usually unilateral, but may extend contralaterally, upward into the thorax, or downward into the thigh along the fascia of the psoas muscle.

The bacterial isolates reflect the origin of the infection, with mixed aerobic and anaerobic organisms from bowel and single aerobic organisms such as *E. coli,* Proteus sp., or *S. aureus* from the kidney.

Clinical features are often nonspecific, with fever, chills, anorexia, weight loss, weakness, and pain in the lower abdomen, flank, or back. Urinary tract symptoms may precede a perinephric abscess. Many patients are not seen until weeks after initial onset of symptoms. A mass may be palpable in the abdomen, flank, or upper thigh, and extension of the thigh on the affected side may worsen the pain (psoas sign). Rectal examination may detect a presacral abscess.

Anemia and neutrophilia may be present with abnormal urinalysis (white cells, red cells, albumin) in the patient with pyelonephritis. Plain abdominal radiographs often show an indistinct psoas shadow, an abdominal mass, extraintestinal gas, or an air-fluid level. Intravenous pyelography can demonstrate displacement of the ureter or kidney. Ultrasonography and computed tomography allow more accurate localization of the retroperitoneal abscess and can be used to guide diagnostic percutaneous needle aspiration. Radionuclide scanning with gallium or indium-labeled neutrophils are often used as well.

Adequate surgical drainage is essential, together with initial broad-spectrum antibiotic therapy such as gentamicin or tobramycin with clindamycin, chloramphenicol, metronidazole, or cefoxitin. Modification is based on results of Gram's stain, culture, and susceptibility testing of material obtained from needle aspiration or at surgery. Mortality is directly related to delay in diagnosis, inadequate surgical drainage, and the severity of the underlying disease.

ANNOTATED BIBLIOGRAPHY

Correia MD, Conn HO. Spontaneous bacterial peritonitis in cirrhosis: endemic or epidemic? Med Clin North Am 1975;59:963–982.

Demonstrates the increasing incidence of spontaneous bacterial peritonitis in cirrhotic patients in one institution. The most common bacterial isolates were *E. coli* and *Klebsiella* sp., with very high mortality despite appropriate therapy.

Ferrucci JT, van Sonnenberg E. Intraabdominal abscess: radiological diagnosis and treatment. JAMA 1981; 246:2728–2733.

Ultrasonography and computed tomography are highly accurate in detection and localization of intraabdominal abscess and have been successfully used to guide percutaneous catheter drainage. Radionuclide imaging requires more time to complete the investigation and is less specific.

Gorbach SL, McGowan K. Comparative clinical trials in treatment of intra-abdominal sepsis. J Antimicrob Chemother 1981;8(Suppl):95–104.

A review of the bacteriology and therapy of intraabdominal sepsis. Polymicrobial infection reported in most studies, with the *B. fragilis* group as the most predominant anaerobic isolate.

Harding GKM, Buckwold FJ, Ronald AR, et al. Prospective randomized comparative study of clindamycin, chloramphenicol, and ticarcillin, each in combination with gentamicin in the therapy for intra-abdominal and female genital tract sepsis. J Infect Dis 1980;142:384–393.

No significant difference in the cure rate was noted among the three regimens. Among the aerobic and anaerobic isolates, *E. coli* and the *B. fragilis* group respectively were the most common. The side effects of the regimens are also reported.

Hau T, Ahrenholz DH, Simmons RL. Secondary bacterial peritonitis: the biologic basis of treatment. Curr Probl Surg 1979;16:2–65.

Comprehensive review of the bacteriology, pathogenesis, and management of secondary bacterial peritonitis. Pathogenesis, diagnosis, and management of intraabdominal abscess are also included.

Johnson WC, Gerzof SG, Robbins AH, Nabseth DC. Treatment of abdominal abscesses: comparative evaluation of operative drainage versus percutaneous catheter drainage guided by computed tomography or ultrasound. Ann Surg 1981;194:510–520.

Percutaneous catheter drainage of intraabdominal abscesses guided by ultrasonography or computed tomography is at least as efficacious as operative drainage, and has fewer complications.

Pitcher WD, Musher DM. Critical importance of early diagnosis and treatment of intraabdominal infection. Arch Surg 1982;117:328–333.

Higher morbidity and mortality occur with delay in diagnosis and definitive therapy for intraabdominal infection.

Rubin J, Rogers WA, Taylor HM, et al. Peritonitis during continuous ambulatory peritoneal dialysis. Ann Intern Med 1980;92:7–13.

In these patients peritonitis was most often due to gram-positive organisms — staphylococci and streptococci. The cell count of peritoneal fluid was a dependable indication of infection, while Gram's stain was less helpful. Intraperitoneal antimicrobic therapy was successful.

Singh MM, Bhargava AN, Jaian KI. Tuberculous peritonitis: an evaluation of pathogenetic mechanisms, diagnostic procedures and therapeutic measures. N Engl J Med 1969;28:1091–1094.

Primary focus of infection is most often undetected and diagnosis more readily made with peritoneal biopsy. Antituberculous therapy highly effective.

Snyder SK, Hahn HH. Diagnosis and treatment of intraabdominal abscess in critically ill patients. Surg Clin North Am 1982;62:229–239.

Radiologic diagnosis is much improved with the use of ultrasonography, computed tomography, and radionuclide scanning. Percutaneous aspiration and drainage are frequently successful, particularly in the critically ill patient.

14 GASTROENTEROCOLITIS AND ENTERIC FEVER SYNDROMES

Thomas J. Louie

In North American communities acute diarrheal disease is second only to upper respiratory illness as a cause of absenteeism from school and work. Despite the prevalence of this condition, morbidity and mortality are low. Poor socioeconomic status, poor public health facilities, and malnutrition are major factors promoting morbidity and mortality in underdeveloped countries. This chapter discusses the pathogenesis, major clinical syndromes, and an approach to the diagnosis and management of diarrheal diseases.

PATHOGENESIS

The pathogenesis of acute infectious diarrhea is based primarily on three factors acting alone or in combination.

Increased Microbial Challenge

Small inocula of pathogenic organisms may be handled by host defenses; larger inocula may overcome these natural barriers. Conditions that allow for a higher microbial burden include poor socioeconomic conditions (crowding, poor sanitation, inadequate water supply) and inadequate personal hygiene. Thus the young and the economically disadvantaged populations are most susceptible.

Decreased Host Resistance

Host resistance can be impaired by destruction of the normal gastric acid barrier, reduction of peristalsis, impairment of colonization resistance (ablation of the normal microbial flora), or by underlying diseases including malnutrition.

Normal gastric acid secretion provides the host with a "portable autoclave." At a pH of 1.5, over 99.9% of ingested organisms are killed within 30 minutes. Very few organisms (fewer than 1000/ml) are recovered from gastric secretions in the normal fasting state. Hypochlorhydria or achlorhydria allows ingested organisms to persist and enter the small bowel. Thus the infecting inoculum of *Vibrio cholerae* can be reduced from 10^8 to 10^4 organisms if 2 gm of sodium bicarbonate are used to neutralize gastric acid. Patients with hypochlorhydria are more susceptible to or have more severe disease when challenged by *Salmonella* sp., *Giardia lamblia,* or helminths.

Intestinal motility is required to maintain absorptive processes and the normal indigenous microflora, and may be an important mechanism of elimination of pathogens. In experimental animals, enteric infections are most easily established by using drugs that inhibit peristalsis. Also, it has also been shown that use of diphenoxylate hydrochloride with atropine (Lomotil) to control diarrhea is associated with prolongation of symptoms of shigellosis and intestinal carriage of the organism.

The presence of normal enteric flora competitively inhibits the establishment of exogenous organisms in the gastrointestinal tract. Thus alpha-hemolytic streptococci inhibit oropharyngeal colonization by beta-hemolytic streptococci and coliform organisms. In experimental animal models, antibiotic therapy suppresses the normal flora and reduces the size of the inoculum required to produce colonization and infection by *Salmonella* species. Clearance of intestinal pathogens is associated with restoration of the normal microflora.

Prior to the acquisition of normal immune status in the gastrointestinal tract, neonates may be more susceptible to pathogenic microorganisms. At birth, the mucosa of the gastrointestinal tract is sparsely infiltrated with inflammatory cells. In association with the acquisition of the normal intestinal microflora, the mucosa is infiltrated with polymorphonuclear leukocytes, plasma cells, lymphocytes, and macrophages, and Peyer's patches develop. This normal immune response is absent in experimental germ-free animals. In the normal host, the response maintains an equilibrium between the host and the intestinal flora. In addition, specific coproantibodies, which may be bactericidal, may promote opsonization, prevent bacterial adherence, or neutralize virus particles that are absent in immunologically naive hosts. Passively acquired colostral antibodies and diminished likelihood of environmental contamination reduce the incidence of diarrheal disease in breast-fed infants.

Microbial Virulence Factors

Virulence of microorganisms has been measured by epidemiologically linking the isolation of microorganisms with clinical illness, by reproducing disease in animals and humans by microbial challenge, and by measuring immunologic responses to infection. Knowledge of pathogenic mechanisms of disease is continually being refined and it is hoped that microbial virulence factors will ultimately be identified at a molecular level. At the present time, microbial virulence factors have been broadly classified as adherence factors, toxins that affect a variety of in vitro and in vivo experimental systems, or even quite crudely as invasive factors (e.g., Vi antigen of *S. typhi*). Examples of each are discussed within the clinical entities.

PHYSIOLOGIC DISTURBANCES IN DIARRHEAL DISEASE

An understanding of fluid dynamics in the gastrointestinal tract is essential as a framework for understanding the physiologic consequences of diarrheal disease. In the average adult, oral daily fluid intake is approximately 1.5 liters. In addition, salivary, gastric, biliary, and pancreatic secretions contribute 7 to 8 liters to the intestinal lumen. Only 150 gm of feces (75% to 85% water) are excreted per day, however, indicating that at least 98% of the fluid secreted into the intestinal lumen is reabsorbed. In fact, intestinal absorption is much more efficient. In addition to the 10 liters of ingested or secreted fluid, there is a massive bidirectional fluid flux in the small bowel that is thought to exceed 50 liters per day. Normally, reabsorption from the lumen exceeds secretion into the gut lumen. Relatively small shifts in the balance of secretion into and reabsorption from the lumen lead to diarrheal disease. Fluid that is not reabsorbed in the small bowel is discharged into the large bowel. However, the large bowel is only able to resorb between two and three liters of fluid per day. Thus small bowel diarrhea occurs when the volume of effluent exceeds the capacity of the colon to resorb it.

Broadly speaking, there are three major clinical complexes based on physiologic disturbances — small bowel diarrhea, large bowel diarrhea, and penetrating disease typified by enteric fever syndromes (Table 14.1). Small bowel diarrhea is characterized by a large volume of watery diarrhea associated with crampy periumbilical pain. Usually the infection does not damage the mucosa and consequently, fecal leukocytes are infrequently found. Most often the disease is mediated by enterotoxins produced by bacteria, or by viruses and protozoa (*G. lamblia*). Bowel movements are usually less frequent than in large bowel disease and are not associated with tenesmus (lower colonic or rectal pain).

Large bowel diarrhea, which is typified by the dysenteric syndrome, is associated with invasion of the colonic mucosa. Usually it is characterized by frequent small volume bowel movements, an inflammatory exudate with pus cells in the stool, and tenesmus.

Some types of organisms (e.g., *Salmonella* sp. and *Yersinia* sp.) may produce disease by penetrating the mucosa of the distal small bowel to infect the reticuloendothelial system. The classic example of this is typhoid fever. Thus assessment of major physiologic disturbances may provide etiologic clues and may guide therapeutic intervention.

ACUTE INFECTIOUS DIARRHEAL SYNDROMES

Noninflammatory Syndromes

From the foregoing discussion, it is apparent that different diarrheal syndromes tend to be produced by different groups of etiologic agents. Clinical assessment may

TABLE 14.1. Three Types of Enteric Infections

	Small Bowel Diarrhea	*Large Bowel Diarrhea*	*Penetrating Disease*
Illness	*Watery Diarrhea*	*Dysentery*	*Enteric Fever Syndrome*
Direct examination of stool			
Fecal leukocytes	Uncommon	Common	Variable, usually mononuclear
Bloody diarrhea	Uncommon	Common	Variable
Diarrhea	Large volume Less frequent Tends to dehydrate Periumbilical cramps	Small volume Very frequent Less chance of dehydration Hypogastric cramps and tenesmus	Variable Variable Dehydration uncommon Cramping variable
Proctosigmoidoscopy	Normal	Colitis	Normal
Agents	Enterotoxigenic gram-negative bacilli Viruses (epithelial replication) *Giardia lamblia*	*Shigella* *Campylobacter* (also involve small bowel?) *Salmonella* Invasive *E. coli*	*Salmonella* *Yersinia*

be helpful in establishing the agents. The most common causes of noninflammatory diarrhea and their important clinical features are outlined in Table 14.2. Since these agents are not invasive, fever and clinical toxicity are not prominent features. Because of the small bowel involvement, each of these disease entities may produce significant dehydration. Assessment of the extent of dehydration and initiation of oral rehydration with glucose (or sucrose)/electrolyte fluid is of paramount importance. With serious dehydration (4% to 8% body weight depletion), thirst, decreased skin turgor, muscle cramps, sunken eyes, reduced peripheral pulses, and decreased urine output are observed. More severe dehydration leads to mental obtundation and circulatory collapse.

With the exception of giardiasis, all of these illnesses tend to be self-limited in the absence of antimicrobial therapy, again emphasizing the importance of fluid replacement and symptomatic treatment. No specific therapy is available for the viral illnesses, and antibiotic administration may be useful in limiting the severity of the bacterial illnesses (Figure 14.1).

Rotavirus Gastroenteritis

Rotavirus gastroenteritis is an important cause of nonbacterial gastroenteritis because of its worldwide distribution and high prevalence, and because it primarily affects infants and young children who are more susceptible to develop dehydration and its complications. This is the most common cause of nonbacterial diarrhea in the winter months in temperate climates, and accounts for 60% of cases of gastroenteritis in hospitalized patients. In tropical climates the disease appears to occur frequently throughout the year.

The virus is 70 nm in diameter, and possesses icosahedral symmetry; its wheel-like appearance is produced by the arrangement of the 32 capsomeres that form its outer shell. Three species-specific outer shell glycoprotein antigens have been identified. The inner core contains double-stranded RNA and several glycoprotein antigens that are group specific (common to other rotaviruses). Two antigenically distinct serotypes of human rotavirus are identified, and may account for repeated infections. Morphologically identical viruses have been identified as diarrheal agents in calves, piglets, monkeys, mice, foals, and sheep.

The incubation period is usually 48 to 72 hours. The majority of cases of rotavirus infection are characterized by sudden onset of vomiting, low-grade fever, and watery diarrhea. Vomiting usually occurs at the onset, may last for up to 48 hours, and may be of sufficient severity to cause dehydration. Diarrhea may persist for one to two weeks. The peak prevalence of disease occurs in infants aged 6 to 18 months. Infection may be

TABLE 14.2. Essential Features of Etiologic Agents and Clinical Features of Noninflammatory Diarrhea

	Etiologic Agent	Pathology/ Pathogenesis	Predominant Clinical Features	Predominantly Affected Age Group	Seasonality	Diagnosis	Treatment
Rotavirus diarrhea	70-nm double-stranded RNA virus, at least 2 serotypes	Replication in enterocytes, blunted villi	Incubation period 48–72 hrs Diarrhea may persist for 7–10 d 90% of children ≥3 yrs have antibody	6–18 mo	Winter months in temperate zone; nonseasonal in tropics	Direct electron microscopy $>10^6$ particles/gm stool	Symptomatic Rehydration with oral glucose-electrolyte solution
Parvovirus-like diarrhea	20- to 27-nm single-stranded DNA virus (Norwalk, Montgomery, Hawaii, Ditchling agents)	Replication in enterocytes, blunted villi	Incubation period 24–48 hrs Illness lasts 24–48 hrs Secondary attack rates of 30%	School-age children and adults	Year-round as outbreaks	Immunoelectron microscopy $<10^6$ particles/gm stool	Self-limited Rehydration if required
Giardiasis	*G. lamblia* trophozoite 12–16 μm long × 5–12 μm wide ventral suction discs	Attachment to enterocytes, pathogenesis unknown; cysts transmit disease	Incubation period 7 d Periumbilical cramps, flatulence, foul-smelling stools, steatorrhea Diarrhea tends to be persistent (50% >1 week) Disease more severe in hypochlorhydria or IgA-deficient patient	All ages	Year-round outbreaks, day-care centers; endemic worldwide	Stool examination for cysts and trophozoites	Metronidazole, 250 mg tid × 7 d for adults, 5 mg/kg tid × 7 d for children Quinacrine hydrochloride, 100 mg tid × 2 mg/kg tid × 7 d for children Furazolidone, 2 mg/kg qid × 7 d, pediatric suspension

Enterotoxigenic *E. coli* diarrhea (turista)	*E. coli* containing plasmids directing production of enterotoxins	Intestinal colonization and production of enterotoxins, which increase secretion of fluids and electrolytes by activating adenyl cyclase	Small bowel diarrhea cholera-like illness	All ages	Year-round	In vitro assessment of enterotoxin production by *E. coli* Tests not widely available Diagnosis based on exclusion of other causes and clinical features	Rehydration*: Prevention by trimethoprim/sulfamethoxazole, 160/800 mg po qd or doxycycline, 100 mg po qd Bismuth subsalicylate (Pepto-Bismol), 60 cc po qid daily
V. cholerae Cholera	*V. cholerae*	Same as for enterotoxigenic *E. coli*	Explosive small bowel diarrhea, dehydration	All ages	Year-round	Isolation of organism	Tetracycline, 500 mg qid $\times$ 5 d

*Rehydration: po 20 gm glucose (or 40 gm sucrose), 4 gm NaCl, 4 gm $NaHCO_3$, 1 gm KCl per liter of water. IV 5 gm NaCl, 4 gm Na HCO_3, 1 gm KCl per liter sterile water.

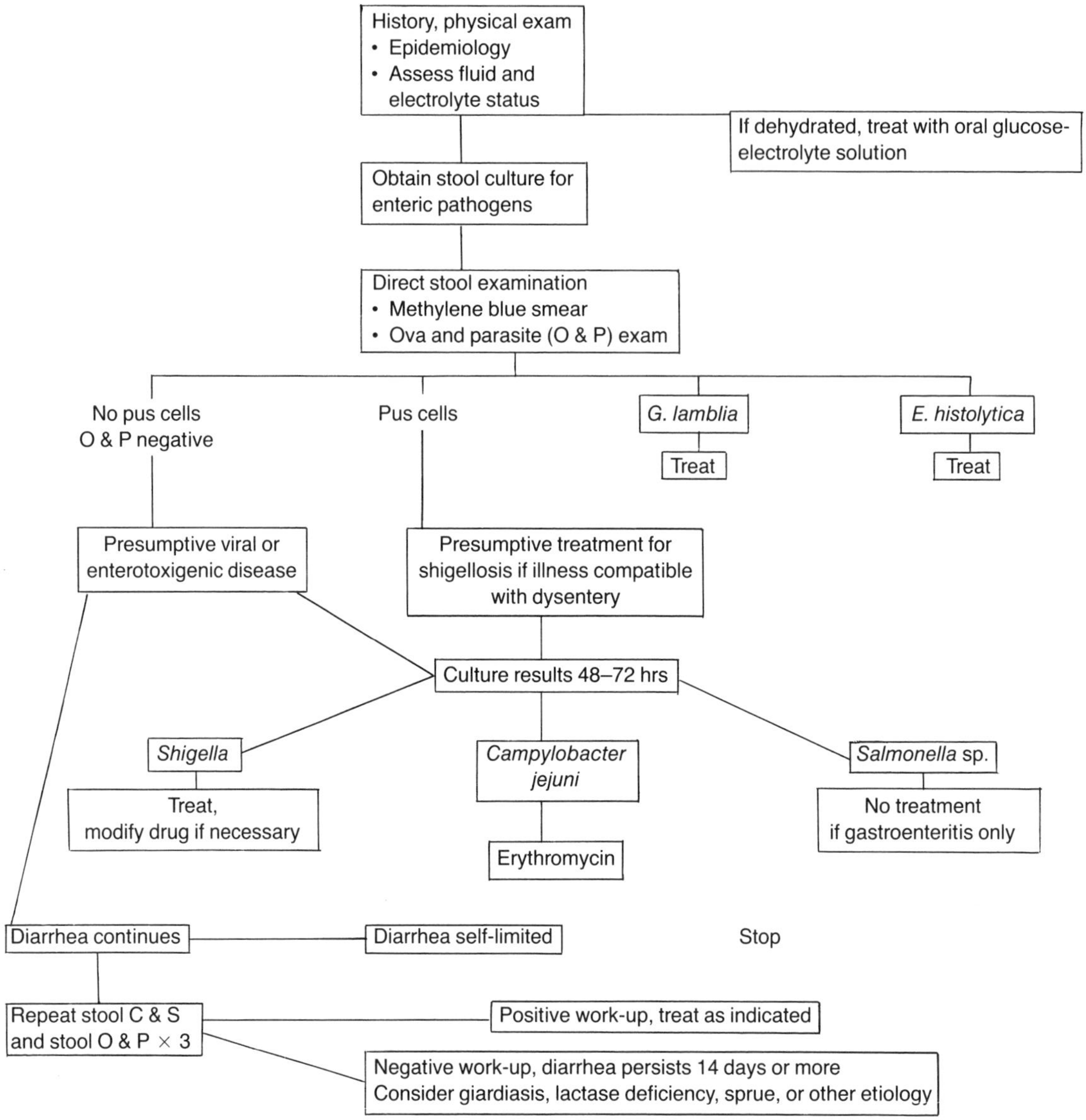

FIGURE 14.1. Algorithm for the treatment of acute infectious diarrhea.

more likely to occur at this time because of a decline in maternally acquired antibodies and withdrawal of the protective effect of colostral antibodies in breast milk. Ninety percent of children under 3 years of age have antibodies to rotaviruses. Infection is less frequently documented and is milder or asymptomatic in older children and adults. Older persons often are secondarily infected in households where childhood illness is present. Upper respiratory illness including rhinitis, pharyngitis, and cough in association with diarrhea is seen in 20% to 40% of cases. Infection is presumed to occur by way of fecal-oral transmission.

The virus replicates in the jejunal and ileal enterocytes. Sloughing of affected enterocytes and their replacement by immature crypt enterocytes results in blunted villi, temporary disaccharidase deficiency, and impairment of glucose-sodium transport. Diarrhea is not mediated by activation of cyclic nucleotides as in enterotoxigenic diseases. Most commonly, direct microscopy of fecal supernatants has been used for the diagnosis, since most patients have no fewer than 10^6 virions per gm of feces.

Since antiviral chemotherapy is not available, oral rehydration is the mainstay of therapy, which is successful in 90% of patients; the remaining patients require parenteral rehydration. Most field studies have been conducted with glucose-electrolyte solutions as used for rehydration of patients with enterotoxic disease. Sucrose can be substituted for glucose with equivalent results.

Gastroenteritis Caused by Parvovirus-like Agents

Illness characterized by acute onset of nausea and vomiting, with or without diarrhea, in school-age children or adults is usually described in reported outbreaks of parvovirus-like gastroenteritis. Low-grade fever, headache, and myalgias generally accompany the intestinal illness. The incubation period is only 24 to 48 hours and illness is equally brief, lasting only one to two days. In contrast to rotavirus infection in temperate zones where disease is seasonal (winter), parvovirus-like disease occurs year-round. Illness is uncommon in children under 3 years of age; however, serosurveys have shown that antibodies are present in half of the population in the fifth decade of life. Transmission of disease is thought to occur by fecal-oral spread, and secondary attack rates may approach 30%. Water and shellfish have been implicated as vehicles of transmission in several outbreaks.

The etiologic agent(s) have not been fully identified as parvoviruses. The viral particles are 20 to 27 nm in diameter, possess icosahedral symmetry, and contain single-stranded DNA. Physiochemical characteristics suggest that these agents are similar to parvoviruses. The types of parvovirus-like agents have been described by their associated outbreaks: Norwalk agent (Ohio, 1968), Montgomery agent (Montgomery County, Maryland, 1971), Hawaii agent (Honolulu, 1971), and Ditchling agent (Ditchling, England, 1975). The Norwalk and Montgomery agents have been shown to be antigenically similar in cross-challenge studies, whereas the Hawaii agent is antigenically dissimilar, since infection with Montgomery or Norwalk agent does not render the patient immune to infection with the Hawaii agent.

Results of intestinal biopsies show blunted villi, shortened microvilli, dilatation of the endoplasmic reticulum, dilated mitochondria, and increased intercellular spaces between enterocytes. These changes are accompanied by transient decreases in the activity of brush border enzymes and malabsorption of xylose and lactose.

Since the number of virions seen in the stool is lower than that seen with rotavirus infection, immunoelectron microscopy is required for diagnosis. Convalescent sera containing specific antibody are used to agglutinate and concentrate viral particles.

No specific therapy is recommended since the disease is self-limited, since it affects a host that is less susceptible to dehydration, and because diarrhea may not be a prominent feature. Handwashing and hygiene may be important in preventing transmission of disease.

Other Viral Enteric Pathogens

At the present time, enteroviruses are not considered to be common causes of diarrheal illness. Numerous viruses have been found in diarrheal stools without a proven etiologic relationship to the illness: coronavirus, adenovirus, astrovirus, minireovirus, minirotavirus, and calciviruses. Additional studies are required to determine the pathogenic potential of these agents.

Giardiasis

Intestinal infestation with the protozoan *G. lamblia* is extremely common and is distributed worldwide. The organism is a flagellate that has both a trophozoite and a cyst stage. The disc-shaped 12 × 7-μm trophozoite with its eight flagella and internal organelles creates an appearance of a face with eyebrows, moustache, and beard.

Infection occurs by ingestion of as few as 10 cysts. The cysts originate from the alimentary canal of humans or other mammals. Contaminated water may be a vehicle for transmission. In several studies in tropical countries, up to two-thirds of the sampled population excreted cysts. Once ingested, the cysts pass through the gastric barrier and excyst in the duodenum and jejunum. Using its ventral suction discs, the trophozoite adheres to duodenojejunal enterocytes and produces diarrheal illness by as yet undefined means. The organism encysts as it is passed down the intestinal tract.

Studies have shown that *Giardia* infestation is associated with lactase and peptidase deficiency, vitamin B_{12} malabsorption, and bacterial overgrowth in the small bowel. Patients with hypochlorhydria or IgA deficiency may have more severe illness.

The incubation period is approximately one week, although a larger inoculum could shorten the incubation period. Acute onset of foul-smelling, watery diarrhea, abdominal cramps and distention, nausea, and flatulence are the most prominent features. Fever and vomiting are unusual. Fecal leukocytes are not usually seen. Approximately half of the infections last longer than one week and the illness may persist for up to a month, resulting in steatorrhea and weight loss. Symptoms may improve and the patient may have intermittent bouts of diarrhea.

In the acute diarrheal stage, trophozoites and cysts may be found in the diarrheal effluent. With chronic diarrhea, however, cysts are more likely to be found. At least three stool examinations should be obtained over a period of days to rule out the disease. In some instances, several stool examinations over a period of four to five weeks may be required for diagnosis. Although it is commonly stated that one-quarter to one-third of cases may not be detected by stool examination, proper stool handling and processing will provide the diagnosis in over 95% of cases according to a recent study.

There are three treatment regimes: (1) metronidazole (Flagyl), 250 mg three times a day in adults, or 5 mg per kg three times a day in children for seven days; (2) quinacrine hydrochloride (Atabrine), 100 mg three times a day for those over 8 years of age, or 2 mg per kg three times a day in children; and (3) furazolidine (Furoxone), 2 mg per kg four times a day as a pediatric suspension. The last is useful in children because it is well tolerated. Approximately 10% to 20% of patients develop nausea, epigastric cramps, or a metallic taste while taking metronidazole. Side effects of quinacrine include gastrointestinal upset, headache, fever, rash, toxic psychosis, hemolytic anemia, and rarely, hepatic necrosis. With each regimen a treatment course is successful in 80% to 90% of cases.

Enterotoxigenic Diarrheal Diseases

Enterotoxins that are manufactured by gram-negative bacteria cause diarrhea by increasing the secretory fluid flux in the small intestine. The best studied diseases are cholera and enterotoxigenic *Escherichia coli* diarrhea. Bacterial enterotoxins are exotoxins elaborated by intact bacteria in the lumen of the gut or in broth cultures. Release of the toxin depends on diffusion or transport through the bacterial cell wall and not on cell lysis. In general, enterotoxins are heat labile (inactivated by heating to 60° C for 30 minutes), sensitive to pronase but resistant to trypsin, not dialyzable, inactivated by acid pH, and extremely potent in small doses.

Once ingested, the organism must colonize the small bowel and elaborate the enterotoxin, which is composed of an active moiety, an inactive linkage unit, and several binding fragments. The binding fragments adhere to ganglioside GM_1 on the enterocyte membrane, after which the toxin enters the cell. The active fragment activates adenylate cyclase, which in turn converts adenosine triphosphate (ATP) into cyclic adenosine monophosphate (cAMP). It is postulated that cAMP activates a protein kinase that phosphorylates a membrane protein and stimulates secretion of fluid and electrolytes. *Escherichia coli* heat labile (LT) enterotoxin is similar to the cholera toxin in structure and function. It is thought that the cholera toxin is encoded by chromosomal DNA, whereas plasmid DNA is responsible for production of *E. coli* enterotoxin.

Cholera

Cholera used to occur worldwide. Since the early nineteenth century there have been six pandemics; however, in the past 20 years the disease has been endemic only in Southeast Asia and northern Africa.

Vibrio cholerae is a gram-negative, comma-shaped organism that on subculture becomes a bacillus. It is oxidase positive and grows best in an alkaline media from pH 9 to 9.6. Specialized culture media such as thiosulfate citrate bile salt agar are required for isolation. There are three serotypes: AB or Ogawa, AC or Inaba, and ABC or Hikojima. All share a group-specific O antigen abbreviated as A, with secondary antigens abbreviated as B and C that are type specific. Most of these strains do not possess soluble hemolysins, and are referred to as classic biotypes. The El Tor biotype, named after a quarantine camp in Egypt, refers to strains possessing the hemolysin. As compared to the classic biotypes, the El Tor biotype is associated with prolonged intestinal carriage after infection and is able to survive a longer time in water. These properties may facilitate new outbreaks of disease.

The clinical features of cholera are primarily vomiting at onset and small bowel diarrhea, with loss of water and electrolytes from the intravascular and extracellular spaces of the body into the gut lumen. As compared to electrolytes in the serum, the diarrheal effluent

TABLE 14.3. Electrolyte Composition of Diarrheal Stools, Oral and Intravenous Replacement Solutions (mEq/L) for Cholera

Substance	Na^+	Cl^-	K^+	HCO_3^-	*Glucose*
Stool					
Adult	135	100	15	45	—
Child	105	90	25	30	—
Oral solution*	90	80	20	30	111
IV solution†	134	99	13	48	Optional

*WHO solution, 3.5 gm NaCl, 2.5 gm Na HCO_3, 1.5 gm KCl, glucose 20 mg/L (or sucrose 40 gm/L).

†Dacca solution (5/4/1) = 5 gm NaCl, 4 gm $NaHCO_3$, 1 gm KCl/L.

contains similar amounts of sodium and chloride, but excessive amounts of potassium and bicarbonate (Table 14.3). Patients become volume depleted, hypokalemic, and acidotic. Severely affected patients may die from shock in less than a day. Mucous flecks and watery diarrheal effluent give rise to the description, rice-water stools.

Treatment involves prompt replacement of volume and electrolytes orally in less severely affected patients; restoration of volume and electrolytes intravenously in those who have diarrheal stools greater than 100 ml per kg per 24 hours or greater than 7 liters per day in adults; correction of electrolyte imbalance; and antibiotic therapy with tetracycline, 250 mg every six hours for five days, or ampicillin in similar dosage. Treatment with antibiotics shortens the duration of diarrhea. Glucose is added to the oral electrolyte solutions to facilitate reabsorption, since the reabsorptive capacity of the small bowel is unaffected by enterotoxin-induced diarrhea. Prevention is based on developing and maintaining public health sanitation. Vaccines are protective only up to six months.

Enterotoxogenic E. coli

Travelers have a 50% to 70% chance of developing acute watery diarrhea (see also Chapter 27). In 1956 it was found that *E. coli* isolated from patients with cholera-like illness was able to cause fluid secretion in ligated rabbit ileal loops. Subsequently it has been shown that travel to areas outside of one's native residence may result in the colonization of the small bowel with enterotoxin-producing strains of *E. coli.* On stool cultures, these strains cannot be differentiated from nontoxin-producing strains. In vitro and in vivo animal tests for enterotoxin are required for identification of toxin production. Once ingested, toxigenic organisms first must be able to adhere to the brush border of the enterocyte. Adherence (colonization) is mediated by one of two colonization-factor antigens. Two types of enterotoxins may be produced, alone or together: a heat-labile cholera-like enterotoxin (LT) and a heat-stable enterotoxin (ST). In contrast to LT, ST is of low molecular weight, is nonantigenic, activates cyclic guanosine monophosphate (GMP), and is of rapid onset (minutes instead of two to three hours).

Traveler's diarrhea is often clinically recognized as noninvasive watery diarrhea. The most commonly used term is "turista," although there are many unflattering euphemisms that reflect the indignation of the victim. Although half of the cases are caused by enterotoxigenic *E. coli,* other etiologic agents are *G. lamblia, Campylobacter jejuni, Salmonella* sp., *Shigella* sp., and *E. histolytica. Aeromonas hydrophila* has also been recently recognized as a cause of diarrhea in travelers.

Most patients are affected approximately one week after arrival in the foreign country. The disease usually resolves within a week. Treatment is rehydration as in cholera. Bismuth subsalicylate (Pepto-Bismol) has been found to bind LT enterotoxin and may reduce the severity of diarrhea; however, the large doses required may be inconvenient for the traveler and may induce salicylate poisoning in infants and young children. Although diphenoxylate hydrochloride with atropine (Lomotil) or opiates may relieve symptoms, these drugs can worsen inflammatory processes such as shigellosis. Thus the cornerstone of treatment is adequate hydration with glucose-electrolyte solution, with the realization that the disease is self-limited. Antimicrobial therapy with agents such as trimethoprim/sulfamethoxazole may shorten the course of illness.

Prevention may be difficult, but can be attempted by avoiding exposure to sources of infection. Salads, raw fruits, vegetables, and untreated water have been implicated as sources. Water should be boiled or decontaminated with halides. Prophylactic sulfonamides and doxycycline have been shown to be effective in preventing disease in short-term (four-week) studies. Ingestion of antimicrobials may suppress the normal microbial flora, thereby reducing resistance to colonization with other organisms. Travelers receiving longer-term prophylaxis have been shown to have increased susceptibility to salmonellosis.

Enteropathogenic E. coli *Diarrhea*

Epidemiologic evidence suggests that outbreaks of infantile diarrhea in nurseries are associated with isolation of certain serotypes of *E. coli*. On the basis of O (somatic) and B (capsular) antigenic analysis, the following are the 14 most commonly identified enteropathogenic *E. coli* (EPEC) serotypes isolated from infantile diarrhea outbreaks: 0111:B4, 055:B5, 026:B6, 0127:B8, 086:B7, 0119:B14, 0125:B15, 0126:B16, 0128:B12, 020:B7, 044:K74, 0:114, 0:142, and 0:158. The mechanism of production of diarrhea is unknown and the disease is included here because of its noninflammatory features. Most patients are under 4 months of age, although disease may occur in children up to 2 years of age. Absence of a normal intestinal flora, altered intestinal immunity, congenital diseases, and prematurity may be predisposing factors.

Onset is often insidious, with the development of listlessness, irritability, and poor feeding over three to six days. Vomiting and fever are infrequent, and stools are watery and without mucus, pus, or blood. Patients may respond to oral neomycin or polymyxin therapy. Without supportive therapy and adjunctive antibiotic therapy, dehydration and complicating superinfection such as otitis media, pneumonia, bacteremia, or peritonitis can occur.

Inflammatory Gastroenteritis

Infections that damage the intestinal mucosa usually elicit an acute inflammatory response. Polymorphonuclear leukocytes are often seen in the diarrheal effluent. In the past, dysentery was the prototype syndrome typifying inflammatory diarrheal illness. Dysentery, a clinical syndrome recognized since biblical times, is characterized by frequent small-volume bowel movements accompanied by mucus and blood with associated tenesmus. Following the identification of *Shigella dysenteriae* in 1896, shigellosis became synonymous with the term *bacillary dysentery*. This designation recognized that shigellae and amebae were the two etiologic agents responsible for this syndrome. In the past two decades, improvements in microbiology have expanded the spectrum of known etiologic agents. Thus organisms such as *C. jejuni,* invasive strains of *E. coli, Yersinia enterocolitica,* and *Vibrio parahemolyticus* have joined *Salmonella* sp., *Shigella* sp., and *E. histolytica* as pathogens that tend to cause inflammatory diarrhea.

In addition to the larger number of etiologic agents, the clinical spectrum of disease has expanded. Whereas dysentery is associated with colonic disease, new agents such as *C. jejuni* and old agents such as *Shigella* sp. may produce both small and large bowel disease.

The etiologic agents, clinical spectrum, diagnosis, and therapy of inflammatory diarrhea are outlined below and summarized in Table 14.4. Salmonellosis, shigellosis, and campylobacteriosis are the most common causes of inflammatory diarrheal disease in both developed and less-developed nations. Because of their importance, these entities are emphasized in the following discussion.

Salmonellosis

Because of the different clinical syndromes produced by *Salmonella* sp., salmonellosis is discussed in the section Penetrating Pathogens (see page 232).

Shigellosis

Shigellosis continues to be one of the most common causes of inflammatory diarrhea, although *Campylobacter* enteritis is seen as frequently in some centers. After ingestion of an infectious inoculum (10 to 100 bacteria), the incubation period varies from one to four days. Bacteria multiply rapidly in the small bowel to counts of 10^{7-9} colony-forming units (CFU) per ml of gut fluid. Abdominal pain and diarrhea occur in nearly all patients, fever is present in one-third to one-half, and hematochezia in 40%. Enterotoxin production by strains of shigellae is thought to account for watery diarrhea initially seen in some cases. Better recognized is the dysenteric syndrome in which shigellosis is a nonpenetrating superficial mucosal infection confined to the colon. In the acute phases, bacterial counts approach 10^9 CFU per gm of stool; with recovery from illness, bacterial counts rapidly decline. Despite fever and toxemia, bacteremia is uncommon in patients over 2 years of age. The duration of illness is usually five to seven days, although it may persist for two to three weeks in a minority of cases.

Complications of shigellosis include severe dehydration, febrile convulsions, septicemia (particularly in neonates), rarely, bacterial keratoconjunctivitis that may be due to autoinoculation, postinfectious arthritis, which is more common in those who are HLA-B27-positive, and the hemolytic uremic syndrome.

Shigellae are divided into four groups: A (*S. dysenteriae*), B (*S. flexneri*), C (*S. boydii*), and D (*S. sonnei*). Within groups A, B, and C there are 38 different serotypes, whereas there is only a single serotype in group D. At the present time group D organisms are prevalent in industrialized countries and group B organisms are more common in less-developed countries. The prevalence and antimicrobial susceptibility of strains in each locale may vary from time to time, the precise reasons for which are unknown. *Shigella dysenteriae,* the Shiga bacillus, produces more serious disease, which if untreated, has a mortality of 20%. In contrast, *S. sonnei* infections are thought to be more benign.

The reservoir for organisms is in the human gastrointestinal tract, since animal and environmental reservoirs have not been identified. Thus fecal-oral contamination is the mode of transmission of disease. Outbreaks involving common sources such as contaminated water are infrequently reported. The low infectious inoculum required to cause disease explains the high secondary attack rate of 20% to 60% within households, particularly in those under 2 years of age.

Seasonal variations of shigellosis differ depending upon geographic area. In Canada and Scotland the disease tends to occur year-round, whereas it is more common in the summer or late fall in the United States. In tropical countries it peaks during the hot and rainy season.

In contrast to *Salmonella* gastroenteritis in which treatment with antibiotics is not useful and may prolong carriage, treatment of shigellosis with antibiotics is important in shortening the period of fecal excretion and in aborting the course of illness. Treatment with antibiotics may therefore prevent secondary cases. Since prevalent strains and antimicrobial susceptibilities vary in different geographic areas, no specific recommendations can be given with regard to therapy. Nevertheless, trimethoprim, 160 mg plus sulfamethoxazole, 800 mg twice a day in adults, or trimethoprim, 10 mg per kg, plus sulfamethoxazole, 50 mg per kg per day as a suspension in two divided doses in children, is now commonly used to treat shigellosis, since most strains are sensitive to the combination (abbreviated TMP/SMZ). Patients should be treated for at least five days; however, widespread use may also induce TMP/SMZ-resistant strains. In areas where most endemic strains are sensitive, ampicillin is the drug of choice. Amoxicillin (Amoxil) is not to be used because it is ineffective. Tetracycline should only be used in older children (over 8 years of age) because of dental staining. Aminoglycosides given orally (e.g., neomycin) or intravenously are not effective.

Additional therapeutic considerations are emergency treatment of shock, dehydration, and acidosis, and management of convulsions. Over-the-counter antidiarrheal preparations are of unproved benefit.

Adequate hygiene, maintenance of sound public health policies and practices, isolation of patients, and prompt therapy are required to control or prevent the spread of infection. Infected food handlers should not be permitted to work until three negative stool cultures, obtained on consecutive days, are reported. Hand washing is important to break the fecal-oral chain of infection.

Campylobacter *Enteritis*

Campylobacter fetus is a short, motile, nonspore-forming, spiral-shaped, gram-negative rod that has a single unipolar or bipolar flagellum. The organism is different from *Spirillum* and *Borrelia* organisms, which have multiple flagella. Previously *C. fetus* was named *Vibrio fetus;* in 1963 it was renamed since it differed from *Vibrio cholerae* in that it did not ferment carbohydrates, was more fastidious in its growth requirements, and guanine plus cytosine (C+C) content was different. There are three subspecies of *C. fetus: fetus, intestinalis,* and *jejuni* (abbreviated *C. jejuni*). While all three have been isolated in animals, only the last two are thought to be pathogenic in humans.

Until 1977, most human infections were caused by the subspecies *intestinalis*. This organism was identified as an uncommon cause of bacteremia, cellulitis, meningitis, septic thrombophlebitis, and endocarditis, and was rarely implicated in localized infections including arthritis, peritonitis, and pulmonary infections. Diarrhea has been reported in septicemic conditions with this organism, but without recovery of the bacterium from stool cultures.

In 1972 it was shown that filtration of diarrheal stools with a 0.65-μ filter allowed the recovery of *C. jejuni* in 5% of specimens. At the present time, the organism is recovered using selective blood based media containing trimethoprim, vancomycin, and polymyxin to suppress the normal enteric flora (*C. jejuni* is resistant to these antibiotics). Cephalothin and amphotericin B have been added in some situations as well. With incubation at 37° or 42°C in a microaerophilic environment containing 5% to 6% oxygen and 10% carbon dioxide, the organism can be detected on 24- or 48-hour cultures. The organism survives one to three days in diarrheal specimens. Swabs should be sent in specialized transport media (e.g., Cary-Blair), since exposure to room air reduces recovery of the organism. With these improved culture techniques, *C. jejuni* has been recognized as an important cause of infectious diarrhea, rivaling shigellosis in prevalence.

The infectious inoculum may be as few as 500 organisms. Signs and symptoms include an influenzalike prodrome characterized by anorexia, myalgias, and malaise. Fever, periumbilical pain, and diarrhea ensue. It is suspected that both large and small bowel infections may account for the clinical findings. Polymorphonuclear leukocytes are found in the stool of 80% of patients and the diarrheal effluent becomes bloody in 50% after four to six days of illness. Untreated, the mean duration of illness is 6 days with a range of 1 to 21 days.

The drug of choice is erythromycin since 99% of isolates are susceptible. Since antibiotic therapy is usually initiated after four to six days of illness, erythromycin has not been shown to shorten the duration of illness. Treatment rapidly eradicates intestinal carriage in several days, however, whereas without treatment intestinal carriage persists for approximately two weeks. Tetracycline is an alternative drug, although 10% of strains are resistant.

Although avian and mammalian species are suspected sources of infection, the epidemiology of this disease remains to be defined.

Invasive E. coli *Diarrhea*

Invasive *E. coli* diarrhea is uncommonly diagnosed, the last serious outbreak occurring in the early 1970s, related to imported cheese. These strains possess O antigens that are similar to those found in *Shigella* serotypes. Most commonly, these belong to O groups number 28, 112, 115, 124, 136, 143, 144, 147, and 152. Otherwise the serotypes are indistinguishable from noninvasive strains. Invasiveness can be tested using the guinea pig conjunctival sac (Sereny test); keratoconjunctivitis develops one week after inoculation.

Vibrio parahemolyticus *Gastroenteritis*

Currently, *V. parahemolyticus* is the most common cause of food poisoning in Japan, where raw seafood is commonly consumed. Illness occurs 9 to 25 hours after ingestion of poorly cooked fish or shellfish. Most cases are reported in coastal areas, on cruise ships, or in patients who have been on vacation abroad. Diarrhea may be explosive and watery or may be a dysenteric syndrome with blood and pus. Superficial ulceration of the large bowel mucosa is seen on proctosigmoidoscopic examination. The colitis syndrome may be associated with abdominal cramps, nausea, vomiting, headache, and fever. Generally the illness is self-limited, lasting three to four days. No specific therapy is recommended. Strains that are beta-hemolytic on a special medium are called Kanagawa-positive, and are pathogenic in humans, whereas nonhemolytic strains are nonpathogenic. Thiosulfate citrate bile salt sucrose medium, which is also used in the isolation of *V. cholerae,* is used to identify the organism in stool cultures. Since this syndrome is associated with the ingestion of seafood, the physician should suspect the illness on epidemiologic grounds and alert the microbiology laboratory to perform special cultures.

Antibiotic-related Diarrhea

Penicillins, cephalosporins, macrolides (particularly clindamycin), tetracycline, and chloramphenicol have been the agents most frequently implicated as inducing antibiotic-associated diarrhea and colitis. Between 0.5% and 2% of patients treated with these drugs develop colitis. Diarrhea may develop at any time during antibiotic therapy or several weeks later. Rarely, TMP/SMZ, and metronidazole, have been implicated as predisposing agents.Aminoglycosides, of themselves, are unlikely to predispose to the development of *C. difficile* diarrhea.

Antibiotic therapy suppresses the normal enteric flora and promotes colonization with exogenous strains or overgrowth of endogenous strains of *Clostridium difficile*. Most strains have been found to be toxigenic, producing both an enterotoxin responsible for the diarrhea and a cytotoxin that alters the morphology of tissue culture cell monolayers. It is uncertain whether the cytotoxin measured in vitro is important in producing disease. Cytotoxin titers in fecal filtrates of patients with diarrheal illness usually are positive in dilutions of 1 in 4000 or greater. Intestinal carriage of the organisms, usually in the absence of detectable cytotoxin, has been identified in 5% to 30% of asymptomatic persons not receiving antimicrobial agents. Diagnosis and therapy are summarized in Table 14.4.

In neonatal intensive care units, up to 40% of infants have been found to be colonized with *C. difficile*, usually in association with high titers of cytotoxin but without diarrheal illness. Recently it has been shown that fetal intestinal cells are not affected by the cytotoxin, possibly accounting for the paradoxical clinical findings.

TABLE 14.4. Diagnosis and Therapy of Acute Inflammatory Diarrheal Illnesses

Infection	*Diagnosis*	*Treatment**
Shigellosis	Stool cultures, antigenic analysis, and antimicrobial susceptibility testing	Trimethoprim/sulfamethoxazole, 160/800 mg po bid × 7 d Ampicillin, 250–500 mg po, qid × 7 d
Salmonella gastroenteritis	Stool cultures, antigenic analysis	Self-limited illness, no treatment
Campylobacter enteritis	Direct-phase-contrast microscopy of diarrheal effluent Culture on selective medium	Erythromycin, 250 mg qid × 5–7 d
V. parahemolyticus gastroenteritis	Culture on TCBS medium	Self-limited illness, no treatment
Antibiotic-associated colitis	Proctosigmoidoscopy +/− biopsy Culture on CCFA medium Toxin testing on tissue culture cell monolayers	Withdraw inducing antibiotic if possible Metronidazole 250 mg po q6h × 7–14 d Vancomycin, 125–500 mg po q6h × 7–14 d 20% of patients may relapse, require retreatment with vancomycin followed by cholestyramine, 4 gm po, tid × 5 d to bind toxin (do not use vancomycin and cholestyramine concurrently)
Intestinal amebiasis	Ova and parasite examination Undermined ulcers on proctosigmoidoscopy	Asymptomatic cyst passer, nonendemic area Diloxanide furoate (Furamide), 500 mg po tid × 10 d Diiodohydroxyquin, 650 mg po tid × 21 d Tetracycline, 250 mg po qid × 7 d as an adjunct to diiodohydroxyquin Symptomatic, nondysenteric Metronidazole, 500 mg po tid × 5 d followed by diiodohydroxyquin, 650 mg po tid × 21 d Symptomatic, dysenteric Metronidazole, 750 mg po tid × 10 d plus diiodohydroxyquin, 650 mg po tid × 21 d

*Adult dosages reported here.

Other Less Common Causes of Invasive Diarrhea

Balantidium coli is the only ciliate parasite that is pathogenic for humans. The reservoir is in pigs. Like *E. histolytica,* this organism excysts in the small bowel and invades the terminal ileum and colon. Although it may produce an appendicitis-like syndrome, the dysenteric syndrome with rectosigmoid ulceration and heaped-up ulcers up to 3 cm in diameter occurs more commonly. Secondary bacteremia may complicate local disease. Unlike amebic dysentery, the organism does not invade distant organs. On sigmoidoscopy the margin of the ulcer can be scraped and examined for the ciliated trophozoites or cysts. Pigs are usually infected with *B. suis,* a similar type of organism that is pathogenic for animals but not for humans.

Schistosomiasis may cause acute bloody diarrhea, abdominal pain, and weight loss when adult schistosomes, usually *S. japonicum* or *S. mansoni,* migrate into the wall of the large bowel where they deposit their eggs. This usually occurs three to eight weeks after the cercarial form of the organism penetrates the skin. Pus, blood, and ova are found on fecal examination. Associated findings include leukocytosis, fever, and eosinophilia.

Male homosexuals sometimes develop purulent gonococcal proctitis. Proctosigmoidoscopy may show an erythematous, friable mucosa in the rectal vault. Abscesses or fistulas may be formed. Discharge is often copious, purulent, and associated with tenesmus. However, two-thirds of patients who have anorectal infection are asymptomatic.

The clinical features of acute necrotizing enterocolitis (NEC) in the newborn include apneic spells, vomiting, abdominal distention, and occasionally, bloody diarrhea. Most affected infants are less than 1 week of age. The predisposing clinical associations are prematurity, maternal infection such as chorioamnionitis, exchange transfusions through the umbilical vein, and use of hypertonic infant formulas. Necrosis and sloughing of the intestinal mucosa and intestinal perforation usually at the terminal ileum often occur. Extraintestinal gas may be found in the wall of the intestine (pneumatosis intestinalis), in the portal system, or in the peritoneal cavity. Shock and septicemia supervene. Untreated, infection may be fatal in over 50% of patients; the use of parenteral antibiotics with or without oral antibiotics has reduced mortality to 20%. Gram-negative bacilli including *E. coli, Klebsiella* sp., *Pseudomonas* sp., *Salmonella* sp., and *Clostridium butyricum* have been implicated as pathogens.

Prevention includes avoiding predisposing factors and taking careful infection control measures to prevent colonization of these infants with hospital organisms.

Necrotizing enterocolitis in adults (enteritis necroticans) is thought to be caused by ingestion of poorly cooked foods contaminated with alpha- and beta-toxin-producing *C. perfringens* type C. It is a fulminant necrotizing small bowel infection characterized by segmental gangrene and intestinal perforation. *Darmbrand,* a word signifying "firebowels," referred to epidemic disease seen in northern Germany after World War II. *Pig-bel* is applied to the illness incurred by New Guineans after they ingest inadequately cooked pork.

Penetrating Pathogens

Enteric pathogens may penetrate the intestinal mucosa without producing serious mucosal injury and proliferate in the lamina propria. Since there is limited mucosal damage, the diarrheal effluent may contain fewer inflammatory cells. If the infection is not contained within the submucosal lymphoid follicles, infection may spread to the regional lymph nodes and into the systemic circulation.

Salmonella *Infections*

The major clinical forms of *Salmonella* infection along with the clinical features, diagnosis and therapy are summarized in Table 14.5. The American classification divides the organism into three species: *S. typhi, S. choleraesuis,* and *S. enteritidis*. The species *S. enteritidis* includes over 1900 serotypes. Each serotype is written after the species name as follows: *S. enteritidis* serotype *typhimurium, S. enteritidis* serotype *newport,* and so on. In many other countries, the serotypes of *S. enteriditis* are given species status, such as *S. typhimurium,* or *S. newport*. Regardless of the nomenclature used, all *Salmonella* organisms are serotyped on the basis of their O and H antigens, which are universally recognized. The O antigen profiles are used to classify species into 9 serogroups A through I, with groups A through E containing fewer than 40 serotypes but accounting for greater than 90% of human infections.

Salmonella organisms can be grouped into three ecologic divisions according to host specificity: (1) serotypes that are adapted to human or primate hosts, such as *S. typhi* and organisms producing paratyphoid fevers; (2) serotypes adapted to nonhuman hosts, such as *S. choleraesuis* (porcine) and *S. dublin* (equine); and (3) serotypes that are not adapted to any specific host. Most are in the last category.

Salmonellae continue to rank with shigellae and *C. jejuni* as the most common causes of acute infectious diarrhea. In developed countries, most cases are nontyphoidal. Organisms originate from the intestinal flora of domestic animals and from contamination of animal byproducts. In underdeveloped countries, typhoid and paratyphoid infections continue to be prevalent.

After the ingestion of an infectious inoculum (10^6 to 10^9 organisms), organisms must pass the gastric barrier, proliferate in the small bowel lumen, and penetrate the ileal mucosa. Diarrhea may be produced by activation of prostaglandins and adenylate cyclase. Microorganisms proliferate in lymphoid follicles in the small intestinal submucosa. In most cases of *Salmonella* gastroenteritis, infection does not extend beyond the submucosa and illness is self-limited.

In immunologically compromised hosts, infection may not be contained and systemic spread occurs. Thus, *Salmonella* infections complicated by bacteremia are more common in the very young and in the very old who have underlying diseases. In particular, bacteremia and reticuloendothelial system infection are frequently seen in patients with hematologic disease,

TABLE 14.5. Salmonella Infections

Disease Syndrome	*Most Common Organism(s)*	*Clinical Features*	*Diagnosis*	*Treatment*
Asymptomatic carriage (colonization without illness)	Nontyphoidal *Salmonella*	Asymptomatic (probable low inocula ingested)	Usually not diagnosed, stool cultures taken for other reasons	Nil, enteric precautions
Gastroenteritis (accounts for majority of *Salmonella* infections in North America and Western Europe)	Nontyphoidal *Salmonella,* esp. *S. typhimurium*	Accounts for 10–15% of food poisoning outbreaks, primarily in the summer and early fall Nausea, vomiting, diarrhea, and abdominal pain Clinical spectrum ranges from mild small bowel diarrhea to dysenteric infection Low-grade fever for several days, transient bacteremia in 1–4%	Stool culture isolation and serologic identification	Nil, disease usually self-limited, enteric precautions
Bacteremia	*S. choleraesuis* *S. typhimurium* *S. heidelberg*	Endovascular infection and sustained bacteremia with metastatic infections (10%) in immunocompromised hosts, patients with valvular heart disease, and atherosclerotic aorto-iliofemoral arterial disease Extravascular metastatic infections, esp. osteomyelitis Meningitis, esp. in neonates	Blood, stool cultures, specific tests for organ dysfunction	Removal of intravascular focus Systemic antimicrobial therapy as per enteric fever syndrome Therapy for 4–6 wks, surgical intervention may be necessary as well.
Enteric fever syndrome	*S. typhi* *S. paratyphi* A *S. schottmülleri* (*paratyphi B*) *S. hirschfeldii* (*paratyphi C*)	Gradual-onset febrile illness with nonspecific symptoms Prolonged febrile course 2–4 weeks, sustained bacteremia Hepatosplenomegaly and lymphadenopathy	Blood, urine, stool, bone marrow, and rose spot cultures. Widal test is nondiagnostic but 4-fold increase in 0 antigen titers occurs in 40–60% of patients	Chloramphenicol, 50 mg/kg/d IV/po × 2–4 wks Ampicillin, 100–150 mg/kg/d IV × 2–4 wks (Amoxicillin, 4–6 gm/d po) Trimethoprim, 320–640 mg/ sulfamethoxazole, 1600–3200 mg po or IV b.i.d. × 2 wks

TABLE 14.6. Clinical Pathologic Events in Untreated Typhoid Fever

	Incubation Period 14 ± 7 Days	*Week 1 (proliferation in reticuloendothelial system)*	*Weeks 2–3 (established disease)*	*Weeks 4–5 (convalescence)*
Pathogenic events	Ingestion, luminal proliferation penetration, transient bacteremia	Proliferation in lymphoid follicles and reticuloendothelial system, septicemia	Bacteremia, reticuloendothelial hyperplasia, metastatic infection, focal necrosis of lymphoid follicles	Host immunity Healing
Clinical features	Diarrhea 10% of patients	Flulike illness — headache, myalgia, anorexia, malaise, cough, pharyngitis, diarrhea, or constipation	Toxemia, prostration, pneumonia, bronchitis, hepatosplenomegaly, anemia, leukopenia, rose spots, relative bradycardia	Recovery Relapse (5–10%)
Fever	− to ±	+ + to + + +	+ + + +	+ to + +
Cultures				
Blood	—	80–90% +	80–90% +	—
Stool culture	Transiently +	—	75% +	50% +
Urine	—	—	25% +	10%
Marrow	—	—	80–90% +	10%
Biopsy of rose spots	NA*	NA	60% +	NA
Widal test	−	20% +	50% +	75% +

*NA = not applicable.

for example, sickle cell hemoglobinopathy, hemolytic anemias, leukemia, or lymphoproliferative disorders. Infections associated with hemolysis, especially malaria and bartonellosis, predispose to serious *Salmonella* infections. Increased susceptibility to bacteremia may occur because underlying diseases interfere with reticuloendothelial system clearance mechanisms.

Certain serotypes such as *S. choleraesuis, S. typhimurium,* and *S. heidelberg* have a proclivity to produce primary bacteremias, and where opportunities exist, may set up secondary intravascular (e.g., infection of atherosclerotic blood vessels or abnormal heart valves) or metastatic infections (e.g., osteomyelitis, meningitis, splenic abscess, or soft tissue infection). The clinical course of these bacteremias is unlike that of the enteric fever syndrome since the onset is sudden, the hectic febrile course may last several days to weeks, and the organism is rarely isolated from the stool.

Finally, enteric fever syndromes are produced by organisms that seem to be adapted to and are more pathogenic to the human host. After the initial intestinal infection and transient asymptomatic primary bacteremia, *S. typhi* replicates within macrophages in the reticuloendothelial system and lymphoid follicles, ultimately producing a secondary bacteremic phase. The stages and clinical findings of typhoid fever are outlined in Table 14.6.

Although gastroenteritis is the most commonly recognized type of salmonellosis, asymptomatic carriage following the ingestion of low inocula of organisms is suspected to be a common occurrence. In most instances intestinal carriage is transient. In cases of gastroenteritis, 10% of patients eliminate the organism by 2 weeks, 60% by 4 weeks, 90% by 10 weeks, and 95% by 20 weeks. Antibiotic therapy has been shown to prolong intestinal carriage.

The therapeutic regimens are listed in Table 14.5. Effective therapy of enteric fever results in defervescence and symptomatic improvement in three to five days. Therapy reduces mortality of untreated disease from 12% to 1% and reduces the frequency of intestinal perforation and hemorrhage from approximately 10% to 2%. Although most strains of *Salmonella* organisms are susceptible to aminoglycosides and cephalosporins in vitro, in vivo effectiveness has not been demonstrated and use of these agents is discouraged.

Yersiniosis

Yersinia enterocolitica and *Y. pseudotuberculosis* are both nonlactose-fermenting, urease-positive, gram-negative bacteria that are characteristically motile at 22°C but nonmotile at 37°C. Compared with other enteric organisms, they are unique in that they are also able to grow at 4°C. This differential temperature growth may be useful for isolating the organism. There are 34 serotypes of *Y. enterocolitica,* of which types 03 and 08 are most commonly isolated in North America. There are five serotypes (I through V) of *Y. pseudotuberculosis,* with type I strains most frequently causing human infection.

Virulence factors in *Y. enterocolitica* include guinea pig conjunctival invasion (positive Sereny test), invasion of animal intestinal mucosa, and the production of a heat-stable enterotoxin in some strains. Tissue invasion evokes a granulomatous tissue reaction.

Most cases of *Y. enterocolitica* infection are sporadic and the reservoir in nature is not well investigated. Contact with animals and ingestion of meat, seafoods, and dairy products are possible sources of infection. Wild and domestic mammals serve as reservoirs for *Y. pseudotuberculosis.*

Patients with *Y. enterocolitica* infections can appear to have one of the following diseases:

1. Acute enterocolitis accounts for two-thirds of cases. Fever, inflammatory diarrhea, and abdominal pain last for one to three weeks. Most patients are less than 5 years of age.
2. Mesenteric adenitis and acute terminal ileitis may be different spectra of the same illness, causing fever, right lower quadrant pain, and leukocytosis. The syndrome is indistinguishable from acute appendicitis and is seen most commonly in adolescents as a self-limited disease.
3. Postinfectious polyarthritis generally occurs in adults who are HLA-B27-positive. The migratory polyarthritis involves both weight-bearing and small joints and may persist for months.
4. Erythema multiforme and erythema nodosum.
5. Septicemia affects patients with underlying disease, including diabetes, anemia, cirrhosis, and malignancy, and in elderly debilitated patients. Septicemia may result in abscesses in the reticuloendothelial system, osteomyelitis, or meningitis.

Yersinia pseudotuberculosis infection in humans usually has the features of mesenteric adenitis. Diagnosis of yersiniosis is based on isolation of the organism and serology.

Disease is self-limited in most cases and antibiotic therapy is usually not recommended. However, patients with septicemia or clinically severe disease may benefit from antibiotic therapy. Most strains of *Y. enterocolitica* are resistant to penicillins and cephalosporins, whereas *Y. pseudotuberculosis* is sensitive to ampicillin and cephalosporins. Chloramphenicol and aminoglycosides may be effective against both organisms.

FOOD POISONING SYNDROMES

Outbreaks of food poisoning are defined as illness experienced by two or more persons eating the same food, when epidemiologic data suggest food as the source of illness. One case of botulism or of chemical food poisoning may constitute an outbreak, however. It is estimated that less than 1% of instances of food poisoning is reported to public health agencies. Most cases are of brief duration, self-limited, and escape medical attention.

Of the reported outbreaks, 65% are caused by bacteria and account for 90% of affected persons. Twenty-five percent are the result of chemical poisonings, but account for 5% of affected persons. Parasites including *Trichinella spiralis, Diphyllobothrium latum, Toxoplasma gondii,* and aniskidae are responsible for 8% of outbreaks affecting 3% of food poisoning cases; and viruses, primarily hepatitis A, account for the remaining few. Between 1970 and 1974, 456 outbreaks affecting 15,000 persons were reported and investigated in the United States. Less than half were etiologically confirmed. Of those that were unconfirmed, incubation periods ranged from 1 hour to 14 hours. This suggests that these outbreaks were either staphylococcal in origin (incubation period 1 to 7 hours) or due to *Clostridium perfringens* (incubation period 8 to 14 hours). There were 13 fatal cases, half of them due to botulism.

The clinical features and etiologic agents of ten food poisoning syndromes are summarized in Table 14.7. Syndromes are categorized on the basis of clinical features and time of onset of illness after ingestion of food. The first three represent gastrointestinal upset in afebrile patients due to enterotoxin that is either preformed or produced in vivo. Febrile gastrointestinal illness is produced by previously discussed invasive or penetrating bacterial pathogens. The remaining five gastrointestinal syndromes are associated with neurologic findings, including botulism, scombroid fish poisoning, and three types of dinoflagellate toxin poisoning.

Staphylococcal Food Poisoning

Five antigenically distinct, heat-stable enterotoxins (A to E, molecular weight 28,000 to 35,000 daltons) are produced by *S. aureus*. Contamination of food, primarily from human sources and conditions promoting growth of bacteria, leads to the production of preformed enterotoxin in food. Illness begins one to six hours after ingestion of food. Nausea and abdominal

TABLE 14.7. Syndromes of Food Poisoning

Symptoms (onset)	*Etiology*	*Pathogenesis*	*Reservoir*	*Foods*
Nausea and vomiting (1–6 hrs)	*S. aureus*	Preformed enterotoxin type *A*,B,C,*D*,E (MW 28,000–35,000) heat-stable Vagal stimulation of emetic center Enterotoxin effect	Food workers, nasal carriage, local infections esp. hands	Ham, poultry, salads, pastries (high-protein foods)
	B. cereus (short incubation)	Preformed enterotoxin	Soil contamination	Cereal, rice, custards
Abdominal cramps, diarrhea (8–16 hrs)	*B. cereus* (long incubation)	In vivo production of enterotoxins	Soil contamination	Cereal, rice, custards
	C. perfringens	In vivo production of enterotoxins	Feces, soil, animal carcass contamination	Poultry
Abdominal cramps, diarrhea (16–72 hrs)	Enterotoxin-producing *E. coli* or *V. cholerae*	Colonization → enterotoxin → adenylcyclase activation	Fecal contamination	Unwashed fruits and fresh vegetables, water
Abdominal cramps, diarrhea, fever (16–72 hrs)	*Salmonella*	See text	Poultry, domestic animals	Eggs, poultry, milk, meat
	Shigella	See text	Hand-spread, oral-fecal from humans	
	V. parahemolyticus	See text	Seafood, seawater	Fish
	Invasive *E. coli*	See text	?	Imported
	Campylobacter fetus ss *jejuni*	See text	? Poultry, domestic animals	Source to be determined
	Yersinia	See text	Dogs, domestic animals	Meat, unpasteurized milk
Abdominal cramps, fever (mesenteric adenitis) (16–72 hrs)	*Y. enterocolitica, Y. pseudotuberculosis*	Lymphatic invasion, terminal ileitis	Animals, dairy products	Meat, unpasteurized milk

TABLE 14.7. continued

Symptoms (onset)	*Etiology*	*Pathogenesis*	*Reservoir*	*Foods*
Nausea, vomiting, diarrhea, followed by neurologic syndrome of sequential descending weakness and paralysis (6 hrs–8 d)	*C. botulinum*	Preformed toxin A,B,E (MW 150,000) Binds to neuromuscular junction and prevents release of acetylcholine Toxin production by bacteriophage *C. botulinum* growth in vivo in intestine of infants may be a cause of sudden infant death syndrome	Soil	Acid foods prevent spore germination Heat-labile, heating to 100°C × 10 min or 80°C × 30 min inactivates toxin Type A,B toxin-producing strains also produce enzymes that spoil food
Histamine-like toxicity: flushing headache, dizziness, abdominal cramps, nausea, vomiting, urticaria, bronchospasm (½ hr)	Scombroidea	Bacterial contamination of fish flesh, decarboxylation of histadine to histamine-like substance with >100 mg/gm flesh	Scombroidea Tuna, mackerel, skipjack, bonito	Scombroidea Tuna, mackerel, skipjack, bonito
Nausea, vomiting, diarrhea followed by numbness, paresthesia, palsies, respiratory failure lasting days–weeks (1–6 hrs)	Ciguatera toxin poisoning	Dinoflagellate (*G. toxicus*) toxin accumulates in scavenger fish flesh	Red snapper, barracuda, grouper, amberjack (35° N–S latitude)	Larger fish (>2.5 kg) more likely to be toxin positive
Paresthesias and paralysis (5 min–4 hrs)	*Gonyaulax catanella* (west coast) *G. tamarensis* (east coast)	Dinoflagellate toxins Heat-stable saxitoxin-produced and concentrated in bivalve mollusks Blocks sodium influx of nerve action potentials	Scallops, clams (seasonal: May–October)	Scallops, clams
Paresthesias (5 min–4 hrs)	*Gymnodinium breve* (Florida)	Dinoflagellate toxin	Bivalve mollusks	Bivalve mollusks

cramps are followed by vomiting and diarrhea. Fever is absent and illness lasts only four to six hours.

An etiologic diagnosis is established by demonstrating enterotoxin and isolation of 10^6 organisms or more per gram of food or vomitus. Phage typing may be useful in large outbreaks.

Treatment is supportive. Since the toxin is not heat inactivated, avoidance of food contamination and proper refrigeration are required to prevent disease.

Bacillus cereus *Food Poisoning*

Two syndromes are produced in *B. cereus* poisoning: a short incubation illness similar to staphylococcal food poisoning and a longer-incubation illness that is clinically indistinguishable from *C. perfringens* food poisoning. In the former, preformed toxin produces nausea and vomiting; diarrhea is not prominent. Fried rice from Chinese restaurants has been implicated, since previously cooked rice may become contaminated and flash frying does not inactivate the toxin. In the latter syndrome, in vivo production of enterotoxin that activates adenyl cyclase is thought to produce disease. Illness is self-limited.

C. perfringens *Food Poisoning*

In vivo production of enterotoxin and diarrhea are facilitated by a mechanism independent of adenyl cyclase activation. Food poisoning with *C. perfringens,* a self-limited illness, is characterized by nausea (30%), vomiting (10%), abdominal cramps, and diarrhea. Absence of fever and systemic toxicity support the diagnosis. Contaminated meat or meat products are major vehicles of infection. Most cases are presumptively diagnosed, since cultures showing 10^5 or more organisms per gram of food and stool, and serotyping of isolates are required for definitive diagnosis.

Botulism

Botulism is the most serious type of food poisoning, since it is potentially fatal. Persistence of *C. botulinum* spores and subsequent conversion to vegetative bacilli lead to the production of a neurotoxin in contaminated food. Seven serologically distinct toxins (A to G) are produced, but only toxins A, B, and E are commonly involved in human disease. Boiling for 10 minutes or heating for 30 minutes at 80°C will destroy the toxin and vegetative forms, although spores will survive. Inactivation of toxin prevents illness. Rarely, colonization of the intestinal tract and in vivo production of toxin may prolong disease. Absorbed toxin binds to the neuromuscular junction and prevents acetyl choline release. Adrenergic fibers are spared.

After an episode of nonspecific acute gastroenteritis that may pass unnoticed, illness usually begins six hours to eight days after ingestion of the toxin. Nausea and vomiting are present in only one-third of patients with type A or B disease, but are common in type E poisoning. The cardinal features of botulism are descending paralysis and progressive respiratory weakness, unexplained postural hypotension, dilated unreactive pupils (adrenergic effect), and dry mouth. The sensorium is normal and the patient is afebrile. Blockage of cholinergic fibers accounts for dry mouth, ileus, and urinary retention. Ptosis and extraocular muscle paralysis may occur.
stituted presumptively. The diagnosis is confirmed by demonstrating toxin in the serum, gastric contents, and stool, and by isolating the organism in food. Electromyographic findings supportive of botulism include prolonged post-tetanic facilitation, muscle fibrillation, and small-amplitude, polyphasic motor unit potentials of increased number and brief duration.

Treatment consists of administration of polyvalent (equine) antitoxin intravenously and intramuscularly, supportive care in an intensive care setting, and elimination of unabsorbed toxin by enemas. Guanidine hydrochloride, an experimental drug that enhances the release of acetyl choline, may partially reverse the neuromuscular junction blockade. Treatment has reduced mortality from 60% to 25%.

Fish and Shellfish Chemical Intoxication

In addition to heavy metals, mushrooms, and other chemical intoxicants, seafoods are now recognized as frequent causes of food poisoning.

Bacterial contamination of fish flesh containing histadine and its decarboxylation into a histamine-like substance is thought to produce the clinical findings in scombroid food poisoning. *Proteus* and *Klebsiella* species have been implicated. This self-limited illness is extremely rapid in onset and is as short-lived, lasting less than four hours.

Ciguatera toxin poisoning and paralytic shellfish poisoning are produced by the concentration of dinoflagellate toxins from the food chain. Ciguatera toxin is the most common cause of chemical food poisoning in the United States, occurring several times more frequently than scombroid or paralytic shellfish poisoning. The term "cigua" refers to the turban-shelled snail, *Cittariam pica,* which produced illness in sixteenth-century Spanish explorers in the West Indies. Large, bottom-dwelling, reef scavengers, such as red snapper and grouper, concentrate a toxin derived from a photosynthetic dinoflagellate *Gambierdiscus toxicus*. In one study the toxin was present in the flesh of 69% of red snapper weighing 2.8 kg or more. Concentrations are higher in internal organs. In severe disease, cranial nerve paralysis and respiratory failure may occur and persist for several weeks. Most cases occur in Hawaii, Florida, and seacoast cities. Treatment is supportive.

Paralytic shellfish poisoning occurs with the ingestion of bivalve mollusks (scallops and clams) that have concentrated toxins derived from dinoflagellates. Proliferation of dinoflagellates, usually in the months from May until October, creates the so-called red tide. Appearance and taste of the mollusks are not affected. Poisoning causes paresthesias of the face, lips, and extremities, and less commonly, paralysis, since the toxin interferes with nerve conduction by altering sodium flux in axons. As the intoxication is fatal in 8% of untreated cases, supportive therapy and catharsis to eliminate the toxin are the mainstays of treatment.

In summary, food poisoning caused by bacteria can be controlled by adequate cooking, refrigeration, and hygiene. Chemical intoxications are most difficult to treat since the toxins are not inactivated by heat. Periodic monitoring of mollusks for toxin and avoiding the ingestion of scavengers may reduce the risk of chemical intoxication from seafoods.

AN APPROACH TO ACUTE INFECTIOUS DIARRHEA

Figure 14.1 is an algorithm for the diagnosis and treatment of acute infectious diarrhea. While the clinical features, epidemiology, and initial laboratory examination may suggest specific etiologic agents, definitive microbiologic data are required for diagnosis and management. Numerous pathogens can produce the same syndrome, and a single pathogen can produce several clinical syndromes.

Most diarrheal illnesses are self-limited. Therefore in many instances an etiologic diagnosis may not be required. Efforts should be made to identify situations where intervention is required. Foremost is assessment and therapy of fluid and electrolyte imbalance. The major advance in the past ten years has been the recognition that oral rehydration is effective and should be pursued early in the course of management.

Techniques for isolation of pathogens have improved such that well-equipped laboratories can identify 60% to 70% of pathogens as compared to a 20% to 25% identification rate ten years ago. The management of acute infectious diarrhea is continuing to evolve with improved methods of diagnosis and treatment.

ANNOTATED BIBLIOGRAPHY

Bartlett, JG. Antibiotic-associated pseudomembranous colitis. Rev Infect Dis 1979;1:530–539.
A historical review and clinical-laboratory data leading to the definition of antibiotic colitis as an infectious disease.

Blacklow NR, Cukor G. Viral gastroenteritis. N Engl J Med 1981;304:397–406.
The current status of viral gastroenteritis is reviewed.

Blaser MJ, Reller LB. Campylobacter enteritis. N Engl J Med 1981;305:1444–1452.
A recent update emphasizes clinical features.

Carpenter CCJ. The pathophysiology of secretory diarrheas. Med Clin North Am 1982;66:597–610.
An overview of etiologic agents and general pathophysiologic events of enterotoxin-mediated diarrhea.

Fekety R. Recent advances in management of bacterial diarrhea. Rev Infect Dis 1983; 5(2):246–257.
An update of current developments on several bacterial pathogens, particularly *C. difficile*.

Hornick RB, Greisman SE, Woodward TE, Dupont HL, Dawkins AT, Snyder MJ. Typhoid fever: pathogenesis and immunologic control. N Engl J Med. 1970;283:686–691; 739–746.
An excellent review with historical perspectives.

Vantrappen G, Agg HO, Geboes K, Ponette E. Yersinia enteritis. Med Clin North Am 1982;66:639–653.
A review of clinical features of yersinia enterocolitis.

Withers NW. Ciguatera fish poisoning. Ann Rev Med 1982;33:97–111.
Clinical features and origins of ciguatera toxin are discussed.

Wolfe MS. Giardiasis. N Engl J Med 1978;298:319–321.
A review of the clinical features of giardiasis.

Woodward TE, Smadel JE. Management of typhoid fever and its complications. Ann Intern Med 1964; 60:144–157.
A review of complications including relapse, intestinal perforation and hemorrhage, and mortality.

15 HEPATITIS

D. Lorne J. Tyrrell and M. John Gill

The usual reaction of the liver to injury is an acute inflammatory response called hepatitis. This nonspecific reaction to a challenge causes the differential diagnosis of hepatitis to be both large and varied. In most developed countries, toxins are a significant and major cause of hepatitis. Alcohol abuse, industrial toxin exposure, and even drug therapy are common causative factors. Fortunately, in the majority of these cases, removal of the toxic challenge causes the hepatitis to resolve, although residual damage in the form of cirrhosis may persist.

The infectious causes of hepatitis are nearly as numerous as the toxic causes. Bacterial, fungal, viral, parasitic, rickettsial, and spirochetal infections have all been implicated directly or indirectly. In most cases the hepatitis is mild and is only one feature of a disseminated systemic infection that is relatively easy to diagnose. Acute disease with its elevations of hepatic enzymes such as serum aspartate aminotransferase (AST, SGOT) and serum alanine aminotransferase (ALT, SGPT) is usually the marker of a small group of viral infections — hepatitis A (HAV), hepatitis B (HBV), and non-A, non-B hepatitis (NANB). Leptospirosis, Q fever, and syphilis may also produce significantly elevated hepatic enzymes, but usually other features characteristic of the infection facilitate diagnosis. Infections with the Epstein-Barr virus and cytomegalovirus can cause the mononucleosis syndrome, one feature of which is mild to moderate hepatitis. Diagnosis of these infections is often suggested by serology and characteristic clinical features.

The three infections — HAV, HBV, and NANB — differ from the other infectious causes of hepatitis in that their pathogenicity is primarily targeted to the liver. The identification in 1965 of a definitive serologic marker, hepatitis B surface antigen (HBsAg), stimulated both interest and research into all causes of hepatitis, and HBV has become the focus of study as it is endemic throughout the world, its sequelae can be fatal, and it is readily transmissible by blood products. The recent identification of HAV has led to a better understanding of this as a second major cause of hepatitis. Despite the encouraging progress made over the last two decades, many problems still remain to be solved, such as identifying the causative agents of NANB hepatitis, developing effective treatment for HBV carriers, and producing and employing efficient vaccines.

HEPATITIS A

Etiology

The hepatitis A virus has both the linear genome of single-stranded RNA and the four major polypeptides characteristic of the enterovirus genus in the picornavirus group. Electron microscopic examination shows its diameter to be 27 nm. The virus is difficult to culture, but recently it has been successfully grown using primary explant cell cultures from marmoset livers or cells from normal fetal rhesus monkey kidney. The principal value of culturing HAV is to develop vaccine, and is as yet of no practical value in the early diagnosis or management of HAV infections.

Epidemiology

Hepatitis A is endemic worldwide. Localized outbreaks are frequently reported, but the exact incidence is unknown. Serologic and epidemiologic surveys suggest that the infection must frequently be subclinical. In developing countries, most (80% to 90%) of the adult population has antibodies to HAV, whereas in the industrialized nations, about 20% of the adult population has antibodies. In communities where housing and hygiene are poor, many children acquire HAV at an early age, but the infection is often anicteric and subclinical. In industrialized countries where housing and hygiene are good, most children are not exposed to HAV and it is more usual to see the infection in adults.

It is transmitted by the fecal-oral route with an incubation period of three to five weeks. As persistent infections or long-term carrier states with HAV do not occur and since there is no known animal reservoir, the virus can only be maintained by transmission from acutely ill patients to susceptible individuals. The virus can be detected in the feces by immune electron microscopy or radioimmunoassay, with highest concentrations noted in feces during the late stages of the incubation period. Little or no virus is detectable by the time the serum transaminase levels peak or jaundice is evident. Low levels have been detected for up to 16 days after the onset of icterus, but this is unusual. The virus has not been demonstrated in respiratory secretions and is found only rarely in urine samples. Viremia is short-lived, and percutaneous transmission of HAV is not a factor in its epidemiology.

Most HAV infections are spread by close personal contact but it is clear that some epidemics are the result of food- or water-borne virus. Some outbreaks have been reported to be secondary to raw sewage contamination of shell fish.

Pathophysiology

Hepatitis A virus enters the body by ingestion. It is resistant to acid digestion and it reaches the blood stream after the primary intestinal infection. The target organ of infection is the liver, where HAV has been identified replicating in the cytoplasm of hepatocytes. Large numbers of HAV particles can be detected in the feces beginning about two weeks after exposure and continuing until serum transaminase levels peak. The histologic and immunologic evidence for HAV replication is limited to the liver. Lymphocyte and histiocyte infiltration with periportal necrosis and focal degeneration may be seen on pathologic examination of liver tissue.

Clinical Manifestations

Hepatitis A infections are frequently subclinical. Icteric cases usually have acute onset with anorexia, nausea, vomiting, fatigue, and malaise. Some patients experience myalgias, arthralgias, and alterations of taste and smell during the prodrome. Late in the prodrome and a few days prior to onset of clinical jaundice, patients may develop right upper quadrant discomfort, darkening of urine, and clay-colored stools. The icteric phase of HAV infections is variable and lasts for a few days to a few weeks. The disease is milder in children than in adults. In children, serum transaminase levels usually return to normal within three weeks of the onset of the icteric phase while in adults the illness may be more prolonged. In one study of HAV infection in adults, 50% had elevated serum transaminase levels at 4 weeks and 8% at 16 weeks. By 24 weeks, all patients had normal levels. Most infections are self-limited and fulminant hepatitis is rare. No instances of persistent infection with HAV have been reported. In a small number of cases, aplastic anemia may develop as the hepatitis resolves. The anemia is often refractory to current drug therapy and may result in death.

Diagnosis

The serum transaminases (AST and ALT) are the first liver function tests to become abnormal in hepatitis and they usually peak before the onset of jaundice. Peak values of serum transaminases are often greater than ten times the upper limit of normal. Serum bilirubin is elevated and it is usually divided equally between indirect and direct fractions. Alkaline phosphatase can be normal or mildly elevated. In HAV infections, mild lymphocytosis and atypical lymphocytes may be present in peripheral blood.

A specific diagnosis can be made by demonstrating IgM antibodies to HAV. A fourfold rise of these antibodies between acute and convalescent sera also confirms the diagnosis.

Immune electron microscopy or radioimmunoassay can be used to demonstrate HAV in fecal specimens. This is not practical for routine diagnosis, since in most cases, the HAV antigen disappears from fecal specimens with the onset of jaundice.

Treatment

There is no specific therapy for hepatitis A and treatment is symptomatic. Some patients with severe infection may require hospitalization but most can be managed at home. All patients should be considered infectious for approximately 14 days after the onset of jaundice. They do not require strict isolation, but do require enteric isolation, with gloves being worn by health care personnel handling fecal or soiled material. Patients should be instructed in careful hand washing, and they should not handle food for others. Household contacts should receive immune prophylaxis (see below).

Prophylaxis

The prevention of HAV depends on the use of immune serum globulin (ISG). Postexposure prophylaxis is provided by ISG, 0.01 to 0.02 ml per kg intramuscularly. The earlier ISG is given, the more effective the prophylaxis. The frequency of icteric disease can be reduced by about 80% with postexposure prophylaxis. The accepted indications for use of ISG include household contacts, institutionalized patients with poor hygiene, and epidemics where a common food or water source is contaminated with HAV.

Preexposure prophylaxis is indicated for susceptible individuals traveling to or residing in highly endemic areas. They require 0.01 ml per kg every four to six months, with the indications for ISG determined by the anticipated duration and type of exposure. Prophylaxis is not indicated if the exposure is brief and the usual tourist facilities are provided, but if travelers plan excursions outside these facilities, ISG should be given.

Although a vaccine does not exist, the ability to culture the hepatitis A virus in some cell culture systems should facilitate the development of an effective one soon.

HEPATITIS B

Etiology

Hepatitis B is caused by a DNA virus from the new family of hepadnaviruses. There are at least four viruses in this family, all with common properties, although only one member, HBV, infects humans. These viruses exist in many forms in the circulation of the host animal. Hepatitis B surface antigen (HBsAg) may be present in the circulation as either 22-nm spherical or tubular forms. The infectious form, known as the Dane particle, has a diameter of 42 nm and a lipid-containing outer layer (envelope) that contains the HBsAg.

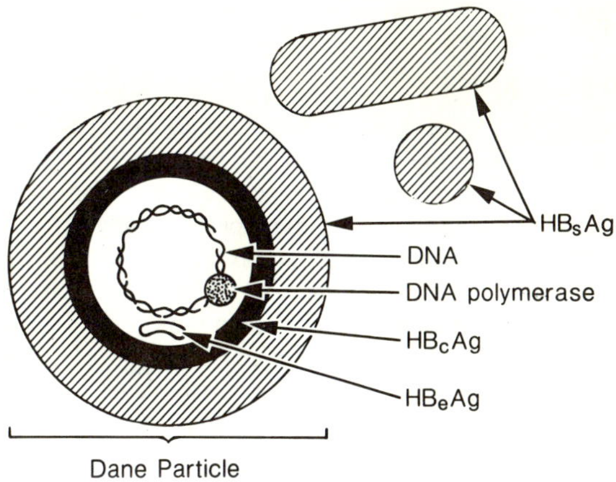

FIGURE 15.1. Schematic diagram of HBV.

The envelope can be removed by detergents, leaving the nucleocapsid that consists of the core antigen (HBcAg), e antigen (HBeAg), small circular DNA (1.6×10^6 daltons), and a DNA polymerase (Figure 15.1). The ratio of Dane particles to the 22-nm particles of HBsAg can vary greatly.

All HBsAg-positive body fluids should be considered potentially infectious, but the degree of infectiousness differs. In the serum of some patients, only the spherical and tubular structures containing HBsAg are present, with no evidence of Dane particles. The blood products of these persons are unlikely to be infectious. In contrast, when Dane particles, HBeAg, or DNA polymerase can be readily identified, the blood products are highly infectious. Electron microscopic identification of Dane particles and determination of DNA polymerase activity in HBsAg-positive serum are technically possible but not practical ways of estimating the degree of infectivity of these fluids. Immunologic detection of HBeAg is at present the best practical means of determining this, but the technique may be replaced by new ones such as blot hybridization, which detects HBV DNA in biologic fluids.

At least 10 different strains of HBV have been defined by identification of the antigenic determinants of HBsAg. These strain differences may be of value in epidemiologic studies. As they all share one antigen called the *a* determinant, this simplifies immunologic screening procedures for HBsAg-positive fluid and also provides a basis for vaccine development.

Epidemiology

Like HAV, HBV is endemic worldwide. Accurate statistics on the incidence of infections are not available, as many cases are subclinical, but from serologic studies it is estimated that 200,000 new cases per year occur in the United States. Of these, approximately 150,000 patients remain anicteric, 10,000 require hospitalization, and 250 die from fulminant hepatitis. Between 6% and 10% of young adults with acute HBV infection become chronic carriers. In more than 25% of these chronic carriers, chronic active hepatitis develops, progressing frequently to cirrhosis and sometimes to hepatoma. In the United States approximately 4000 people die from HBV-induced cirrhosis per year, with a further 800 deaths resulting from HBV-induced hepatoma.

The HBV carrier plays the key role in the epidemiology of infection. A carrier is defined as a person who is HBsAg positive on two occasions at least six months apart. Using this criterion, it is estimated that there are approximately 170 million carriers in the world. The HBV carrier rate varies from 0.01% to 20% depending upon the population sampled. In North America 0.1% to 0.3% of volunteer blood donors are carriers, and rates are much higher in certain subpopulations such as drug abusers, homosexuals, immunosuppressed patients and those undergoing hemodialysis, and persons with Down's syndrome. In Africa, Asia, and Oceania, the carrier rates may be as high as 20%. In these geographic regions the incidence of hepatoma is much higher and in many countries it is one of the most common malignancies.

Transmission of HBV requires contact with biologic fluids from carriers or patients with acute disease. In carriers, the highest concentrations of HBV are found in the blood or serous fluids, with lower concentrations present in other fluids such as saliva, semen, and breast milk. Transmission is most common by the percutaneous route with contaminated needles during accidental needle pricks, drug abuse, hemodialysis, use of blood or blood products, and procedures such as acupuncture, tattooing, or ear piercing. Arthropod-borne infections may also occur by the percutaneous route. Transmission can occur with HBsAg-positive fluids contaminating open wounds or mucous membranes, and this is believed to be the mode of infection in sexual partners, household contacts, and institutionalized children.

There are many unknown factors associated with the development of the carrier state, but some risk factors are apparent. If HBV is transmitted from HBsAg-positive mothers to infants, the risk of the infant becoming a carrier is high. Similarly, the carrier state is more likely to develop after anicteric hepatitis than after icteric infection. Some evidence suggests that the carrier state is more likely to be associated with a low initial infecting dose of HBV. For example, it is more frequent after percutaneous puncture with contaminated needles than after transfusion with HBsAg-positive blood.

Pathophysiology

Hepatocytes can be stained using immunofluorescence for either HBsAg or HBcAg. The HBV replicates only in hepatocytes, and during acute infections almost all hepatocytes are infected. In persistent infection, the numbers of cells supporting the synthesis of HBsAg always exceeds the number of cells synthesizing HBcAg. This in part explains why the HBsAg particles in blood may exceed the number of Dane particles by a large ratio.

In an acute self-limited infection after exposure to HBV, HBsAg can be detected at 6 to 12 weeks, while clinical hepatitis is not apparent until 10 to 16 weeks. In most cases the blood becomes negative for HBsAg by 20 weeks. Anti-HBs may develop early in infection even while HBsAg is still present. More commonly, however, anti-HBs appears in the serum only after the disappearance of HBsAg. This interval without either HBsAg or anti-HBs results in the concept of the serologic window in HBV infections. Serum samples taken during the window are positive for anti-HBc, however as antibody to core develops relatively early in infection and remains positive for months to years. The HBeAg and viral DNA polymerase are two markers of the Dane particle that can be detected in the serum of patients during late incubation and early clinical illness. Under normal circumstances, these markers remain in the serum for only a few weeks. The disappearance of HBeAg may be followed by the development of anti-HBe (Figure 15.2).

Unfortunately, not all patients follow the relatively uneventful course of HBV infection described above. Between 5% and 10% of patients develop persistent infection. In them, HBsAg is detected in the blood for more than 20 weeks, and usually for years. Anti-HBc is present in all persistent carriers and remains elevated. Anti-HBs is not detectable and in most cases it is prob-

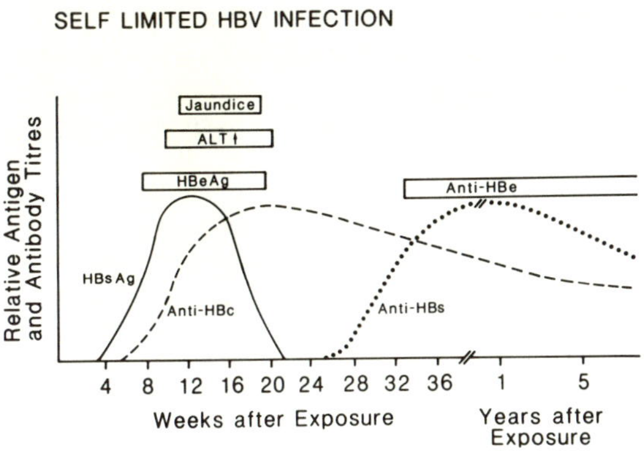

FIGURE 15.2. Self-limited HBV infection.

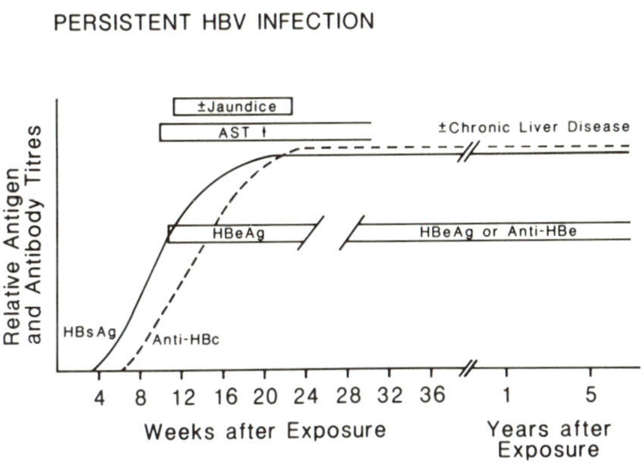

FIGURE 15.3. Persistent HBV infection.

ably not produced (Figure 15.3). Some patients may develop immune complexes in their serum as a result of some anti-HBs in the presence of excess HBsAg. Persistent carriers may have either HBeAg or anti-HBe. The biologic fluids of patients with anti-HBe are of lower infectivity.

The natural history of HBsAg carriers is incompletely defined. It appears that a small percentage may clear their antigen annually, suggesting that carriage is self-limited in certain cases rather than lifelong.

In 1977, a new antigen called *delta* was detected by immunofluorescence in the liver of several patients who were HBsAg carriers. Since then delta has only been identified in HBV carriers. It is distinct from HBV and has an RNA genome coated with HBsAg. Delta has both defective and interfering properties. Not only does the delta agent require HBV to provide helper function for its expression, it interferes with HBV replication. The presence of delta usually signifies aggressive disease with a poor prognosis.

Clinical Manifestations

The incubation period ranges between 4 and 20 weeks and is related both to the size of initial infecting dose of HBV and to host factors. Many patients do not develop an icteric phase after HBV infection, but are detected later as patients with anti-HBs but no previous history of infection. Others may have manifestations of the chronic carrier state and HBsAg-positive serum.

Acute HBV hepatitis usually follows a course similar to acute HAV infections. The illness has a spectrum from mild to very severe or even fatal. Symptoms include anorexia, nausea, headache, malaise, and fever. The urine becomes dark and the stools pale as jaundice develops. On examination, the most common findings include scleral icterus and generalized tenderness in the right upper quadrant. The liver may be tender on palpation as well as on percussion, and splenomegaly is occasionally present. Some patients with HBV develop circulating immune complexes with features resembling serum sickness, such as skin rashes, urticaria, arthralgias, and arthritis of distal joints. Polyarteritis nodosa and membranous glomerulonephritis have been associated with chronic HBV infection.

Diagnosis

The most striking laboratory abnormality is the markedly elevated serum transaminase levels with normal or slightly elevated levels of hepatic alkaline phosphatase. Serum bilirubin, both direct and indirect, is usually elevated, and urinalysis may reveal the presence of bilirubin.

A specific diagnosis of HBV hepatitis is usually made by identifying HBsAg in the serum during acute infection. In difficult cases, increasing titers of anti-HBs or anti-HBc confirm a recent HBV infection and differentiate from HAV or NANB infections in the chronic HBsAg carrier.

Treatment

Patients with acute HBV infections are usually treated symptomatically with bedrest, restricted dietary protein, and elimination of hepatotoxins such as alcohol. Various drugs have been tried without success to treat severe acute infections. Corticosteroids initially appeared promising, but in controlled trials failed to show any benefit. Although some studies have shown that endogenous interferon is inadequate during fulminant viral hepatitis, a beneficial effect from administering exogenous interferon has not been demonstrated in a controlled clinical trial. Unfortunately, no therapy has been found that can prevent acute HBV infection from developing into chronic hepatitis in some patients.

Patients with chronic acute hepatitis (CAH) and a negative HBsAg respond well to steroids. If the CAH is due to HBV, however, steroids with or without other immunosuppressants not only fail to improve the clinical state, but increase the titers of viral markers during therapy.

The antiviral agents adenine arabinoside (ara-A) and adenine arabinoside-5′-monophosphate (ara-AMP) have been used either alone or in combination with human leukocyte interferon to treat CAH due to HBV. In these open trials some patients have shown serologic improvement, with 25% to 30% losing the HBV DNA polymerase from the blood. Significant numbers of patients treated in this manner have encountered drug toxicity, with muscle pains, tremor, ataxia, bone marrow suppression, and gastrointestinal symptoms. This therapy needs further evaluation in randomized controlled trials before its benefit can be ascertained fully.

Prophylaxis

Hepatitis B infections can be reduced by (1) identifying chronic carriers and employing appropriate blood isolation procedures, (2) passive immunization after exposure with either immune serum globulin (ISG) or hyperimmune serum globulin (HBIG), and (3) active immunization with vaccine in high-risk groups.

Hospitalized chronic carriers do not require isolation, but precautions are required in handling their biologic fluids, particularly blood. Postexposure prophylaxis is of proved value. After needle-stick injuries from known HBsAg carriers, HBIG reduces seroconversion from 25% to 5.6% and clinical hepatitis from 6% to 1.4%. The value of ISG depends upon its anti-HBs titer, which can vary from one lot to another. Its use is adequate for postexposure prophylaxis when there is low to moderate risk.

Administration of HBIG has been shown to decrease seroconversion in infants born to HBsAg-positive mothers. A regimen of HBIG administration at birth, together with the HBV vaccine is advised. HBIG is also suggested for sexual partners of patients with acute HBV infection. If HBIG is unavailable, ISG at a dose of 0.2 ml per kg should be used. To be effective, both should be given as soon as possible after exposure, and ideally within 48 hours. For further discussion of HBIG, see Chapter 8.

HBV Vaccine

Several vaccines have been developed that are noninfectious but sufficiently antigenic to produce a protective immune response to HBV. The vaccine developed by Hilleman and his associates at Merck Sharpe and Dohme is licensed both in Canada and the United States. It is unique since it is prepared by purifying HBsAg from the sera of HBV carriers. The blood is ultracentrifuged to separate HBsAg from Dane particles. The HBsAg is sequentially treated with pepsin at pH 2 and 8 M urea. Then it is subjected to gel filtration and treated for 72 hours at 36°C with formalin 1:4000. The final product is adsorbed onto aluminum hydroxide, which serves as an adjuvant. These steps inactivate any contaminating Dane particles and ensure that the vaccine is noninfectious.

In animal studies and in clinical trials, over 90% of vaccine recipients produced sufficient titers of anti-HBs to prevent HBV infection. The vaccine can also be used simultaneously with HBIG in passive-active immunization in postexposure prophylaxis analogous to the approach used in rabies vaccination. The vaccine is given in three doses, the initial dose and two boosters at one and six months. Each 1-ml dose contains 20 μg of purified HBsAg. Persons receiving hemodialysis treatment and immunosuppressed patients should receive 2-ml (40-μg) doses. In children under 10 years of age, 0.5-ml (10-μg) doses are sufficient. The vaccine should be stored at 2° to 8°C, but not frozen, as this destroys its potency.

Carriers of HBsAg and patients having anti-HBs do not require vaccination; however, the cost effectiveness of prevaccination screening is debatable. It depends on three variables: the prevalence of immune individuals in the group to be screened, the cost of serologic screening, and the cost of the vaccine. It is generally safe to assume that prescreening is cost effective in high-risk groups such as homosexuals, users of illicit drugs, prisoners, and mentally retarded persons in institutions. In the intermediate-risk group such as health care workers, prescreening programs are of marginal benefit. For groups with a low prevalence of immunity but who will be exposed to high risks of HBV infection, such as students of dentistry, nursing, laboratory technology, and medicine, prescreening is not cost effective.

Use of the vaccine is determined primarily by the risk of infection and its cost. It is currently being used primarily to immunize high-risk individuals in industrialized nations, but the greatest benefit will be in areas of the world where HBV infections are common. In these countries, long-term application of vaccine may decrease the chronic carrier rates with an associated decrease in chronic liver disease and primary hepatocellular carcinoma. As less expensive vaccine will almost certainly be available in the near future, the goals are realistic.

Vaccine recommendations for susceptible individuals who are at a substantial risk of exposure to HBV are listed below:

1. Preexposure vaccination
   - Health care workers — medical, dental, laboratory, nursing, and support groups with exposure to blood or blood products
   - Clients and staff of institutions for the mentally retarded
   - Patients undergoing hemodialysis
   - Homosexually active males
   - Users of illicit injectable drugs
   - Recipients of factor VIII or factor IX concentrates
   - Household contacts and sexual partners of HBV carriers
   - Inmates of long-term correctional institutions
2. Postexposure vaccination (often used with HBIG)
   - Infants (at birth) born to HBsAg-positive mothers
   - Sexual contacts of patients with acute HBV
   - Health care workers who have received needlestick injury

There has been some concern that the hepatitis vaccine might act as a mode of transmission for the agent responsible for acquired immune deficiency syndrome (AIDS). This concern has arisen due to failure to identify the causative agent and also from the fact that some of the HBsAg-positive paid donors for the vaccine are male homosexuals. However, all available evidence points to the safety of the vaccine. First, the three inactivation steps used in preparation of the vaccine inactivate all known infectious agents. Second, a careful review of vaccine and placebo recipients in the original trial in New York homosexuals has shown no increased incidence of AIDS in the vaccine recipients. A second review of 15,000 vaccine recipients carried out by the Centers for Disease Control has also failed to show any increased risk of AIDS, and currently the vaccine is believed to be completely safe.

NON-A, NON-B HEPATITIS

Initial evidence for the presence of a non-A, non-B (NANB) cause for viral hepatitis came from epidemiologic studies of posttransfusion hepatitis. The distribution of cases with a peak incidence around 48 days after exposure was incompatible with either HAV or HBV as being the sole cause. As sensitive serologic diagnostic tests for both those infections became available, a group of patients with hepatitis but without evidence of HAV or HBV infections was clearly identified. Both clinical and experimental evidence suggests that several agents rather than one are responsible for NANB hepatitis. This, of course, creates difficulties in defining the epidemiology and clinical features of the disease, as well as in designing appropriate methods of prevention and treatment. Despite the considerable research that has been undertaken to determine the agents responsible for NANB hepatitis, their identity remains elusive, as do appropriate screening tests to limit transmission.

Epidemiology

With the introduction of routine screening of blood donors for HBV, the prevalence of posttransfusion hepatitis has decreased by about 80%, but still poses a significant risk due to the presence of NANB. These infections are responsible for 90% to 95% of posttransfusion hepatitis. Several studies have shown that the risk of acquiring NANB hepatitis varies with the source of the blood. With volunteer donors, the disease occurred after transfusion in 6% to 7% of recipients, while with paid donors it occurred in 17% to 35% of recipients. The prevalence of NANB hepatitis in recipients of blood donated voluntarily from healthy adults implies that a significant number of people may be asymptomatically infected.

There is considerable evidence that NANB hepatitis can be transmitted without exposure to blood products. Between 10% and 50% of sporadic cases of hepatitis in the United States fit the criteria of NANB disease, although no exposure to blood products or drug abuse has been documented. In some outbreaks, the clinical picture is indistinguishable from HAV infection with a proposed fecal-oral route of transmission. Cases of NANB hepatitis after either transfusions or fecal-oral transmission have been documented in many countries, indicating NANB agents are found throughout the world. Table 15.1 outlines some of the comparative features of HAV, HBV, and NANB.

TABLE 15.1. Comparative Features of Viral Hepatitis

Factor	*Hepatitis A*	*Hepatitis B*	*Non-A, Non-B Hepatitis*
Etiology	RNA virus	DNA virus	Agents unknown
Main route of transmission	Fecal-oral	Parenteral	Fecal-oral and parenteral
Carrier state	No	Yes	Yes
Progression to chronic disease	No	Yes	Posttransfusion common; Fecal-oral rare
Usual range for incubation (wks)	3–5	4–20	5–10

Clinical Manifestations

Several studies have attempted to define the incubation period for NANB hepatitis after a blood transfusion. Although in most cases abnormal liver function tests are first detected between 5 and 10 weeks, the extremes of range are 2 to 26 weeks. This wide range could be a manifestation of several different agents causing the same condition.

The clinical course of NANB hepatitis is usually benign and is indistinguishable from that of HBV or HAV infections. Less than 30% of patients become jaundiced and the diagnosis is usually made by elevations in serum transaminase levels. One-third of patients have marked enzyme elevations, but only a small number develop fulminant hepatitis. The disease acquired by fecal-oral transmission has not been associated with any chronic sequelae; however, when it develops after parenteral transmission it has an even greater tendency than HBV to develop into chronic hepatitis. Although chronic hepatitis is common, progression to cirrhosis occurs less frequently than with HBV infections. As in HBV infections, the risk of developing chronic hepatitis appears to be related to the severity of the initial NANB infection. An acute nonicteric episode of NANB hepatitis is more likely to progress to chronic hepatitis than is an acute icteric infection. Various studies have documented prolonged elevation of enzymes in 10% to 60% of patients after acute disease. Healthy adults may carry the NANB agents and thus act as the source of hepatitis after a transfusion.

Some studies have demonstrated that patients can suffer from more than one episode of NANB hepatitis. This has been confirmed in studies with a chimpanzee model, and adds further weight to the belief that a variety of agents causes the disease.

Prevention and Treatment

Patients with recognized NANB hepatitis should be excluded from donating blood. Furthermore, it would appear wise to use standard blood and enteric pathogen isolation procedures when these patients are hospitalized. Some studies have documented a reduction in posttransfusion NANB hepatitis if ISG is given together with the blood products, but the exact role of ISG in prophylaxis has still to be clarified. Immune serum globulin is indicated in needle-stick injuries from known persons with NANB hepatitis. No drug is effective in treating the acute disease, but steroids may be beneficial in cases that have progressed to chronic hepatitis.

Unfortunately, no sensitive and specific tests have been devised to screen potential blood donors for NANB hepatitis. Although it has been advocated that donors with minor elevations of hepatic ALT be excluded, such screening would be expensive and exclude some donors without disease. This idea has not gained general acceptance.

GRANULOMATOUS HEPATITIS

Etiology

The demonstration of granulomata in a biopsy of liver tissue is a nonspecific histopathologic finding. Granulomatous hepatitis is present in 3% to 10% of liver biopsies performed in most general hospitals. In the majority of cases, it is a manifestation of a systemic disease; however, it can be a feature of a primary liver disease such as primary biliary cirrhosis or alcoholic cirrhosis. Occasionally it is a reaction to a disease that is neither hepatic nor granulomatous. Many infectious agents can act as a foreign body in the liver and stimulate an immunologic reaction, as can noninfectious causes. A list of some causes of granulomatous hepatitis is below:

1. Infectious causes
   - Bacteria — mycobacteria, brucellosis, melioidosis
   - Fungi — coccidioidomycosis, histoplasmosis
   - Viruses — Epstein-Barr virus, cytomegalovirus
   - Parasites — *Toxocara canis* or *catis, Ascaris*
   - Rickettsia — *Coxiella burnetii*
   - Spirochetes — *Treponema pallidum*
2. Noninfectious causes
   - Sarcoidosis
   - Neoplasms — Hodgkin's disease
   - Hypersensitivity disorders — berylliosis, drugs
   - Primary hepatic disease — primary biliary cirrhosis
   - Miscellaneous

In most series, tuberculosis is the most common infectious cause, while the major noninfectious causes include sarcoidosis and drug hypersensitivity reactions.

Clinical Features

Although granulomatous hepatitis is a manifestation of a systemic disease, the primary infection may be inapparent and the clinical symptoms nonspecific. A fever of unknown origin is a relatively common feature. Fatigue, chills, abdominal pains, and weight loss also occur relatively frequently. These symptoms probably reflect the high frequency of tuberculosis as a cause of granulomatous hepatitis. Hepatomegaly, splenomegaly, and lymphadenopathy have all been found on physical examination but are not indicative of any particular cause of granulomatous hepatitis.

Diagnosis

The laboratory findings in granulomatous hepatitis are nonspecific. An elevated erythrocyte sedimentation rate and elevations of hepatic alkaline phosphatase and transaminases commonly occur, although clinical jaundice is rare. Anemia is found in over 70% of patients. A careful review of the histopathology of the liver biopsy may indicate the cause of the granuloma but frequently it is nonspecific. Appropriate staining of the biopsy tissue for microorganisms can provide the diagnosis in some cases; however, this has a relatively low sensitivity and samples must be cultured for fungi, bacteria, mycobacteria, and viruses. Serology should also be reviewed, since in some infections such as syphilis it may provide the diagnosis.

Therapy

Treatment of granulomatous hepatitis should be delayed until a definitive diagnosis of the underlying cause has been made. Then it should be directed toward that disease.

Successful treatment of the systemic disease usually leads to improvement of the granulomatous hepatitis. In a minority of patients no diagnosis is made. In such cases, if the clinical conditions warrant, an empiric trial of antituberculous therapy can be instituted. If there is no clinical response noted after two months, steroids may be added and isoniazid continued if the patient's skin test was positive.

Summary

Various systemic infectious and noninfectious diseases cause most cases of granulomatous hepatitis. Tuberculosis and sarcoidosis are the most common, accounting for 50% to 60% of cases. Achieving a diagnosis is important and it usually requires a comprehensive workup.

CHRONIC HEPATITIS

Chronic hepatitis is defined as a continuing inflammation of the liver initiated by viruses, drugs, or unknown toxins which may eventually progress to cirrhosis and liver failure. The hallmark of the disease is a persistent elevation of serum transaminase levels over a period of six months. The classification of the various forms of chronic hepatitis is complex and will remain unclear until the etiology for all the forms has been defined. A working classification based on the histopathologic appearance of the liver biopsy divides chronic hepatitis into (1) chronic persistent and (2) chronic active, mild, or severe categories. The exact classification is important as it determines patient management.

Chronic Persistent Hepatitis

Chronic persistent hepatitis (CPH) in most if not all cases is the result of infection with HBV or NANB agents. Its histologic appearance shows mononuclear cells infiltrating the portal areas of the liver lobule, but there is no erosion of the limiting plate or extension of inflammation into the lobule. There is minimal fibrosis and no evidence of cirrhosis, although some evidence of hepatocyte regeneration is common. The condition rarely progresses to cirrhosis, portal hypertension, or liver failure. It is a benign disease and does not require therapy.

Chronic Active Hepatitis

Chronic active hepatitis (CAH) is an aggressive disease that requires not only careful monitoring but often, therapy. Patients with CAH have features of abnormal liver function for longer than six months. The disease frequently progresses to cirrhosis, portal hypertension, and liver failure. Biochemical evidence for severe CAH includes AST activity of 5 or 10 times normal with a twofold increase above the normal gamma globulin level. Biopsy of liver tissue is diagnostic and shows portal inflammation with destruction of hepatocytes in the liver lobule (piecemeal necrosis) and erosion of the limiting plate. Connective tissue septa extending from the portal zones into the lobules accompanied by evidence of liver regeneration are common. Chronic active hepatitis can be caused by viruses and drugs but may be of unknown etiology. Some of the numerous drugs that have been implicated include oxyphenisatin, nitrofurantoin, methyldopa, diphenylhydantoin, acetaminophen, and isoniazid. Fortunately, removal of the offending agent reverses the disease.

In patients with severe CAH from causes other than HBV, cirrhosis develops in 33%. The use of systemic corticosteroids in non-HBV CAH has resulted in a 10-year survival of 63% in the steroid-treated group compared to 27% in the placebo-treated group. Corticosteroids improved the median survival from 3.3 years in the control group to 12.2 years in the treated group.

The use of corticosteroids to treat CAH resulting from HBV infection is controversial. Controlled trials are difficult, as it usually is a slowly progressive disease with a duration of 10 to 20 years before the complications of cirrhosis are noted. The fluctuation of disease activity makes an assessment of therapeutic agents particularly difficult; however, most studies have failed to show the benefit of prolonged corticosteroid use in HBV-induced CAH. Other forms of therapy with antivirals have been discussed earlier in this chapter.

One form of CAH called lupoid or plasma cell hepatitis usually begins in childhood or early adolescence. Most patients are female (70% to 80%) and the disease begins abruptly. There is commonly no history of the patients receiving blood or blood products, using illicit drugs, or being exposed to patients with hepatitis. Jaundice, hepatomegaly, and splenomegaly are the usual symptoms. Other features may include ascites, amenorrhea, clubbing of digits, arthritis, or arthralgias. Routine blood tests show that most patients have elevated AST (often over 1000 IU/L), hypoalbuminemia, hypergammaglobulinemia, and mild eosinophilia. Immunologic tests often show antinuclear and smooth muscle (antiactin) antibodies. Corticosteroids, with or without the addition of azathioprine, are of clear benefit in these patients, and disease activity can be readily followed by monitoring serum transaminase levels. The doses of prednisone and azathioprine should be tapered eventually to a level sufficient to keep the AST to twice the upper limit of normal. In these patients, evidence of disease activity usually disappears in one to three years and therapy can then be stopped safely.

ANNOTATED BIBLIOGRAPHY

Centers for Disease Control. Inactivated hepatitis B virus vaccine. Recommendations of the immunization practices advisory committee. Ann Intern Med 1982;97:379–383.

A succinct summary of the appropriate indications for hepatitis B vaccine.

Klatskin G. Hepatic granulomata: problems in interpretation. Ann NY Acad Sci 1976;278:427–431.
Review of the etiology of the hepatic granulomata found in 565 consecutive biopsies of liver tissue at Yale University.

Lam KC, Lai CL, Trepi C, Wu PC. Deleterious effect of prednisone in HBsAg-positive chronic active hepatitis. N Engl J Med 1981;304:380–386.
Study demonstrates the ineffectiveness of prednisone in HBsAg-positive patients with chronic active hepatitis.

Mosley JW. Epidemiology of HAV infection. In: Vyas HN, Cohen SN, Schmidt R, eds. Viral hepatitis: a contemporary assessment of etiology, epidemiology, pathogenesis and prevention. Philadelphia: Franklin Institute Press, 1978.
Review of the epidemiology of HAV in industrialized and nonindustrialized nations.

Robinson WS. The enigma of non-A, non-B hepatitis. J Infect Dis 1982;145:387–394.
A comprehensive discussion of many of the important features of this disease.

Szmuness W, Stevens DE, Harley EJ, et al. Hepatitis B vaccine: demonstration of efficacy in a controlled clinical trial in a high-risk population in the United States. N Engl J Med 1980;303:833–841.
This early trial demonstrated the efficacy of vaccination in preventing hepatitis B in New York homosexuals.

16 URINARY TRACT INFECTION

Michel G. Bergeron

Urinary tract infection, which can be defined as the presence of significant numbers of microorganisms in properly collected urine, is one of the most commonly observed infections in clinical practice. Moreover, it is estimated that up to 40% of nosocomial infections originate in the urinary tract.

The last 25 years of clinical, microbiologic, and animal investigations have broadened our understanding of urinary tract infections; these include better defined diagnostic criteria for new clinical entities such as the acute urethral syndrome, reevaluation of classic diagnostic criteria based on colony counts of midstream urine for a urinary tract infection, supplementation of standard diagnostic tools with newer techniques to differentiate between lower and upper tract infections, and the introduction of shorter courses of therapy in the treatment of cystitis.

Etiology

The common organisms isolated in the various syndromes are shown in Table 16.1. *Escherichia coli* is still the most frequently isolated agent in cystitis, pyelonephritis, and prostatitis; several other Enterobacteriaceae are also responsible for a large number of cases. *Staphylococcus saprophyticus* (coagulase-negative) is now considered a common cause. Enterococci, *Proteus* sp., *Klebsiella* sp., and *S. aureus* are often isolated in cases of pyelonephritis in patients with renal calculi. These last two, as well as other Enterobacteriaceae, *Pseudomonas* species, and fungi are often hospital acquired and observed in patients who undergo urologic manipulation or have obstruction.

Chronic catheterization results in colonization of the urinary tree with a mixed flora. This is often quite resistant as a result of selection by numerous courses of antibiotic therapy.

Anaerobes, which do not survive easily in the urine, are very rarely responsbile for urinary tract infections. Viruses, especially adenovirus, have been incriminated as the cause of hemorrhagic cystitis most commonly observed in the pediatric age group.

Bladder infection associated with low-count bacteriuria (>10^5 coliforms/l of midstream urine) may be detected in a significant number of patients suffering from urinary tract infection and may be responsible for the symptoms associated with the acute urethral syndrome of women. *Chlamydia trachomatis* and, to a lesser extent, *Ureaplasma urealyticum* (T-strain *Mycoplasma*) also appear to play a major role in the urethral syndrome. Other organisms, for example, coagulase-negative staphylococci and fastidious gram-positive bacteria such as corynebacteria and lactobacilli, have also been recovered in some of these patients but are probably not pathogenic for the urinary tract. *Trichomonas vaginalis* and *Candida* organisms may also cause the acute urethral syndrome of women.

Epidemiology

Approximately 20% of all females will have at least one episode of urinary tract infection at some time during their lives, whereas males are rarely affected before the age of 45 years. Urinary tract infection in the different age groups is often asymptomatic.

During the first few months of life, the prevalence of bacteriuria is actually higher in boys than it is in girls, and averages about 1%. Thereafter, between the ages of 4 months and 5 years, the prevalence in females increases and averages 4.5% compared to 0.5% in boys.

TABLE 16.1. Etiology of Urinary Tract Infections

Acute Urethral Syndrome	*Cystitis-Pyelonephritis*	*Prostatitis*
Chlamydia	*E. coli* (80%)	*E. coli* (80%)
Ureaplasma	Staphylococci	*Proteus* sp.
Enterobacteriaceae (low-count cystitis)	*Klebsiella* sp.	*S. faecalis*
	Proteus sp.	*Klebsiella* sp.
	S. faecalis	*Enterobacter* sp.
Staphylococci?	*Pseudomonas*	*Pseudomonas* sp.
Trichomonas?	*Candida*	*Serratia* sp.
Candida?		*Chlamydia*
		Ureaplasma

Listings in approximate order of frequency.

From the age of 5 years to adulthood, the prevalence in males is very low and varies between 0.03% to 0.1% at 45 years of age. In men older than 60 years, the prevalence is higher and varies between 1% and 4% and may reach up to 10% and 12% in very elderly patients. In girls between 5 to 16 years old, the frequency is 1%, and one-third of the subjects are asymptomatic; between 16 and 45 years, prevalence increases to 4%. Although the occurrence is identical in pregnant and non-pregnant women, infections are generally more serious in pregnancy and up to 40% of women with bacteriuria diagnosed early in pregnancy develop pyelonephritis if the infection is untreated. Also, in contrast with bacteriuria in school-age girls and women, spontaneous remissions are rarely observed during pregnancy. Up to 12% of elderly women are affected by urinary tract infection.

One percent of ambulatory patients who have a single catheterization become infected, while the same procedure performed in hospitalized patients induces infection in up to 10% of subjects. One hundred percent of patients become infected or colonized within the first week of continual urinary catheterization.

The prevalence of urinary tract infection is higher in women of lower socioeconomic status and in women who had either symptomatic or asymptomatic bacteriuria in childhood.

The prevalence of urinary tract infection in diabetics is no greater than in non-diabetic patients; however, diabetic patients and those suffering from structural abnormalities or neurologic problems are at a greater risk of developing severe illness.

PATHOPHYSIOLOGY

For the most part, the Enterobacteriaceae organisms that cause urinary tract infection originate from the intestinal flora and contaminate the vaginal vestibule or the anterior urethra and reach the urinary tract by the ascending route. Rarely, hematogenous spread from another focus of infection results in pyelonephritis. This mode of infection is to be suspected in young children, especially boys, and in adults following *S. aureus* or *Salmonella* bacteremias. Gram-negative bacteremias, in contrast, rarely are the cause of a urinary tract infection.

Several factors, including colonization of the urethra, structural anomalies of the urinary tract, disturbed local defences, and bacterial virulence, are important pathogenetically.

Colonization of the Urethra

Under most circumstances, the anterior portion of the urethra is not colonized with Enterobacteriaceae. Newborns are an exception, and a few days following birth, colonization with *E. coli* and enterococci can be observed. Colonization diminishes with increasing age, and is absent in children older than 5 years. In childhood and the reproductive period of life, the majority of women are not colonized by Enterobacteriaceae in their urethral or periurethral region; however, 50% of postmenopausal women and 80% of females with recurrent urinary tract infections are colonized in these areas. In fact, patients with recurrent cystitis are not only more frequently colonized than healthy persons, they are more heavily colonized with enterococci and *E. coli* for a much longer time.

In healthy women, the usual aerobic flora recovered in the anterior urethra includes lactobacilli, corynebacteria, staphylococci, and streptococci, while peptococci, clostridia, bacteroides, and fusobacteria constitute the anaerobic microorganisms recovered from this area. Hormonal factors may modify the bacterial ecology of the periurethral region.

The rate of colonization of the male urethra is very low, and diphtheroids, coagulase-negative staphylococci, and *Mycobacterium smegmatis* are considered normal microflora.

Structural Anomalies

The short urethra of the female offers only a limited barrier to bacteria ascending from the vaginal introitus and periurethral region to the bladder. Local urethral trauma, caused, for example, by sexual intercourse, further enhances urethral contamination. The observation that the incidence of urinary tract infection in women without a history of sexual intercourse is identical to that observed in men further supports the role of urethral trauma in the pathogenesis.

Obstruction of urine flow and incomplete emptying of the bladder resulting from congenital anomalies, such as bladder neck obstruction and urethral stricture, and acquired anatomic abnormalities, including cystocele, diverticula, prostatic hypertrophy, and neurogenic bladder, favor bacterial colonization and overdistention of the bladder that may interfere with local defenses. Foreign bodies, including catheters or calculi, located in the bladder or in the kidney also favor the development of chronic infections.

Vesicoureteral reflux, resulting from congenital or anatomic anomalies of the urinary tract, is probably the single most important factor responsible for the development of abnormal renal function in the first few years of life.

Disturbed Local Defenses

A specific adherence of urinary pathogens to urogenital epithelium is probably one of the most important factors in the pathogenesis of recurrent urinary tract infection. Urinary pathogens do not uniformly adhere to genitourinary epithelium from healthy individuals, but cells from patients with recurrent urinary tract infection appear to be more receptive to these bacteria. Moreover, specific receptors on epithelial cells may favor the attachment of bacteria to their surface. There also appear to be lower levels of antibodies in the vaginal secretions of patients with recurrent urinary tract infections than in healthy controls, which probably predisposes to colonization.

In men, any change in the bactericidal properties of prostatic secretions increases the probability of invasion of the urinary tract. In fact, prostatic secretions are normally bactericidal against several gram-positive and gram-negative bacteria.

Although urine easily supports the growth of Enterobacteriaceae, it inhibits the growth of anaerobes. The relatively poor vascular supply and hypertonic environment of the medulla tends to impair local host defenses, including leukocyte migration, phagocytosis, and complement activity, and enhances bacterial seeding and the development of cell-wall-deficient bacteria in this area.

Urinary antibodies directed against bacterial antigens or pili also appear to play a protective role in lower and upper tract infection by either preventing adhesion or by having a cidal effect on bacteria in the urinary tract.

Bacterial Virulence

Serotypes 1, 5, 6, 50, and 75 of *E. coli* are the pathogens most frequently recovered in the infected urinary tract. This distribution probably reflects the fact that these serotypes are the predominant microorganisms recovered in the gut flora. Several components of the bacterial surface structure relate to virulence. Pili or fimbriae, rigid polypeptide structures that project from the bacterial wall, are responsible for the attachment of *E. coli* to the epithelial surface of the urinary tract. The *E. coli* recovered from patients with pyelonephritis and acute cystitis were found to have a better adhesive capacity than bacteria isolated from patients with asymptomatic bacteriuria or noninfected persons. The pathogenic role of pili was further confirmed by the fact that antibody directed against them could prevent the development of pyelonephritis in animals. Although the exact mechanism of virulence of the capsular polysaccharide antigens is uncertain, they may determine resistance to phagocytosis and serum bactericidal activity.

The role of the O antigen, a lipopolysaccharide, in the pathogenesis of pyelonephritis, has not been clearly defined. It is probably responsible, however, for local inflammation and may be associated with the decrease in ureteral peristalsis observed in infected patients. Antibody against the O antigen plays a protective role against ascending and systemic experimental pyelonephritis, and interferes with bacterial adhesion.

Enzyme production by microorganisms, especially the production of urease by *Proteus* sp., is another virulence factor that may result in alkalinization of the

TABLE 16.2. Clinical Manifestations of Urinary Tract Infections

Acute Urethral Syndrome	*Cystitis*	*Pyelonephritis*		*Prostatitis*	
		Acute	*Chronic*	*Acute*	*Chronic*
Frequency	Frequency	Frequency	Asymptomatic	Frequency	Asymptomatic
Dysuria	Dysuria	Dysuria	Relapsing infection	Dysuria	Dysuria
Urgency	Urgency	Urgency		Urgency	Perineal discomfort
Urethral pain	Suprapubic pain	Fever		Fever	Relapsing infection
	Turbid, malodorous urine	Flank pain		Perineal pain	Nontender prostate
		Tender or normal kidney on palpation		Tender prostate	

urine. This favors the production of magnesium ammonium phosphate stones, which further favor bacterial colonization.

CLINICAL MANIFESTATIONS

The clinical manifestations of the various syndromes are summarized in Table 16.2. It is often difficult to distinguish clinically among the acute urethral syndrome, cystitis, pyelonephritis, and prostatitis. Up to one-half of patients with significant bacteriuria may be asymptomatic, but if symptoms and bacteriuria are present, it is estimated that half of the subjects will have upper tract infections. In contrast, the presence of dysuria, frequency, and urgency does not necessarily signify that the patient has a urinary tract infection.

Several clinical indicators including age and the presence of an underlying disease are also of great help to the clinician. Most complicated infections with concurrent bacteremia or septic shock occur in young children, diabetics, older men, or patients with structural abnormalities; this fact should be kept in mind when these patients are examined. Papillary necrosis and renal abscess should also be suspected if lumbar pain and fever persist after apparently effective therapy.

Cystitis

Cystitis may be acute, chronic, or recurrent. Patients with acute cystitis usually complain of the sudden onset of frequency, dysuria, urgency associated with suprapubic pain, and turbid, malodorous urine. On physical examination, the bladder may be sensitive to palpation and the urethra may be inflamed. Systemic manifestations including fever are usually absent. The presence of fever should suggest the possibility that the infection is localized in the kidney or prostate. Also, cystitis seldom occurs as an isolated infection in men.

Chronic cystitis is a less commonly encountered entity. It causes similar but less severe symptoms that can be observed in older patients if residual urine is present. Tuberculosis and schistosomiasis of the bladder may also be associated with a chronic cystitis syndrome.

Recurrent cystitis usually occurs in girls or young women. Although sometimes associated with sexual intercourse, in most cases there is no specific predisposing factor. These infections usually recur within a few days or weeks.

Acute Urethral Syndrome

The acute urethral syndrome is seen in females and is characterized by frequency, dysuria, and urgency without suprapubic tenderness. In patients with vaginitis, similar symptoms are often present, but these patients usually have a vaginal discharge and complain of vulvar burning. Patients suffering from urethritis may describe their pain as localized at the urethral orifice. The urine of patients with urethral syndrome may be of normal appearance.

Acute Pyelonephritis

High fever and flank pain strongly suggest the presence of pyelonephritis. Most patients also have manifestations of cystitis. Nausea, vomiting, and diarrhea or constipation usually occur in severe cases, especially if septicemia or shock is present. On physical examination, the kidney may or may not be tender on palpation. Occasionally, the patient will have right upper quadrant pain mimicking acute cholecystitis or pain radiating from the back to the inguinal region simulating renal stone. Symptoms of both cystitis and pyelonephritis may resolve spontaneously without therapy. If pyelonephritis occurs in men or is accompanied by bacteremia, one should suspect obstruction caused by urologic abnormalities or renal stones.

Chronic Pyelonephritis

Most patients suffering from chronic pyelonephritis are either asymptomatic or have repeated episodes of acute urinary tract infection. Symptoms are those of cystitis or of acute pyelonephritis. Physical examination usually does not reveal any abnormality between acute episodes.

Prostatitis

A soft, exquisitely tender prostate upon palpation in association with fever and perineal pain is diagnostic of acute prostatitis. This classic triad is often incomplete and symptoms compatible with cystitis may be the only clue to diagnosis. Patients may also complain of low back pain and testicular discomfort. Occasionally, some patients suffering from chronic prostatitis may have recurrent episodes of cystitis and complain of perineal discomfort, although the examination of the prostate is often normal.

DIAGNOSIS

Readily available diagnostic tests in urinary tract infection are summarized in Table 16.3.

Urine Collection

One of the most crucial parts of the investigation of urinary tract infections is collection of the urine specimen. The midstream collection is a simple procedure that is reliable as long as the method is carefully explained and followed by the patient. After proper cleaning of the periurethral region, the urine should be sampled directly from the stream, approximately at mid-time during micturition. Suprapubic puncture is a reliable technique in children or older patients who are unable to void properly and avoid contamination. Urethral catheterization should be avoided as much as possible, since it may result in urine contamination or infection.

Microscopic Urine Examination

The microscopic examination, although useful, is often unreliable. White blood cell casts suggest pyelonephritis. The presence of one or two bacteria per high-power (oil) field of unspun urine on Gram's stain usually signifies at least 10^8 bacteria per liter of urine.

Urine Culture

The interpretation of urine cultures is dependent upon the presence or absence and types of symptoms experienced by the patient. The conventional diagnostic criterion of greater than 10^8 bacteria per liter ($>10^5$/ml) of urine is still applicable for most patients with urinary tract infections, but recent studies have shown that the urine of at least one-third of women with acute dysuria may have smaller colony counts. In this respect, the criterion of more than 10^5 organisms per liter ($>10^2$/ml) of midstream urine appeared to be a very sensitive and fairly specific diagnostic test for the presence of lower tract disease (acute urethral syndrome and cystitis) in one series of patients. These recent observations need further confirmation, however, before new standards are applied universally in diagnosis. It is also important to remember that bacterial counts of fewer than 10^8 organisms per liter ($<10^5$/ml) of a midstream urine can be observed in some patients with pyelonephritis and acute prostatitis, although the majority have counts greater than this. Any number of bacteria is usually of significance if specimens are obtained by suprapubic puncture.

Mixed cultures almost always signify contamination and must be repeated.

Dip-slide tests or other quantitative methods may be very useful and much less expensive than routine urine culture in the management of acute noncomplicated infections.

In patients with the acute urethral syndrome, cultures for *C. trachomatis* and *U. urealyticum* may be requested but are usually not available.

TABLE 16.3. Readily Available Diagnostic Tests for Urinary Tract Infections

Procedures	*Findings*	*Interpretation*
Microscopic urine examination	Pyuria (>10 WBC/hpf)	Unreliable (20% false positive, 30% false negative) as only test
	WBC casts	Suggestive of pyelonephritis
	Gram's stain	
	2 bacteria/hpf	Infection ($\geq 10^8$ bacteria/l)
	No bacteria	Significant infection in 20% of cases
Urine culture*	$\geq 10^8$ bacteria/l in 1 sample of midstream urine	True infection in: Most symptomatic patients; 95% asymptomatic men; 80% asymptomatic women
	$\geq 10^8$ bacteria/l in 2 samples	95% asymptomatic women
	$\leq 10^8$ bacteria/l in 1 sample from suprapubic puncture	95% all patients
	10^7–10^8 bacteria/l in 1 sample by catheterization	50% all patients
	$\leq 10^7$ bacteria/l	Contamination or acute urethral syndrome
	Mixed infection ≥ 2 microorganisms	Contamination
	$>10^5$ bacteria/l of midstream urine	May provide optimal sensitivity and specificity for diagnosis of infection
IVP	Normal	Acute pyelonephritis or noninfected kidney
	Kidney swelling, decreased nephrographic density	Acute pyelonephritis
	Pelvis and ureter dilation	Acute pyelonephritis, eliminate obstruction
	Atrophic, scarred irregular kidney	Chronic pyelonephritis
	Abnormal calyces and papilla	Papillary necrosis
Voiding cystourethrography	Vesicoureteral reflux	Functional or anatomic obstruction of lower urinary tract
	Bladder neck-urethral obstruction	

*Disc sensitivity dealt with in the Treatment section. Dip-slide tests may be used for ambulatory patients.

In men suffering from urinary tract infection, the Stamey procedure, which includes cultures of a urethral sample (initial 10 ml of urine), bladder sample (midstream collection), and prostatic sample (expressed prostatic secretions and/or postmassage urine), is useful in distinguishing among urethritis, cystitis, and prostatitis, respectively.

Radiologic Investigation

An intravenous pyelogram (IVP) must be done if obstruction of the urinary tract is suspected. Although in the acute phase of infection one may see kidney swelling or decreased nephrographic density, the IVP may be essentially normal in acute pyelonephritis. Unless obstruction is suspected, an IVP is usually carried out after symptoms disappear. This procedure should be performed with care in diabetics and may be dangerous in patients with multiple myeloma if patients are dehydrated prior to the examination.

A voiding cystourethrogram is most useful in children younger 5 years of age, but may in any age group allow the detection of anatomic or functional abnormalities such as vesicoureteral reflux or lower urinary tract obstruction.

TABLE 16.4. Selected Diagnostic Tools To Differentiate Upper vs Lower Urinary Tract Infection

Procedures	*Advantages*	*Disadvantages*
Ureteral catheterization	Reliable Selective detection of unilateral or bilateral kidney infection	Invasive procedure
Bladder washout	Good correlation with ureteral catheterization	Invasive technique Does not distinguish among left, right, or bilateral infection Results equivocal in 10–29% of patients
Antibody-coated bacteria (ACB test)	Relatively good correlation between ACB test and kidney infection in adults	Limited availability Tedious technique Interpretation difficult: 25% false negative in adults Positive in prostatitis and falsely positive in urine contaminated by fecal flora, in urinary infection caused by gram-positive cocci, *Pseudomonas,* yeast. Negative in early infections and often negative in children
Gallium 67 scan	Good correlation with ureteral catheterization and bladder washout	May become a useful test
Serum antibody to Tamm-Horsfall protein	Present in pyelonephritis	Still investigational
Serum C-reactive protein	Elevated in pyelonephritis	Still investigational

Since most urologic studies are not cost effective in females with uncomplicated infection, these tests should be limited to patients with suspected mechanical or anatomic anomalies, kidney or bladder stones, pyelonephritis, patients with several recurrences of urinary tract infection, or in those who do not seem to respond to appropriate antibiotic therapy.

Specific Tests

Selected diagnostic tests to differentiate between upper and lower urinary tract infections are summarized in Table 16.4. As noted, the differentiation may be difficult. Ureteral catheterization and bladder washout procedures are reliable but are invasive and time consuming. The detection of antibody-coated bacteria (ACB) by direct immunofluorescence is a relatively reliable noninvasive test. The procedure takes considerable time (1½ hours), however, and is not available in all centers. Interpretation of test may be difficult, and false negative results are seen in up to 25% of cases of pyelonephritis in adults and the majority of children with pyelonephritis, the latter likely being due to a poor antibody response. Conversely, positive results are observed in persons with prostatitis and in contaminated urine specimens.

Gallium scan, serum antibody to Tamm-Horsfall protein, and serum C-reactive protein are promising tests under investigation.

TREATMENT

General Principles

The main objective of therapy is to eradicate the invading microorganism whether it is superficially implanted in the bladder or deeply seeded in the prostate or renal parenchyma. Occasionally, especially when unremovable foreign bodies (e.g., stones) are present in the urinary tract, it is impossible to cure the infection. Ther-

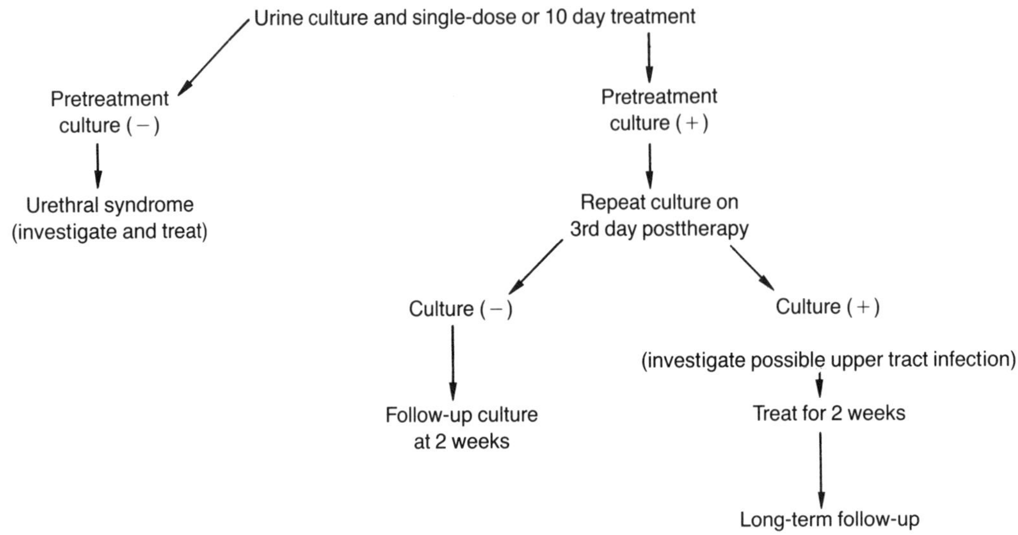

FIGURE 16.1. Management of acute lower urinary tract infections in women.

apy is then aimed at controlling the infection to prevent dissemination and is suppressive only. These two forms of therapy (eradicative and suppressive) should be distinguished from prophylactic therapy, which is aimed at preventing frequent recurrent infections.

Proper management includes knowledge of the exact localization of the infection, the presence or absence of structural abnormalities or foreign bodies, and the microorganism involved and its susceptibility to antibiotics. Knowledge of the bioavailability of antimicrobial agents at the site of infection, side effects, and cost of the drugs should also be considered by the physician. Follow-up, which is probably inadequate in 50% of cases, is crucial to the proper management of these patients.

Although no one approach to the management of UTI can be recommended to the clinician who is confronted daily with a complex and heterogenous patient population, guidelines for the management of acute lower urinary tract infections in women are proposed in Figure 16-1.

Drug Susceptibility

Sensitivity testing of antimicrobials in general is based on normally attained serum levels, the exceptions being the sulfonamides and nitrofurantoin. The latter is almost exclusively used in urinary tract infections. The concentrations of antibiotics reached in the urine are usually 10 to 100 times higher than those observed in the serum, and therefore patients may respond to therapy even in the presence of an apparently resistant microorganism, as determined by sensitivity testing. Under these circumstances, the clinical response and the results of follow-up cultures prevail over sensitivity testing. Some experienced investigators even suggest that susceptibility tests are not needed for the management of acute uncomplicated urinary tract infection and that it should be used only for patients with recurrent or complicated infection.

Intrarenal Pharmacokinetics of Antimicrobials

Minimal information is generally available on the intrarenal distribution of antibiotics in humans, so that most of our knowledge is based on animal experimentation (Table 16.5). There are notable differences in the distribution and persistence of different antibiotics in the kidney parenchyma, and both the serum and urine levels are poor predictors of what happens in the renal tissue, especially the medulla where bacterial growth is the highest in pyelonephritis. Moreover, the mere presence of infection may modify the intrarenal pharmacokinetics of antimicrobial agents. For example, aminoglycosides have the capacity to accumulate in the infected parenchyma in concentrations up to 100 times

TABLE 16.5. Diffusion of Antibiotics in Kidney Parenchyma

High Medullary Levels	*Intermediate Medullary Levels*	*Low Medullary Levels*
(10– ≥100 times serum levels)	*(≤10 times serum levels)*	*(Identical or lower levels than in serum)*
Aminoglycosides (Gentamicin, tobramycin, netilmicin) Persist in kidney up to 6 mo after cessation of therapy	Penicillins (Penicillin G, ampicillin, carbenicillin) Persist in kidney for a few hrs	Sulfamethoxazole Persist in kidney for 24 hrs
Trimethoprim Persist in kidney for a few hrs	Cephalosporins (Cephalothin, cefazolin, cefoxitin) Persist in kidney for a few hrs	Tetracyclines Persist in kidney for a few hrs

Urinary levels will be 10 to ≥100 times higher than in the serum for most antibiotics.

higher than those observed in the serum, and persist in concentrations above the minimum inhibitory concentration for most gram-negative bacteria for more than six months after a week or two weeks of therapy. Trimethoprim also concentrates in all parts of the kidney and reaches levels of up to 20 times those observed in serum, but in contrast with aminoglycosides, trimethoprim has a very short half-life in the kidney. The penicillins and cephalosporins also have shorter half-lives in the renal tissue, and reach medullary concentrations that are up to 10 times higher than those observed in serum. Sulfonamides penetrate renal tissue poorly, and are found in lower concentrations than in the serum while tetracycline concentrations are usually identical in both kidney and serum. Several factors, including the state of hydration, shock, the use of diuretics, and binding to tissues, influence the pharmacokinetics of antibiotics in the kidney.

The prostate is a very selective organ with respect to antibiotic uptake. Only trimethoprim, erythromycin, and to a lesser extent, some tetracyclines are highly concentrated in nonacutely inflamed prostatic tissues. The new quinolone antibiotic, norfloxacin, presently under investigation, also penetrates into prostatic tissue.

Antibiotic Treatment and Prophylaxis

See Table 16.6.

Acute Urethral Syndrome

Therapy for acute urethral syndrome is identical to that for urethritis in men. After gonococcal infection is excluded, chlamydiae and to a lesser extent, *U. urealyticum* are the most common agents in this disease. Since most laboratories are not equipped to isolate these organisms, tetracycline, which is effective for both, is the treatment of choice.

Pregnant women with urethritis can be treated with erythromycin, but the efficacy of this therapy in this population has not yet been defined. Consideration should be given to the treatment of sexual partners.

Cystitis

One recent advance in the therapy of acute cystitis is the use of a single, effective, large dose of antibiotic. In fact, regimens that produce high concentrations of drug in the bladder, which is only superficially infected, result in rapid killing of bacteria. These regimens are effective as long as no obstruction is present. Single-dose therapy is not expensive, results in minimal side effects, does not disturb bowel and periurethral flora, and often allows the early detection of renal infection. After single-dose treatment, patients with pyelonephritis usually have a relapse of infection within two or three days. Therefore, those in whom upper tract disease is suspected are not candidates for single-dose therapy. Such treatment is particularly useful, however, in young women with lower tract infections with no anatomic dysfunction who have been symptomatic for less than five days, and who can be followed up easily for test of cure (Figure 16.1).

Single doses of several antibiotics including amoxicillin, sulfonamides, the combination of trimethoprim and sulfamethoxazole (TMP/SMZ), and kanamycin have been advocated as effective therapy in cystitis. Amoxicillin and sulfisoxazole are the usual antibiotics. Seven or ten days of therapy with several of these agents, as noted in Table 16.6, can be given but is more

TABLE 16.6. Antibiotic Therapy

Diseases	*Choices of Therapy*		*Relapse or Reinfection*
Acute urethral syndrome	Etiology unknown Tetracycline, 500 mg qid × 7 d	If etiology known, adjust therapy to etiology	Same treatment, investigate and treat sexual partner
Acute cystitis	Amoxicillin, single 3-gm dose Sulfisoxazole, single 2-gm dose TMP/SMZ, 480 mg/2400 mg (single dose)	Sulfisoxazole, 1 gm qid × 7 d* Amoxicillin, 250 mg qid × 7 d* TMP/SMZ, 160 mg/800 mg bid × 7 d*	Relapse: eliminate prostatitis, pyelonephritis, obstruction, and treat like pyelonephritis
Recurrent infection	Prophylaxis, TMP/SMZ, 40 mg/200 mg nightly, or 3×/wk × 6 mo	Nitrofurantoin, 50 mg nightly × 6 mo or antibiotics after sexual intercourse	Reinfection: treat like acute cystitis
Asymptomatic infection	Treat children, young women, pregnant women, or men as for acute cystitis	Older patients: do not treat	
Severe pyelonephritis (should be hospitalized)	Ampicillin, 1 gm q6h IV preferably associated with gentamicin, tobramycin, or netilmicin, 1.0–1.5 mg/kg q8h IV until clinical improvement. Followed by amoxicillin or TMP/SMZ for a total of 14 d	TMP/SMZ, 160 mg/800 mg, or cephalothin, 1 gm q6h, or other cephalosporins preferably associated with aminoglycosides until clinical improvement. Followed by cephalexin or TMP/SMZ for a total of 14 d	Relapse: same medication for 6 wks
Acute prostatitis	TMP/SMZ, 160 mg/800 mg bid × 30 d	Ampicillin, 1 gm q6hIV associated with aminoglycosides until clinical improvement. Followed by TMP/SMZ bid for a total of 30 d	Investigate for complicating factors (stones) and treat for 3 mo
Chronic prostatitis	TMP/SMZ, 160 mg/800 mg bid × 12 wks	Tetracyclines for 12 wks	Retreatment or prostatectomy

*Some investigators recommend from 3 to 10 days of therapy.

expensive and may result in more side effects. At the present time, more investigations are needed to recommend strongly either single-dose or longer courses of therapy.

Recurrent Cystitis

Most patients with recurrent urinary tract infections are reinfected with new bacteria each time. Each episode of cystitis can be treated with a single dose of antibiotic, or long-term prophylaxis with trimethoprim/ sulfamethoxazole or nitrofurantoin. The prophylactic regimens are limited to patients with closely spaced recurrent infections or who have at least three to five episodes of urinary tract infection per year. When infection appears to be related to sexual intercourse, a single dose of antibiotic taken after intercourse, when effective, is preferred to long-term prophylaxis.

Recurrent infections with the same microorganism (relapse) necessitates a thorough investigation, especially for upper tract disease, and should be treated aggressively. (See Table 16.6.) Rarely, for example in patients with kidney stones, chronic treatment with mandelamine will be used.

Asymptomatic Bacteriuria
In the presence of asymptomatic urinary tract infection, treatment should be limited to patients who are at high risk of developing serious complications. These include men, young children, and young or pregnant women. In these populations, one should eliminate the possibility of a bladder abnormality or prostatic or upper tract involvement. Patients with structural abnormalities that are not correctible with surgery, neurologic problems, indwelling catheters, or those in the older age group do not usually respond to therapy. If they do respond, they often become reinfected with more resistant organisms. Routine antibiotic treatment in these populations is thus not recommended.

Pyelonephritis
In contrast to the innovative approaches described with lower tract and recurrent infection, therapy of pyelonephritis is still for the most part empiric. Most patients with acute pyelonephritis should be hospitalized. For them, parenteral therapy with ampicillin, cephalosporin, aminoglycoside, or trimethoprim/sulfamethoxazole until clinical improvement is evident, followed by oral therapy for a total of 14 days, usually is effective. If the infection relapses, longer courses of 6 to 12 weeks may be necessary.

Chronic pyelonephritis requires long-term oral therapy (minimum of six weeks) based on antimicrobial sensitivity. If structural abnormalities are present, surgical correction should be considered.

In pregnancy, acute pyelonephritis is a serious illness that should be treated with hospitalization and parenteral antibiotics. Penicillins and cephalosporins are potentially less toxic than the aminoglycosides in this setting.

Prostatitis
The treatment of acute or chronic prostatitis is presented in Table 16.6. In the acute phase, most antibiotics diffuse easily, but as inflammation subsides, it is necessary to use drugs that have a better rate of penetration. In this respect, trimethoprim/sulfamethoxazole or trimethoprim alone is the preferred and most effective form of therapy. A minimum of 30 days is usually required to sterilize the acutely inflamed prostate, whereas 3 months may be necessary for the treatment of chronic prostatitis. After relapse, another three months of therapy is usually indicated. Complicating factors such as stones or foreign bodies should be eliminated. Prostatectomy with antibiotic coverage has been used but should be the last resort in the treatment of chronic prostatitis.

Urinary Catheter-associated Infections
The urine of patients with urinary catheters can be cultured intermittently, but patients should not receive antibiotics that allow the selection of resistant strains. Therapy should be administered if patients are symptomatic with localized or systemic sepsis. Initial antibiotic treatment can be based on previous surveillance cultures and modified accordingly when cultures are available prior to therapy.

Follow-up

An important aspect of the management of patients with urinary tract infection is careful follow-up, both clinically and with cultures to detect recurrence. The type of evaluation will vary depending upon the population studied. In patients with acute cystitis, follow-up cultures (routine or dip-slide) can be done on day three post therapy and repeated in 2 weeks. If the culture is still positive on day two or three after single-dose therapy, the patient should be investigated for pyelonephritis and be given appropriate treatment. Failure to respond to any treatment regimen in 48–72 hours necessitates a repeat culture. If cultures are negative at two weeks after a single dose or standard 7- to 10-day course of antibiotic therapy, no further investigation or follow-up is necessary. Patients with the acute urethral syndrome with low bacterial counts (less than 10^5/l) require only one follow-up culture if symptoms disappear. If the initial urine culture is negative (possibly *C. trachomatis* or *U. urealyticum* infection), no follow-up culture is necessary if there is a treatment response. Patients with pyelonephritis and men suffering from prostatitis should have their urine cultured at regular intervals for up to two years (for example, at 1 week, and 1, 3, 6, 12, and 24 months) after cessation of therapy. Children less than 5 years old, diabetic patients, or patients with a structural abnormality of the urinary tract should probably have periodic urine cultures for more than two years after pyelonephritis. Patients with asymptomatic bacteriuria, if not in a high-risk group, probably do not need regular urine cultures.

PROGNOSIS

Most lower urinary tract infections in women are of no major consequence medically, but cause major discomfort that usually results in time lost from work. Even without therapy, symptoms disappear spontaneously in a few days, but improvement is rapid if antibiotic therapy is given. In pregnant women, pyelonephritis is a common complication of asymptomatic or symptomatic lower tract disease and should be approached aggressively. Asymptomatic bacteriuria in children or adults without obstruction or structural or functional anomalies of the urinary tract should not result in renal failure but may predispose to recurrent episodes of infection. Recent work suggests that asymptomatic urinary tract infection in the elderly may be associated with a lower survival rate in this population.

Acute pyelonephritis after lower urinary tract infection or urologic manipulation may be associated with septicaemia and shock, but once these acute complications have been controlled, there is no evidence to suggest that renal impairment follows. Two other serious complications of acute pyelonephritis include renal or perirenal abscess and papillary necrosis (necrotizing papillitis), the latter especially in diabetics. A renal abscess develops as the acute inflammatory process progresses to an area of suppuration initially in the renal medulla, usually as a result of impaired drainage from obstruction in the urinary tract. From its intramedullary location, the abscess can extend to the cortex and perirenal space, rupture into the retroperitoneum, or extend through fistulization into other areas including the subdiaphragmatic space, or even the pleura, to produce an empyema. Emphysematous pyelonephritis as a result of gas-producing Enterobacteriaceae organisms may also result from a renal abscess. With papillary necrosis, the papilla can slough and cause further obstruction of the urinary tract.

Cortical or perirenal abscess may also result from hematogenous seeding (usually *S. aureus*) or direct spread to the kidney from a contiguous source of infection. The diagnosis of renal abscess should be suspected when there is a lack of clinical response of pyelonephritis with five days of appropriate antimicrobial therapy. The disease may also have a more insidious onset, and cause fever of unknown origin with some flank and abdominal pain. Occasionally a mass may be felt in the flank. The urine usually demonstrates pyuria and the causative organism can be cultured in the majority of cases of intramedullary abscess and papillary necrosis. In patients with complete obstruction of the urinary tract, cortical abscesses, or perirenal abscesses due to hematogenous or contiguous spread, there is a greater chance for the urine to be normal. Additional studies including an intravenous pyelogram, ultrasound, and computerized tomographic scan will usually detect the abscess, the last two examinations being particularly sensitive. Because patients with these complications are usually quite ill, empiric therapy with a combination of an aminoglycoside with either ampicillin or a cephalosporin is usually begun before definitive microbiology is known. Surgical treatment is generally required to relieve obstruction or remove the abscess. In the case of several small abscesses, antibiotic therapy alone may be effective and should be considered prior to nephrectomy.

Chronic renal failure is an uncommon sequel to urinary tract infection. Infection may play an important role, however, in renal failure developing in diabetic patients, children or adults with structural abnormalities, obstructive uropathy, or neurogenic bladder.

Urinary tract infection in the male population is usually an index of prostatic or renal involvement. Prostatitis is a cumbersome and often very difficult disease to treat, and relapses are common.

ANNOTATED BIBLIOGRAPHY

Bergeron MG, Bastille A, Lessard C, Gagnon PM. Significance of intrarenal concentrations of gentamicin on the outcome of experimental pyelonephritis in rats. J. Infect Dis 1982;145:91–96.

Persisting high levels of gentamicin in infected renal parenchyma long after cessation of therapy was shown to play a significant role in the treatment of experimental pyelonephritis.

Harding, GKM, Ronald AR. A controlled study of antimicrobial prophylaxis of recurrent urinary infection in women. N Engl J Med 1974;291:597–601.

Trimethoprim/sulfamethoxazole was shown to be more effective than sulfamethoxazole alone or methenamine mandelate in preventing reinfections of the urinary tract in females.

Kunin CM. Detection, prevention, and management of urinary tract infections. Philadelphia: Lea & Febiger, 1979.

Practical book covering most aspects of urinary tract infections.

Mulholland S. Lower urinary tract antibacterial defense mechanisms. Invest Urol 1979;17:93–97.

Review of the role of vaginal and urethral flora and of bladder defense mechanism on the development of urinary tract infections.

Naeye RL. Causes of the excessive rates of perinatal mortality and prematurity in pregnancies complicated by maternal urinary tract infections. N Engl J Med 1979;300:819–823.

Women who had pyuria and bacteriuria close to the time of delivery had an increased incidence of amniotic fluid infections. The presence of UTI seems to make already compromised fetuses more vulnerable.

Rubin RH, Fang LST, Jones SR, et al. Single-dose amoxicillin therapy for urinary tract infection. Multicenter trial using antibody-coated bacteria localization technique. JAMA 1980;244:561–564.

For lower urinary tract infection, single-dose amoxicillin was shown to be of equal efficacy to standard therapy with trimethoprim/sulfamethoxazole or ampicillin.

Schiff M, Glickman M, Weiss RM, et al. Antibiotic treatment of renal carbuncle. Ann Intern Med 1977;87:305–308.

Renal carbuncles in six of seven young males were successfully treated with long-term administration of penicillinase-resistant antibiotics without surgical exploration.

Silverblatt FJ, Cohen LS. Antipili antibody affords protection against experimental ascending pyelonephritis. J Clin Invest 1979;64:333–336.

Rats passively immunized with rabbit antipili serum were protected against *E. coli* pyelonephritis.

Stamm WE, Running K, McKevitt M, Counts GW, Turk M, Holmes KK. Treatment of the acute urethral syndrome. N Engl J Med 1981;304:956–958.

In women with acute urethral syndrome and pyuria, tetracycline was shown to be effective treatment.

Thomas V, Shelokov A, Forland M. Antibody-coated bacteria in the urine and the site of urinary tract infection. N Engl J Med 1974;290:588–590.

Classic article suggests that the immunofluorescence test can be useful in distinguishing infection of the kidney from infection of the bladder.

17 SEXUALLY TRANSMITTED DISEASES

William R. Bowie

Sexually transmitted or transmissible diseases (STD) remain a major, and probably growing, problem. The number of pathogens that are recognized to have sexual transmission either as a major or a minor means of spread continue to increase because of better understanding of the etiology of STD syndromes and recognition of new agents (Table 17.1). Classic discussions of STD have tended to focus on specific organisms, but in practical terms, physicians must usually recognize and manage a syndrome, and the knowledge of the specific etiology may not be available until later, and possibly never. This chapter focuses on a syndromic approach, as follows:

1. Most important syndromes
   - Urethritis
   - Vaginitis
   - Cervicitis
   - Epididymitis
   - Endometritis, salpingitis
   - Genital ulcers
   - Acquired Immune Deficiency Syndrome (AIDS)
2. Other syndromes
   - Enteritis
   - Anorectal disease
   - Frequency, dysuria
   - Hepatitis
   - Balanoposthitis
   - Bartholinitis
   - Pharyngitis
   - Infestations
3. Important sequelae
   - Involuntary infertility
   - Ectopic pregnancy
   - Cervical dysplasia and cancer
   - Reactive arthritis
   - Fetal consequences
   - Infection in infancy

EPIDEMIOLOGY

For most of the STD, rates of disease are maximal between the ages of 15 and 24 years. These are the ages for greatest frequency of gonorrhea and chlamydial infections, which are presumably related to sexual practices resulting in increased exposure to these pathogens. Relative rates of different pathogens over time fluctuate with sexual practices, ease of diagnosis of the infection, and effectiveness of management modalities. Thus diseases such as Herpes simplex virus (HSV), which recur and cannot be eradicated, assume a relatively greater role in older age groups. In addition, within certain populations, the patterns may differ. Among homosexual and bisexual men, the peak rates of disease occur in some older persons. For example, since one-half to two-thirds of primary, secondary, and early latent syphilis in developed countries is seen in homosexual and bisexual men, this results in a shift toward higher peak rates in older age groups.

In general, well-recognized risk factors for the presence of STD include early age of onset of sexual activity, early age of first pregnancy, increased number of pregnancies, increased number of sexual partners in the person's lifetime but especially recently, past history of STD, presence of genital symptoms in the patient or partner, and in some situations, the type of contraception used.

ETIOLOGY AND CLINICAL MANIFESTATIONS

Urethritis

Urethritis is suggested by the presence of urethral discharge, burning on urination, or an itch at the end of the urethra. The classic findings are urethral discharge and

TABLE 17.1. Sexually Transmitted Pathogens

Sexual Transmission a Major Means of Spread	*Sexual Transmission One Means of Spread*
Bacteria	Bacteria
Chlamydia trachomatis	*Shigella* sp.
Neisseria gonorrhoeae	*Campylobacter jejuni*
Treponema pallidum	?*Yersinia* sp.
Gardnerella vaginalis	?*Salmonella* sp.
Ureaplasma urealyticum	
Mycoplasma hominis	
Hemophilus ducreyi	
Calymmatobacterium granulomatis	
Group B streptococci	
Viruses	Viruses
Herpes simplex	Hepatitis B
Genital wart	Hepatitis A
Molluscum contagiosum	Cytomegalovirus
Protozoa	Protozoa
Trichomonas vaginalis	*Entamoeba histolytica*
	Giardia lamblia
	Ectoparasites
	Phthirus pubis
	Sarcoptes scabiei
	Yeasts
	Candida albicans

inflammation of the urethral meatus. Clinical diagnosis requires demonstration of an increased number of polymorphonuclear leukocytes (PMN) in urethral material. When urethritis is present, if *Neisseria gonorrhoeae* is detected, gonorrhea is diagnosed. If gram-negative intracellular diplococci are not seen on Gram's stain and *N. gonorrhoeae* is not cultured, nongonococcal urethritis (NGU) is diagnosed. The most important causes of NGU are *Chlamydia trachomatis* (30% to 50%) and *Ureaplasma urealyticum* (30% to 40%). In 20% to 30% of men with acute, untreated NGU, neither organism is recovered and the etiology is usually not apparent. In the 30% to 40% of men who have persistent or recurrent urethritis after a seven-day course of tetracycline for NGU, approximately 20% have *U. urealyticum* recovered, but the cause is not usually apparent in the rest. Very infrequently, *Trichomonas vaginalis* or herpes simplex virus is identified in urethral material. Yeasts and *Gardnerella vaginalis* are very infrequent causes of urethritis, but occasionally there can be a PMN response in conjunction with balanitis. The distinction between gonorrhea and NGU is helpful for management, but the presence of urethritis is only an indirect indicator of the presence of pathogens. Because urethral gonorrhea and chlamydial infections are frequently asymptomatic, absence of urethritis does not exclude infection with these agents. Furthermore, *C. trachomatis* infection is often present concurrently with gonorrhea, being recovered from 0% to 11% of heterosexual men without urethritis, approximately 20% of heterosexual men with gonorrhea, and 5% to 10% of homosexual men with gonorrhea. Most of the men with gonorrhea and urethral chlamydial infection go on to develop postgonococcal urethritis (PGU) if treatment of gonorrhea does not eradicate *C. trachomatis*.

Compared to men with NGU, symptoms in men with gonococcal urethritis tend to be marked and acute. Discharge in gonococcal urethritis is often green or yellow, while in NGU it is often clear or mucoid, and may only be present in the morning or noted as staining on underpants. This has important clinical significance and indicates the need for careful examination. Frequently, men complain of genital symptoms, but abnormalities cannot be detected on examination. Such men should be evaluated in the morning prior to voiding. Approximately half will have urethritis, usually nongonococcal.

Epididymitis

Complications of urethritis in men are unusual, with epididymitis occurring in fewer than 1%. Epididymitis causes painful unilateral or bilateral scrotal swelling, often in association with urethritis, pain in the groin, and fever. In the past, most epididymitis was considered to be idiopathic, especially in younger men. Recent studies show that there are two distinct groups of causes. In older men, men with urologic structural or functional abnormalities, and possibly in homosexual men, infection is usually caused by coliforms or pseudomonads, that is, typical urinary tract pathogens. In contrast, among younger or sexually active men without urologic structural abnormalities, *C. trachomatis* and *N. gonorrhoeae* are the major causes. Careful examination of many of these men demonstrates urethritis.

TABLE 17.2. Clinical and Rapid Laboratory Features in the Differential Diagnosis of Vaginitis

	Normal	G. vaginalis	*Yeasts*	T. vaginalis
Symptoms				
Vaginal discharge	±	+	±	+ +
Genital irritation	−	−	+ +	+ +
Fishy odor	−	+ +	−	−
Signs				
Thin, homogeneous discharge	−	+ +	−	−
Curdy discharge	±	−	+ +	−
Vulvar erythema	−	−	+ +	+
pH	<4.5	>4.5	<4.5	5.5–6.0
Vaginal Gram's stain	GPR*	GVR†	Fungi	*T. vaginalis*
Wet mount				
Epithelial cells	+ +	Clue cells	+ +	+ +
Polymorphonuclear leukocytes	±	+	+ +	+ +
Trichomonas vaginalis	−	−	−	+ +
Potassium hydroxide preparation				
Fungi	−	−	+	−
Amine odor	−	+ +	−	−

*Gram-positive rods.
†Gram-variable rods.

Vaginitis

Women with vaginitis characteristically have one or more of the following symptoms: vaginal discharge, itch, odor, external dysuria, and introital pain with sexual intercourse (Table 17.2). The three major causes are *T. vaginalis,* yeasts, and *G. vaginalis*. *Gardnerella vaginalis* produces disease in conjunction with vaginal anaerobes and the infection is now called bacterial vaginosis. The frequency of *T. vaginalis* infection may be diminishing, but *G. vaginalis* is very prevalent. Both yeasts and *G. vaginalis* are frequently isolated from women without any evidence of infection, and these patients should not be treated. When recovered from women with objective evidence of vaginitis, however, these organisms are usually considered to be pathogens. In general, symptoms correlate poorly with objective evidence of disease. This is especially the case with *G. vaginalis*-associated vaginitis.

Classically, with *T. vaginalis* vaginitis women have discharge and itch. On examination there is often a frothy green or yellow discharge with intense vaginal erythema. Women with yeast vaginitis complain of itch and introital erythema, but not vaginal discharge. On examination, however, a thick "curd-like" discharge is present in addition to erythema of the vagina, and often erythema, edema, and excoriation of the introital region (vulvitis). Generally, *G. vaginalis*-associated vaginitis produces discharge and an unpleasant fishy odor. On examination there is a thin, homogeneous, adherent discharge in the vagina, often extending to the introitus. The discharge has a milklike consistency.

Cervicitis

Uncomplicated infection of the cervix is often asymptomatic, and unless discharge is very profuse, it may not be noted. The major causes of cervicitis are *C. trachomatis, N. gonorrhoeae,* and HSV. Possible causes include *M. hominis,* Enterobacteriaceae, *T. vaginalis,* and *G. vaginalis*. Very unusual causes are *Treponema pallidium* and *Calymmatobacterium granulomatis*. Women with uncomplicated genital tract gonorrhea are usually infected in the cervix and/or urethra. Rectal infection is also frequent, but most such women are infected in the cervix or urethra. Among those with a history of gonorrhea or contact with a male with gonorrhea, 40% to 60% have concurrent *C. trachomatis* infection. Lower genital tract infection with this organism is often present in 30% to 60% of partners of males with NGU. In STD clinics, *C. trachomatis* is seen one to three times as frequently as gonorrhea, but it is noted up to ten times as frequently in private practice and student health services. It has been isolated from 2% to 30% of pregnant women in North American studies. Among women with *C. trachomatis* lower genital tract infection, approximately 40% have both cervical and urethral infection, 40% have cervical infection alone, and 20% have urethral infection alone.

Manifestations of gonococcal and chlamydial infections in women are almost identical. Women with *C. trachomatis* or *N. gonorrhoeae* lower genital tract infection are often asymptomatic. When symptoms do occur, they might not necessarily suggest cervical infection, or they may be due to concurrent infection with other agents. Women might note vaginal discharge, external or internal dysuria, vaginal bleeding after intercourse or in the middle of the menstrual cycle, heavier periods than normal, or lower abdominal pain. The symptoms of herpes are discussed subsequently.

On examination, women with positive cervical cultures for *C. trachomatis* or *N. gonorrhoeae* often have no apparent disease; however, many have abnormalities. Presence of mucopurulent cervicitis is strongly associated with recovery of *C. trachomatis* or *N. gonorrhoeae*. Mucopurulent cervicitis is suspected by the presence of endocervical mucopus, edema in an area of ectopy, or both. Mucopus is defined as a green or yellow appearance of endocervical secretions when viewed on a cotton-tipped swab. Ectopy is the extension of normal cervical columnar epithelium out onto the ectocervix. With infection, the ectopy often becomes erythematous, edematous, and friable.

Endometritis, Salpingitis, and Perihepatitis

Infection that ascends from the cervix can invade the endometrium, spread to involve the fallopian tubes, and spread further to cause pelvic peritonitis or perihepatitis. Endometritis may be quite frequent with cervical *C. trachomatis* and *N. gonorrhoeae* infections. Ascending infection probably occurs in approximately 10% of women infected with either agent. The rates are higher in young women. The major known causes of acute salpingitis are *C. trachomatis, N. gonorrhoeae, M. hominis,* Enterobacteriaceae, and anaerobes including actinomyces. The relative importance of the different causes varies somewhat with severity of the symptoms, history of prior episodes of salpingitis, and use of an intrauterine device. The presence of *N. gonorrhoeae,* Enterobacteriaceae, and anaerobes is more frequent in clinically severe infection associated with tubal abscesses. Salpingitis due to sexually transmitted pathogens often arises after dilatation and curettage, insertion of intrauterine devices, therapeutic abortions, and in the late postpartum period. The Fitz-Hugh–Curtis syndrome is most often caused by *C. trachomatis,* but *N. gonorrhoeae* is also an important cause.

Symptoms suggestive of endometritis in addition to cervicitis include midcycle bleeding or bleeding after sexual intercourse, abnormally heavy periods, and lower abdominal pain. These symptoms in conjunction with fever and more severe abdominal pain are in keeping with salpingitis. If right upper quadrant pain is present, Fitz-Hugh–Curtis syndrome should be considered.

On examination, there may or may not be evidence of cervical infection. Cervical motion, palpation of the uterus, and palpation of the adnexa usually result in pain. An adnexal mass may be detected in more severe cases. The sensitivity of symptoms and signs as indicating salpingitis is low. Even in studies in which women with symptoms suggestive of salpingitis routinely undergo laparoscopy, and hence clinicians can constantly evaluate their clinical acumen, only two-thirds of those with evidence of lower genital tract infection, bilateral lower abdominal pain of less than three weeks duration, and abdominal tenderness on bimanual examination have salpingitis. About one-quarter have no pathology detected, and the rest have other conditions, including those necessitating surgical intervention such as acute appendicitis and ectopic pregnancy. If diagnostic criteria are made more stringent, by requiring an erythrocyte sedimentation rate greater than 15 mm per hour, rectal temperature above 38°C, and a palpable adnexal mass, 96% of women with all the criteria have acute salpingitis. It is clear, however, that most cases of salpingitis would not be recognized using these criteria.

Since recent studies indicate that late sequelae such as involuntary infertility can arise in women with little or no prior evidence of salpingitis, the criteria for consideration of salpingitis must be made less rather than more stringent.

Women with gonorrhea or anaerobic infections are generally thought to have clinically severe disease. In a study performed in Sweden, in a population in which anaerobic salpingitis is not usually seen, women were categorized as having chlamydial, gonococcal, and nonchlamydial, nongonococcal salpingitis. Women with chlamydial salpingitis appeared to have a clinically more benign condition, with gradual onset and temperatures below 38°C. In contrast, elevated erythrocyte sedimentation rates were more frequent in chlamydial salpingitis, and at laparoscopy disease was as severe with *C. trachomatis* as with *N. gonorrhoeae,* and mild disease was more frequent in women in whom neither organism was detected.

Enteritis and Proctocolitis

Infections of the small and large bowel and the rectum are being recognized with increasing frequency, especially in homosexual and bisexual men. These have often been labeled the "gay bowel" syndrome. The most frequent infective causes are shown in Table 17.3 according to typical findings. There are two very distinct means of acquiring infection, and the disease produced and etiology vary accordingly. The causes of enteritis are typical causes of small or large bowel infections spread by the fecal-oral route. With the exception of increased frequency in homosexual men and the frequent concurrent presence of several potential pathogens, disease manifestations are not particularly different in this group as compared to those who acquire the disease by conventional means. With the major exception of *G. lamblia,* most of the causes of enteritis can also involve the rectum; however, the major route of acquisition of anorectal infection is by inoculation of pathogens into the rectum by rectal intercourse. Coexistent with the infections, there may be evidence of traumatic lesions.

Symptoms of enteritis include increased frequency and looseness of bowel movements, occasionally with blood or mucus, cramping, and possibly fever. More chronic symptoms, especially mild cramping and a bloated sensation, are especially seen with *G. lamblia.* Proctitis symptoms are often acute in onset, and include pain with defecation, tenesmus, and blood in or on the feces. External lesions may be seen. Rectal discharge is frequent with *N. gonorrhoeae, C. trachomatis,* and HSV. Physical examination may reveal external lesions suggestive of HSV, *T. pallidium,* warts, or molluscum, and erythema and discharge in the anal canal. Anoscopy or sigmoidoscopy may show erythema, friability, and discrete lesions.

TABLE 17.3. Major Infective Causes of the "Gay Bowel" Syndrome

Symptoms	*Bacteria*	*Parasites*	*Viruses*
Enteritis	*Shigella* *Campylobacter* *Yersinia* *Salmonella*	*Giardia* *Entamoeba*	—
Perianal growths	Syphilis	—	*Molluscum* Warts
Ulcers	Syphilis	—	Herpes
Proctitis	*Neisseria* *Chlamydia* *Shigella* *Campylobacter* *Salmonella*	*Entamoeba* *Enterobius*	Herpes

Genital Lesions

Both men and women can have genital lesions. Most frequently encountered are HSV, syphilis, genital warts, molluscum, scabies, and traumatic lesions. Much less frequent causes are *Hemophilus ducreyi,* lymphogranuloma venereum (LGV), and granuloma inguinale. Syphilis, HSV, *H. ducreyi,* and LGV infections often demonstrate lymphadenopathy as a dominant finding. In contrast to other syndromes, infections with these organisms often have fairly characteristic signs and symptoms, and an adequate, although not conclusive, etiologic diagnosis may be made on the basis of the findings (Table 17.4). The relative importance and etiologies of genital ulcers vary dramatically geographically. They account for 20% to 70% of patient visits in Southeast Asia and Africa, but only 3% to 4% of visits in North America and Europe. Chancroid, syphilis, and to a lesser extent, granuloma inguinale and lymphogranuloma venereum are major causes of genital ulcer disease in the former areas, whereas HSV

TABLE 17.4. Major Features of Genital Ulcer/Lymphadenopathy Syndrome

Factor	*HSV*	*T. pallidum*	*H. ducreyi*	*LGV*	*C. granulomatis*
Usual incubation (days)	2–7	14–42	3–5	10–14	?
Ulcers					
Number	Many	1	1–3	≤1	≥1
Painful	Yes	No	Yes	No	No
Initial appearance	Vesicle	Papule	Variable	Variable	Papule
Eventual appearance					
Irregular shape	No	No	Yes	No	Yes
Margins	Flat	Raised	Undermined	Flat	Raised
Base	Red	Smooth	Gray	—	Beefy
Induration	No	Yes	No	No	Yes
Constitutional symptoms	Yes — primary No — secondary	No — primary Yes — secondary	No	No — primary Yes — secondary	Rare
Lymph nodes					
Number	Multiple	Multiple	Single	Matted	Rare
Tender	Yes	No	Yes	Yes	
Bilateral	50%	Usual	Rare	40%	
Fluctuance	No	No	Yes	Yes	
Duration of ulcers/nodes	Weeks Recur	Months	Weeks	Transient	Months

and syphilis are the major causes in Europe and North America.

Herpes Simplex Virus

In North America and Europe, HSV is a major cause of genital lesions in heterosexual men and women and the number of infected individuals is increasing. Genital herpes may be due to both types I and II viruses. Type I usually causes herpes labialis, but is recovered from approximately 20% of genital herpes. Infections have a marked tendency to recur and the majority of individuals have one or more recurrences. This might be less in patients who have type I infection, or have type II infection when there is preexisting antibody to type I. Initial episodes tend to be most severe, especially in women. The characteristic lesions of HSV are painful and begin as fluid-filled vesicles that become pustular, then rupture to leave small ulcers, eventually scab over (if in a dry region), and heal without scarring. Tender regional lymphadenopathy often develops. With the episodes, many individuals experience a prodrome of up to 24 hours in duration, during which there may be symptoms of burning or itching at the site, or pains that may radiate, especially into the legs. The duration of new lesion formation tends to last 10 to 12 days in initial herpes and 4 to 6 days in recurrent episodes. Additional features in men include urethral discharge or dysuria in one-third of initial infections and 10% of recurrent episodes. Fever is unusual. In women, the initial episode is often very severe with fever, marked dysuria, and vaginal discharge. The cervix is almost always involved with initial but not subsequent episodes. Occasionally, with both sexes there may be symptoms or signs of meningitis or urinary retention.

Syphilis

Until recently, the number of cases of syphilis was decreasing yearly. There has been a recent increase, which is readily attributable to an increased number of infections in homosexual men. In North America, approximately two-thirds of infectious syphilis is identified in homosexual or bisexual men, a group at high risk for numerous other infections. Syphilis can be separated into primary, secondary, early latent, late latent, and tertiary stages. The primary infection is noted at the site of inoculation. This is usually on the genitalia or mouth in heterosexual men or women, but anorectal infection is frequent in homosexual men; however, lesions can be anywhere. Classically, the primary lesion or chancre arises one to six weeks after contact and is a firm, nontender ulceration with a heaped-up margin. Usually there is associated regional nontender lymphadenopathy. Atypical features of lesions are frequent. The primary lesion then heals without scarring. Four to six weeks after inoculation, secondary disease becomes apparent, usually with nonspecific systemic symptoms such as malaise and fever. Over 90% of patients have a rash; typically it is macular or maculopapular, but can become pustular with time. It can be anywhere on the body, but has a predilection for the palms and soles. Diffuse lymphadenopathy is frequent. Oral lesions and condylomata lata may also arise. The manifestations of secondary syphilis can wax and wane, and the lesions can appear for up to two years. In the secondary stage, manifestations such as iritis, meningitis, involvement of the second through eighth cranial nerves, or hepatitis may occur. The diagnosis is often missed in these patients. After the second stage heals, the condition enters a latent stage without clinically apparent disease. In early latency, variably defined as one to two years postinfection, the patient is still infectious. After this time, the stage of late latency, infectivity falls dramatically; however, the treponemes persist. Approximately one-third of patients will develop tertiary lesions with neurosyphilis, cardiovascular syphilis, or gummata.

Lymphogranuloma Venereum

Lymphogranuloma venereum is caused by 3 of the 15 forms of *C. trachomatis* — L_1, L_2, and L_3. Classically, LGV is considered to have three stages, and is the only *C. trachomatis* infection that typically produces multisystem involvement and constitutional manifestations. The primary stage, which is usually transient or missed, consists of a painless vesicle, papule, or ulcer on the genitalia that forms days to three weeks after exposure. In homosexual men, or women, a primary anorectal infection with proctitis may occur. Within two to six weeks after exposure, the secondary stage develops with constitutional symptoms and regional lymphadenopathy. Initially discrete, the nodes become matted with overlying redness and erythema, and they may become fluctuant and drain. In addition, there may be fistulas involving the rectum, bladder, or vagina. In a small proportion of patients, a tertiary stage may arise due to progressive involvement or secondary to fibrosis and abnormal lymphatic drainage. These can result in fistulas, strictures, elephantiasis, and local swelling or ulcers.

Chancroid

Hemophilus ducreyi produces an infection that in endemic regions, for example, Africa or Southeast Asia, and in outbreaks in nonendemic regions can be relatively easily recognized. In contrast, apparently typical episodes occurring in nonendemic regions at other times are often due to HSV, sometimes with concurrent *H. ducreyi* infection.

From 1 to 14 days, but on average 3 to 5 days, after contact, one or more painful lesions arise. The initial appearance ranges from a macule to a pustule, but not a vesicle. The lesions rapidly enlarge to result in irregular ulcers that can be several centimeters in diameter. The base is often gray or even necrotic, and the edges are often undermined. Induration is not present. There is usually one large matted inguinal mass with overlying erythema. Fluctuance or even suppuration often occurs. In contrast to LGV, constitutional symptoms are rare. In contrast to HSV, relapses are unusual, although reported.

Donovanosis

Donovanosis, or granuloma inguinale, is rarely seen in developed countries, but occurs in Southeast Asia. The incubation period is longer than for the previously described genital lesions. One or more lesions slowly grow from a papule to a regular, but sharply defined, indurated lesion that is raised and has a beefy appearance without necrotic exudate. Pain, inguinal lymphadenopathy, and constitutional symptoms are rare. The lesions can persist over a long period of time and result in significant ulceration.

Condyloma accuminatum

Condyloma accuminatum, or genital warts, caused by a human papillomavirus are one of the most common genital infections. In North America, infection is seen more often in women than in men and is reported more frequently than HSV. The incubation period is two to three months, and in the absence of treatment, lesions tend to persist for years. They are especially likely to develop in moist regions or when there is prior vaginal discharge. Single or grouped lesions typically occur on the penile shaft in heterosexual men, the shaft and the perirectal region of homosexual men, and the introitus, vagina, cervix, or perirectal region of women. Warts are raised, fleshy, pointed, firm lesions several millimeters in diameter. They may attain very large size, especially during pregnancy. They are not associated with lymphadenopathy or constitutional symptoms. Although usually painless, they can cause dyspareunia and rectal pain.

Acquired Immune Deficiency Syndrome

Since 1979, a devastating and apparently new syndrome has been recognized primarily in homosexual and bisexual men. The number of reported cases is presently doubling every six months. The etiology is still uncertain, (although there is strong evidence for human T-cell leukemia virus) but is probably transmitted in a manner similar to hepatitis B. The major groups at risk are homosexual and bisexual men, intravenous drug users, hemophiliacs, and to a much smaller extent, individuals in close contact to high-risk groups or those receiving blood products from them. Possibly related to AIDS is a chronic, diffuse lymphadenopathy syndrome frequently seen in homosexual men. As part of AIDS, there is progressive impairment of T-lymphocyte function. Laboratory correlates are impaired lymphocyte blast transformation to antigens, impaired ability to make new antibodies, and a marked decrease in the number of helper T cells so that the ratio of helper to suppressor T cells is markedly diminished. Affected individuals generally have one of two major but not mutually exclusive problems. The first is a particularly aggressive form of Kaposi's sarcoma with skin or mucosal lesions, weight loss, lymphadenopathy, and fever. This is probably ultimately fatal, although one-year survival is usually 80%. Other unusual malignancies are also being recognized. The second problem is a marked predisposition to numerous infections not normally seen in other than severely immunocompromised individuals. Examples include pneumonia, intracranial infections, and diarrhea. The major pathogens are *Pneumocystis carinii,* cytomegalovirus, *Toxoplasma gondii, Candida* and other yeasts, typical and atypical mycobacteria, severe herpes infection, and cryptosporidium. These infections are particularly aggressive and are relatively resistant to available therapies. The fatality rate is almost 50% in individuals with these opportunistic infections.

Other Conditions

Other conditions can be caused by sexually transmitted pathogens; of these, hepatitis is very important. Both hepatitis A and hepatitis B infections are very frequent among homosexual or bisexual men, and hepatitis B can be transmitted heterosexually. In homosexual and bisexual men, anorectal intercourse is a major risk factor for acquisition of hepatitis B. Cytomegalovirus, a cause of non-A, non-B hepatitis, is also prevalent, especially in homosexual or bisexual men.

Symptoms of pharyngitis are increased in those who practice orogenital contact. *Neisseria gonorrhoeae* is isolated at greater frequency from the pharynx of such persons, but most gonococcal pharyngeal infections are asymptomatic, and most individuals who engage in orogenital sex and have pharyngitis do not have *N. gonorrhoeae* infection.

Bartholinitis, or infection of the Bartholin's glands in the posterolateral aspect of the vaginal introitus, is most often due to *N. gonorrhoeae,* but other pathogens such as *C. trachomatis* have been isolated.

Reactive Arthritis

Transient or persistent arthritis sometimes follows infections, most typically viral or enteric bacterial infections. In association with urethritis, which is usually nongonococcal, reactive arthritis arises significantly more often in HLA-B27-positive individuals. Sometimes there is a full-blown picture of Reiter's syndrome with urethritis; arthritis especially of the knees, heels, and digits; iritis; and often skin or oral lesions. Infection with *C. trachomatis* is strongly correlated with Reiter's syndrome, but an etiologic role has not yet been proved.

As part of disseminated gonococcal infection, there can be a polyarthritis with negative synovial fluid cultures, and a monoarthritis or oligoarthritis with positive synovial fluid cultures.

Cervical Dysplasia and Carcinoma

Cervical dysplasia and carcinoma have the epidemiologic characteristics of STD, and with the exception that a history of smoking is correlated with increased risk of cancer, most of the risk factors for cancer are also risk factors for acquiring STD. Several studies show a strong association between the presence of dysplasia and carcinoma, and infection with HSV, *C. trachomatis,* or human papillomaviruses. None of these studies has demonstrated causality, however.

Sequelae in Pregnancy

The STD can have deleterious effects on reproductive ability, pregnancy, the postpartum period, and infants. Infertility on the basis of functional or structural tubal abnormalities occurs on average in 20% of women who have had acute salpingitis, and the risk rises with the number and severity of episodes. There is mounting evidence that *U. urealyticum* infection may very occasionally produce involuntary infertility. If real, this should be potentially reversible because *U. urealyticum* can be eradicated. This organism may also be a cause of recurrent spontaneous abortions in the first half of pregnancy. Late pregnancy losses can be due to *T. pallidum.* The role of sexually transmitted pathogens in causing premature delivery and low-birth-weight infants requires further evaluation. Both *U. urealyticum* and *M. hominis* can cause early postpartum fever; *C. trachomatis* may be a cause of late postpartum endometritis, analogous to acute salpingitis.

Infections of infants are significant problems when the mothers are infected with *C. trachomatis, N. gonorrhoeae, T. pallidum,* HSV, CMV, or group B streptococci. Silver nitrate ocular prophylaxis prevents transmission of most gonorrhea, but if not used or if it fails, the infant is at risk for rapidly blinding ophthalmia, or even sepsis and death. Silver nitrate has no efficacy against *C. trachomatis,* and 60% to 70% of exposed infants demonstrate serologic or culture evidence of infection. Since on the average 2% to 6% of pregnant women are infected with *C. trachomatis,* this is potentially a huge problem. Approximately one-half of infected infants develop mild conjunctivitis, 10% to 20% develop a chronic afebrile pneumonia, and the rest have asymptomatic nasopharyngeal or rectal carriage, or antibody without positive cultures. *Treponema pallidum,* especially if acquired in the last trimester, can cause intrauterine death, stillbirth, or congenital syphilis. Also, HSV has the potential to produce severe sequelae or death. When vaginal delivery occurs through infected genitalia, approximately 40% of infants are affected, with death and severe sequelae occurring in most of the survivors. Fortunately, despite the ever-increasing number of women with genital HSV infection, infection of infants is very rare, perhaps occurring in 1 of 3000 deliveries. Cytomegalovirus infection is frequent, but not usually noticed in the mother or the infant. Cognitive impairment arising years later is relatively frequent. Gross birth defects and death also occur. Group B streptococcal colonization of pregnant women is quite frequent, perhaps being present in at least one-third of pregnant women. Approximately 10% of infants become colonized and under 1% develop meningitis or sepsis, which is fatal in approximately 30% of cases.

DIAGNOSIS

It is apparent that sexually transmitted infections have numerous features. Clearly a high index of suspicion is required. In some cases, consideration of a STD is obvious, for example, with a vaginal or urethral discharge. In other situations, for example, midcycle bleeding, the urethral syndrome, or reactive arthritis, the possibility is less obvious. In other situations, such as meningitis, acute urinary retention, or acute right upper quadrant abdominal pain, STD may not be considered at all. Also, it is the rule rather than the exception that if one STD is suspected or diagnosed, there is a strong possibility that others may be present. In many cases, confirmation of the syndrome and often the etiology can be accomplished by relatively simple clinical and laboratory tests.

Clearly a first step in diagnosis requires a careful history and physical examination. Unfortunately, many physicians have difficulty obtaining a good sexual history. A good argument can be made for always knowing the sexual preference of a patient, but in dealing with possible STD symptoms, it is mandatory. The sites to be examined and cultured, and the relative likelihood of different pathogens being present are clearly related to sexual preference and practices. For example, rectal gonorrhea in a heterosexual male virtually never occurs, whereas it is a frequent problem in homosexual or bisexual men who practice anorectal intercourse. The possibility of sexual activity must be considered in any age group, but especially from the early teens on. Among sexually active individuals, it is important to know if there is a monogamous relationship or whether there have been additional partners, especially in the months preceding the examination.

If approached in a forthright manner, most patients

are quite willing to discuss their sexuality. Questions that can be asked include: "When did you last have sexual intercourse? Do you have a steady partner? When did you last have sexual intercourse with someone other than your present partner?" If the person has a steady partner, one asks, "To your knowledge, does your partner have other partners?" Often by this time the person's sexual preference is obvious, but it is still reasonable to ask men if they have ever had sexual intercourse with males. If the answer is yes, then the number of partners and type of sexual activity should be ascertained.

In addition to current symptoms, a past history of STD should be obtained. In men, as a minimum, a history of prior gonorrhea, urethritis, syphilis, and genital lesions should be sought. In women, questions regarding a history of gonorrhea, chlamydial infection, cervicitis, pelvic inflammatory disease (including after-abortion, intrauterine device insertion, or delivery), trichomoniasis, warts, and HSV, and urethritis or other diseases in male partners should be asked.

Diagnosis of Syndromes

The diagnosis of urethritis requires the demonstration of increased numbers of PMNs in a urethral discharge or from a smear of an endourethral swab. The presence of a mean of four or more PMNs in each of five oil-immersion (× 1000) fields of a stained smear correlates with urethritis. For optimal results, the examination for a urethral exudate should be performed after as long an interval as possible without voiding. If discharge is not present spontaneously, the penis should be stripped from the base to the meatus three or four times in an attempt to express a discharge. Methylene blue or Gram's stain of the discharge is useful in distinguishing rapidly between gonococcal and nongonococcal urethritis; the presence of intracellular diplococci has a high positive predictive value for the diagnosis of gonococcal infection and is most helpful from an immediate therapeutic standpoint. In addition, all discharges should be cultured for *N. gonorrhoeae*. Although culture for *C. trachomatis* is usually not routinely done, the best yield is obtained with an endourethral swab passed 3 to 4 cm into the urethra rather than a culture of the discharge only.

When a discharge is not present either in symptomatic patients or asymptomatic contacts, an endourethral swab should be done, stained, and cultured at least for *N. gonorrhoeae*. Culture for *C. trachomatis* and/or other suspected pathogens in urethritis such as *Ureaplasma urealyticum* will depend upon the facilities available.

An additional diagnostic test for urethritis is examination of the urine sediment in the first 10 ml of voided urine. The presence of 15 or more PMNs in one or more high-power fields of the sediment correlates with urethritis.

The diagnosis of epididymitis is primarily clinical, but other possibilities such as torsion of the testicle and malignancy must be considered and be excluded if there is any doubt about the diagnosis. To establish the etiology of epididymitis, men should be examined and secretions be cultured for urethral pathogens as above, a Gram's stain should be performed on uncentrifuged urine to look for urinary tract pathogens, and the urine should be cultured for urinary tract pathogens. An epididymal aspirate can be performed for cultures for *N. gonorrhoeae, C. trachomatis,* and urinary tract pathogens.

The cause of vaginitis can often be suspected by the history and physical examination. Vaginal discharge should be mixed with saline to detect motile trichomonads and clue cells suggestive of *G. vaginalis*-associated infection. Clue cells are epithelial cells studded with small bacteria so that they look dirty and have an obscured margin. On Gram's stain, the epithelial cells are covered with gram-variable coccobacilli, and often there are sheets of similar organisms between cells. The Gram's stain, and a potassium hydroxide preparation in which discharge is mixed with 10% potassium hydroxide, should also be examined for yeasts. All these organisms can be cultured on appropriate media. Identification of yeasts or *G. vaginalis* in the absence of symptoms or signs is not an indication for treatment, but identification of *T. vaginalis* is.

Diagnosis of cervical infection is much more difficult. The presence of mucopurulent cervicitis strongly suggests infection; however, in many cases, this can only be suspected on epidemiologic grounds. A Gram's stain of cervical secretions showing typical gram-negative diplococci is only 60% sensitive for the diagnosis of cervical gonorrhea, but is quite specific. For both *N. gonorrhoeae* and *C. trachomatis* endocervical swabs should be obtained for culture. The yield in diagnosis of lower genital infection with both organisms is enhanced by culturing the urethra and rectum as well. All such cultures are indicated in high-risk groups, but cervical culture alone is probably adequate for screening.

Infection of the uterus or fallopian tube must initially be suspected on clinical grounds. Investigations for lower genital tract infection are indicated, but even if they are positive, they do not establish the diagnosis or the etiology of the upper genital tract infection. Ideally, all women with possible salpingitis should have laparoscopy to confirm that the fallopian tubes are inflamed, and to obtain cultures. The sensitivity of these cultures is not well established. Cul-de-sac aspiration appears to carry some organisms from the vagina. Cultures of pooled pelvic secretions obtained at laparoscopy should have better predictive value for aerobes and anaerobes, but are poor for *C. trachomatis*. For culture of *C. trachomatis,* swabs from inside the lumen of the fallopian tube or biopsies of tubal tissue are most sensitive. Since infertility is one of the consequences of salpingitis, however, biopsies are contraindicated. More data are required for assessment of the value of endometrial cultures in lieu of tubal cultures, but it is possible that they will be quite useful. Laparoscopy is definitely indicated when the woman is sick and the diagnosis is in doubt, or when she does not improve after 48 to 72 hours of appropriate antimicrobial therapy.

Diagnosis of the cause of enteritis requires standard diagnostic procedures. These include direct examination of stool for parasites and culture for bacterial pathogens. Occasionally, biopsies of specimens of small bowel are required for *G. lamblia*. Diagnosis of the cause of anorectal infection should include the above studies as well as Gram's stain of rectal discharge or an anal swab to detect gram-negative diplococci, rectal swabs for culture for *N. gonorrhoeae* and *C. trachomatis,* and syphilis serology. If lesions are detected either directly or by anoscopy or proctoscopy, they should be studied by darkfield and with HSV cultures as well. Biopsies of lesions may occasionally be useful in establishing the diagnosis.

Determining the etiology of genital ulcers or lymphadenopathy syndromes requires examination of the lesion by Gram's stain, darkfield, Tzanck preparation, or direct studies for HSV antigens, as well as culture for HSV and *H. ducreyi*. The darkfield examination should be repeated on three separate occasions. Serology should be performed for syphilis and LGV. Fluctuant buboes should be aspirated and cultured for aerobes, including *H. ducreyi* and *C. trachomatis*. Other non-STD causes must also be considered. Diagnosis of genital warts is usually made clinically, but can be made by Papanicolaou smear or biopsy.

At the moment, AIDS is a clinical diagnosis because laboratory abnormalities can often be found in individuals without AIDS.

Diagnosis of Specific Organisms

Cultures for *N. gonorrhoeae* should either be plated directly onto enriched media or else placed in a suitable transport media for rapid delivery to an experienced laboratory. Under optimal conditions, sensitivity is good for urethral specimens, but for single cultures from other sites it may be no better than 90%. With delay in transit, cultures can become falsely negative. The concentration of vancomycin in antimicrobial-containing plates will suppress or prevent growth of some isolates. If penicillinase-producing *N. gonorrhoeae* (PPNG) is a local problem, or if the patient is suspected on epidemiologic or clinical grounds to have a PPNG isolate, isolates should be tested for beta-lactamase production. In addition to PPNG, there are increasing numbers of isolates with relatively high minimum inhibitory concentration to penicillin that are not caused by beta-lactamase production.

Diagnosis of *C. trachomatis* infections usually requires culture. Optimal results require that epithelial cells rather than exudates be cultured, that the correct transport media be used, that the specimen be quickly inoculated onto cell culture or else frozen at −70°C, that the laboratory have good quality control, and that the cultures be examined for evidence of inclusions by experienced individuals. Under ideal circumstances, the yield may be as high as 90% to 95%. In other than research situations, results are likely to be considerably less reliable. If the laboratory is not experienced in recognizing inclusions in culture, there is a definite possibility of false positive as well as false negative results. In general, serology has little useful role for diagnosis of sexually transmitted *C. trachomatis* infections. The exceptions are LGV, infant pneumonia, and possibly pelvic inflammatory disease. There are now several nonculture systems that purport to identify chlamydial antigens or elementary bodies directly from smears. If these systems live up to their promise, they will greatly facilitate management of chlamydial infections when cultures are not feasible.

For diagnosis of HSV, the yield by any direct or culture technique is best at the vesicle stage and declines rapidly thereafter so that late ulcers or scabs are usually culture negative. In contrast to most viruses, HSV grows rapidly in culture and more than 50% of cultures are positive within 36 to 48 hours after inoculation. Tzanck preparations show multinucleated giant cells with intranuclear inclusions in approximately 60% of early lesions. Fluorescent antibody or immunoperoxidase-conjugated antibody detects HSV antigens somewhat more often. In general, serology has no role in the diagnosis of HSV infections.

For syphilis, darkfield examinations of lesions often show typical spirochetes at the primary and secondary stages, but not later stages. Prior use of oral or topical antimicrobials or other topical agents significantly interferes with the reliability of the studies. Serology is the most important means of making a diagnosis. Nontreponemal tests (automated reagin test, ART; venereal diseases research laboratory, VDRL) usually become positive within one month of infection, are positive in 75% of primary syphilis, and are always positive in secondary syphilis. In general, the titer correlates with disease activity in primary or secondary syphilis, but can become negative in late latent or tertiary disease despite persistence of treponemes. It usually becomes negative or falls to stable low titers after appropriate treatment. False positive reactions with nontreponemal tests are frequent with numerous other infections or diseases. These reactions are usually transient. Treponemal tests, for example, the microhemagglutination-*T. pallidum* (MHA-TP) or the immunofluorescent antibody-absorbed (IF A-ABS) test is used as confirmation with reactive nontreponemal tests. They remain positive for life, even if infection is eradicated. When late consequences of syphilis, for example neurosyphilis, are considered, a negative nontreponemal test does not exclude syphilis and a treponemal test must be ordered. The fluorescent treponemal antibody absorption (FTA-ABS) test has the added advantage that it becomes positive more quickly than nontreponemal tests, so that it is useful in primary syphilis (80% positive). The MHA-TP becomes positive less quickly, but is otherwise similar to the FTA-ABS test in terms of sensitivity and specificity.

TREATMENT

Detailed treatment recommendations from the Centers for Disease Control have recently been published. They concentrate on the syndromic approach and also include recommendations for treatment of specific infections once recognized. Several principles must always be remembered. First, even if infection with one agent is specifically diagnosed, treatment must often be directed against other major causes of the syndrome because they could be present concurrently. For example, in patients with gonorrhea, *C. trachomatis* is often present. Treatment with a penicillin or spectinomycin does not reliably eradicate concurrent *C. trachomatis* infection and leaves the patient at risk for other sequelae. Second, since STD do not arise de novo, there has to be at least one partner with infection. Consequently, sex partners should be treated, in general, with similar regimens. Treatment of only the index cases is of little benefit if the person becomes reinfected from an untreated partner. Third, an apparently normal examination in a partner does not exclude the possibility of infection and the need for treatment. Indeed, there is an increased likelihood that the source contacts will be asymptomatic, because if they had been symptomatic, they might have sought medical attention on their own. Fourth, whenever possible, tests of cure cultures are indicated after an appropriate interval. For *N. gonorrhoeae,* this is three to five days after the end of treatment. For *C. trachomatis,* it is three to six weeks after the end of treatment.

Tetracyclines have a very important role in the treatment of STD. They are active against *C. trachomatis;* most isolates of *N. gonorrhoeae* (but not most PPNG), *U. urealyticum,* and *M. hominis;* and *T. pallidum.* Seven days of tetracycline, 500 mg orally four times daily, or doxycycline, 100 mg orally twice daily, are regimens of choice for NGU, PGU, mucopurulent cervicitis, and uncomplicated chlamydial infections in nonpregnant patients. In compliant patients they are also recommended for uncomplicated gonococcal infection, either alone or in conjunction with single-dose treatments with aqueous procaine penicillin G, 4.8 million U intramuscularly, plus probenecid, 1 gm by mouth; ampicillin, 3.5 gm, or amoxicillin, 3 gm orally, plus probenecid, 1 gm by mouth; spectinomycin, 2 gm intramuscularly; cefoxitin, 2 gm intramuscularly, plus probenecid, 1 gm orally; or cefotaxime, 1 gm intramuscularly. Whenever PPNG are diagnosed or suspected, one of these last three regimens should be used as single-dose therapy. Tetracyclines alone are not reliable for PPNG and rectal gonorrhea in men. An alternative for the treatment of NGU and chlamydial infection, but not gonorrhea, is erythromycin base, 500 mg four times daily for seven days. During pregnancy if this dosage cannot be tolerated, erythromycin base, 250 mg four times daily for 14 days, can be tried.

For complicated infections such as epididymitis and acute salpingitis, a minimum of 10 days of one of the tetracycline regimens should be used. This should be adequate for *C. trachomatis* and most isolates of *N. gonorrhoeae*, and could be used alone for epididymitis due to sexually transmitted agents. For acute salpingitis, however, additional therapy is indicated because tetracyclines alone are not adequate against all the major causes, which include *C. trachomatis, N. gonorrhoeae, M. hominis*, Enterobacteriaceae, and anaerobes including actinomyces. Most women with salpingitis should be hospitalized for treatment. The Centers for Disease Control suggest that hospitalization should strongly be considered when the diagnosis is uncertain, surgical emergencies such as appendicitis and ectopic pregnancy have not been excluded, if a pelvic abscess is suspected, severe illness prevents outpatient management, the patient is pregnant, the patient is unable to follow or tolerate an outpatient regimen, the patient has failed to respond to outpatient therapy, or clinical follow-up 48 to 72 hours after the start of therapy cannot be arranged. For inhospital treatment, the best regimen is probably cefoxitin, 2 gm intravenously every six hours, plus doxycycline, 100 mg intravenously (or orally if intravenous doxycycline is not available) every 12 hours. Alternative regimens that could be less active against some of the causes are either (1) clindamycin, 600 mg intravenously every six hours, plus gentamicin or tobramycin, 2 mg per kg intravenously, as a loading dose followed by 1.7 mg per kg every 8 hours, or (2) metronidazole 1 gm intravenously every 12 hours, plus doxycycline, 100 mg intravenously every 12 hours. After initial resolution, oral therapy can be used to complete a 10- to 14-day course. The Centers for Disease Control recommend use of doxycycline, 100 mg orally twice daily, to complete 10- to 14-day therapy. The author adds metronidazole, 500 to 750 mg orally three times daily, as well. If therapy is initiated with an outpatient regimen, in addition to doxycycline with or without metronidazole, a standard single-dose regimen for gonorrhea can be used as well. With either oral or intravenous therapy, if there is not improvement within 48 to 72 hours, laparoscopy is indicated. The efficacy of these more aggressive regimens in decreasing late sequelae of involuntary infertility, ectopic pregnancy, and chronic pelvic pain has yet to be established.

Treatment of vaginitis is often unsatisfactory. Results are best with *T. vaginalis*. The drug of choice is metronidazole given either as a single 2-gm oral dose or as 250 mg three times daily for seven days. Both regimens are 85% to 95% effective. Infection with relatively resistant isolates appears to be increasing in frequency. This can often be cured with high-dose metronidazole, 750 mg three times daily orally plus 500 mg twice daily intravaginally, given for 10 days. *Gardnerella vaginalis*-associated infections are also best treated with metronidazole, but results are less satisfactory. The usual dosage is 500 mg twice daily orally for seven days. Most women improve on this regimen, but approximately 15% will have recurrent infections, and only some of these will be cured by a repeat course. Ampicillin or tetracycline, 500 mg four times daily for seven days, is considerably less effective.

Numerous regimens are available for treatment of genital yeasts. Nystatin, intravaginally once daily for 7 to 14 days, results in rates of failure of 30% to 40% by one month posttreatment. Six- or seven-day regimens of intravaginal miconazole or clotrimazole produce rates of failure of 10% to 20% by one month posttreatment. Rates of failure are slightly higher with three-day regimens of econazole, miconazole, or clotrimazole. Unfortunately, when one intravaginal imidazole fails, others often do. Intravaginal boric acid, 600 mg once daily for 7 to 14 days, sometimes succeeds when nitroimidazoles fail. Oral ketoconazole in a variety of regimens is more convenient to use, but also results in rates of failure of 10% to 20% by one month after treatment. In general, little is gained by the treatment of sex partners unless they are symptomatic. Treatment of women with recurrent or persistent episodes is unsatisfactory. Use of oral nystatin for patients and their sex partners has not enhanced results. Sometimes long-term or monthly cycles of treatment will result in cure.

Treatment of genital lesions depends upon the etiology. For HSV, of marketed antivirals, only acyclovir appears of benefit, and then only for primary initial infection treated within six days of onset of symptoms. Topical 5% acyclovir ointment applied every three hours, six times daily for seven days, or oral acyclovir, 200 mg five times daily for five days, is effective. Intravenous acyclovir accomplishes the same goals, but is not generally practical. All of these regimens shorten viral shedding and the duration of disease, but do not prevent recurrences. In addition to medical therapy, patients should be given factual information about HSV. Women should be encouraged to have yearly Papanicolaou smears and if they become pregnant, to inform their physicians about their history of genital HSV. Abstention from intercourse when symptoms are present should be stressed.

For treatment of syphilis, penicillins are the preferred antimicrobial, but in those allergic to penicillin, tetracycline hydrochloride is used. Recommended penicillin regimens are benzathine penicillin G, 2.4 million units intramuscularly at a single session, for early syphilis (primary, secondary, or latent syphilis of less than one year's duration), and benzathine penicillin G, 2.4 million units intramuscularly once weekly for three doses, for syphilis longer than one year's duration except for neurosyphilis. For neurosyphillis, prior to using the three-dose benzathine penicillin regimen, (1) no additional penicillin; (2) aqueous crystalline penicillin G, 12 to 24 million units daily intravenously for 10 days; or (3) aqueous procaine penicillin G, 2.4 million units per day, plus probenecid, 500 mg four times daily per day, both for 10 days, can be given. For those allergic to penicillin, tetracycline hydrochloride, 500 mg four times daily, should be given for 14 days for early syphilis and for 30 days for syphilis of more than one year's duration.

For LGV and chancroid, buboes should be aspirated in an attempt to avoid spontaneous drainage and to obtain material for culture. For LGV, at least 14 days of tetracycline, 500 mg orally four times daily, or alternatively, 14 days of doxycycline, 100 mg twice daily; erythromycin, 500 mg four times daily; or a sulfonamide, should be given. Systemic symptoms usually respond quickly, buboes less quickly, and late complications poorly or not at all. Late complications may require surgery. For chancroid, single-dose treatment with spectinomycin, 2 gm intramuscularly; ceftriaxone, 250 mg intramuscularly; or trimethoprim, 640 mg and sulfamethoxazole, 3200 mg (eight tablets), by mouth, are effective. Better-studied regimens that are effective are erythromycin, 500 mg orally three times daily for seven days, or trimethoprim, 160 mg with sulfamethoxazole, 800 mg (two tablets) twice daily for five days.

Granuloma inguinale is best treated with trimethoprim, 160 mg with sulfamethoxazole, 800 mg (two tablets) twice daily for 14 days. An alternative regimen is tetracycline, 500 mg four times daily for 14 days.

Treatment of genital warts is poorly evaluated and no treatment is entirely satisfactory. Anogenital warts have been associated with cancer, and podophyllin may be carcinogenic, so that cryotherapy, electrosurgery, or surgical removal may be preferable. Podophyllin is contraindicated for intraurethral warts, during pregnancy, and possibly for anorectal and cervical warts. When used, podophyllin, 10% to 25% in compound tincture of benzoin, is applied carefully to the lesion avoiding normal tissue. It is then thoroughly washed off in one to four hours. It is applied weekly for up to four doses. If warts persist, alternative therapy should be used. Urethral warts have been treated with intraurethral 5% 5-fluorouracil or thiotepa.

PREVENTION AND CONTROL

Adequate control of STD requires many improvements. In general, diseases that are readily diagnosed and treated, for example, *N. gonorrhoeae, C. trachomatis,* and *T. pallidum,* should be theoretically controllable. Diseases where both diagnosis and treatment are suboptimal, for example, genital warts, will be controlled less well. When treatment fails to prevent recurrent disease, for example, HSV, the control will probably be very poor. In all STD, when deficiencies in disease recognition and management occur, control efforts will be even less optimal. From the point of view of the health care delivery system, the major effort must be placed on education, disease recognition, provision of adequate diagnostic facilities for diagnosis and screening, use of appropriate treatment, contact tracing of symptomatic and asymptomatic contacts, and appropriate follow-up.

For individuals, there should be a minimal level of education stressing the facts that (1) mucosa-to-mucosa contact transmits organisms that are sometimes pathogens, (2) sexually transmitted pathogens can be present without symptoms, (3) development of genital symptoms should prompt a visit to a health care deliverer and cessation of sexual activity, and (4) sexual intercourse with an untreated partner may result in reinfection. Since vaccines are unlikely to be available for most STD in the near future, additional preventive measures are indicated. Most important is the use of barrier, contraceptive methods such as condoms and diaphragms, and spermicidal agents when having sexual intercourse with a casual contact. Condoms probably diminish the spread of and spermicidal agents are inhibitory to most sexually transmitted pathogens. Individuals may be wise to ask prospective partners about a past or present history of genital tract disease. In most cases this will be difficult, and will not reliably exclude the risk of acquiring a STD. Prophylactic tetracyclines decrease the risk of acquisition of several STD, but their use is not advocated.

ANNOTATED BIBLIOGRAPHY

Amsel R, Totten PA, Spiegel CA, et al. Nonspecific vaginitis. Diagnostic criteria and microbial and epi-

demiologic associations. Am J Med 1983;74:14–22.
This study critically analyzes the clinical and microbiologic features that support the diagnosis of bacterial vaginosis, and differentiates it from normal vaginal secretions and other causes.

Berger RE, Alexander ER, Harnisch JP, et al. Etiology, manifestations, and therapy of acute epididymitis: prospective study of 50 cases. J Urol 1979;121:750–754.
A study prospectively evaluating 50 men with acute epididymitis, using history, examination, and cultures for aerobes, anaerobes, *Neisseria gonorrhoeae, Chlamydia trachomatis,* and *Ureaplasma urealyticum.*

Bowie WR. Nongonococcal urethritis. Urol Clin North Am 1984;11:55–64.
This is a discussion of the etiology and therapy of nongonococcal urethritis. It also contrasts the features differentiating nongonococcal from gonococcal urethritis.

Brunham RC, Paavonen J, Stevens CE, et al. Mucopurulent cervicitis: the ignored counterpart in women of urethritis in men. N Engl J Med 1984;311:1–6.
This study evaluates the clinical and microbiologic features of cervicitis.

Centers for Disease Control. Sexually transmitted diseases: treatment guidelines, 1982. Rev Infect Dis 1982;4:S729–S746.
This is a relatively detailed outline of treatment regimens for most of the sexually transmitted disease syndromes, with brief discussions of the advantages and disadvantages of different regimens when several choices are available.

Chapel TA, Brown WJ, Jeffries C, et al. How reliable is the morphological diagnosis of penile ulceration? Sex Transm Dis 1977;4:150–152.
This study performed by venerealogists with good diagnostic support shows that herpes is the most frequent cause of identified genital ulceration in this American study, but that in almost half of the cases diagnosis could not be established. Furthermore, the microbiologic results did not always support the clinical diagnosis.

Corey L, Adams HG, Brown ZA, Holmes KK. Genital herpes simplex virus infections: clinical manifestations, course, and complications. Ann Intern Med 1983;98:958–972.

Corey L, Holmes KK. Current concepts in diagnosis, therapy, and prevention. Ann Intern Med 1983;98:973–983.
These two articles described features of genital herpes simplex virus infection in great detail.

Holmes KK, Eschenbach DA, Knapp JS. Salpingitis: an overview of etiology and epidemiology. Am J Obstet Gynecol 1980;138:893–900.
A very good summary of salpingitis.

Quinn TC, Stamm WE, Goodell SE, et al. The polymicrobial origin of intestinal infection in homosexual men. N Engl J Med 1983;309:576–582.
This study thoroughly investigated a relatively large group of homosexual men with the so-called gay bowel syndrome and correlates clinical and microbiologic features.

Schachter J. Chlamydial infections. N Engl J Med 1978;298:428–435, 490–495, 540–549.
A detailed discussion of many of the diseases caused by *C. trachomatis,* and of treatment.

Taylor-Robinson D, McCormack WM. The genital mycoplasmas. N Engl J Med 1980;302:1003–1010, 1063–1067.
A discussion of the current role of mycoplasmas in genital tract disease.

18 OSTEOMYELITIS AND SEPTIC ARTHRITIS

Edward D. Ralph

OSTEOMYELITIS

Osteomyelitis is an infection of bone involving the cortex and/or the marrow cavity. Because of differences in symptoms, treatment, and prognosis, osteomyelitis has been traditionally classified clinically as either acute or chronic. Acute refers to the initial episode of the infection and chronic to disease characterized by relapses.

Etiology

The etiology of osteomyelitis by age groups is summarized in Table 18.1. As noted, a few bacteria are the causative agents for most cases. Rarely, insidious forms of osteomyelitis are caused by mycobacteria (*Mycobacterium tuberculosis, M. bovis,* and atypical mycobacteria) and fungi ·(candidiasis, blastomycosis, coccidioidomycosis).

The most common organism isolated is *Staphylococcus aureus,* which is found in approximately 50% to 60% of cases in adults. In about 10% of cases, *Streptococcus* species, including *S. pneumoniae* and *S. pyogenes* are isolated, and the remaining 20% to 40% of cases are caused by gram-negative bacilli (*Escherichia coli*). These last bacteria are becoming increasingly important in bone infections. Anaerobic bacteria are important in polymicrobial infections producing osteomyelitis, although they are less common as single causative agents.

In children, *S. aureus* accounts for 80% to 90% of cases, with *Hemophilus influenzae* also common in early childhood.

Epidemiology

In addition to age as a significant epidemiologic factor determining the likely causative organism. certain patient groups are at higher risk for osteomyelitis with specific organisms (Table 18.2). The increase in nonstaphylococcal osteomyelitis (gram-negative rods, anaerobes) can be attributed to the growing importance of peripheral vascular disease with ischemic tissue infections and the use of prosthetic joints and internal fixation.

The epidemiology of mycobacterial and fungal osteomyelitis is that of the pulmonary form of the infection (see Chapter 12). Candidal osteomyelitis is seen in patients with candidemia secondary to intravascular lines, antibiotic treatment, and/or immunosuppression.

Pathophysiology

Oseteomyelitis is often classified pathophysiologically as resulting from hematogenous spread, direct inoculation, spread from an adjacent focus, or associated with peripheral vascular disease.

Osteomyelitis secondary to hematogenous seeding occurs primarily in the metaphyses of long bones, especially the femur, tibia, and humerus. With a bacteremia, organisms are deposited in this area because of the exceptionally slow blood flow and poor phagocytic activity of the lining cells of the arterioles, capillaries, and venous sinusoids in the metaphyses. A history of trauma to the bone involved precedes osteomyelitis in up to 25% of patients. Trauma presumably predisposes to infection by increasing the blood flow to the traumatized area and allowing seeding out through disrupted

TABLE 18.1. Etiology of Bacterial Osteomyelitis in Various Age Groups

Age	*Organisms*
Neonates (≤2 mo)	*S. aureus* Group B streptococci Gram-negative rods (*E. coli*)
Children (3 mo–4 yrs)	*S. aureus* *S. pyogenes* *H. influenzae*
Children (5–15 yrs)	*S. aureus*
Adults	
16–30 yrs	*S. aureus*
>30 yrs	*S. aureus* *Streptococcus* sp. Gram-negative rods (*E. coli*) Anaerobic bacteria

TABLE 18.2. Etiology of Bacterial Osteomyelitis in Specific Epidemiologic Settings

Epidemiologic Feature	*Organisms*
Hematogenous spread	
Intravenous drug abuse	*S. aureus* Gram-negative rods (*Pseudomonas aeruginosa*)
Central venous line Hemodialysis catheter	*S. aureus*
Vertebral osteomyelitis	*S. aureus* Gram-negative rods (*E. coli*, *Proteus* sp.)
Sickle cell disease	*Salmonella* sp.
Direct inoculation or spread	
Postoperative	*S. aureus* Gram-negative rods
Internal fixation, prosthetic joints	*S. aureus* Coagulase-negative staphylococci Gram-negative rods
Human bites	Anaerobes
Dental/sinus infections	Anaerobes *S. aureus* *Streptococcus* sp.
Peripheral vascular disease (diabetes, elderly)	*S. aureus* Anaerobes Gram-negative rods

vessels. It may also simply draw the patient's attention to the tender, infected area.

The presence of multiplying bacteria in bone produces a local acute inflammatory response with edema and polymorphonuclear luekocytes. This causes swelling and compromises the blood supply, producing a local area of ischemia that may ultimately lead to the development of a piece of necrotic bone (sequestrum). Because of the rigid structure of bone, the infection tracks out through the bony canals to the periosteum, usually producing some degree of elevation or an actual abscess under the periosteum. Subsequent perforation of the periosteum and development of a sinus tract to the skin is unusual in acute osteomyelitis but is common in chronic infection. The infection stimulates osteoblast activity, with new bone formation (involucrum) surrounding the infection and sequestrum. With treatment, the evolving process may be interrupted at any stage, with minimal bony changes occurring or progress to a chronic infection with a sequestrum, reactive sclerotic bone changes, and a chronically draining sinus typical of chronic osteomyelitis. A secondary bacteremia from the focus of osteomyelitis may occur with seeding of other tissues (including other bones and joints).

Vertebral osteomyelitis (also referred to as discitis) is an infection of the disc space and adjacent vertebral bodies that usually results from hematogenous spread of infection and has unique features. The organisms may be deposited by way of the nutrient artery to the vertebrae, supporting ligaments, or intervertebral disc, or through the extensive system of venous plexuses, especially those interconnecting the pelvis and the vertebral column. Infections of the prostate, bladder, and pelvis could therefore be transported directly to the vertebral column, especially the lumbrosacral area. The infection probably begins most often in the vertebral body in the subchondral plate area because of the rich vascular supply, and then spreads through the cartilaginous plate or through ligaments into the disc and ultimately the adjacent vertebral body. The proximity of the infection to the spinal cord and the possibility of an epidural abscess make it potentially a very serious infection. The abscess may compress the cord directly or interfere with the blood supply and cause cord ischemia. Vertebral osteomyelitis may also result from direct inoculation following surgery or invasive radiologic procedures (e.g., discogram).

Osteomyelitis arising from inoculation (surgical or nonsurgical trauma) or spread from an infected focus (sinusitis) can occur in any bone and may arise either through penetration of the periosteum with initial involvement of the cortical bone, or as an outward extension from the deeper cortical bone or marrow cavity. The presence of foreign bodies in bone such as prosthetic joints or internal fixation devices provide a favorable milieu for infections that are very difficult to eradicate once established.

Peripheral vascular disease predisposes to osteomyelitis usually in the lower extremities and especially the feet. Gangrene, minor trauma with ulceration (often unrecognized due to neuropathy), and subsequent soft tissue infection with seeding of bone is the usual sequence of events. Tissue ischemia provides a good environment for organism multiplication and diminishes the transport of antibiotics to the area.

Tuberculous osteomyelitis from lymphohematogenous spread produces a granulomatous lesion, usually with accompanying arthritis, and affects the vertebrae (Pott's disease) as well as the joints and bones of the lower extremities most commonly. Fungal osteomyelitis (candidiasis, blastomycosis, coccidioidomycosis) also produces a granulomatous lesion.

Clinical Manifestions

Acute osteomyelitis may occur with sudden or insidious onset. Bacterial osteomyelitis resulting from hematogenous spread usually is associated with the signs and symptoms of a bacteremia, localized pain in the bone involved, and an acute inflammatory reaction in the surrounding soft tissue. In other cases (e.g., tuberculosis), the systemic manifestations are often minimal and the only findings are those caused by the infection locally. Chronic (recurrent) osteomyelitis is almost always associated with fewer systemic symptoms and less severe local symptoms and signs, although there often is increasing erythema, mild pain, and increased drainage from a sinus tract, if present, in the skin. An underlying osteomyelitis should be suspected when a cellulitis or skin ulcer fails to heal or recurs after treatment.

Vertebral osteomyelitis (discitis) may occur also either suddenly with fever, severe back pain of a few days' duration or of gradually increasing severity, and minimal systemic symptoms. There is usually no evidence of overlying soft tissue involvement, although paraspinal muscle spasm is often present and tenderness may be elicited by deep palpation or percussion of the spinal processes of the involved vertebrae. Unfortunately, because low back pain is a very common symptom in many patients seeking medical attention, early cases of osteomyelitis can be easily overlooked.

Osteomyelitis associated with internal fixation devices or prosthetic joints is usually slow in onset and should be suspected if there is persistent pain at the site after surgery, purulent drainage from the wound, failure of bony union with internal fixation, and loosening of a prosthesis with pain.

Diagnosis

The diagnosis of osteomyelitis in long bones is based on the clinical features of pain and tenderness in the bone with an associated inflammatory reaction in the overlying soft tissue. Since the location of osteomyelitis in the metaphysis is in close proximity to a joint, this disease must be differentiated from acute arthritis either of infectious or noninfectious etiology. To distinguish the two entities, gentle joint movement through a limited range of motion is usually possible with osteomyelitis but not with acute arthritis.

A "sympathetic" effusion may occur in a joint with adjacent osteomyelitis but is not associated with the exquisite pain seen in bacterial arthritis. In infants less than 1 year of age and in the adult, a focus of osteomyelitis may extend from the metaphysis into a joint, also producing bacterial arthritis.

Cellulitis of the soft tissues must also be differentiated from the acute inflammatory reaction produced by an underlying osteomyelitis. Characteristically, cellulitis is more painful to touch superficially and is usually associated with regional lymphadenitis. Less acute cases of osteomyelitis must be differentiated from osteogenic sarcoma, Ewing's tumor, and a fracture.

The diagnosis of chronic osteomyelitis is less difficult, although in long-standing cases the rare development of a malignancy in the area may mimic an acute exacerbation or occur concurrently.

In acute osteomyelitis, blood for three cultures should be drawn. They are positive in up to 60% to 70% of cases of hematogenously spread infection, but a much lower rate of bacteremia is present in osteomyelitis secondary to spread from an adjacent focus or direct inoculation. Also, in chronic osteomyelitis blood cultures are rarely if ever positive. X-ray examination of the bone at initial examination may show no abnormalities but evidence only of soft tissue swelling, which is detected clinically. An early change, however, is the development of periosteal elevation, but definite x-ray changes of lytic lesions may not occur for two to three weeks. Sclerotic changes may not appear until one month following onset of infection.

Isotopic scans, including pyrophosphate, which detects bone remodelling with osteoblast activity, and gallium, which detects an inflammatory reaction in bone are usually positive within three to five days of onset of infection. They may be helpful in distinguishing between osteomyelitis and septic arthritis. Rarely, false negative scans do occur. In suspected vertebral osteomyelitis (discitis), tomograms or computerized tomographic (CT) scan of the involved area may detect disease missed by plain x-rays and even isotopic scans.

Open surgical procedures or closed bone biopsy may be necessary if blood cultures are negative in acute osteomyelitis and there is a poor response to empiric therapy tailored to the particular epidemiologic setting. In vertebral osteomyelitis (discitis), direct needle aspiration of the disc space, under radiologic control, should be attempted if blood cultures are negative. All joint effusions, if present, should be aspirated, stained, and cultured (see under Arthritis).

In cases of acute osteomyelitis secondary to direct spread, cultures of the initial septic focus may be helpful. In chronic osteomyelitis in particular, with sinus tract drainage, culture of the external drainage may prove misleading, especially in cases where *S. aureus* is not isolated. In these circumstances, cultures taken at the time of surgical debridement are very important. Otherwise, certain pathogenic organisms within bone may be missed and conversely, external contaminants erroneously considered as important. It is obvious that to devise a therapeutic regimen, the significant pathogens must be identified.

Anaerobic organisms should be sought routinely with blood cultures and also in cases of osteomyelitis where anaerobes are common isolates such as in patients with diabetes mellitus and peripheral vascular disease where there is poor tissue perfusion resulting in tissue hypoxia.

In suspected cases of unusual forms of osteomyelitis caused by mycobacteria and fungi, biopsies, special stains, cultures, and serology should be ordered where appropriate.

Treatment

Acute forms of osteomyelitis usually respond to antibiotic therapy alone if instituted early, and this therapy is summarized in Table 18.3. In patients who fail to respond to treatment after 72 hours, an open surgical procedure for drainage of loculated pus or debridement of infected tissue may be indicated. Moreover, at this time, cultures of bone currettings or pus can be done for diagnostic purposes, and antibiotic therapy modified accordingly.

In general, antibiotics should be started as early as possible, intravenously or intramuscularly, at high doses. Bone infections are much more difficult to eradicate than soft tissue infections, probably as a result of the presence of organisms in ischemic areas of bone that are relatively inaccessible to antibiotics. The optimal duration of treatment is variable, depending upon the organism, but usual regimens consist of parenteral antibiotics for at least three weeks after defervescence, followed by oral therapy for an additional two weeks, which usually results in a six-week therapeutic course. A useful test for following the response, in addition to clinical signs and symptoms, is the erythrocyte sedimentation rate (ESR), which usually begins to fall within one week of starting appropriate therapy. It should be within or close to normal range at the end of the treatment period. Shorter courses of antibiotic of one week parenterally followed by two to three weeks orally have been successful, but unless there are compelling reasons against it, the longer course is recommended.

With vertebral osteomyelitis, immobilization of the spine by body cast, brace, or Stryker frame has commonly been employed; however, bedrest alone and analgesics are usually sufficient for pain control. Neurosurgical opinion should be sought immediately if abnormal neurologic signs are present or appear during treatment.

The treatment of chronic osteomyelitis is more prolonged and usually requires both a surgical and medical approach. The chronicity of the process has led to the development of sequestra, loculated pus, and/or sinus tracts that all require extensive debriding for cure. This is combined first with intensive antibiotic therapy parenterally for at least one month, usually followed by three months of oral therapy. In some cases, because of the extent of osteomyelitis, total debridement is not possible and such patients may require long-term suppressive antibiotic therapy or periodic treatment for acute exacerbations. Such difficult cases emphasize the importance of the aggressive treatment of acute osteomyelitis, which is more amenable to cure. In chronic osteomyelitis caused by *S. aureus*, fusidic acid, 500 mg q8h po or IV in combination with a penicillin or cepha-

TABLE 18.3. Initial Antimicrobial Treatment of Selected Bacterial Osteomyelitis or Arthritis

Organism	*Antimicrobial*
S. aureus	
Penicillinase producing	Cloxacillin, 2 gm q4h IV* Cefazolin, 1 gm q6h IV Vancomycin, 1 gm q12h IV
Nonpenicillinase producing	Penicillin G, 3 MU q4h IV Cefazolin, 1 gm q6h IV Vancomycin, 1 gm q12h IV
H. influenzae	
Nonpenicillinase producing	Ampicillin, 50 mg/kg q4h IV†
Penicillinase producing	Chloramphenicol, 20 mg/kg q6h IV Trimethoprim, 5 mg/kg with sulfamethoxazole, 25 mg/kg q6-12h IV
N. gonorrhoeae	
Nonpenicillinase producing	Penicillin G, 2 MU q4h IV Cefazolin, 1 gm q6h IV Tetracycline, 1.5 gm po (loading dose), plus 500 mg q6h po
Penicillinase producing	Cefoxitin, 1 gm q6h IV Spectinomycin, 2 gm q12h IM
S. pneumoniae	Penicillin G, 1 MU q4h IV Cefazolin, 1 gm q8h IV Clindamycin, 600 mg q6h IV
E. coli‡	Ampicillin, 2 gm q4h IV Cefazolin, 1.5 gm q6h IV Gentamicin/tobramycin, 1.5 mg/kg q8h IV
Ps. aeruginosa‡	Gentamicin/tobramycin, 1.5 mg/kg q8h IV, plus ticarcillin/piperacillin, 50 mg/kg q4h IV Amikacin, 7.5 mg/kg q12h IV, plus ticarcillin/piperacillin, 50 mg q4h IV

*Dosage based on 70-kg patient with normal renal function.

†In milligram per kilogram for dosages in children.

‡Antimicrobial used depends upon results of susceptibility testing.

losporin may be more effective than the beta-lactam alone.

Osteomyelitis in patients with poorly perfused areas (diabetics and patients with peripheral vascular disease) and skull infections often requires early surgical treatment. Amputation, for example, of digits, often prevents a long drawn-out hospital course of antibiotic treatment that ultimately fails.

In osteomyelitis associated with fracture, union of the fracture appears necessary for ultimate eradication of the infection. Therefore internal or external fixation is often performed in conjunction with antimicrobial therapy until the fracture has undergone union, and then the fixation devices are removed. In this setting, only with removal of the foreign material can a cure ultimately be effected. Osteomyelitis associated with prosthetic joints usually requires removal of the prosthesis and debridement for cure. After removal, the type and duration of antibiotic treatment are controversial: a prolonged course of antibiotics may be given (several months to a year in duration) followed by reinsertion of a new joint if technically feasible. A newer alternative approach is a short course (two weeks) of parenteral antibiotics followed by insertion of the prosthesis with cement containing antibiotic. This technique, if effective in the long term, has obviously major advantages.

Aggressive treatment of a wound infection overlying a prosthetic joint or internal fixation device often is successful in preventing osteomyelitis as a complication. This would include parenteral treatment rather than oral medication initially, and careful follow-up to exclude osteomyelitis. Duration of treatment usually is two to four weeks.

Treatment of tuberculous and fungal osteomyelitis is similar to that described for pulmonary disease (see Chapter 12).

Prognosis

Acute osteomyelitis caused by *S. aureus, H. influenzae,* and streptococcal species has a very good prognosis if appropriate antibiotic therapy is instituted early and disseminated infection is not present. In contrast, osteomyelitis caused by gram-negative enteric organisms or associated with compound fractures and foreign bodies carries a much less favorable prognosis with a greater predisposition to becoming chronic. A persistently elevated sedimentation rate in a patient with osteomyelitis suggests continuing infection if other causes can be excluded.

In vertebral osteomyelitis, clinical and radiologic resolution may be very slow as the adjacent vertebrae become sclerotic and fuse. Pain relief usually is quite dramatic with treatment but may not be complete until fusion. Persistent pain in an area of vertebral osteomyelitis may be helped with formal surgical fusion.

Chronic osteomyelitis carries a much poorer prognosis for complete cure than the acute infection. The duration of disease appears to correlate directly with the difficulty in ultimately eradicating it, and likely reflects the presence of extensive sequestra formation. Aggressive surgical debridement coupled with newer, more effective antibiotics against gram-negative organisms may improve the overall cure rate.

Prophylaxis

No specific prophylaxis is available for hematogenously spread osteomyelitis, but early recognition and treatment of bacteremias will reduce the possibility of metastatic spread to bone. Soft tissue infections, especially those seen in diabetics and patients with peripheral vascular disease, if treated early will reduce the frequency of osteomyelitis from direct spread. Prophylactic antibiotics, usually cephalosporins or penicillinase-resistant penicillins, have reduced the frequency of infections with prosthetic or internal fixation devices. Also, prophylaxis of compound fractures with a cephalosporin or an aminoglycoside in combination with an antistaphylococcal penicillin (cloxacillin) is usually given.

INFECTIOUS ARTHRITIS

Infectious arthritis is an infection of the synovium, usually with secondary involvement of the joint space and cartilage. Septic arthritis usually refers specifically to an acute bacterial infection.

Etiology

The common etiologies of bacterial arthritis in various age groups are listed in Table 18.4. Overall, the most common cause is *S. aureus,* although cases due to *Neisseria gonorrhoeae* may be as frequent in certain populations. In contrast to osteomyelitis, anaerobic bacteria are distinctly unusual causes of septic arthritis.

TABLE 18.4. Etiology of Bacterial Arthritis in Various Age Groups

Age	*Organisms*
Neonates (≤2 mo)	*S. aureus* Group B streptococci Gram-negative rods (*E. coli*)
Children (3 mo–4 yrs)	*H. influenzae* (type b) *S. aureus* *S. pyogenes*
Children (5–15 yrs)	*S. aureus*
Adults	
16–30 yrs	*N. gonorrhoeae* *S. aureus*
>30 yrs	*S. aureus* *S. pneumoniae, S. viridans* Gram-negative rods (*E. coli*) *N. gonorrhoeae*

Other infectious causes include mycobacteria (*M. tuberculosis, M. bovis,* and atypical mycobacteria), systemic mycoses including sporotrichosis (*Sporothrix schenkii*), candidiasis, histoplasmosis, blastomycosis, and coccidioidomycosis, and viruses, including rubella, hepatitis B, and less commonly, Epstein-Barr, herpes simplex, and cytomegalovirus.

Postinfectious arthritis as seen in Reiter's syndrome may follow *Salmonella, Shigella,* and *Yersinia* gastroenteritis, and *Chlamydia trachomatis* genital infections, but no organisms are cultured from the joint and the inflammatory response is probably immunologic in etiology.

Epidemiology

The epidemiology of bacterial arthritis caused by hematogenous spread reflects the relative incidence of bacteremias in the various age groups involved (Table 18.4). For example, although *S. aureus* causes infection in all age groups, in children between 3 months and 4 years, *Hemophilus influenzae* (type b) occurs as commonly as *S. aureus,* while in the 15- to 30-year-old age group, gonococcal infection is the most common.

Staphylococcus aureus infections predominate in the older adult population, often occurring in the setting of established joint disease such as osteoarthritis or rheumatoid arthritis, or in patients with underlying diseases such as diabetes mellitus. Gonococcal arthritis, as part of the syndrome of disseminated gonococcal infection (DGI), occurs more commonly in females, probably because of the increased prevalence of asymptomatic genital infection. Also, patients lacking the terminal components of the complement system are predisposed to DGI.

Intravenous drug abuse is associated with unusual causes of septic arthritis including *Pseudomonas aeruginosa*.

Infections following joint surgery and instrumentation, and involving prosthetic joints are usually due to coagulase-negative staphylococci, *S. aureus,* or gram-negative rods, the last usually resistant to the prophylactic antibiotic used.

Tuberculous arthritis, although a rare disease, is one of the more common types of extrapulmonary tuberculosis and should be suspected in high-risk groups. Fungal arthritis caused by *Candida* (or *Torulopsis*) species is being seen more frequently in immunosuppressed or debilitated hospitalized patients who have usually received extensive antibiotic therapy. Patients living in indigenous areas of specific fungal infections (e.g., histoplasmosis, coccidioidomycosis) are at risk for this type of infectious arthritis. Sporotrichal arthritis is rare but has a worldwide distribution and tends to occur in patients exposed to soil and vegetative matter, for example, farmers, gardeners, and florists.

Rubella arthritis is most common in females and there is a high frequency of postvaccinal arthritis in postpubertal women. Arthritis associated with hepatitis B infection should be suspected in patients who are at high risk, including intravenous drug abusers, medical and paramedical personnel handling blood products and involved in hemodialysis, and male homosexuals. The actual prevalence of viral arthritis, because of the usual transient nature of the illness, may be higher than reported.

Pathophysiology

Most bacterial arthritis results from hematogenous spread with seeding out of bacteria in the synovium. Bacterial multiplication produces an acute inflammatory reaction in the synovium, including the production of excessive purulent synovial fluid that accumulates in the joint space. The metabolic products and toxins of bacteria, the low pH of the joint fluid, and lysozymes from leukocytes resulting from the inflammatory reaction, all combine to cause cartilage destruction and stimulate pannus formation. The degree of articular cartilage destruction depends upon the infecting bacterium (for example, *S. aureus* produces rapid destruction; *N. gonorrhoeae* produces minimal to moderate destruction), the duration of the arthritis, previous joint disease (e.g., rheumatoid arthritis), and individual host differences. With severe destruction of the articular cartilage, bone formation is stimulated, with ankylosis of the joint. Very rarely, osteomyelitis in the adjacent bone can result. Dissemination of the infection from the septic joint to other parts of the body can also occur.

Two other routes of infection causing septic arthritis are (1) inoculation of the joint space with organisms at the time of trauma, surgery, insertion of prosthetic joints, arthroscopy, and injection of therapeutic agents (e.g., steroids); and (2) extension of a focus of osteomyelitis to the joint in neonates (through perforating blood vessels through the epiphyseal plate from the metaphysis) and adults (no epiphyseal plate and anastomoses between metaphyseal and epiphyseal blood vessels).

Mycobacterial and fungal arthritis arise from lymphohematogenous spread of the organisms from a distant focus (usually pulmonary) and is characterized by granuloma formation in the synovium and insidious joint destruction. Candidal arthritis can result from disseminated candidiasis in immunosuppressed patients and those with indwelling central lines. Occasionally, sporotrichal arthritis will arise from direct inoculation of the organism with trauma to a joint or direct spread from a skin lesion. Viral arthritis from hematogenous spread is associated with a predominantly mononuclear cell infiltrate in the synovium and minimal or no joint destruction.

Clinical Manifestations

Bacterial arthritis from hematogenous spread usually occurs acutely as a monoarticular infection (rarely as an oligoarticular disease) affecting the large joints mainly (knee, hip, ankle, and shoulder) with systemic manifestations of bacteremia. There are inflammatory changes in the affected joint and surrounding soft tissues with swelling, erythema, and pain at rest, which is greatly aggravated with even minimal movement of the joint. If there is no obvious swelling of the joint, an effusion usually can be detected.

Gonococcal arthritis is often a biphasic illness in which the patient initially has evidence of a systemic bacteremia with polyarthralgias or polyarthritis often affecting large and small joints, and characteristic vasculitic skin lesions (petechial, pustular, or necrotic) usually on the extremities, typical of disseminated gonococcal infection. This particular phase of the illness is then followed within days by a monoarticular arthritis affecting the large joints (knee, wrist, or ankle). Although such a pattern is often seen, in many cases the bacteremic and arthritic components are inseparable.

Bacterial arthritis may be a complication of another focus of infection, and therefore in severely ill obtunded patients, an infected joint should not be overlooked. Also, in patients with underlying joint disease (e.g., rheumatoid arthritis or systemic lupus erythematosus), exacerbations of arthritis must be suspected of having an infectious cause until proved otherwise.

Pain and loosening of a prosthesis are clinical features of an infection of a prosthetic joint, which may occur within a month or years after its insertion. The infection is an osteomyelitis at the contact point of the prosthesis and the bone (see page 287).

Viral arthritis is usually polyarticular and can affect both large and small joints. It is seen in conjunction with other manifestations of the viral infection either concurrently or several weeks later. Hepatitis B arthritis usually occurs prior to jaundice and is associated with an urticarial rash. Fungal and mycobacterial arthritis are usually insidious in onset and associated with less acute joint symptoms. An exception is acute arthritis caused by *Candida* or *Torulopsis* species, occurring usually as a complication in an immunocompromised host.

Diagnosis

Acute infectious arthritis must be differentiated from noninfectious arthritis including gout, pseudogout, hemarthrosis, rheumatoid arthritis, and Reiter's syndrome. Septic bursitis (olecranon or prepatellar area) may also simulate septic arthritis, but joint movement is not very painful and a cellulitis is often present. Blood for three cultures should be drawn, and results will be positive in approximately 50% of cases. Any other lesion (e.g., skin lesions) should be cultured as a possible source of bacteremia. In addition, when gonococcal arthritis is suspected, pharyngeal, urethral, anal canal, and endocervical cultures should be done. A gonococcal complement fixation test is often positive in disseminated gonococcal infection and may be helpful when other cultures are negative. Cultures of sexual contacts of patients with suspected DGI may also aid in the diagnosis.

A complete blood count usually demonstrates polymorphonuclear leucocytosis (reflecting sepsis), normal or mildly decreased hemoglobin, and invariably an elevated ESR.

The most important aspect of diagnosis is early aspiration of the joint and examination by Gram's stain (and other appropriate stains for mycobacteria and fungi as indicated), and culture on various media for bacteria, mycobacteria, and fungi; cell count, glucose and protein concentration, and crystals (uric acid and calcium pyrophosphate) (Table 18.5). It is important to remember that definitive diagnosis depends upon a positive Gram's stain and/or culture, or the presence of specific crystals; the other variables, although helpful, are not diagnostic.

Radiologic examination of the joint may show only soft tissue swelling and distention of the joint space. Narrowing of the joint space usually is a late finding and results from destruction of the cartilage. Bony changes with ankylosis are also seen only late in the reparative phase after a particularly serious bacterial arthritis or during the course of a more chronic insidious arthritis such as that caused by mycobacteria or fungi. Another rare, late finding would be evidence of an osteomyelitis occurring secondary to destructive septic arthritis.

Isotopic scans may be helpful in differentiating osteomyelitis that produces a sympathetic effusion from septic arthritis. A pyrophosphate scan may show a slightly increased uptake in the region of the joint, which differs from the intense uptake in bone seen in osteomyelitis. In contrast, a gallium scan may demonstrate increased uptake in the joint compared to the bone scan, substantiating the diagnosis of septic arthritis, rather than osteomyelitis.

Viral arthritis is usually diagnosed on the basis of the systemic illness and joint fluid characteristics. Rarely are viruses cultured from the joint fluid. Isolation of virus from other sites may be helpful, however, and viral serology may also confirm, in retrospect, the clinical suspicion of viral arthritis.

Cultures of synovial fluid, especially synovial biopsy material, for mycobacterial species and fungi are indicated in suspected cases, and serology for coccidioidomycosis and histoplasmosis may be helpful. *S.*

TABLE 18.5. Usual Synovial Fluid Characteristics in Patients with Bacterial, Viral, Mycobacterial, and Noninfectious Inflammatory Arthritis

	Bacterial	*Mycobacterial*	*Viral*	*Inflammatory*
Appearance	*Turbid/Purulent*	*Slightly Turbid*	*Clear/Slightly Turbid*	*Turbid*
Cell count	>25,000	>10,000	<25,000	<25,000
% polymorphonuclear cells	>75	>50	<50	>50
Stain of fluid	Gram's stain positive ≃ 50%	Acid-fast stain positive ≃ 30%	Negative	Negative
Culture of fluid	Positive (up to 90%)	Positive 80%	Positive (rare)	Negative

schenckii is usually cultured successfully from synovium or synovial fluid, although stained smears of the fluid are usually negative.

Treatment

Acute bacterial arthritis is a medical emergency and therefore should be considered a possible diagnosis in any patient with an acute arthritis. The two most important aspects of treatment of this condition are (1) early decompression of the joint and removal of the potential cartilage-destructive fluid by needle aspiration or open surgical drainage and (2) aggressive antimicrobial therapy. Most joints can be aspirated, repeatedly as necessary, without an open surgical procedure. For the hip joint, however, because of the difficulty of aspiration, open drainage is necessary. That procedure is recommended also for any joint that is difficult to aspirate because, for example, of multiple loculations of pus. A poor response to appropriate antibiotic treatment and needle aspiration indicates the strong need to consider surgery. Adequate drainage of the joint is therefore both therapeutic and provides diagnostic material.

Antibiotic treatment is begun immediately and is determined by the clinical picture and initial Gram's stain results. Various antibiotic regimens for different etiologies of septic arthritis are shown in Table 18.3. Where the Gram's stain is negative, choice of drug is determined by the patient's age and the most likely pathogens. These empiric regimens usually include an antistaphylococcal penicillin (beta-lactamase-resistant) or cephalosporin because *S. aureus* is a common pathogen in most age groups. Additional antibiotics are added as necessary. All drugs are given initially parenterally. The response to treatment can be followed by culturing joint fluid if repeated aspirations are done.

Duration of therapy is determined by the response of the individual patient but as a general rule, antibiotics are given intravenously or intramuscularly for at least one week after the patient becomes afebrile and until the erythrocyte sedimentation rate is declining. Oral therapy is then usually continued for two to four weeks. Gonococcal arthritis usually responds after a few days of treatment, while arthritis caused by *S. aureus* and especially gram-negative enteric rods usually is slower to respond. Supportive measures including splinting of the affected joint and analgesics for pain relief are also used as required.

Because the majority of antibiotics diffuse well into the synovial fluid, instillation of antibiotics directly into septic joints is not necessary and should be discouraged because of possible complications. These include a chemical synovitis as a result of the usually high concentrations of antibiotics instilled and also the possibility of introducing a secondary pathogen into the joint. Irrigation of the joint with nonantibiotic-containing fluids has been done to cleanse the joint cavity mechanically to eliminate substances associated with dissolution of articular cartilage. Although the technique appears theoretically valid, it is difficult to prove its efficacy. If used, it should be for 48 hours or less to reduce the possibility of superinfection.

Treatment of septic arthritis associated with prosthetic joints is described on page 289 in the discussion of osteomyelitis.

The treatment of tuberculous arthritis is similar to that of pulmonary tuberculosis, as described in Chapter 12. Fungal arthritis is usually treated with amphotericin B, as described on page 77, with total doses between

1.5 and 2.5 gm. Amphotericin B by intravenous injection or irrigation may be necessary if response is poor with systemic drugs alone. Optimal intraarticular concentrations are not known, but 10 mg per liter should be adequate. Ketoconazole, a new antifungal agent, at a dose of 200 to 400 mg per day, may prove an efficacious alternative in certain types of fungal arthritis, but clinical experience is limited. Surgical treatment is often required in fungal arthritis. Viral arthritis is treated symptomatically.

Prognosis

Complications and sequelae of septic arthritis vary depending upon the infecting organism, the presence of preexisting joint disease, the immunocompetence of the host, and the time of institution of appropriate therapy. Gonococcal arthritis carries a good prognosis, whereas arthritis caused by other organisms, especially gram-negative rods, may be very difficult to eradicate and is associated with a high frequency of residual joint destruction. Patients with underlying joint disease such as rheumatoid arthritis have a poorer prognosis. Delay in appropriate surgical and medical therapy also worsens the prognosis, especially with respect to residual joint complications.

Tuberculous arthritis generally responds favorably to therapy, but considerable joint destruction generally has occurred prior to diagnosis. Fungal arthritis is often very difficult to treat, usually because of the toxicity of amphotericin B, the prolonged duration of treatment required, and poor host defenses. Viral arthritis has a very good prognosis without sequelae.

Prophylaxis

No specific prophylactic measures are available, although aggressive treatment of bacteremias and fungemias prevent septic arthritis as a complication. Penetrating wounds to joints should be surgically debrided and treated with prophylactic antibiotics to cover the most likely pathogens in particular epidemiologic settings. Prophylaxis should also be given at the time of prosthetic joint insertion; usually a cephalosporin or penicillinase-resistant penicillin is used.

ANNOTATED BIBLIOGRAPHY

Bayer AS, Guze LB, Scott VJ, Choi C, Tillman DB. Fungal arthritis. I–V. Semin Arthritis Rheum 1978;8:142–150; 1979; 8:200–211; 1979;9:66–74, 145–151, 218–227.

Comprehensive review of the major fungal causes of septic arthritis and synovitis including *Candida* organisms, *Coccidiodes, Sporothrix,* blastomycetes, cryptococci, and *Histoplasma.*

Brogadir SP, Schimmer BM, Myers AR. Spectrum of gonococcal arthritis-dermatitis syndrome. Semin Arthritis Rheum 1978;8:177–183.

Retrospective review of 104 patients with the gonococcal arthritis-dermatitis syndrome in which the classically described biphasic nature of the disease is questioned and the tenosynovitis and periarthritis syndrome is stressed.

Davidson PT, Horowitz I. Skeletal tuberculosis. a review with patient presentations and discussion. Am J Med 1970;48:77–84.

Illustrative cases emphasizing (epidemiologic and clinical) clues to the early diagnosis of skeletal tuberculosis.

Goldenberg DL, Cohen AS. Acute infectious arthritis: a review of patients with non-gonococcal joint infections (with emphasis on therapy and prognosis). Am J Med 1976;60:369–377.

Clinical and laboratory features of 59 patients with infectious arthritis emphasizes host factors, antimicrobial regimens, medical versus surgical treatment, and prognosis.

Hyer FH, Gottlieb NL. Rheumatic disorders associated with viral infection. Semin Arthritis Rheum 1978;8:17–31.

Clinical manifestations and laboratory features of viral arthritis associated with etiologic agents including hepatitis B, common childhood viruses (rubella, mumps, varicella, erythema infectiosum), and other viruses (infectious mononucleosis, echovirus, adenovirus, and arbovirus).

Lewis RP, Sutter VL, Finegold SM. Bone infections involving anaerobic bacteria. Medicine 1978;57:279–305.

Comprehensive review of the literature and authors' experience with 23 patients with mixed anaerobic-aerobic infections.

Sapico FL, Montgomerie JZ. Pyogenic vertebral osteomyelitis: report of nine cases and review of the literature. Rev Infect Dis 1979;1:754–776.

Detailed analysis of a total of 318 cases of vertebral osteomyelitis regarding etiology, epidemiology, clinical manifestations, diagnosis, and therapy.

Sharpe JT, Lidsky MD, Duffy J, Duncan MW. Infectious arthritis. Arch Intern Med 1979;139:1125–1130.

Review of 113 patients with bacterial arthritis (gonococcal and nongonococcal) over a 14-year period, with emphasis on etiology, joint involved, host characteristics, and prognosis.

Waldvogel FA, Medoff G, Schwartz MN. Osteomyelitis; a review of clinical features, therapeutic considerations and unusual aspects. N Engl J Med 1970;282:198–206, 316–322.

Concise, excellent review of osteomyelitis with 170 references.

Waldvogel FA, Vasey H. Osteomyelitis: the past decade. N Engl J Med 1980;303:360–370.

Update on the original paper emphasizing newer aspects of microbiology, diagnosis, and therapy.

19 INFECTIONS OF THE SKIN AND SOFT TISSUE

M. Ian Bowmer

The skin forms a major barrier against infection. The keratinized epithelium is a relatively impenetrable surface, and the constant desquamation of cells creates a mechanical cleansing system. These factors, plus the production of a low surface pH (approximately 3.0) through the hydrolysis of sebum triglycerides to free fatty acids, help to ensure a relatively constant bacterial flora on the skin. These organisms are moderately avirulent and maintain an ecologic balance that suppresses more pathogenic organisms.

Despite many homeostatic factors, the normal flora of the skin is quite variable. Predominant bacteria are staphylococci, coryneforms, and micrococci, but their relative distribution varies from one anatomic site to another; *Staphylococcus* species are predominant around the nares and facial areas and *Micrococcus* species are isolated more peripherally. These organisms have very low pathogenicity and, except for some of the coryneforms, are rarely associated with significant skin infection. More pathogenic bacteria such as *S. aureus* and *Streptococcus pyogenes* do reside on the skin surface episodically and for varying periods of time. Individuals often carry these organisms on the mucosal surfaces, especially the nasopharynx. During outbreaks of streptococcal infection, disease-free individuals can be shown to have streptococci as part of their skin flora. Personnel working in hospitals are particularly susceptible to increased frequency of *S. aureus* carriage on the skin and nasopharynx — perhaps up to 25% are carriers. Other organisms, such as gram-negative aerobic rods, are unusual skin flora except in individuals in the hospital environment. The skin also acts as a transient carrier of many nonbacterial microorganisms, including viruses and fungi. Mouth-to-hand-to-hand contact is recognized as a major transmission mechanism of rhinovirus, but this agent is presumably a transient passenger on the skin surface. Fungal organisms, such as dermatophytes and *Candida,* are so commonly isolated on the skin surface that they could be considered normal flora, but they are associated with both mild and clinically significant infections.

For any of these organisms to cause skin infections, there must be some break in the integrity of the barrier mechanism. Small cuts are a major source of infection, but penetration of hair follicles and sweat glands with obstruction by sebum or desquamating cells forms the other major entry site.

This chapter deals with the common microbial skin infections. Each section describes the clinical entity in order of frequency usually seen in general practice. Emphasis is placed on the clinical description since, for the most common conditions, the etiologies often overlap and they can be discussed as a group. Secondary infections are discussed in other sections of the book dealing with the primary problem (e.g., pseudomonal bacteremia, ecthyma gangrenosa). Infections associated with burns are discussed in Chapter 24.

PRIMARY BACTERIAL SKIN INFECTIONS

The most useful classification of bacterial skin and subcutaneous tissue infection is a clinical one based on the morphologic appearance of the lesion. This approach provides the most helpful initial clues to diagnosis, although therapy must be directed toward the specific etiologic agent. The simplest approach is to consider whether the skin lesions are focal or diffuse, superficial or deep. Considerable overlap occurs, since many infections can affect the superficial skin surface, subcu-

TABLE 19.1. Clinical Features of Bacterial Infections of the Skin and Soft Tissues

Lesion	*Primary Clinical Feature*	*Predominant Etiology (other organisms)*
Focal		
Folliculitis	Red indurated papules involving hair follicle	*S. aureus* (*P. aeruginosa*)
Acne	Red pustular papules involving sebaceous glands	*Propionibacterium acnes, P. granulosum*
Furuncle, carbuncle	Red indurated perifollicular abscess	*S. aureus*
Impetigo	Tender or pruritic oozing, crusted surface inflammation	*S. pyogenes* (group A) (*S. aureus*)
Bullous impetigo	Bullae that exfoliate	*S. aureus*
Paronychia	Purulent collection in nail bed	*S. aureus*
Ecthyma	Inflamed papule with ulcerated or necrotic center	*S. pyogenes* (group A) (*P. aeruginosa*)
Anthrax	Edematous papule with central vesicle	*Bacillus anthracis*
Diffuse superficial		
Cellulitis	Diffuse, red skin with linear streaking	*S. pyogenes* (group A) *S. aureus* (*H. influenzae*)
Erysipelas	Diffuse, red skin with sharply raised margins	*S. pyogenes* (group A)
Erysipeloid	Painful, raised reddish purple lesion with central clearing	*Erysipelothrix rhusiopathiae*
Seal finger	Painful, indurated reddish purple skin on extremities	Unknown
Erythrasma	Brown, scaling erythema in crural areas	*Corynebacterium minutissimum*

taneous tissue, and even fascia and muscle layers. Numerous bacterial species, either individually or in combination, can cause diseases with similar clinical manifestations.

Folliculitis

Folliculitis is an inflammatory eruption that involves hair follicles. It causes an erythematous, raised papule frequently associated with a central pustule (Table 19.1). The most common etiologic agent (Table 19.2) is *S. aureus,* although *Pseudomonas aeruginosa* has been a cause of folliculitis in patients who have had exposure in whirlpool baths. In that situation, the lesions are more restricted to truncal surfaces.

Folliculitis is the most common skin infection. It occurs frequently in the second and third decades of life and is precipitated either by occlusion of the follicle or minor trauma. Sycosis barbi, a severe folliculitis of the beard area, is associated with shaving. In these situations, not only is there trauma to the epidermis, but the hair shaft is severed below the skin surface and regrowth is associated with further trauma. Other shaved areas, such as axillae and legs, are potential sites for folliculitis. The diagnosis is made on the basis of clinical manifestations, localization to the hair follicle, and a history of predisposing trauma.

Although the etiology can be confirmed by removing the superficial crust and sending swabs of the serous exudate to the bacteriologic laboratory, this is usually unnecessary. Treatment is cleansing of the skin and soaking with either warm water or saline compresses to remove any crusts. For those infections associated with shaved areas, shaving should be discontinued until there is complete healing. Resolution of the folliculitis usually occurs within five to seven days.

Acne

Acne is a focal inflammatory lesion involving the pilosebaceous structures. It produces opened or closed comedones or inflammatory papules, and may progress to pustules and nodules. Acne begins just before or at puberty; it is felt that the gonadotropin surge occurring at this time increases circulating and tissue androsterones. This in turn causes sebaceous hypertrophy, and the lipid and follicular keratinization provides a base for the lipase-producing diphtheroids, *Propionibacterium acnes* and *Propionibacterium granulosum*, to produce potentially irritating, medium-chain, free fatty acids. Recently, electron microscopy studies have shown a keratinization defect in the infundibular portion of the sebaceous follicle. Occurring on the sebaceous-rich areas of the face, shoulders, and chest, acne affects 85% to 100% of adolescents.

Diagnosis

Diagnosis is made purely on the basis of clinical manifestations. The presence of comedones or pustules involving pilosebaceous areas, predominantly the face, are characteristic. When this occurs in adolescence the diagnosis is rarely in doubt. Similar manifestations in older persons may not suggest acne, but facial and anterior chest distribution and its association with the use of steroids should alert the physician to the diagnosis.

Treatment

Treatment includes topical measures to open sebaceous follicles and to reverse the hyperkeratosis so that plugs can be easily expelled and prevented from reforming. Topical agents include retinoic acid, which is believed to act directly on the keratinocytes and can be applied in 0.5%, 0.025%, and 0.01% gels or creams. Salicylic acid in 5% or 10% concentrations increases desquamation. The side effects from these drugs include local irritation, hypersensitivity, and burning sensation. Benzoyl peroxide and topical antibiotics have been used to decrease the population of propionibacteria and therefore reduce the surface levels of free fatty acid. Five percent and 10% solutions can be used, but the higher concentrations cause some irritation, and a small percentage of patients develop contact dermatitis. Topical antibiotics shown to be effective are clindamycin and the tetracyclines.

For moderate to severe acne, tetracycline and erythromycin administered orally have been shown to be effective and safe. High-dose tetracycline hydrochloride, 2 gm per day for 6 to 12 weeks, with subsequent reduction of the dose, is an effective treatment but may cause dyspepsia and, in some cases, may cause photosensitization or central nervous system side effects. All tetracyclines are contraindicated in pregnancy. An effective alternative is erythromycin in the same dosage.

Other factors that have been found helpful in the treatment of acne include vitamin A, oral retinoic acid (isotretinoin), and dietary control with reduced intake of soft drinks, chocolate, milk and milk products, fatty foods, and iodides. With the combined approach to therapy, most patients can control the degree of skin lesions. Limiting factors may be their tolerance of oral antibiotics. Most patients tend to have mild to moderate disease that resolves with age. Severe acne may result in permanent scars, and cosmetic surgery should be considered in these patients. Oral retinoic acid is contra-indicated during pregnancy.

Furuncles and Carbuncles

Furuncles are deeper and more serious perifollicular abscesses. Carbuncles extend into the subcutaneous fat and usually involve multiple follicles. Drainage of a carbuncle therefore occurs along the course of more than one hair follicle. The etiology is invariably *S. aureus*. Both furuncles and carbuncles occur in all age groups but are more common in the second and third decades. Their usual site is exposed skin undergoing friction and maceration, with carbuncles more frequent in the head and neck region and over the thighs. Very frequent recurrence of furuncles or carbuncles should raise the suspicion of an underlying disease, including immunosuppression, neutrophil dysfunction, or diabetes mellitus. Obesity may also play a role, facilitating infections in moist intertriginous zones.

Diagnosis

The diagnosis of a furuncle or carbuncle can be made with certainty in any patient with a focal perifollicular abscess. Fever and leukocytosis may be present when the lesions are large or complicated by extension of infection into the surrounding skin or when bacteremia occurs. Bacteremia may be precipitated by manipulation of the lesion, including any drainage procedure. Lesions about the nose and upper lip should be considered particularly dangerous since regional spread of the infection may extend into the cavernous sinus.

Treatment

In early lesions, nonspecific therapy with warm compresses aids in the localization and drainage of the lesion. The presence of associated cellulitis or location in the facial region is an indication for systemic antistaphylococcal antibiotic treatment. Antibiotic therapy should also accompany any surgical manipulation of the lesions.

Since the majority of community-acquired *S. aureus* may produce penicillinase, the drug of choice is a semisynthetic penicillin such as cloxacillin or erythromycin in penicillin-allergic patients (for dosage see Table 19.2). Since these lesions are abscesses, surgical drainage is necessary if they are fluctuant.

TABLE 19.2. Etiologic Agents of Skin Infections

Lesion (Organisms)	Drug	Therapy: Adults	Therapy: Children
Bacterial			
Acne, moderate to severe	Tetracycline HCl	1–2 gm/d po 6–12 wks	
(Propionibacterium acnes)	Erythromycin		7.5 mg/kg po qid
(*P. granulosum*)			
Furuncle, with cellulitis	Cloxacillin	500 mg po qid × 7–10 d	7.5 mg/kg po qid × 7–10 d
(*S. aureus*)			
Impetigo	Phenoxymethyl penicillin	600 mg po qid × 7–10 d	7.5 mg/kg po qid × 7–10 d
(Group A streptococci)	Penicillin G (inpatient)	1 MU IV q4h (acute phase)	400,000/kg IV q4h
(*S. aureus*)	Erythromycin (penicillin-allergic patients)	500 mg po qid × 7–10 d	7.5 mg/kg po qid × 7–10 d
Paronychia	As for furuncle		
Ecthyma	As for furuncle		
(Group A streptococci)			
Cutaneous anthrax	Benzyl penicillin	4×10^6 IV q4h × 10 d	
(*Bacillus anthracis*)	Tetracycline HCl (penicillin-allergic patients)	500 mg po qid × 10 d	
Cellulitis	Cloxacillin	Moderate — 500 mg po qid × 10 d	7.5 mg/kg po qid × 10 d
(*S. aureus*)		Severe — 1 gm IV q4h (acute phase)	15 mg/kg IV q4h (acute phase)
	Erythromycin (penicillin-allergic patients)	500 mg po qid × 10 d	7.5 mg/kg po qid × 10 d
(*H. influenzae*)	Ampicillin	1 gm IV q4h	100 mg/kg/d
	Trimethoprim/sulfamethoxazole	2 tablets po bid	Trimethoprim, 6 mg/kg/d
			Sulfamethoxazole, 30 mg/kg/d divided into 2 equal doses
Erysipelas	As for impetigo		
(Group A streptococci)			
Erysipeloid	As for impetigo		
(*Erysipelothrix rhusiopathiae*)			
Seal finger	Tetracycline	500 mg po qid × 7 d	
(Unknown)			

Erythrasma (*Corynebacterium minutissimum*)	Erythromycin	500 mg po qid × 7 d	7.5 mg/kg po qid × 7 d
Necrotizing cellulitis (Streptococci)	Penicillin	2 MU IV q4h	
(*S. aureus*, gram-negatives)	Cloxacillin	1 gm IV q4h	
(Clostridia, anaerobes)	Tobramycin	1.5 mg/kg IV q8h	
	Metronidazole		30 mg/kg/d
Lymphangitis (Group A streptococci) (*S. aureus*)	Phenoxymethyl penicillin	As for cellulitis	
	Erythromycin		
	Cloxacillin		
Tularemia (*Francisella tularensis*)	Streptomycin	0.5 mg IM q12h × 10 d	
Fungal			
Tinea pedis	Topical clotrimazole (mild)		
	Griseofulvin (severe) or	0.5–1 gm po daily	10 mg/kg/d
	ketoconazole	200 mg po bid × 10–14 d	
Tinea cruris	Topical clotrimazole	As above	
Tinea barbae	Griseofulvin	As above	
Sporotrichosis	Saturated solution potassium iodide*	5 gtt in milk daily, increasing 5 gtt/d to 120 gtt/d	
Candida	Topical clotrimazole	As above	
Others			
Warts	10–50% podophyllin, topical application once daily		
Pediculosis	Gamma benzene hexachloride, 1 topical application		
Scabies	As for pediculosis		
	10% thiabendazole, 1 topical application		
Cutaneous larva migrans	Thiabendazole 15%, topical application	25 mg/kg/d	

*Toxicity may occur (lacrimation, salivation, parotid swelling, gastrointestinal symptoms). In that case, stop medication and reinstate at lower dosage. Acneiform rash is not an indication for discontinuation.

Recurrent folliculitis and furunculosis, especially in hospital employees, may become a major clinical problem. Most of these patients, especially adults, do not have an underlying host defense defect and are not diabetic. They may, however, carry *S. aureus* in the nasopharynx or on the perineum. In the latter form of colonization, the use of an antistaphylococcal cleansing agent such as hexachlorophene or chlorhexidine can be effective in reducing the number of organisms. Regular changes of clothing, especially underwear, should be recommended, and it is best to use cotton underclothing that promotes reduction in moisture and maceration. The nasopharyngeal carrier state has also been temporarily eradicated by using local applications of an antistaphylococcal antibiotic ointment, such as bacitracin. The instillation of a low-virulence strain of *S. aureus* (ATCC 502)* into the nares has been reported to interfere with colonization by high-virulence strains. Recurrent carrier states are usually hard to eradicate completely, however, and most measures work for only short periods of time. Removal of the employee from the work environment for 10 to 14 days often eradicates the carrier state. A one-week course of rifampin plus cloxacillin by mouth may also be tried since it terminates the carrier state in some individuals.

Impetigo

Impetigo is a common superficial infection characterized by two clinically distinct entities. The first and more common is a focal inflammatory lesion associated with thick crusts, and the second is a less erythematous lesion but tender exfoliation.

In the majority of patients, the etiology is *S. pyogenes*. Mixed infections with group A streptococci and staphylococci also occur, and less frequently *S. aureus* alone may be the etiologic agent. Impetigo occurs predominantly in patients under the age of 20 years and is prevalent during all times of the year, but more so in the late summer and early winter. Peak prevalence occurs during the first three years of school, and important in its pathogenesis is a history of close contact with an infected person or of trauma.

Usually the initial lesion begins as a superficial, raw, circular, discharging area with a defined spreading edge and yellow crusting. The lesion may be associated with significant pruritus. The common sites of occurrence are the upper trunk, face, and head. The bullus form usually has a yellow exudate, and the surface of the bullae may slough easily when touched.

Diagnosis

The diagnosis is usually made clinically, but cultures of the exudate should be obtained, especially in atypical cases. Alternative diagnostic techniques such as measurement of antistreptolysin O titres are less useful in patients with streptococcal skin disease than in those with pharyngitis. Increased diagnostic sensitivity has been obtained by using anti-DNAse B and antihyaluronidase measurements, but these may be positive in only 60% of patients.

Differential diagnosis includes herpes simplex and herpes zoster, and the early erythematous lesions may resemble fungal infections. Crusting, however, is usually present only in true impetigo.

Treatment

Although penicillin is the drug of choice, there is no definite evidence that systemic treatment on diagnosis will prevent subsequent glomerulonephritis, and there is often a delay in seeking medical attention for mild infections. For mild impetigo, general nonspecific measures such as warm saline soaks to remove the crusts, frequent changes of clothing and bed linen, and separate towels and washcloths for the patient are usually all that is recommended. It is not known whether the use of penicillin prevents the spread of disease either in the patient or to close family members. Penicillin also seems to be equally effective in patients with staphylococcal or streptococcal impetigo. Therefore its precise role in therapy is somewhat unclear since, as stated previously, the majority of *S. aureus* organisms are penicillin-resistant. Oral penicillin in divided doses for 10 days is an acceptable alternative form of therapy. In penicillin-allergic patients, erythromycin in divided doses for 10 days is effective. In severe impetigo, benzathine penicillin is the parenteral drug of choice.

Other Focal Infections

Bullous impetigo is due to *S. aureus*. The lesions usually occur in the newborn and in younger children, be-

*American Type Culture Collection, strain number 502.

ginning as vesicles and turning into flaccid bullae filled with yellow fluid. The skin easily sloughs from the bullae or the bullae rupture, forming light brown crusts. Evidence exists that *S. aureus* produces an exfoliative exotoxin that is responsible for the separation of the epidermis. *Staphylococcus aureus* can be isolated from the lesions, and polymorphonuclear leukocytes can be seen on smear of the exudate. When the organism has been specifically isolated, a semisynthetic penicillin such as cloxacillin, or erythromycin in penicillin-allergic patients, should be used.

Paronychia are purulent focal infections in the region of the nail bed with associated erythema and severe pain in the terminal phalanx. The etiology is *S. aureus*. This infection is most common in late childhood and early teenage years and is associated with trauma to the cuticle of the nail. Treatment includes surgical drainage and antibiotic treatment as for furuncles, especially if there is cellulitis or fever.

Ecthyma is an uncommon focal bacteriologic skin lesion consisting of an inflammatory papule with a punched-out necrotic center. The most common pathogenesis is secondary infection of a preexisting superficial lesion such as an insect bite. In these circumstances, the etiology is usually group A streptococci, but these skin lesions can be produced secondarily to pseudomonal bacteremia. Treatment may be local for infected insect bites but the underlying disease and bacteremia must be treated in cases due to *Pseudomonas* infection.

Cutaneous anthrax is another uncommon focal skin infection and is caused by *Bacillus anthracis*. The diagnosis should be considered when patients have focal skin lesions and a history of contact with sheep, imported raw wool or unprocessed wool products, or other animal products potentially contaminated with the spores of *B. anthracis*. The lesion is usually painless and occurs in the area of exposure to the infectious spores (frequently the face and upper trunk). Beginning as a papule, it enlarges with a central vesicle surrounded by red-brown pitting edema. There is often associated malaise and a low-grade fever. As the lesion evolves, the center becomes hemorrhagic, vesicular, and eventually necrotic with scar formation.

The treatment of choice is benzyl penicillin, 4 million units intravenously every four hours or, in penicillin-allergic patients, tetracycline, 2 gm per day in divided doses for 10 days. Excision and debridement should be avoided in these patients because it increases the possibility of bacteremia.

Diffuse Bacterial Skin Infections

Cellulitis is the most common diffuse skin infection, characterized by the spread of erythema, which can involve the deeper subcutaneous tissue. It frequently originates in areas of local trauma. In the early stages, pain may not be a major complaint, but there are usually associated regional lymphadenopathy, fever, and chills. The most common etiologic agents are group A streptococci and *S. aureus*. Other streptococci, including Lancefield groups B and C, have been implicated, and *Hemophilus influenzae* causes a similar clinical picture, especially in younger children. The cellulitis associated with *H. influenzae* spreads less rapidly and has a darker erythema than the gram-positive cellulitis; however, the two are frequently indistinguishable. *Hemophilus influenzae* should be considered in the differential diagnosis, especially in younger children and in patients who respond poorly to penicillin therapy. It occurs in all age groups but is more common in childhood and early adulthood and in patients with underlying acquired host defense defects, such as hyperglycemia and lymphatic obstruction.

Diagnosis

The diagnosis is based on clinical features, but bacteriologic cultures can be obtained by injecting either nonbacteriostatic saline or Ringer's lactate solution intradermally into the cleansed advancing edge of the cellulitis. Aspiration of this fluid and inoculation into blood culture bottles provides the highest isolation rate but still only identifies the condition in less than half of patients. Blood cultures should also be done in patients with severe disease, since associated bacteremia may exist.

Treatment

The treatment of choice is penicillin or, in penicillin-allergic patients, erythromycin. The initial treatment of any cellulitis is directed toward the most common causes, which are streptococci and *S. aureus*. When the clinical appearance is typical of a streptococcal cellulitis such as erysipelas, or of a penicillin-sensitive cellulitis such as erysipeloid, benzyl penicillin is the treatment of choice. If the etiology is unknown or *S. aureus* cannot be ruled out, a semisynthetic penicillinase-resistant penicillin such as cloxacillin, orally in mild cases and intravenously in more severe cases, should be instituted. If the etiology is subsequently proved to be streptococcal, benzyl penicillin can be substituted. In situations where there is a history of contact with sea water or marine mammals, other etiologies, including marine vibrios, should be suspected. If *H. influenzae* is isolated, ampicillin or, in cases of penicillinase-producing *Hemophilus,* trimethoprim/sulfamethoxazole can be used.

Resolution of the cellulitis is usually rapid, within four to seven days. Progression of disease during therapy or delayed resolution indicates either organisms resistant to the antibiotics used or the presence of local factors that might delay healing. Penicillinase production is the most usual mechanism of resistance in this infection, and the presence of less common organisms such as *H. influenzae* should also be considered. Local changes delaying healing include blockage of lymphatics by extensive edema, involvement of superficial veins, and local suppurative collections or foreign bodies.

Erysipelas is a less common but clinically distinct form of cellulitis and is pathognomic for group A streptococci. It is characteristically located on the face, especially the malar and paranasal areas, and is a deep red inflammatory process with a very distinct, raised, advancing edge. Involvement of the subcutaneous lymphatics causes the skin to be indurated and have a *peau d'orange* appearance. This clinically characteristic form of cellulitis is usually seen more frequently in adults, and is generally accompanied by fever and leukocytosis.

Erysipeloid is also an uncommon form of cellulitis and is due to *Erysipelothrix rhusiopathiae*. It occurs in patients who have had contact with salt water, salt water fish, shellfish, or sea mammals, for example, dolphins and whales. Adults are most commonly affected. The lesions tend to be peripheral, involving the hands and fingers, and characterized by a raised, painful inflammation, the advancing edge being erythematous and the center of the lesion frequently less so or completely clear.

Seal finger is a painful, purple-red, indurated cellulitis seen in persons who handle seals, their pelts, and seal meat. Of unknown etiology, it is most common in Norway and Newfoundland during the spring seal hunt, and has also been described in persons working with seals in captivity. A slowly progressive, very painful violaceous cellulitis usually affects the skin over the fingers or thumbs. There can be an associated arthritis of the small joints, and extension can occur into the palmar fascia. There are few or no systemic findings.

Erythrasma is a less common superficial mild cellulitis caused by an anaerobic bacterium, *Corynebacterium minutissimum*. Occurring in all age groups, it differs from the previous clinical entities in that it causes a spreading patch of brown erythema often with superficial scaling. It is located primarily in the genital and crural areas and is mildly pruritic. The diagnosis can be confirmed by its characteristic coral red fluorescence under Wood's light.

Diagnosis

Diagnosis of all types of cellulitis is made initially on the basis of the clinical features and in certain cases, a history of unusual exposure. Confirmation of an etiologic agent should be attempted by culturing an aspirate from the advancing edge of the cellulitis as described above, but this is often unsuccessful. When fever and chills are present, blood cultures are indicated and may yield the etiologic agent.

Treatment

In patients with a history of exposure to marine mammals it should be noted that erysipeloid responds to penicillin. Seal finger and rarer forms of cellulitis associated with marine vibrio organisms will not respond to penicillin or penicillinase-resistant penicillins. Therefore, in these patients, physicians should consider tetracycline, 500 mg orally every six hours for 10 days, which is the treatment of choice for seal finger. A rapid response after failure on penicillin, together with the appropriate history, confirms the diagnosis. The organism that causes erythrasma is resistant to penicillin but sensitive to erythromycin.

DIFFUSE DEEP INFECTIONS

Necrotizing Cellulitis and Fasciitis

These are infections that involve subcutaneous tissue and, as the terms suggest, tissues deep to the skin such as fascia and muscle (Table 19.3). The terminology is somewhat confusing since some of the processes describe the pathologic lesion while others describe a potential etiologic agent. The clinical syndromes, especially in the early stages, may be difficult to distinguish and there may be considerable overlap. The etiology of all these diseases is frequently multiple, including both

TABLE 19.3. Major Clinical Features of Deep Diffuse Infections

Disease	*Onset*	*Pain/Swelling*	*Gas/Odor*	*Systemic*	*Organism*
Necrotizing cellulitis					
Anaerobic	Gradual to rapid	Mild/moderate	+ + + +/foul	Moderate	*Bacteroides* sp. Peptostreptococci Peptococci
Synergistic	Acute	Severe/moderate	+ +/foul	Severe	Anaerobes + *E. coli*, *Klebsiella* sp., *Enterobacter* sp.
Necrotizing fasciitis	Acute	Severe/severe	+ +/foul	Usually severe	Mixed anaerobes, streptococci, aerobic gram-negatives
Clostridial anaerobic cellulitis	Gradual	Mild/moderate	+ + + +/occ. foul	Minimal	*C. perfringens*
Myonecrosis	Acute	Severe/severe	+ +/sometimes sweet	Severe	*C. perfringens*

anaerobic and aerobic bacteria acting synergistically, such as *S. aureus,* streptococci, and aerobic gram-negative organisms in association with anaerobic gram-negative organisms such as *Bacteroides fragilis* and *B. melaninogenicus,* or anaerobic gram-positive organisms such as *Clostridium perfringens*. The many terms that have been used to describe these deep forms of cellulitis include necrotizing fasciitis, progressive synergistic gangrene, necrotizing cellulitis, streptococcal gangrene, and infected vascular gangrene. All these clinical entities involve extensive cellulitis with necrosis of subcutaneous tissue and usually the presence in tissue of gas either clinically or radiologically. The infections frequently originate around necrotic devitalized tissue, including puncture wounds, diabetic and decubitus ulcers, and areas of vascular insufficiency. Mixed aerobic and anaerobic agents should also be suspected when cellulitis arises in the perirectal or perineal areas or close to mucosal surfaces in the oral pharynx. This may follow alimentary tract surgery.

True gas gangrene or clostridial myonecrosis is not actually a skin infection, although it may be secondary to penetrating skin trauma. It is summarized in Table 19.3.

Diagnosis

The diagnosis should be suspected in patients with skin infections associated with vascular insufficiency, either as a result of local processes such as trauma or systemic processes such as diabetes mellitus or atherosclerosis. Clinical clues suggesting the possibility of anaerobic organisms are the presence of a foul-smelling purulent exudate or evidence of gas in the tissue, with palpable or audible crepitus. It should be kept in mind, however, that certain aerobic organisms are able to produce gas, and gas in tissues may also be secondary to trauma. Laboratory confirmation can be obtained by aspirating material, which should be cultured anaerobically. Anaerobes should also be suspected if organisms identified in the exudate on Gram's stain cannot be isolated on culture, assuming that the patient was not taking antibiotics that might have suppressed their growth.

Treatment

Treatment includes both appropriate antibiotic therapy and adequate debridement of devascularized tissue. Antibiotics should be directed toward both aerobic gram-positive and gram-negative organisms as well as anaerobes. Penicillin, or cloxacillin if penicillin-resistant gram-positive organisms such as *S. aureus* are suspected, plus an aminoglycoside such as gentamicin or tobramycin would be appropriate for gram-positive and aerobic gram-negative organisms. The latter play a less important role except in patients with perialimentary tract lesions. *Clostridium perfringens* and *B. melaninogenicus* are penicillin sensitive. *Bacteroides fra-*

gilis is penicillin resistant, and either clindamycin or metronidazole is effective against this group of organisms (Table 19.2).

It needs to be emphasized that antibiotic therapy alone is ineffective and should always be accompanied by surgical debridement of all devitalized tissues associated with the site of infection. The prognosis depends not only on early recognition of mixed infection, but on adequate surgical debridement.

Lymphangitis

Lymphangitis is an inflammation of the lymphatic channel in the deeper subcutaneous tissue. It is usually caused by *S. aureus* or streptococci and rarely by atypical mycobacteria. This disease occurs in all age groups and is most frequent in individuals who are subject to minor trauma or those who have recurrent fungal infections, especially in areas such as between the toes and intertriginous sites. Atypical mycobacteria cause predominantly nodular lesions along the lymphatics, and the erythematous streaking of classic lymphangitis is less obvious.

Diagnosis

These patients have a history of exposure to swimming pools or of contact with fish tanks and tropical fish. The diagnosis is based on clinical signs and symptoms. Linear red streaking on the skin with involvement of the regional lymph nodes is usual, but diffuse erythema can involve an entire limb. There may be peripheral edema associated with the inflammatory process and the site of origin of infection is often not visible. Fever, chills, and leukocytosis are not uncommon, and a bacteremia may be present at the time of initial examination, so blood for cultures should be taken. Laboratory confirmation by culture of aspirates from sites of local inflammation may only be helpful if the lesion is advanced. The diagnosis of atypical mycobacteria usually requires both the history of exposure and an excisional biopsy for acid-fast staining and culture.

Treatment

Presumptive treatment should be directed against penicillinase-producing staphylococci, so cloxacillin is the drug of choice. It should be administered orally in mild cases and intravenously in severe cases.

In chronic lymphangitis or in those clinical situations where the lymphangitis does not respond to usual antibiotic therapy, less common causes of lymphangitis should be considered, including tularemia and atypical mycobacteria. With the latter, local excision may be all that is necessary if only one or two granulomas are present. Patients with more extensive disease may require rifampin and ethambutol. These organisms are often resistant to isoniazid, but may be sensitive to tetracyclines.

Tularemia

Tularemia involving the skin is characterized by significant lymphadenopathy that may precede the lymphangitis streaking along the affected limb. *Francisella tularensis* is the causative organism and there is usually a history of exposure to rabbits or small mammals such as muskrats during the summer and fall seasons. There may be only a history of exposure to animal ticks, however. The lymphangitis is painful and may originate quite peripherally. The lymph node may become fluctuant even after treatment, and drain spontaneously.

In patients with tularemia, confirmation by culture may be too great a hazard in the general laboratory. The diagnosis can be confirmed by serial rise in agglutinating antibodies. A single titer greater than 1 in 80 is also considered diagnostic. If the patient's serology is negative initially, repeat serology should be performed after 10 to 14 days. Streptomycin is the treatment of choice for tularemia (Table 19.2). The lesions can drain spontaneously and slowly resolve over a number of weeks. A repeat course of streptomycin may be necessary if the lesion shows no improvement during initial therapy.

FUNGAL SKIN INFECTIONS

Fungal infections of the skin, like those caused by bacteria, may be focal or diffuse. Superficial fungal infections, including the dermatophytoses, tinea versicolor, and candidiasis, which are the subjects of this section, are the most prevalent skin infections. In North America, it has been estimated that 10% of the population is infected. Therefore a fungal etiology should always be suspected when patients have a mild inflammatory skin infection, especially if it is located in intertriginous zones, interdigital webs, or the nail bed. These infections have a worldwide distribution and can occur in all age groups. There are many clinical infectious syndromes associated with these dermatomycoses and even more antifungal agents presently available. Therefore laboratory diagnosis is essential to confirm the etiology and to choose appropriate therapy. This section concentrates on identifying clinical syndromes and choosing a limited number of agents for therapy.

Focal lesions may mimic bacterial folliculitis. They may be wartlike or appear to be red, boggy nodules called kerion. The latter are more chronic and on biopsy, tissue specimens often show granuloma formation. The presence of an immune response to the fungal agent can also change the clinical picture. When cell-mediated immune responses are active, there may be few fungal elements, but an intense reaction with bright erythema and tenderness. When cell-mediated immunity is compromised there may be abundant fungi but very mild erythema and chronic dermatitis. Individuals in whom cell-mediated immunity is expressed respond much better to therapy and have fewer relapses.

Dermatophytoses or *tinea* fungal infections are superficial and confined to the dead stratified corneum of hair and nails. The genera *Microsporum, Epidermophyton,* and *Trichophyton* are responsible for tinea infections, and fewer than 10 species cause more than 95% of them. These organisms belong to the class Hyphomycetes, which also includes *Sporothrix schenckii* and *Blastomyces dermatitidis*. The fungi are nourished by keratin and inhibited by chemicals from sweat, sebaceous follicle material, and surface fatty acids. This may explain the presence of tinea infections throughout life, with occasional spontaneous resolutions at puberty when the sebaceous glands are hypertrophying. It may also explain the increased number of infections on the soles and palms, which lack sebaceous glands.

The clinical picture of the dermatophytoses infections is related to the anatomic area involved. This is because the keratinizing cornified skin varies from one anatomic site to another. One species, such as *Trichophyton rubrum,* may produce very different clinical signs and symptoms, depending on the infected site. The opposite is also true; namely, many different species may cause similar changes in the same anatomic site such as the foot. The other clinical factor that is important is the portion of the integument involved. Selection of therapy may depend on whether the nails, hair follicles, or glabrous areas of skin are involved. Therefore it is appropriate to consider site rather than etiology in discussing the various clinical manifestations and therapy.

Tinea pedis may affect the web space and may be vesicular, or it may appear as hyperkeratosis. In web space infections and the hyperkeratotic form, topical therapy may be effective, and topical imidazoles such as clotrimazole or miconazole are the drugs of choice. When the vesicular form occurs, topical therapy may aggravate the already tender and weeping lesions, and systemic therapy should be considered.

Tinea corporis may be acute and focal or chronic and extensive. When the skin is acutely inflamed, the use of topical imidazoles is effective. When the lesions are chronic and weeping or when there is extensive involvement of the body surface, oral therapy with griseofulvin or ketoconazole is essential.

Tinea capitis may also be acute and inflammatory or chronic or dry and scaling, the latter indicating a lack of fungal specific cell-mediated immunity. The acute inflammatory type is commonly misdiagnosed as a papilloderma, a condition that may coexist and complicate therapy. Griseofulvin is again the treatment of choice.

Tinea cruris is an intertriginous infection with a more intense inflammation that generally occurs on the edge of the lesion. There are usually no satellite lesions and topical therapy with an imidazole agent is effective.

Tinea barbae is an infection of the beard hair and may be misdiagnosed as a bacterial infection. Topical medications are usually of little value, and systemic antifungals such as griseofulvin or ketoconazole may be required.

Tinea versicolor is a scaling fungal infection of the skin over the thorax and the trunk. This is usually speckled brown, and scraping of the skin removes fine scales and reveals normal skin underneath. A Wood's light examination shows brick-red fluorescence. The causative organism is *Malassezia furfur,* whose short hyphal filaments and clusters of budding forms can be seen under direct microscopic examination. In the presence of small lesions, topical imidazoles may be useful, but for more severe and recalcitrant infections, oral ketoconazole results in more than 95% of patients responding within three weeks.

Sporotrichosis is due to a dimorphic fungus *Sporothrix schenckii* and usually causes small red nodules that extend along the lymphatics, connected by red streaks. These may ulcerate and the patient usually gives a history of contact with thorns, rosebushes, soil, or sphagnum moss.

Candidal infections usually thrive in moist intertriginous areas but can also involve the toes and axillae. Typical intertrigo in the crural area is a densely inflamed, superficial lesion with multiple satellite lesions

TABLE 19.4. Skin Manifestations of Selected Viral and Rickettsial Infections

Skin Lesion	*Pathogen*	*Clinical Disease*
Vesicular rash	Coxsackievirus A16	Hand-foot-and-mouth disease
	Varicella zoster virus	Chicken pox, zoster
Maculopapular rash	Measles virus	Measles
	Rubella virus	German measles
	Coxsackieviruses A9, 16	Hand-foot-and-mouth disease
	Echoviruses 4, 6, 9	Aseptic meningitis
Macular or hemorrhagic rash	*Rickettsia rickettsii*	Spotted fever
	Rickettsia prowazekii	Typhus
Urticaria	Hepatitis B virus	Serum sickness-like illness with hepatitis B

around the periphery. *Candida* along with the dermatophytes may also involve the nail bed. Local clotrimazole therapy may control this, but it does not resolve the problem. Oral ketoconazole may be effective treatment, but at this time no controlled trials have been performed.

The diagnosis of all of these fungal infections requires careful specimen collection and both microscopic and cultural examination. The lesions should be cleansed with saline and then scraped with a scalpel blade to remove the surface cells, which can then be sent for examination. The use of sterile black paper to collect the scrapings is useful since it allows the physician to identify the quantity collected. Examination under high-dry microscopy after the scrapings have been treated with 10% potassium hydroxide to dissolve the keratin allows preliminary identification. This confirms the presence of *Candida* or dermatophytes but does not distinguish between the species. Cultures are especially important when fungal infections are chronic or recurrent and when a noninfectious diagnosis such as hydrosis, neurodermatosis, or atopic and contact dermatitis is being considered.

OTHER SKIN INFECTIONS

A variety of viral and rickettsial infections can manifest as skin lesions in addition to involving other organ systems. Some of these are briefly summarized in Table 19.4.

Warts are focal viral induced tumors caused by a DNA virus of the family Papovaviridae. They are classified as common warts (verrucae vulgaris), flat warts (verrucae plana), plantar warts, and venereal warts (condylomata acuminata). Since they clear spontaneously without scarring, therapy should not be deforming. Topical salicylic acid is the most common therapy for nonvenereal warts and topical podophyllin, 10%, 25%, or 50%, with careful protection of normal skin, provides an effective control for condylomata acuminata.

Several parasitic diseases give a clinical picture of skin infection. They include organisms such as lice, fleas, ticks and mites, cutaneous larva migrans, and fly maggots.

Lice, or Pediculidae, are parasitic for humans and, like fungi, are characterized by the anatomic site in which they settle: corporis, capitis, and pubis. The head louse and pubic louse attach to the hairs in these areas, but the body louse tends to reside attached to fibers of clothing. The parasites have a worldwide distribution and most often affect persons having communal lifestyles. Eradication can be accomplished by application of gamma benzene hexachloride or 25% benzoate creams or lotion to the affected areas. In all cases, personal contacts or sexual partners should be examined and treated if affected, and garments should be washed and cleaned.

Scabies also has a worldwide distribution. The organism, *Sarcoptes scabiei,* lays its eggs in burrows beneath the base of the stratum corneum. They hatch in 72 to 84 hours, emerge, mature, and mate over a 17-day period. They produce intense itching, particularly at night, in the web spaces, penis, and perineal areas. Treatment of scabies is similar to that of pediculosis, although 10% thiabendazole applied topically has also been reported effective.

Miasis is a condition in which the skin serves as a host for certain fly maggots. The lesion is focal, may resemble a furuncle, and the larvae may protrude slightly from the orifice. Surgical excision is the usual therapy.

Cutaneous larva migrans (creeping eruption) is a macerating, highly pruritic skin lesion secondary to larvae of a variety of animal hookworms, with *Ancylostoma braziliense* (a hookworm of dogs and cats) being the most common. The larvae hatch in soil and sandy areas, including children's sandboxes, and penetrate the exposed skin. Any site of the body may be affected, depending on the area in contact with the soil, and all ages are susceptible. The initial symptom is intense pruritus associated with small, raised, erythematous, serpiginous lesions that can move up to 2 cm a day as the larva migrates. There may be single or multiple lesions. Thiabendazole, 25 mg per kg per day, has been shown to be effective in treating cutaneous larva migrans. Topical therapy with thiabendazole, 15% suspended in a hydrosoluble base, can also reduce the pruritus.

Swimmer's itch is the cutaneous response to cercariae of schistosomes (genus *Trichobilharzia*); the adult forms are usually parasitic in birds and small mammals. In North America, the most common schistosome is from migratory birds. The cercariae enter human skin, causing severe pruritus and local erythema. Symptoms resolve spontaneously within 7 to 10 days. Individuals should avoid swimming in contaminated waters.

ANNOTATED BIBLIOGRAPHY

Ferrieri P, Dajani AS, Wannamaker LW, Chapman SS. Natural history of impetigo. Site sequence of acquisition and familiar patterns of spread of cutaneous streptococci. J Clin Invest 1972;51:2851–2862.

A careful study of patterns of spread of infection.

Futsch WC. Therapy of impetigo and furunculosis. JAMA 1970;214:1862–1866.

A concise review of therapy and its rationale.

Hodgkin K. Towards earlier diagnosis in primary care. 4th ed. New York: Churchill-Livingstone, 1978.

A family practitioner's documentation and discussion of his personal practice, pointing out the differences in prevalence of disease entities between hospital and office practice.

Jones HE. Therapy of superficial fungal infection. Med Clin North Am 1982;66:873–893.

A complete review of fungal skin infections, with many references.

Kloos WE, Musselwhite MS. Distribution of *Staphylococcus* and *Micrococcus* species and other aerobic bacteria on human skin. Appl Microbiol 1975;30:381–395.

A microbiologic study of the normal skin flora and its distribution, and a discussion of factors that may influence distribution.

Olsen TG. Therapy of acne. Med Clin North Am 1982;66:851–871.

Very comprehensive, well-referenced review of the current understanding and approach to acne.

20 OCULAR INFECTIONS

David J. McNeely

Primary ocular infections can be classified under four major headings: (1) infections of the lids (blepharitis, hordeolum, chalazion) and lacrimal apparatus (dacryocystitis and dacryoadenitis), (2) conjunctivitis, (3) corneal infections (keratitis), and (4) intraocular infections (endophthalmitis). In addition to primary ocular infections, the eye may be secondarily infected from sinus and central nervous system infections and septicemias because of its close proximity to other structures in the head and the rich supply of intracranial and extracranial blood vessels to the orbit.

INFECTIONS OF THE LIDS AND LACRIMAL APPARATUS

Blepharitis

Blepharitis is a common, chronic, often bilateral inflammation of the lid margins.

Etiology

Staphylococcus aureus and *S. epidermidis* are the organisms cultured most commonly from the lid margins. *Hemophilus duplex* (formerly *Moraxella lacunata*) is recovered from childhood cases of so-called angular blepharitis. In patients who are chronically institutionalized or who have received broad-spectrum antibiotics, gram-negative organisms such as *Pseudomonas aeruginosa* and *Proteus* species are important. Also, after protracted treatment with topical antibiotics, fungi including *Pityrosporon ovale* or *Candida* species may be recovered. The virus of *Molluscum contagiosum* can also cause blepharitis.

Epidemiology

Persons at greatest risk for blepharitis are those who suffer from seborrhea of the eyelashes, scalp, eyebrows, and lateral nares. The disease is also common in debilitated or diabetic patients.

Pathophysiology

The primary problem is seborrhea involving the secretions of the glands of Zeis, which are modified sebaceous glands connected with the hair follicles of the eyelashes. The greasy, scaling secretions obstruct the glands and allow secondary bacterial invasion, similar to that which occurs in acne. With secondary bacterial invasion, ulcers or pustules form along the lid margins. There may be associated conjunctivitis due to the shedding of infected debris under the lid. On careful examination of scrapings of the lid at the base of the lashes, adult forms and eggs of the mite *Demodex folliculorum* have been reported frequently in cases of blepharitis. This mite has also been found with approximately equal frequency in patients without blepharitis, and therefore its role in the pathogenesis of this disease remains uncertain.

Clinical Manifestations

Patients with blepharitis usually have redness, scaling, and itching of the eyelids, with actual loss of the eyelashes in chronic cases. Inasmuch as the disease process is so commonly associated with underlying seborrhea, it often has a chronic history dating back to puberty. If neglected, the reddened lid margins will progress to visible pustules or ulcers. *Hemophilus duplex* blepharitis usually causes a somewhat milder and nonpustular inflammation localized to the medial canthus of the eye. The lesions of the most common viral form of blepharitis, *Molluscum contagiosum,* are small pearllike nodules with an umbilicated center; skin lesions are usually present.

Diagnosis

The diagnosis of blepharitis is made on clinical history and classic appearance of the reddened lid margins. Careful scrapings of the lid margin or swabbing of frank pustules yields material for bacterial and fungal cultures.

Contact dermatitis involving the skin of the lid may mimic blepharitis. This allergic condition is commonly due to a recent change in cosmetics or soaps, or the instillation of intraconjunctival medicines.

Treatment

Therapy consists of frequent warm compresses and careful removal of scales at the lid margin. Although the role of bacterial infection is not entirely clear in this disease, antibacterial ointments and ophthalmic drops, usually containing bacitracin and neomycin, are often used. The ointment is rubbed along the lid margins and the ophthalmic drops are instilled into the conjunctival sac, both applied three or four times a day. In patients in whom staphylococci are continually isolated from blepharitis lesions, the regular use of an antibacterial facial soap may be of some benefit. Conversely, in those patients in whom chronic seborrhea without obvious secondary bacterial infections seems to be the problem, the regular use of an antiseborrheic soap or shampoo containing selenium sulfide may be of some use. If chronic conjunctivitis or frank keratitis develops in the course of therapy, the patient should be referred to an ophthalmologist.

Prognosis

Treatment of blepharitis is often prolonged and the outcome occasionally discouraging. Untreated blepharitis may become a chronic condition, with the subsequent development of hordeola and chalazia.

Prophylaxis

Early diagnosis, good lid hygiene, and adequate treatment of concomitant seborrhea significantly improve the long-term outcome.

Hordeolum and Chalazion

An external hordeolum (sty) is a pyogenic infection of one of the glands of Moll (specialized sweat glands) or Zeis (specialized sebaceous glands) that open onto the anterior skin surface of the lid. An internal hordeolum is an infection of the meibomian gland (modified sebaceous gland) behind the tarsal plate of the lid. Recurrent internal hordeola may result in the formation of a chalazion, a chronic lipogranuloma that occurs in a meibomian gland remnant.

Etiology

The major pathogen is *S. aureus* in all cases with positive cultures. A fairly large number are culture negative.

Pathophysiology

Crusting and obstruction, particularly of the modified sebaceous glands of the lid, are considered the most important predisposing factors in the formation of a hordeolum. Thus many patients with hordeola have an antecedent history of blepharitis.

Clinical Manifestations

A hordeolum is an acutely painful, red, tender swelling on the lid margin. With time, many of these lesions localize and form a typical yellowish head. An external hordeolum, as the name implies, points towards the lid surface or margin. An internal hordeolum, which causes tender swelling of the lid, points toward the inner conjunctival surface. Both lesions may drain spontaneously without medical or surgical treatment.

Diagnosis

The diagnosis of a hordeolum may be made by the acute history and clinical appearance. An attempt should be made to recognize whether the lesion is internal or external. Efforts to isolate a specific etiologic agent from scrapings and cultures of the lid margins are often unsuccessful, despite the established staphylococcal etiology in most cases.

A chalazion is a more chronic and less painful lesion. It often develops subsequent to recurrent episodes of blepharitis and/or hordeola.

Treatment

Management of a hordeolum consists of the application of warm, wet compresses for 15 minutes to the affected lid four times a day. Topical antibiotics (usually a bacitracin or bacitracin-neomycin solution) may be instilled into the conjunctiva in ophthalmologic solutions, especially if there is accompanying blepharitis or secondary conjunctivitis.

Persistence of pain or failure to drain spontaneously are indications for surgical incision and drainage. This can usually be accomplished with local anesthetic as an office procedure in adults. In children, however, a general anesthetic may be required to avoid inadvertent damage to the eye. A chalazion may regress spontaneously but often requires incision and curettage.

Prognosis

While the acute infections usually resolve without sequelae, recurrences of hordeola and subsequent chalazia are not uncommon.

Prophylaxis

Good lid hygiene and management of seborrheic secretions from the specialized lid glands reduce the possibility of recurrence.

Dacryocystitis and Dacryoadenitis

Dacryocystitis is an infection of the lacrimal duct, and dacryoadenitis an infection of the lacrimal sac.

Etiology

The most commonly recovered bacterial agent in these two infections is *S. aureus,* with *Streptococcus pneumoniae* and alpha-hemolytic streptococci isolated less frequently. Rarely, systemic infectious diseases such as tuberculosis and syphilis have been reported to cause chronic dacryocystitis and dacryoadenitis. Epstein-Barr virus may also cause dacryoadenitis as part of infectious mononucleosis.

Pathophysiology

Bacterial dacryocystitis in early infancy is usually secondary to obstruction of a hypoplastic nasal lacrimal duct. In adults, the cause for obstruction is not always clear, although nasal trauma or plugging of the narrow lacrimal duct with epithelial debris and inspissated tears are often cited. The obstructed lacrimal sac becomes colonized with bacteria and then infected.

Systemic infections cause dacryocystitis or dacryoadenitis by bloodstream dissemination.

Clinical Manifestations

Dacryocystitis usually causes a tender swelling at the medial canthus of the eye and is usually more acute and severe in adults than in children. There may be a purulent discharge from the corresponding puncta, and secondary conjunctivitis. Dacryoadenitis produces a tender periorbital swelling in the temporal half of the upper lid.

Diagnosis

The diagnosis of dacryocystitis and dacryoadenitis can be made on the basis of clinical history and physical findings. If the history is acute and there is no associated systemic disease, appropriate material for cultures for bacteria should be taken from the puncta in the medial canthus.

Treatment

Treatment of bacterial dacryocystitis and dacryoadenitis consists of the application of hot compresses and appropriate antibiotics. In infants, topical conjunctival antibiotics are often adequate and spontaneous cannulation of hypoplastic lacrimal ducts often occurs within a week or two. Persistent infections in infants are often successfully managed with a probing of the involved duct and relief of the obstruction.

In adults, systemic antibiotics in the form of oral semisynthetic penicillins or cephalosporins are often necessary in conjunction with topical antibiotics. If warm compresses and antibiotics fail to resolve the process, referral to an ophthalmologist or otolaryngologist should be made.

Prognosis

In most cases, dacryocystitis in the infant is a benign and self-resolving disease. In adults, probing chronically obstructed and infected nasal lacrimal ducts to reestablish normal tear drainage permanently has been notoriously unsuccessful, and chronic tearing and recurrent infections often occur. Occasionally, an extensive surgical procedure (dacryocystorhinostomy) may be undertaken to reestablish normal tear flow into the nasal cavity.

Prophylaxis

No specific prophylactic measures are available.

CONJUNCTIVITIS

The conjunctiva is a thin, transparent mucous membrane that lines the anterior sclera and is continuous over the inner surface of both lids. Infectious conjunctivitis can be classified under five headings: (1) acute purulent, (2) chronic mucopurulent, (3) acute follicular, (4) chronic follicular, and (5) oculoglandular syndromes.

Etiology

The most common etiologic agents responsible for the various types of conjunctivitis are as follows:

1. Acute purulent conjunctivitis (in approximate order of frequency)
   - *S. aureus*
   - *S. pneumoniae*
   - *S. viridans*
   - *S. pyogenes*
   - *H.* sp. *(H. aegyptius)*
   - *Neisseria gonorrhoeae*
   - *H. duplex (Moraxella)*
   - *Neisseria meningitidis*
   - *H. influenzae* type b
   - *E. coli*
   - *Proteus* sp. *(P. mirabilis)*
   - *P. aeruginosa*
2. Chronic mucopurulent conjunctivitis
   - *S. aureus*
   - *H. duplex (Moraxella)*
   - *Candida albicans*
3. Acute follicular conjunctivitis
   - Adenovirus types 3, 4, 8
   - *Chlamydia trachomatis*
   - Herpes simplex
   - Herpes varicella zoster
   - Epstein-Barr virus
   - Newcastle virus
4. Chronic follicular conjunctivitis
   - *C. trachomatis*
   - *Molluscum contagiosum*
5. Oculoglandular conjunctivitis (Parinaud's oculoglandular syndrome)
   - *Francisella tularensis*
   - *Mycobacterium tuberculosis*
   - *Treponema pallidum*
   - Cat-scratch disease
   - *C. trachomatis*
   - *Yersinia pestis*

Epidemiology

Acute Purulent and Chronic Mucopurulent Conjunctivitis

These infections are common in all ages throughout the world. *Staphylococcus aureus* conjunctivitis has no particular seasonal or geographical distribution. Epidemics caused by *S. pneumoniae* or *Hemophilus* species (classically *H. aegyptius*) occur among school-aged children or in family clusters. Outbreaks are often associated with crowding and poor personal hygiene in winter months.

Gonococcal conjunctivitis is most frequently seen in its neonatal form or in sexually active adolescents and young adults. In the neonate, inoculation of the eye occurs during passage through the birth canal, while in the adolescent and adult forms of disease, inoculation from infected urethral, vaginal, or pharyngeal membranes occurs during sexual contact. It has been suggested that in some circumstances, autoinoculation from the patient's own infected genitalia can be the route of an infection. Conjunctivitis due to coliform gram-negative rods usually occurs in debilitated patients, often in those with a preceding history of antibiotic treatment or ocular instrumentation. These pathogens, including *Pseudomonas,* may cause not only conjunctivitis but severe, spreading ocular infections with panophthalmitis and septicemia.

Acute Follicular Conjunctivitis

The acute follicular form of conjunctivitis may occur sporadically or epidemically. Pharyngoconjunctival fever is a contagious adenovirus infection usually spread by aerosol transmission. A number of epidemics have been linked to swimming pools.

Chlamydia trachomatis (immunotypes D to K) causes a sporadic, acute follicular conjunctivitis that is spread by hand contact. Inclusion body conjunctivitis (blenorrhea of neonates) is in fact due to the same species of *C. trachomatis* that causes acute follicular conjunctivitis in older children or adults. This condition can also result from infection with the virus of Newcastle disease that occurs almost exclusively in persons handling live poultry.

Chronic Follicular Conjunctivitis

This disease entity is uncommon in economically developed countries. It is the archetypal form of trachoma disease in the underdeveloped world where different and more sinister immunotypes (A to C) of *C. trachomatis* exist. Trachoma continues to be the most common cause of blindness worldwide.

Oculoglandular Syndromes
Oculoglandular syndromes have a very mixed epidemiology depending upon the etiologic agent ultimately identified.

Pathophysiology

The normal flora of the conjunctiva is variable from person to person and with time in a single individual. The most frequently cultured nonpathogenic commensals are coagulase-negative staphylococci and diphtheroid species. In one study of asymptomatic, unmedicated patients with precataract conditions, over 50% of these older adults were found to have small numbers of coagulase-positive staphylococci or pneumococci in the conjunctiva. In the same population, gram-negative bacilli, especially *Pseudomonas* species, were cultured from asymptomatic conjunctivae in 7%. In another large study, 12% of healthy, asymptomatic young adults were found to have small numbers of fungi in normal conjunctival fluid. *Aspergillus* and *Mucor* species were the most common fungi recovered.

The tears and fluid that wash the conjunctiva are rich in immunoglobulins of both the IgA and IgG fractions. Also bacteriostatic lysozymes in tears make the conjunctival membranes a relatively unfriendly culture medium for many organisms. The development of conjunctivitis after inoculation of an infectious agent onto the conjunctival surface depends, therefore, not only on the virulence of the organism but on the adequacy of host defenses. It is likely that local irritation caused by cosmetics, air pollutants, foreign bodies, or contact lenses plays a role in the production of common forms of bacterial conjunctivitis. Chronic mucopurulent conjunctivitis is usually a bacterial infection associated with chronic blepharitis. It has been suggested that this condition is an allergic reaction to persistent bacterial toxins from the infected lid margins rather than an actual infectious process.

Acute follicular conjunctivitis caused by adenovirus represents infection subsequent to inoculation of virus into the conjunctiva. The virus can only be recovered from involved epithelial surfaces during the symptomatic period. After recovery, there is evidence that type-specific immunity develops. Herpes simplex virus conjunctivitis may represent either a primary infection or relapsing disease process. Herpetic ulcers on the cornea, lid margins, or skin of the mouth and nose may precede or coincide with the development of the conjunctivitis. *Chlamydia trachomatis* produces either an acute or chronic follicular conjunctivitis, and is associated with the presence of intracytoplasmic inclusion bodies in epithelial cells.

Clinical Manifestations

Acute Purulent Conjunctivitis
The onset of acute purulent conjunctivitis is abrupt. The patient complains of severe watering and irritation of the eye and often perceives a foreign body effect. There may be associated photophobia and/or blurring vision in the presence of thick, adhesive, purulent exudate. The patient's eyelids are often adherent and crusted on awakening in the morning. The disease begins unilaterally and inflammation often develops in the other eye within 48 hours. All areas of the conjunctiva are typically hyperemic. There may be petechial hemorrhages present on both the conjunctiva of the inverted lid and the scleral conjunctiva. In children with conjunctivitis due to *Hemophilus influenzae* type b, a bluish tint to the area of infected conjunctiva overlying the sclera has been reported. It is worth mentioning that children with severe forms of *H. influenzae* conjunctivitis may be systemically ill with bacteremia. Metastatic infections such as meningitis or septic arthritis have been reported in this form of conjunctivitis. The purulent conjunctivitis of *Neisseria gonorrhoeae* is described often as hyperacute. The symptoms of this illness progress much more rapidly than other forms of bacterial conjunctivitis. Marked hyperemia and chemosis (edema of the cornea) may be present.

Chronic Mucopurulent Conjunctivitis
This form of conjunctivitis is more insidious in onset. Chronic blepharitis is virtually always present. Thick adhesive morning crusting of the lids is the most common presentation.

Acute Follicular Conjunctivitis
Acute follicular conjunctivitis is variable in signs and symptoms, which are related to the organism producing the infection. In most cases of adenovirus and chlamydial follicular conjunctivitis, the characteristic follicles appear as pale yellow or grey lesions in the conjunctiva, each measuring 0.2 to 2 mm in diameter. Most

cases are unilateral in onset. Pharyngoconjunctival fever, caused by adenovirus, is characterized not only by acute unilateral follicular conjunctivitis but by febrile illness. Pharyngitis, cervical and periauricular lymphadenopathy, and general malaise often are present for part if not all of the 10- to 14-day illness. The acute follicular conjunctivitis of herpes simplex virus may be clinically identified by the association of typical vesicular herpetic lesions on the lid margins and orbital skin. This may be associated with either punctate or dendritic ulcers of the cornea.

Chronic Follicular Conjunctivitis

The archetypal form of this disease is classic trachoma. Fortunately the North American physician is unlikely to see this chronic scarring form of disease with pannus formation in the conjunctiva.

Oculoglandular Conjunctivitis

Oculoglandular forms of conjunctivitis are characterized by unilateral follicular conjunctivitis with marked periauricular and cervical lymphadenopathy malaise and fever. The conjunctival follicles are larger than those of pharyngoconjunctival fever. These granulomatous follicles often have a "yellow-fat" appearance.

Diagnosis

Many noninfectious conditions produce signs and symptoms of conjunctivitis. Irritant chemical exposure, allergic reactions, or the presence of an undetected foreign body should be considered. In cases of severe conjunctivitis with photophobia, chemosis, and eye pain, an ophthalmologist should be consulted early in the investigation. Smears and cultures of the conjunctival discharge should be obtained, whenever possible, prior to treatment. On routine Gram's stain of conjunctival exudates, the predominant inflammatory cell type can be identified. Polymorphonuclear leukocytes suggest a bacterial or, less commonly, fungal etiology. A mixture of polymorphonuclear leukocytes and mononuclear cells suggest a chlamydial infection. Classically, viral conjunctivitis produces a mononuclear cellular response. If bacteria are seen, the predominant population should be noted.

A Giemsa stain should be routinely performed and examined for the presence of typical intracytoplasmic inclusion bodies secondary to chlamydial infection.

Culture specimens of the conjunctiva and lid margin should be obtained prior to the instillation of any topical agents, including anesthetics, into the eye. A sterile, moistened, cotton-tipped applicator should be drawn along the lower lid margin and plated as immediately as possible. Thayer-Martin agar should routinely be employed to isolate *N. gonorrhoeae*.

Viral and chlamydial cultures are not routinely available and are probably indicated only in stubborn cases of complicated conjunctivitis that do not respond to routine treatment.

Treatment

Acute Purulent Conjunctivitis

In the absence of significant local trauma or generalized immunodeficiency, the majority of cases of acute purulent conjunctivitis are ultimately self-limited. Recovery is more rapid with the use of antibiotic therapy, however. For patients who can be treated topically, ointment-based preparations offer most reliable instillation of antibiotics. Unfortunately, ointments may blur vision and therefore ophthalmic antibiotic drops are almost routinely employed in ambulatory patients. "Shotgun" therapy should be avoided if possible and treatment started after appropriate stains and cultures have been done to identify the specific etiologic agent. While many forms of acute purulent conjunctivitis respond well to topical therapy alone, certain of these infections require systemic as well as topical therapy. Because of the risk of panophthalmitis and disseminated systemic infection, *N. gonorrhoeae, S. pyogenes, H. influenzae* type b, and *Pseudomonas* organisms usually require systemic as well as topical therapy. Table 20.1 contains recommendations for topical and systemic therapy for the various bacterial etiologies of acute purulent conjunctivitis. It should be cautioned that chloramphenicol ophthalmic drops have been implicated as causes of fatal bone marrow aplasia. Either sodium sulfacetamide or bacitracin-neomycin ointments are often used empirically when Gram's stain results are equivocal and results of cultures not yet available.

Chronic Mucopurulent Conjunctivitis

Since chronic mucopurulent conjunctivitis often occurs in patients with blepharitis, it is managed by treatment of the latter condition.

Acute Follicular Conjunctivitis

Acute follicular conjunctivitis, if caused by *Chlamydia* (intracytoplasmic inclusion bodies), should be treated

TABLE 20.1. Topical Therapy of Acute Purulent Conjunctivitis

Etiology	*Drug of Choice*	*Alternative(s)*
S. aureus	Bacitracin	Erythromycin estolate, framycetin, gentamicin
S. pneumoniae	Bacitracin	Erythromycin estolate, sodium sulfacetamide
S. viridans	Bacitracin	Erythromycin estolate, sodium sulfacetamide
*S. pyogenes**	Bacitracin	Erythromycin estolate, sodium sulfacetamide
H. aegyptius	Sodium sulfacetamide	Gentamicin, neomycin, tetracycline
*N. gonorrhoeae**	Erythromycin estolate	Tetracycline
H. duplex (*Moraxella*)	Sodium sulfacetamide	Erythromycin estolate, tetracycline
N. meningitidis	Erythromycin estolate	Tetracycline
*H. influenzae**	Sodium sulfacetamide	Gentamicin, neomycin, tetracycline
E. coli	Gentamicin	Framycetin, neomycin, polymixin
P. mirabilis	Gentamicin	Framycetin, neomycin, polymixin
*P. aeruginosa**	Gentamicin	Framycetin, neomycin, polymixin

*Simultaneous systemic antibiotic therapy with appropriate agent(s) is prudent.

with sulfacetamide. Suspected or proven cases of chlamydial inclusion body conjunctivitis that do not rapidly resolve or relapse after topical therapy should be treated with 2–3 weeks of oral tetracycline or sulfa drugs.

Viral conjunctivitis is treated supportively with astringent drops and cold soaks for relief of symptoms. Herpes simplex conjunctivitis should be treated in association with an ophthalmologist. The presence of any associated keratitis demands specific antiviral therapy (topical idoxuridine or vidarabine).

Occuloglandular Conjunctivitis

Patients with various forms of the oculoglandular syndrome should be treated as is appropriate for the systemic infections that cause this unusual form of conjunctivitis.

The use of local anesthetics or steroids in ophthalmic drops is potentially hazardous and should be avoided if possible, in the management of all forms of conjunctivitis.

Prognosis

Most cases of acute purulent conjunctivitis are self-limited. Bacterial conjunctivitis due to agents such as *N. gonorrhoeae, S. pyogenes,* and *H. influenzae* type B require systemic therapy but have a good prognosis.

Acute follicular conjunctivitis caused by various species of adenovirus resolves spontaneously without sequelae over a period of one to two weeks. The course and prognosis of herpetic conjunctivitis depend on the presence or absence of associated keratitis. If hepatitis is present, then a more severe form of herpes infection exists, and chronic and recurrent disease may develop.

Chlamydia-caused inclusion conjunctivitis characteristically resolves more slowly than do bacterial infections. If treatment is delayed or inadequate, the chronic form of disease may develop and necessitate several months of both topical and systemic antibiotics such as sulfonamides or tetracyclines. The prognosis then depends upon the diligence of the physician and the compliance of the patient. The outcome of these chronic forms of follicular conjunctivitis in North America is still good. Trachoma-like illness is distinctly unusual with the immunotypes of *C. trachomatis* organisms extant in North America.

KERATITIS

The cornea is a 1-mm thick, avascular, transparent extension of the sclera. Its exterior surface is lined with stratified squamous epithelium while the internal surface is lined by flat endothelial-like cells.

Etiology

Bacterial Keratitis

Bacterial keratitis, or corneal infection, may be caused by *S. aureus, S. pneumoniae, Ps. aeruginosa, H. du-*

plex (Moraxella lacunata), S. pyogenes, and *N. gonorrhoeae*.

Viral Keratitis

The most common cause of severe corneal ulceration in North America is herpes simplex virus. Other herpesviruses, in particular herpes zoster, can produce a superficial form of keratitis but progression to subepithelial involvement and ulceration is uncommon.

Fungal Keratitis

A variety of fungal pathogens can cause keratitis but the most common in North America are those caused by *Fusarium* species, specifically *Fusarium solanae*.

Epidemiology

Superficial forms of keratitis frequently occur in conjunction with severe bacterial or viral conjunctivitis, and the epidemiology follows the pattern of those diseases. Patients with poor nutrition and poor personal hygiene are likely to progress from conjunctivitis to more severe forms of corneal involvement. Bacterial corneal ulcers commonly develop subsequent to abrasions, foreign body trauma, or corneal burns. Comatose patients in hospital intensive care units who develop desiccated corneas are at particular risk for *Pseudomonas* corneal ulcers.

Pathophysiology

Bacterial Keratitis

The exterior surface of the cornea is lined with stratified squamous epithelium that protects the deeper layers. Therefore even in severe cases of bacterial infections of the conjunctiva and superficial cornea, rarely is there progression to destruction of the corneal epithelium and ulceration. Bacterial infections generally progress to produce corneal ulcers secondary to major or minor trauma that interrupts the superficial epithelial layer of the cornea. This trauma may be obvious, as in the case of a corneal abrasion or foreign body penetration. In other circumstances, interruption of the corneal membrane may be caused by something so apparently benign as a small piece of grit rubbed into the eye. Once bacterial infection gains access to the avascular stroma of the cornea, bacterial proteases cause destruction and ultimate scarring.

Viral Keratitis

Herpes simplex involvement of the cornea may occur in the course of either a primary or recurrent herpes infection. In the primary infection, lesions may remain superficial, producing only a fine, punctate, epithelial keratitis that usually clears in a period of days to weeks without scar formation. In other patients, however, progression during this first infection to the classic deep and spreading dendritic ulcers may occur. Whatever its course, as many as 20% of patients with culture-proved primary ocular herpes have recurrent attacks of herpetic keratitis. The location of the virus during periods of latency is not entirely clear. Inferential evidence suggests that the virus resides in the sensory ganglion of the fifth cranial nerve and spreads centrifugally during periods of reactivation. The recurrent attacks are often characterized by severe corneal edema and necrosis of epithelial cells, with formation of deep branching ulcers.

Fungal Keratitis

The pathophysiology of fungal ulcers is probably very similar to that of bacterial corneal ulcers. It is likely that physical or chemical trauma to the epithelial membranes allows deeper penetration of the fungal pathogens.

Clinical Manifestations

Bacterial Keratitis

The symptoms of most cases of superficial keratitis are related to, or overshadowed by, the accompanying conjunctivitis. In patients with bacterial corneal ulcers, there may be intense local pain and irritation giving rise to the sensation of a corneal foreign body. Blurred vision and the presence of cells in the anterior ocular chamber (hypopyon) should also alert the physician to the possibility of a bacterial corneal ulcer.

Viral Keratitis

Primary herpes simplex ocular infection is usually unilateral and often accompanied by malaise, fever, and viremia. The eye is initially red and irritated, with a watery discharge and typical follicular conjunctivitis. Mucocutaneous vesicular lesions may also be present. Recurrent herpes keratitis often begins with a small row of vesicles in the central cornea. The underlying epithelium is destroyed, producing the classic, dendritic, superficial ulcer pattern. When deeper layers of the interstitial stroma are penetrated, anterior uveitis accompanied by symptoms of pain, tearing, photophobia, and blurred vision often result.

Fungal Keratitis
Fungal keratitis is classically a chronic process. The patient may have no severe localized eye symptoms, but complain only of increased tearing. On examination, the ulcer is often elevated and shaggy in appearance with a surrounding halo of stroma infiltrate.

Diagnosis

The diagnosis of corneal ulcers should be as specific as possible and usually requires the help of an ophthalmologist. The classic ulcer morphology of herpetic or fungal corneal ulcers may be recognized. For suspected bacterial infection, corneal scrapings of the ulcer base are obtained for culture, sensitivity, and cytologic examination. These scrapings should be obtained by an ophthalmologist and transported immediately to the microbiology laboratory.

Treatment

Bacterial Keratitis
Superficial forms of keratitis are treated similarly to the associated conjunctivitis. Bacterial corneal ulcers may be treated with the aggressive application of topical antibiotics, preferably in an ointment base, to assure persistence of active drug over the cornea. At the inception of therapy for an ulcer presumed to be bacterial but before corneal scraping cultures are available, a broad-spectrum antibacterial ointment containing bacitracin, polymyxin, and neomycin is often recommended. Once an etiology has been determined, one should treat the bacterial process with specific antibiotics, as is outlined for bacterial conjunctivitis in Table 20.1. In severe cases of rapidly progressive corneal ulceration, particularly where *S. pneumoniae, N. gonorrhoeae,* or *P. aeruginosa* is suspected or proved, parenteral therapy should be administered as well.

Viral Keratitis
Several agents are now available for the topical treatment of herpes simplex virus keratitis. Once again, they are best used in ointment base applied five to six times a day into the lower conjunctival sac. Idoxuridine, available for many years, was generally effective but often accompanied by ocular discomfort and allergic reactions. In several authors' experience, vidarabine is better tolerated than idoxuridine and may offer a slightly better outcome. Both of these drugs penetrate poorly into deeper stromal layers of the cornea and not at all into the anterior chamber of the eye. In patients with severe stromal involvement and/or uveitis, systemic therapy with intravenous vidarabine is probably indicated. Surgical debridement may be necessary in some cases for removal of corneal scar tissue. This is not generally necessary when superficial dendritic herpetic ulcers are quickly treated.

Fungal Keratitis
Keratomycoses are generally treated with topical antifungal agents including dilute suspensions of nystatin or amphotericin. A number of reports of resistant *Fusarium* infections from the southeastern United States have indicated the worth of a new agent, natamycin (pimaricin) used as a topical 5% optic solution.

Prognosis

The prognosis for superficial keratitis, whatever the etiology, is almost routinely excellent. Primary herpetic keratitis usually heals with little scarring, but treatment does not prevent future recurrence. Unfortunately, in patients with recurrent attacks or in those who are treated late in the course of an individual attack of herpetic keratitis, deep corneal scarring may develop with loss of vision.

Bacterial corneal ulcers if treated early and aggressively have an acceptable response rate. Unfortunately, in elderly and debilitated patients with severe ulcers due to *Pseudomonas* organisms or, less commonly, pneumococci, rapid progression to ocular perforation and loss of the eye may occur despite appropriate treatment. Keratomycoses are often difficult to treat, requiring long courses of topical antifungal antibiotics and often surgical debridement of corneal scar tissue.

INTRAOCULAR INFECTIONS

An infection of the anterior chamber of the eye (aqueous humor) or the posterior chamber of the eye behind the lens apparatus (vitreous humor) is a catastrophic occurrence. Formerly, attempts were made to differentiate infections in these two spaces for the purposes of treatment and prognosis. Today it is recognized that isolated infections of one or other of these anatomic spaces are unusual. Hence the term endophthalmitis is usually employed to describe any intraocular infection. Despite aggressive medical and surgical management of these infections, the outcome is often dismal.

Etiology

Endophthalmitis may arise either secondary to inoculation of organisms intraorbitally or by metastatic blood-borne spread. Endophthalmitis following eye surgery or trauma is most frequently due to *S. aureus, S. epidermidis, E. coli,* or *P. aeruginosa*. On occasion *Candida* species may be introduced postsurgically. Metastatic endophthalmitis may occur in patients with severe systemic infections due to streptococci, *S. pneumoniae, S. aureus,* rarely, enteric gram-negative rods, or *N. meningitidis*. With increasing numbers of immunosuppressed patients suffering *Candida* sepsis, more and more cases of metastatic blood-borne candidal endophthalmitis are reported.

Epidemiology

Most cases of endophthalmitis today occur in patients who have undergone ophthalmologic surgery. Insertion of an intraocular foreign body such as a lens replacement significantly increases this risk.

Pathophysiology

Once viable replicating organisms are introduced into the anterior or posterior chamber of the eye, bacterial toxins mediate a severe inflammatory response. The migration of white cells and the formation of purulent exudates irreparably damage delicate intraocular structures. Even with successful antimicrobial therapy, scarring and retraction of the vitreous routinely result in severe disturbance of vision.

Clinical Manifestations

Most cases of endophthalmitis arise after surgery or penetrating trauma to the eye. In a patient known to have systemic blood-borne infection, one should also be alert to the acute development of metastatic endophthalmitis. The most important clinical features of the condition are severe pain in the eye with hyperemia and swelling of the globe. In postoperative or posttraumatic bacterial infection, these symptoms appear suddenly within 24 to 48 hours and progress rapidly. Blurring of the vision, edema of the cornea, and often lid edema and generalized swelling of the entire orbit are present. This generalized orbital inflammation is often called panophthalmitis. The onset of metastatic fungal ophthalmitis may be very much more insidious and gradual, often taking two weeks to become clinically evident. Early in the development of candidal ophthalmitis, before the lesions break through into the vitreous, focal white lesions appear in the retina and choroid layers.

Diagnosis

Specific etiologic diagnosis of postoperative or posttraumatic endophthalmitis requires bacteriologic samples from the inner chambers of the eye. There is conjecture in the literature as to whether anterior chamber or vitreous aspiration samples should be obtained. It should be emphasized, however, that conjunctival or scleral wound cultures are not adequate to diagnose the agent causing an endophthalmitis. Many cases of metastatic endophthalmitis, whether bacterial or fungal, can be diagnosed by associated positive blood cultures.

Treatment

Patients with endophthalmitis must be immediately hospitalized and treated with maximum doses of parenteral antibiotics. Topical antibiotics are routinely applied to the conjunctival sac but their worth in managing this disease is questionable. It is now well demonstrated that many antibiotics routinely employed in the treatment of serious bacterial and fungal infections do not penetrate intraocular structures well. There is evidence that penicillin and cephalosporin antibiotics do, in fact, penetrate the anterior chamber of the eye in reasonable concentrations, but not the posterior vitreous space.

Given the dismal outcome with systemic and conjunctival antibiotics, various methods of direct instillation have been tried. Subconjunctival antibiotics while easy to administer do not, apparently, penetrate well into the posterior chamber of the eye. Some authors report improved outcome with injection of antibiotics into the sub-Tenon's capsule. Tenon's capsule is the fibrous reflection over the posterior sclera that is continuous with the tendinous insertion of ocular muscles. More recently, with the development of vitrectomy procedures, a small number of patients have apparently been benefited by a combination of vitrectomy aspiration of infected pus in the vitreous space and the direct instillation of small aliquots of semisynthetic penicillins, cephalosporins, and aminoglycosides. Unfortunately, the number of patients so treated is too small to recommend routine vitrectomy drainage and intraocular antibiotic instillation for bacterial endophthalmitis.

Candidal endophthalmitis if diagnosed early, before the choroid and retinal lesions have spread to involve the entire vitreous, should be treated with intravenous amphotericin B. Treatment at this stage is usually accompanied by a reasonably good outcome.

Prognosis

Unfortunately, most patients with endophthalmitis experience severe visual loss. The postinflammatory organization of infected vitreous material often results in contraction and distortion of the eye (phthisis bulbi). Either for cosmetic reasons or because systemic and local antibiotics cannot eradicate continuing infection, many patients require enucleation.

Prophylaxis

Careful sterile technique in the ophthalmologic surgical suite and the use of preoperative and intraoperative topical conjunctival prophylactic antibiotics are of proved worth in reducing postsurgical endophthalmitis. Although many ophthalmologists routinely employ parenteral perioperative prophylactic antibiotics, usually either a semisynthetic penicillin or a cephalosporin, there is a dearth of carefully controlled prospective trials that demonstrate the value of this. Many ophthalmologists use prophylactic parenteral antibiotics in the acute management of penetrating ocular foreign bodies in the hope of preventing subsequent endophthalmitis. It is difficult to condemn short courses in these circumstances, given the relatively poor outcome of treatment of established endophthalmitis.

ANNOTATED BIBLIOGRAPHY

Dawson CR, Hanna L, Wood TR, et al. Adenovirus type 8 keratoconjunctivitis in the United States. Epidemic, clinical and microbiological features. Am J Ophthalmol 1970; 69:473–480.

This article reviews the clinical and laboratory observations made in a series of patients with virus culture proven adenovirus acute follicular conjunctivitis. The potential for epidemic hand to eye transmission in "closed" population groups is highlighted.

Grayston JJ, Wang S. New knowledge of *Chlamydia* and the diseases they cause. J Infect Dis 1975; 132:87–105.

This paper is a comprehensive review of the oculogenital infections now recognized to be secondary to *Chlamydia trachomatis*. The relationship between various immunotypes of *C. trachomatis* and the character and severity of ocular infection is set out.

Laibson PR. Herpes simplex; annual review: cornea and sclera. Arch Ophthalmol 1970; 83:637–655.

The epidemiology, pathogens, clinical presentation, and outcome of *herpes simplex* virus infections of the cornea and sclera are covered in this review article. The concepts of latent neurotropic virus and viral reactivation are succinctly explained.

Perkins R, Kundsin RB, Pratt M, et al. Bacteriology of normal and infected conjunctiva. J Clin Microbiol 1975; 1:147–149.

The results of aerobic and anaerobic cultures from 100 normals and 275 patients with acute purulent conjunctivitis are presented. *Staphylococcus aureus* and various Streptococcal species are the most frequently recovered "pathogens" in cases of acute purulent conjunctivitis.

Peyman GA, Vastine DW, Crouch ER, et al. Clinical use of intravitreal antibiotics to treat bacterial endophthalmitis. Trans Am Acad Ophthalmol Otolaryngol 1974; 78:862–867.

An early but classic paper arguing the need for intraocular antibiotics in bacterial endophthalmitis.

Thygeson P. Complications of staphylococcal blepharitis. Am J Ophthalmol 1969; 68:446–449.

This is a concise review of the acute and chronic complications of staphylococcal blepharitis. The presumed pathogenesis of hordeola and chalazia are outlined.

Wilson LA. Bacterial corneal ulcers. In Duane TD, ed. Clinical ophthalmology. Vol. 4. Hagerstown, Md.:

Harper & Row, 1976:1–19.

This chapter in a standard text of ophthalmology provides an excellent review of the etiology, clinical presentation, and management of this most severe form of bacterial corneal infection. The need for fastidious bacterial cultures and the correct method of obtaining samples are illustrated.

Wilson LA. Bacterial conjunctivitis. In Duane TD, ed. Clinical ophthalmology. Vol. 4. Hagerstown, Md.: Harper & Row, 1976:1–16.

This text chapter is a comprehensive and well illustrated review of the clinical features, microbiology, and antibiotic management of bacterial conjunctivitis.

III SPECIFIC CLINICAL SYNDROMES

21 FEVER OF UNCERTAIN ORIGIN

Thomas J. Marrie

For centuries before the introduction of the thermometer in the 1850s, fever was recognized as a sign of disease. The normal highest daily temperature is widely quoted as 37°C (98.6°F) orally or 37.7°C (99.6°F) rectally. It is not surprising that, as with many other bodily functions, a circadian temperature rhythm is present in humans regardless of geographic region or changes in environment. Changes in daily body temperature vary with age and sex: maximal temperature tends to be lower in elderly persons than in young adults; young women have greater fluctuations from morning to evening than do young men. The normal diurnal variation can range from 35.5°C to 37.8°C orally, with the peak temperature occurring about 6:00 P.M. each day. Many women have peak daily temperatures of 37.8°C during the two weeks prior to start of menstruation.

PATHOPHYSIOLOGY

Before considering fever of uncertain origin, it is appropriate to consider temperature regulation, the mechanism(s) of production of fever, and its beneficial and harmful effects.

Physiologic muscle activity produces the major portion of basal heat production and can serve as an emergency source of heat (a 100% to 200% increase is possible). Exaggerated muscle activity is seen clinically as shivering or rigors. Metabolic activity also produces a small amount of heat as a consequence of the less than perfect conversion of energy to work.

Heat is lost through radiation, evaporation, conduction, and convection, the first two only being under physiologic control. Heat loss by radiation is regulated by cutaneous vasoconstriction and vasodilation; evaporation of 1 liter of sweat results in the loss of 580 calories, and the rate of sweating can be increased up to 3 liters per hour. By this means, body temperature can be lowered 5 to 6°C through the loss of 1% of body weight in water.

The control mechanism appears to be a temperature-sensitive region of the preoptic area of the anterior hypothalamus, which balances heat production and heat loss. Various exogenous pyrogens (microorganisms, antigen-lymphocyte interactions) will induce the production and release of leukocyte or macrophage-endogenous pyrogen. Although phagocytosis is complete in 30 to 40 minutes, endogenous pyrogen is not produced from leukocytes until 4 hours later, indicating that new protein synthesis has to occur. Interaction of sensitized T lymphocytes with an antigen results in the release of a lymphokine, which stimulates monocytes or peripheral macrophages to release endogenous pyrogen. Monocytes produce 20 to 40 times more endogenous pyrogen per cell than the human blood neutrophil. Certain tumors, such as hypernephromas, and spleen cells from patients with Hodgkin's disease have also been shown to release endogenous pyrogen.

The effective moiety of endogenous pyrogen appears to be monomer with a molecular weight of 15,000 daltons and can be measured by a radioimmunoassay. The mechanism whereby endogenous pyrogen resets the thermoregulatory center is still to be elucidated, but the antipyretic effect of inhibitors of prostaglandin synthesis, combined with the knowledge that prostaglandin E_1 (PGE_1) and PGE_2 produce prompt fever when injected into the anterior hypothalamus, and that increased levels of prostaglandins have been measured in the cerebrospinal fluid (CSF) during fever, strongly suggests a major role for these products. Prostaglandin mediated by serotonin and norepinephrine probably increases cyclic adenosine monophosphate (AMP) in the anterior hypothalamus, which stimulates the cells of the thermoregulatory center, producing vasoconstriction (heat conservation), increased muscle activity (increased heat production), and fever. Thus fever can be defined as an elevated thermoregulatory set point.

While very little is known about the precise events leading to resetting of the thermoregulatory center, even less is known about factors responsible for returning the elevated temperature set point toward normal. There may be an endogenous cryogen, a substance that is naturally produced and that both lowers normal body temperature and attenuates fevers. Many fluctuations in body temperature during both health and disease states may involve some interplay between endogenous pyrogens and endogenous cryogens.

The beneficial effects of fever are not clearly defined, but are felt to include:

1. Potentiation of the antiviral actions of interferon.
2. Potentiation and enhancement of the cellular immune responses.
3. Increase in leukocyte mobility.
4. Enhancement of the bactericidal activity of leukocytes.
5. Decreased lysosome stability.
6. Decrease in plasma iron concentration. This effect may be due to endogenous pyrogen. An elevated plasma iron concentration has been shown to result in the increased severity of infections. In vitro decreased plasma iron levels, coupled with an elevation in temperature, results in a significant reduction in the growth rate of various pathogenic bacteria.
7. Increased survival rate (in infected experimental animals).

Many effects of fever may be harmful to the host, including:

1. Nitrogen loss, shifts of iron and zinc, amino acid redistribution from muscle, and a significant increase in caloric consumption to fuel the febrile response.
2. A 13% increase in oxygen consumption plus increase in heart rate of 16 beats per minute for each 1°C rise in body temperature. These two effects may be harmful to the febrile patient with heart disease; however, failure of the pulse rate to increase appropriately in febrile patients is a physical finding that should raise the possibility of factitious fever in a patient with fever of uncertain origin (FUO).
3. Loss of fluid and electrolytes due to increased sweating.
4. Hyperventilation leading to respiratory alkalosis in some patients.
5. Systemic symptoms of malaise, drowsiness, fatigue, and myalgia. Why some febrile patients experience these symptoms and others do not is unknown.
6. Lowered threshold for generalized seizures, especially in children.

Definition

Most febrile illnesses are self-limited. In the majority of instances in which a patient consults a physician because of fever, history and physical findings lead to the diagnosis. A small number of patients manifest persistent fever as their only sign of disease. If the following criteria are fulfilled, a diagnosis of fever of uncertain origin is justified:

1. Illness of longer than three weeks' duration. This eliminates most of the acute, self-limited (usually viral) infectious diseases.
2. Temperature over 101°F (38.3°C) on several occasions. This eliminates the entity of habitual hyperthermia where the temperature elevations are lower.
3. Diagnosis uncertain after one week of study in hospital. This allows completion of the usual laboratory studies made initially in attempts to identify the cause of a febrile illness.

A physician in family practice will probably encounter one such patient every three to four years.

ETIOLOGY

While there are over 100 documented causes of fever of unexplained (uncertain, unknown) origin, a compilation of several series (Table 21.1) shows that infections account for about 40% of all causes, neoplastic diseases 20%, connective tissue diseases 15% and miscellaneous conditions 15%; 10% remain undiagnosed. It is very important to remember that the most frequent causes of FUO are actually common diseases that manifest themselves in an atypical manner.

TABLE 21.1. Categories of Causes of Fever of Uncertain Origin in Different Age Groups

Cause	*Children (%)*		*Adults (%)*	*Elderly Adults (%)*
	<6 yrs	*>6 yrs*		
Infection	60	37	40	36
Neoplastic disease	8	4	20	24
Collagen-vascular disease	8	22	15	25
Miscellaneous	14	16	15	10
Undiagnosed	10	21	10	5

EPIDEMIOLOGY

The causes of FUO in children are different from those in adults. In children younger than 6 years, infection is generally the cause, while in those older than 6 years, infections, juvenile rheumatoid arthritis (Still's disease), or inflammatory bowel disease are the major causes. Tuberculosis and intraabdominal infections, common sources of FUO in adults, are uncommon in children. In elderly adults, giant cell arteritis and intraabdominal abscesses are the most common etiologies.

Data from an study of 347 patients with long-term FUO (75% had fever of more than one year's duration) reveal a different spectrum. One of the most important findings was that 27% were not febrile (i.e., their temperature range was within the normal diurnal variation, but because the peak was above 37°C, both the patients and their primary physicians felt they had a fever) and had no evidence of ongoing disease. No diagnosis could be made despite an extensive work-up in another 29%. Other causes included factitious fever in 9%, idiopathic granulomatous hepatitis in 13%, juvenile rheumatoid arthritis in adults in 9%, (adult-onset Still's disease), and familial Mediterranean fever 4%.

FACTITIOUS FEVER

Factitious fever is discussed first because it should always be considered before one embarks on extensive investigations. Diagnostic clues include the following:

1. Failure of the temperature to follow a diurnal variation
2. Rapid defervescence unaccompanied by diaphoresis
3. Temperatures of 42°C or greater
4. Absence of tachycardia in association with fever
5. Normal physical examination
6. Normal laboratory studies
7. Normal oral and rectal temperatures when these measurements are made under careful supervision

Patients with factitious fever are often medical or paramedical personnel and their methods of producing fever (real or apparent) are ingenious. Switching thermometers, rubbing the thermometer briskly between the fingers, and warming the thermometer with water are obvious and are usually readily detected. There is a linear relationship between oral and urinary temperature and a nomogram has been developed that allows one to confirm or refute the oral temperature by measuring the temperature of the urine. Much more difficult to detect are persons who are infecting themselves by any one of a variety of methods, in which case the above diagnostic clues may not be appropriate.

Case Report

A 31-year-old pediatric nurse was admitted to hospital because of FUO and recurrent polymicrobial bacteremia. Six weeks previously she developed an infection of her right elbow (secondary to trauma) for which she was admitted to a local hospital. The elbow infection resolved but she developed chills and temperatures of 39 to 40°C that persisted for five weeks. Cultures from blood drawn on five occasions over a ten-day period grew (1) diphtheroids and *Staphylococcus epidermidis;* (2) *S. aureus,* diphtheroids, *Bacteroides bivius,* and *Bacteroides* sp.; (3) diphtheroids and *Enterobacter cloacae;* (4) *Fusobacterium symbiosum* and *B. malaninogenicus;* and (5) *Escherichia coli* and enterococcus. All other investigations were negative. On admission to our hospital, she looked well, and parenteral antibiotic therapy that had been started in her local hospital was discontinued. Initially, both she and her husband stated that they had absolutely no emotional problems. In view of the unusual polymicrobial bacteremias and suspected self-infection, a search of the patient's room was done while she was out and revealed a needle and a syringe that contained dried blood. When informed of the suspected diagnosis, the patient's husband admitted to serious problems in their marriage. With the help of a psychiatrist, the patient was confronted with our suspicions and, over the next few days, admitted that she had mixed saliva in her hand and drawn it up in the syringe and then injected it into her intravenous line through the injection port.

This case illustrates the common epidemiologic setting (i.e., a medical or paramedical person) who is otherwise well, and unusual bacteriology (polymicrobial bacteremias) that are seen in self-inflicted infections.

INFECTION

Infection is the most common cause of FUO. The following is a list of infections that should be considered:

1. Common
   - Tuberculosis
   - Infective endocarditis
   - Intraabdominal abscesses
   - Perinephric abscesses
   - Osteomyelitis
   - Biliary tract infections
   - Dental abscesses
   - Cytomegalovirus
   - Epstein-Barr virus
2. Uncommon
   - Q fever
   - Brucellosis
   - Salmonellosis, typhoidal and nontyphoidal
   - Toxoplasmosis
   - Disseminated mycosis (histoplasmosis, coccidioidomycosis, blastomycosis)
   - Tularemia
   - Psittacosis
   - Typhus
   - Relapsing fever
   - Chronic meningococcemia

Tuberculosis

Tuberculosis is a frequent cause of FUO and this may be the initial manifestation of miliary tuberculosis. In such cases, the chest roentgenogram is often negative when the patient is initially evaluated; however, numerous small nodules usually are present when the x-ray is repeated two to four weeks later. Careful examination of the retina for choroid tubercules may be an important clue to the diagnosis. Reports of diagnostic usefulness of liver biopsies in this disease vary, with granulomas being found in 23% to 100% of cases. Biopsies of bone marrow reveal granulomas less frequently (16% to 33%) than liver biopsies, but on occasion may be positive when liver biopsy is negative and are less hazardous. The Mantoux test is negative in up to 40% of patients with miliary tuberculosis. The test is usually positive when repeated after treatment has begun and the patient's clinical and nutritional status have improved.

Tuberculosis of the spine may also cause a FUO some weeks to months before changes can be demonstrated in the vertebrae radiographically or by radionuclide scanning techniques.

Tuberculous peritonitis in the patient with so-called alcoholic hepatitis is a common diagnostic problem. The fever is usually attributed to the alcoholic hepatitis and the ascites is attributed to cirrhosis. In such patients the ascitic fluid should always be aspirated and cultured and, if an exudate is present, a diagnosis of tuberculous peritonitis should be pursued.

The following case report illustrates the atypical manner in which tuberculosis may occur and also demonstrates that all patients with a pleural effusion and FUO should have several pleural biopsies for histology and culture, and the fluid aspirated for chemical analysis, cell count, culture, cytology, and an LE cell preparation. Culture of the pleural fluid alone will diagnose tuberculous pleurisy in about 20% of cases, whereas culture of the fluid and of the biopsy specimen and histology yields a diagnosis of tuberculosis in up to 85% of cases.

Case Report

A 27-year-old male developed a subacute illness characterized by progressive fatigue, decreased energy, anorexia, night sweats (at least twice per week), and a 15-pound weight loss beginning four months prior to admission to hospital. Three weeks before admission, he developed chills and rigors, followed one week later by myalgia, arthralgia, diarrhea (after a course of ampicillin), and a sore throat. Toward the end of the second week of this illness, he developed a dry cough and severe fatigue. A chest roentgenogram showed bilateral pleural effusions. He remained febrile and no diagnosis was made in his local hospital. Therefore he was transferred to our hospital where he was moderately ill, with an oral temperature of 38.6°C and a large right pleural effusion. His abdomen was diffusely tender to palpation. Admission laboratory data included: hemoglobin 127 gm per liter, white blood cell count 5.3×10^9 per liter, with a differential of 90% polymorphonuclear leukocytes, 4% monocytes, an erythrocyte sedimentation rate (ESR) of 90 mm per hour.

Repeat physical examination a few days later revealed free abdominal fluid and a pericardial friction rub. The pleural fluid was aspirated on three occasions over the two weeks and biopsies of the pleura were carried out on each occasion. The pleural fluid contained 5.0×10^9 per liter of white blood cells (53% polymorphonuclear leukocytes, 36% lymphocytes, 11% monocytes), protein concentration of 52 gm per liter, and sugar of 4.6 mmol per liter. His attending physicians felt he had collagen-vascular disease, so prednisone was given for three days before it was discontinued because of concern about tuberculosis. Skin testing with 5 tuberculin units of purified protein derivative-S *Candida,* and trichophyton antigens gave no reaction. A granuloma was found in the third biopsy and eventually *M. tuberculosis* was isolated. The pleural effusion had resolved before therapy with isoniazid and rifampin was begun.

This report illustrates the diversity of the clinical manifestations of tuberculosis and the difficulty in diagnosis, and reaffirms the utility of pleural biopsy.

Infective Endocarditis

Most cases of infective endocarditis do not meet the definition of FUO; however, in nearly all series, this illness remains an important cause of FUO. The diagnosis of infective endocarditis may be difficult when secondary complications such as metastatic infection, immune complex disease, and embolic phenomena become the primary focus of the clinician's attention (see Case Report below). In the setting where endocarditis is suggested and blood cultures are negative (culture-negative endocarditis), the causes given in Chapter 10, page 138 should be considered and the appropriate blood culture media and serologic tests used. In such instances, the laboratory should be advised regarding the possible diagnosis so that the blood cultures can be kept for three weeks and the chocolate agar subculture plates can be incubated in 10% carbon dioxide. This measure combined with careful inspection of blood cultures for granular colonies on the glass at the blood-broth interface should detect slow-growing, fastidious, gram-negative bacteria. Q fever, diagnosed by serologic tests is one of the causes of endocarditis in which immune complex manifestations dominate the clinical picture — arthralgia, clubbing of the fingers, hepatosplenomegaly, glomerulonephritis, very high globulin levels, positive rheumatoid factor, and occasionally, vascular purpura.

Case Report

A 46-year-old female was well until one year prior to admission to hospital. At that time over a three-day period, she developed painful, swollen feet and then fever and hematuria. Trimethoprim/sulfamethoxazole (TMP/SMZ) was prescribed for a presumed urinary tract infection (urine culture was, however, negative), and she felt better. During the next year, she had recurrent episodes of the above illnesses, which responded and then relapsed whenever TMP/SMZ was discontinued. She also developed pains in her calves, thighs, and arms that lasted a few days at a time and rendered the affected part nonfunctional. Six months before admission she had an episode of back pain and from that time, episodes of a petechial rash on her pretibial area and calves. Three months before admission, a red macular lesion developed on her left forearm, a biopsy of tissue from which showed a "sterile abscess." She was seen in consultation by a rheumatologist who diagnosed arthritis and referred her to another center where a diagnosis of interstitial nephritis was made. At that time a mitral insufficiency murmur was described and attributed to mitral valve prolapse. Results of blood cultures were negative.

One month before admission, therapy with a nonsteroidal antiinflammatory drug was begun and three days later she was admitted to her local hospital with acute pulmonary edema. During her four-week stay there she was febrile. Numerous blood cultures were negative, as was a bone marrow culture. The rheumatoid factor was 1:5000.

Physical examination revealed a fit, anxious woman with an oral temperature of 39°C. The fingers were clubbed and a grade IV/VI pansystolic murmur was present at the apex and radiated to the axilla. A grade II/VI systolic ejection murmur was heard along the left sternal border. Hematuria was present, and red cell, white blood cell, and granular casts were noted on microscopic examination of the urine.

The hemoglobin was 128 gm per liter, white blood cell count 10.2×10^9 per liter, with 79% polymorphonuclear leukocytes, 16% lymphocytes, 3% monocytes, and 2% eosinophils.

Blood cultures, including cultures for L forms, grew *Streptococcus morbilorum*. Serial echocardiograms showed no vegetations but revealed systolic prolapse of both the anterior and posterior leaflets of the mitral valve and changes compatible with myxomatous degeneration. Vancomycin therapy was started because of the patient's history of penicillin allergy, but when skin tests were negative for penicillin allergy, penicillin G therapy was instituted. Within three days of starting antibiotics the patient became afebrile.

This patient had the immune complex manifestations of endocarditis. The working diagnosis on admission was culture-negative endocarditis. Why blood cultures in the two other hospitals were repeatedly negative is unknown, although previous antibiotic treatment and low-grade bacteremia associated with well-established immune complex disease may be possible factors.

Intraabdominal Abscess

The only manifestation of intraabdominal abscess, especially in the elderly, may be FUO. The source is often the hepatobiliary tree. Abdominal ultrasound, gallium and indium leukocyte scintigraphy and computed tomography (CT) are available for the assessment of the patient with suspected intraabdominal disease. Lesions less than 1.5 cm in diameter are often missed by gallium scanning. Normal concentration of this isotope in the liver and spleen may make large collections of pus in these areas difficult to identify. Fecal gallium activity, predominantly in the large bowel, may at times cause a false positive finding. Ultrasound is most useful in detecting lesions greater than 3 cm in diameter that are not obscured by overlying bowel gas. In a prospective study comparing CT, abdominal ultrasound, and gallium scanning, no significant difference was found in the ability of the three modalities to differentiate focal from nonfocal sources of sepsis. If any two examinations were used and either was abnormal, the sensitivity increased from 60% to 90%, while the false positive rate increased from 15% to 25%. If focal disease was diagnosed only if two examinations were abnormal, the false positive rate dropped to nearly zero, but the sensitivity fell to below 40%.

Liver abscesses are usually detected by a liver scan using technetium sulfur colloid.

Perinephric abscesses are often associated with high temperature only. The urine sediment is usually normal and flank tenderness may be absent. Eventually, a bulge occurs in the flank, but this may require several weeks. Intravenous pyelography may be normal. Ultrasound examination, CT, and gallium and indium white cell scanning have proved very helpful in making this diagnosis.

Viral Infections

Cytomegalovirus and Epstein-Barr virus infections occasionally pose as FUO, producing an illness greater than three weeks' duration. Atypical lymphocytes should prompt the appropriate serologic tests.

FUO in Returned Travelers

A detailed travel history is always stressed as an important part of the investigation of a patient with FUO. Common causes include malaria, amebiasis (especially amebic liver abscess), toxoplasmosis, trichinosis, and trypanosomiasis. The cause of fever in a returned traveler is usually evident and often manifests itself as an acute illness. Occasionally such patients fulfill the definition of FUO.

Malaria and amebiasis are most commonly overlooked. Malaria can be readily diagnosed by examining thick and thin blood smears. Amebiasis is misdiagnosed as ulcerative colitis on occasion and it is in these instances that serology such as *Entamoeba histolytica* indirect hemagglutination tests are useful. Indeed, every febrile returned traveler with suspected ulcerative colitis should have this test performed; however, amebic liver abscess is more likely to cause FUO.

Trypanosomiasis can be contracted during even brief stays in endemic areas. *Trypanosoma gambiense* is found in West and Central Africa. Fever begins irregularly and is accompanied by an evanescent rash, splenomegaly, and lymphadenopathy. This disease may be readily overlooked and may be present for months as FUO before blood smears are examined. Trypanosomiasis due to *T. rhodesiense* is evident in East and Central Africa. This form of the disease is acute, with a prominent erythematous rash, central nervous system alterations, and high fever. Blood smears are diagnostic.

The visceral form of leishmaniasis, kala azar, is caused by the obligate intracellular protozoan *Leishmania donovani*. It is characterized by a long period of irregular fever, hepatosplenomegaly (this disease is one of the causes of massive splenomegaly), anemia, leukopenia, hyperglobulinemia, and progressive emaciation of the affected host. Kala azar occurs in Asia, Europe, Africa, and Central and South America. Sandflies of the genus *Phlebotomus* are the vectors. The diagnosis is easily confirmed by demonstration of Leishmani bodies within cells obtained by bone marrow aspiration or by liver biopsy.

Finally, it is important to remember that travelers are subject to the same causes of FUO as nontravelers.

NEOPLASTIC DISEASE

Lymphoma (both Hodgkin's and non-Hodgkin's lymphoma) is the most common malignancy that causes FUO. Pel-Ebstein fever is rarely seen. Hypernephroma can have a variety of systemic effects including fever. The following malignancies are noted for causing FUO: hypernephroma, hepatoma, carcinoma of the lung, metastatic carcinoma with primary site unknown, metastatic carcinoma of the thyroid, atrial myxoma, and preleukemia.

In one study, 47 of 6880 patients (0.7%) admitted to a cancer hospital had FUO. Infection was the most common cause, accounting for 57% of the diagnoses, and included localized infections, endocarditis, tuberculosis, and fungal and viral infections. Fever was attributed to the cancer itself in 18 (38%). Six of the seven with FUO and metastatic carcinoma had large liver metastases.

Gallium scanning is useful in the evaluation of patients with possible lymphoma. The false positive rate in patients with known lymphoma is low (below 5%) and about 50% of known disease sites are detected. The size of the lesion influences accuracy, since tumors more than 3 cm in diameter often yield positive results. All abdominal nodal disease visualized by lymphangiography was also positive on gallium scanning.

Lymphangiography is frequently used in the investigation of patients with FUO; however, no studies are available to indicate if the procedure is indicated in the face of a negative gallium scan and no abnormal nodes on computed tomography.

Biopsy of bone marrow is frequently helpful in diagnosing metastatic carcinoma.

Case Report

A 61-year-old male with a three-year history of stable angina pectoris and clinical aortic stenosis was referred for cardiac catheterization. Six weeks prior to admission, he developed fever, chills, night sweats, rigors, malaise, weakness, decreased energy, anorexia, and a 25-pound weight loss. He also complained of pain in his right hip, radiating into his buttock and down his legs, of five months' duration.

On examination he looked chronically ill and had an oral temperature of 38.4°C. There was limitation of straight-leg raising to 35° on the right and 60° on the left. The hemoglobin was 100 gm per liter, white blood cell count 13.3×10^9 per liter, with 66% polymorphonuclear leukocytes, 2% bands, 18% lymphocytes, 12% monocytes, 1% eosinophils, and 1% basophils; ESR was 112 mm per hour, and platelet count 524×10^9 per liter. The alkaline phosphatase was elevated to 217 (normal, 30–104) and lactate dehydrogenase 676 (normal, 117–259).

Infective endocarditis was the working diagnosis. Several blood cultures were negative. The patient remained febrile for the next month.

A bone marrow biopsy revealed metastatic carcinoma; an extensive work-up failed to find the primary source. After treatment with 5-fluorouracil, adriamycin, and mitramycin the patient became afebrile.

The critical test in this patient was his overall assessment. He looked chronically ill, and his back pain with limitation of straight-leg raising and weight loss were suggestive of carcinoma. Since radiographs of his pelvis and spine were negative, we chose a bone marrow biopsy as our initial test, and this revealed the diagnosis.

COLLAGEN-VASCULAR DISEASES

Collagen-vascular diseases that may cause FUO include the following:

1. Vasculitis
   - Polyarteritis nodosa
   - Giant cell arteritis
   - Henoch-Schönlein purpura
   - Serum sickness
   - Wegener's granulomatosis
   - Mixed cryoglobulinemia with vasculitis
   - Lymphomatoid granulomatosis
2. Collagen disease
   - Systemic lupus erythematosus
   - Juvenile rheumatoid arthritis (adult-onset Still's disease)
   - Mixed connective tissue disease
   - Rheumatic fever
   - Ankylosing spondylitis

Systemic Vasculitis

The spectrum of the vasculitides encompasses a group of disorders that *share a common feature of necrotizing inflammation of blood vessels* and *differ in type, size, and location of the involved vessels*. The clinical features vary depending upon the type of vasculitis, but fever is one of the major symptoms of many of these illnesses. Multisystem involvement by vasculitis results in a variety of clinical features, but often nonspecific symptoms such as fever, malaise, myalgia, arthralgia, weakness, and anorexia predominate. Vasculitis usually results from damage to the blood vessels by immune complexes. Under certain circumstances, immune complexes can trigger granuloma formation. Polyarteritis nodosa involves small and medium-sized muscular arteries. Renal involvement is frequent, with glomerulitis occurring in about 30%. The hypersensitivity vasculitides involve small vessels, predominantly postcapillary venules. Skin manifestations (palpable purpura) predominate.

Serum sickness, Henoch-Schönlein purpura, essential mixed cryoglobulinemia, and vasculitis associated with malignancies also involve small vessels. Wegener's granulomatosis consists of necrotizing granulomatous vasculitis of the upper and lower respiratory tracts, glomerulonephritis, and various degrees of disseminated small vessel vaculitis.

Giant Cell Temporal Arteritis

Fever is present in 48% of patients with temporal arteritis and in some may be the only symptom. It is now recognized that this disease is a widely disseminated arteritis involving any large or medium-sized elastic artery. Pathologic abnormalities may be confined to short segments, thereby making results of unilateral arterial biopsies inconclusive in eliminating the diagnosis. If temporal arteritis is suspected, biopsy should be done of both temporal arteries. In each instance it is important that a long segment (4 to 6 cm) be removed and that the pathologist examine serial sections.

Case Report

A 61-year-old female was referred to the neurosurgery service by her family doctor because of headaches. Three months previously she had onset of severe, bitemporal, throbbing headaches. There was associated nausea and decreased appetite. Two months prior to hospital admission her energy decreased and fever and night sweats occurred. There was a weight loss of 20 pounds. Except fever, there were no abnormal physical findings. She was seen in consultation by a hematologist who felt she probably had a lymphoma. Initial laboratory data included: hemoglobin 106 gm per liter, WBC 11.8 $\times$ 10^9 per liter, with 68% polymorphonuclear leukocytes, 26% lymphocytes, 3% monocytes, and 2% basophils; ESR was 128 mm per hour; platelet count 650 $\times$ 10^9 per liter. A chest roentgenogram showed fullness of the left hilum, which on tomography proved to be the left pulmonary artery. Abdominal ultrasound examination showed multiple lesions in the liver consistent with metastases. Subsequent investigations to find the metastases included the following, all of which were normal or negative: barium enema, upper gastrointestinal series and small bowel follow-through, intravenous urography, lymphangiogram, liver spleen scan, bone scan, bone marrow biopsy, liver biopsy, and laproscopy. A gallium scan demonstrated uptake of the isotope in the midabdomen. The latex fixation was positive at 1:1280; LE cells were negative, and antinative DNA antibodies were negative.

At this point, biopsy of the left temporal artery disclosed giant cell arteritis, and prednisone therapy was begun. Throughout her month in hospital, the patient remained febrile (>37.5°C most days).

At follow-up three months later she felt well except for back pain due to an osteoporotic compression fracture of L-2, was afebrile, and her hemoglobin had risen to 147 gm per liter.

The diagnosis should have been made early in the course of her illness, but the suggestion of a chest malignancy and a false positive ultrasound examination led her attending physicians on a search for an occult malignancy. The uptake of gallium in midabdomen probably represented aortitis.

Juvenile Rheumatoid Arthritis in Adults

Adult-onset Still's disease usually occurs in males, some of whom may have had the earliest of their symptoms in childhood but have been asymptomatic for years. Because of the various combinations of polyarthralgia, myalgia, rash, adenopathy, splenomegaly, pleuritis, pericarditis, sore throat, abdominal pain, hepatic abnormalities, and high fever, the diagnosis may be very difficult and simulate other causes of FUO. Therapeutic blood levels of aspirin (25 to 30 mg/dl) may control the fever and result in a rapid reversal of all accompanying abnormalities in some patients. Prednisone, however, may be required in poorly responsive patients. The prognosis is usually unpredictable.

Scleroderma

Fever of uncertain origin in a patient with scleroderma should not be attributed to the disease itself. There appears to be an increased frequency of malignancy in patients with this illness.

Miscellaneous Causes of FUO

Fever of uncertain origin can occur with any of the following conditions: essential oral hyperthermia, pulmonary emboli, drug fever, granulomatous hepatitis, subacute thyroiditis, familial Mediterranean fever, inflammatory bowel disease, sarcoidosis, alcoholic hepatitis, Whipple's disease, and periodic fever.

Essential Oral Hyperthermia

A relatively common cause of low-grade fever in young girls and women is essential oral hyperthermia. The temperature may reach 38°C and be associated with a variety of nonspecific symptoms, but no underlying disease process is found.

Pulmonary Emboli

Fever occurs frequently in patients with pulmonary emboli. Temperatures higher than 39°C and leukocytosis occur early, followed by low-grade fever that may last for up to a week or more. Recurrent emboli result in persistent fever, and when the patient has no respiratory symptoms, a high index of suspicion is needed to obtain a lung scan and diagnose this cause of FUO.

Drug Fever

A careful drug history must be taken when evaluating the patient with FUO. A good rule of thumb is to consider all drugs capable of causing drug fever. The only agents that have not been implicated are digoxin, chloramphenicol, tetracycline, and insulin. Some such as quinidine, penicillin, alpha-methyldopa, procainamide, and cloxacillin are among the most frequent causes of drug fever.

Characteristically, fever develops between 7 and 10 days after starting the drug (if the patient was previously sensitized, fever can occur within 2 to 4 hours), and usually defervescence occurs within 3 to 4 days after it has been discontinued. Defervescence is related to clearance of the drug and its metabolites from the body, hence for some agents such as iodine, fever may not defervesce for two to three weeks after stopping the drug. The patient with drug fever is usually well and occasionally has eosinophilia.

Granulomatous Hepatitis

There are many causes of granulomas in the liver, including tuberculosis, atypical mycobacteria, histoplasmosis, other fungi, brucellosis, Q fever, syphilis, parasites, viruses, sarcoidosis, Crohn's disease, chronic granulomatous disease of childhood, Hodgkin's disease, berylliosis, Wegener's granulomatosis, allergic granulomatosis, reactions to various drugs, primary biliary cirrhosis, and postnecrotic cirrhosis. When all these causes have been excluded, some patients with prolonged fever and noncaseating granulomatous hepatitis respond to corticosteroid treatment. They have fever, chills, sweats, arthralgia, myalgia, asthenia, and weight loss (some also have abdominal pain). Hepatosplenomegaly is frequently present and intermittent jaundice may occur in some patients.

Hormonal Hyperthermia

Subacute thyroiditis is the most frequent endocrine cause of FUO. Hyperthyroidism, adrenal insufficiency, and pheochromocytoma can all cause fever.

Familial Mediterranean Fever

This disorder involves ethnic groups whose origin is in countries bordering the shores of the Mediterranean Sea. It is characterized by episodes of moderate to high fever alone or often in association with diffuse abdominal pain and/or arthritis. Colchicine is effective for reducing acute attacks and for inducing remission of

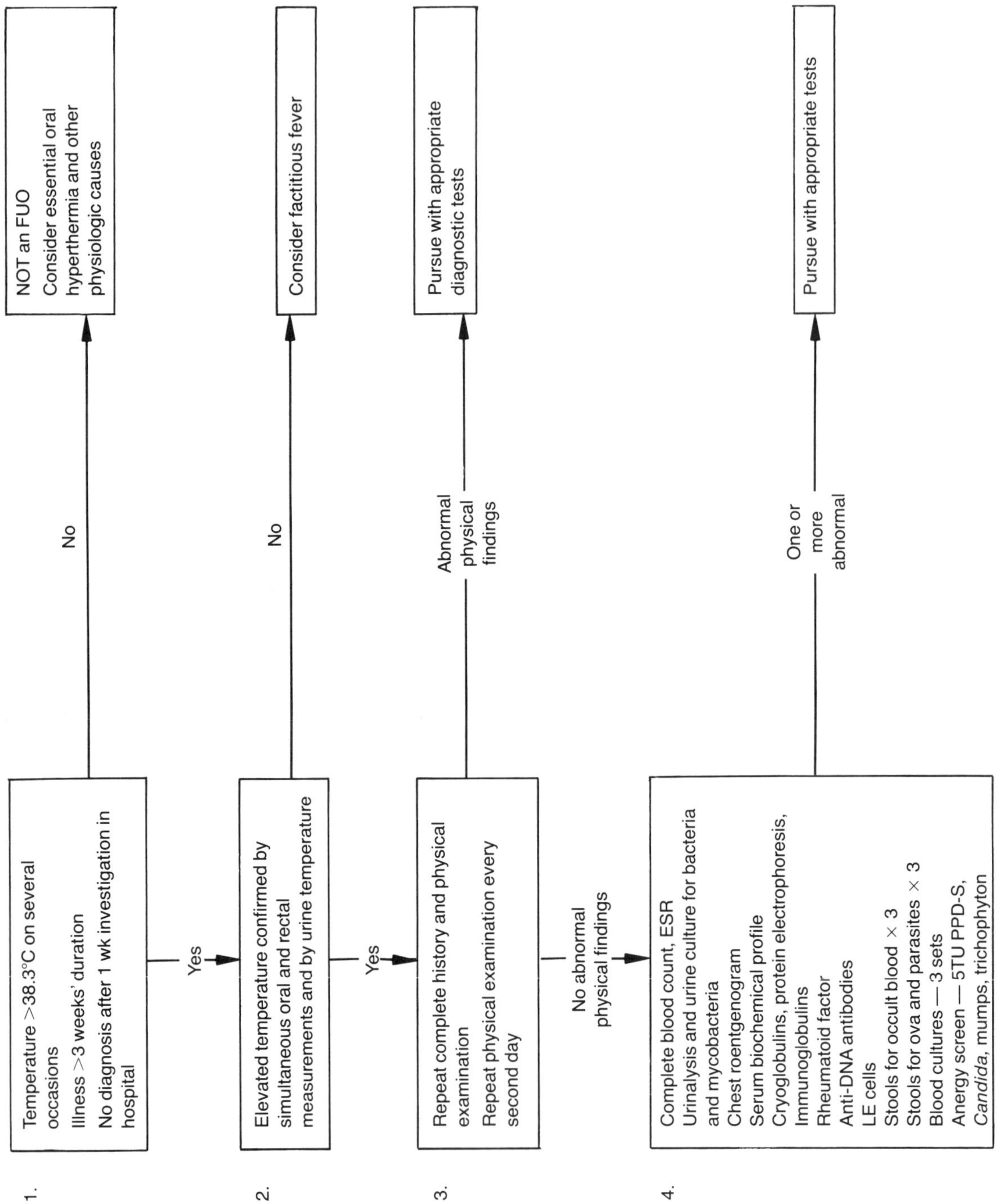
1.
Temperature >38.3°C on several occasions
Illness >3 weeks' duration
No diagnosis after 1 wk investigation in hospital
No
NOT an FUO
Consider essential oral hyperthermia and other physiologic causes
Yes
2.
Elevated temperature confirmed by simultaneous oral and rectal measurements and by urine temperature
No
Consider factitious fever
Yes
3.
Repeat complete history and physical examination
Repeat physical examination every second day
Abnormal physical findings
Pursue with appropriate diagnostic tests
No abnormal physical findings
4.
Complete blood count, ESR
Urinalysis and urine culture for bacteria and mycobacteria
Chest roentgenogram
Serum biochemical profile
Cryoglobulins, protein electrophoresis,
Immunoglobulins
Rheumatoid factor
Anti-DNA antibodies
LE cells
Stools for occult blood × 3
Stools for ova and parasites × 3
Blood cultures — 3 sets
Anergy screen — 5TU PPD-S, Candida, mumps, trichophyton
One or more abnormal
Pursue with appropriate tests

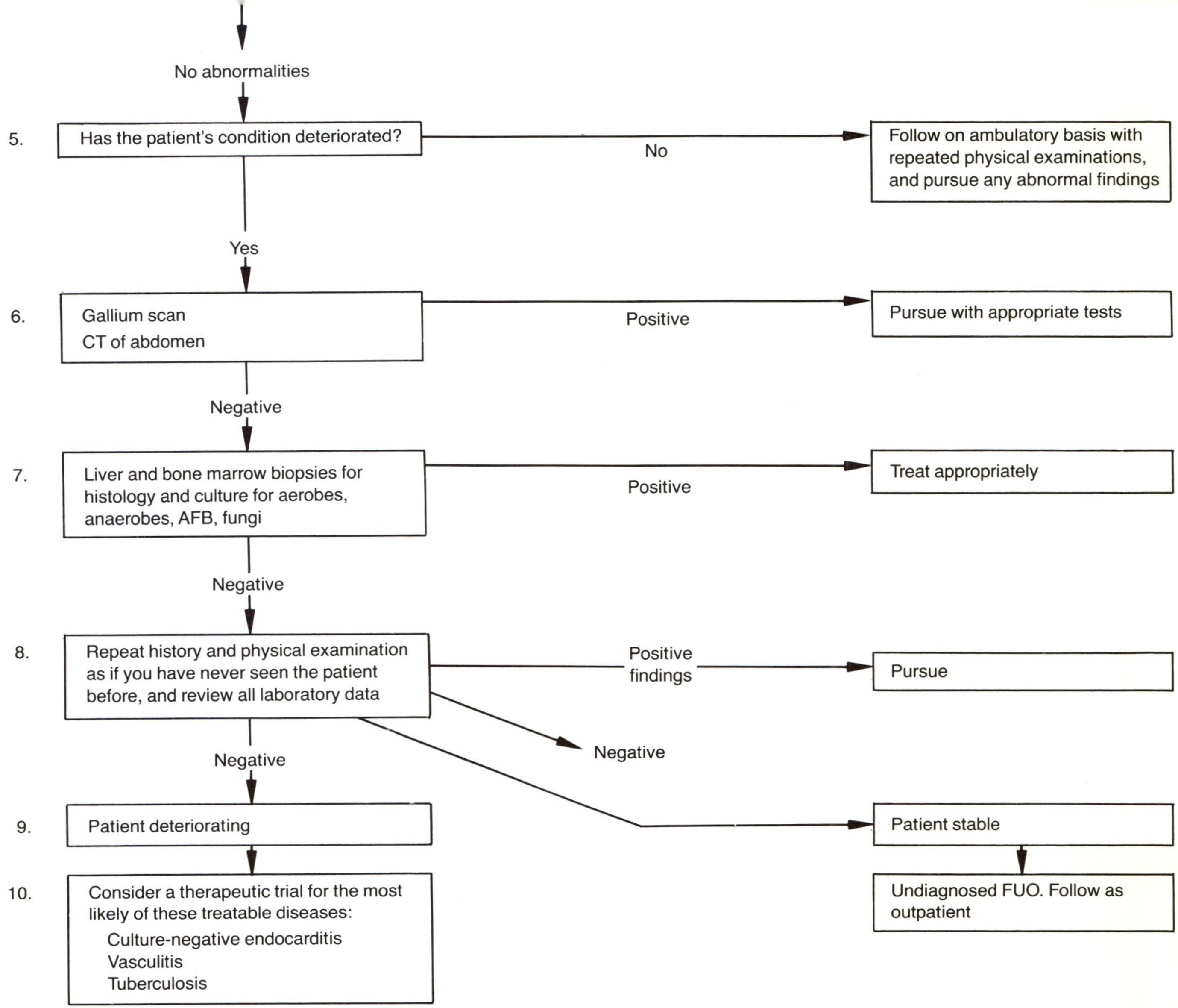

FIGURE 21.1. Algorithm for diagnostic approach to FUO.

the nephrotic syndrome that may complicate this disease.

Inflammatory Bowel Disease

Occasionally the only manifestation of inflammatory bowel disease is FUO. Patients with celiac disease, abdominal pain, and FUO should be carefully investigated for lymphoma of the small intestine.

Occult Dental Infection

Every patient with FUO should have a thorough dental examination, including Panorex roentgenograms. These infections cause nonspecific symptoms such as headaches and myalgia. Mobile teeth or those that are tender to percussion, and gingival swelling and tenderness should be searched for routinely.

Undiagnosed Category

Despite intensive evaluation, some fevers of unknown origin will remain undiagnosed. A prospective study of 347 patients with long-term FUO (most had fever of greater than one year's duration) revealed that 101 (29%) had idiopathic fever with no diagnosis despite well-documented follow-up as long as 16 years. Malignancies accounted for only 11% of the long-term FUOs.

DIAGNOSTIC APPROACH

The initial approach to the persistently febrile patient is one of enthusiasm — a chance to achieve a diagnostic coup. Unfortunately, as test after test is negative, both patient and physician become frustrated (Figure 21.1).

Once the criteria for diagnosis have been fulfilled, it is wise to inform the patient that, on occasion, the investigation can be lengthy and in some instances it is not possible to arrive at a diagnosis. Before embarking on any laboratory tests, one must make sure the patient is febrile. Both rectal and oral temperatures should be recorded simultaneously and the urinary temperature checked. These measures should rule out factitious fever.

The first test is a thorough history and physical examination. An occupational and avocational history should be recorded in detail and particular attention should be directed to foreign travel, past medical history, previous surgical procedures, drug usage including over-the-counter preparations, animal contact, and alcohol intake. Clues detected here may suggest specific tests and avoid a large-scale screening investigation.

During the physical examination, special attention should be directed to the ocular fundi, searching for choroid tubercules and exudates. The teeth should be individually percussed with tongue blade, looking for tenderness. The thyroid must be checked for tenderness; this may be the only clue to subacute thyroiditis. All lymph nodes should be described and any abnormal ones measured and recorded. The liver span should be measured and the liver and Traube's space auscultated for rubs. Heart murmurs should be checked daily. The testicles and epididymis are often neglected in a physical examination and should be examined carefully. All females should have a pelvic examination. Sigmoidoscopy should be included for all patients. Finally, the entire skin, fingernails, and toenails should be carefully examined for petechiae, nodules, and splinter hemorrhages. One of the most useful procedures is to repeat a detailed physical examination every other day.

Screening laboratory tests usually include a complete blood count with differential and erythrocyte sedimentation rate, urinalysis (including careful microscopic examination), chest roentgenogram, electrocardiogram, serum biochemical profile (usually includes calcium, phosphorus, albumin, globulin, serum urea nitrogen, serum glutamic oxaloacetic transaminase, serum glutamic pyruvic transaminase, lactic dehydrogenase, creatinine, alkaline phosphatase, creatine phosphokinase), rheumatoid factor, cryoglobulins, antinuclear antibody, and stool for occult blood and for ova and parasites. Although abnormalities in the results of these tests tend to be nonspecific, they should be scrutinized carefully. For example, the presence of monocytosis would suggest a differential diagnosis of bacterial endocarditis, tuberculosis, brucellosis, inflammatory bowel disease, solid tumor, or Hodgkin's disease.

Three sets of blood cultures (a set is one aerobic and one anaerobic culture) should be done over the first 48 hours in hospital. The laboratory should be advised to hold the blood cultures for three weeks. The other valuable screening test consists of a series of skin tests — Tween 80 stabilized 5 tuberculin unit purified protein derivative-S, *Candida,* mumps, and *Trichophyton.* Demonstration of delayed hypersensitivity to PPD-S or anergy can be very important early clues in the evaluation of patients with FUO.

Investigation from this point on is dictated by the abnormalities found in the screening tests. If results of all the above tests are normal and the patient is clinically well, it is reasonable to follow the patient on an ambulatory basis, repeating physical examination and screening tests from time to time.

The sequence in which diagnostic procedures are carried out must be individualized. As a rule, where possible, tissue should be obtained. For example, a 65-year-old patient with an ESR over 100 should have a temporal artery biopsy early, not two weeks later when all the scans and roentgenographic studies are negative. The key diagnostic tests in one series of patients with FUO were as follows: roentgenographic examinations 27%, biopsy 25%, laparotomy 23%, cultures 19%, clinical course 12%, enzyme determination 9%, serologic tests 6%, liver scan 5%, bone marrow examination 5%, proctoscopy 2%, cerebrospinal fluid examination 1%, and postmortem 1%.

Patients with elevated liver enzymes and/or alkaline phosphatase (5′ nucleotidase elevated) should have a liver-spleen scan and biopsy. All biopsy specimens should be cultured aerobically, anaerobically, for mycobacteria, fungi, and viruses in addition to undergoing histologic examination. If possible, a portion should be frozen for further studies if necessary.

A diagnostic laparotomy should be carried out only if there is some evidence of intraabdominal disease.

In the patient who is deteriorating, the question of a therapeutic trial arises. Antibiotics for tuberculosis or presumed endocarditis, and corticosteroids for vasculitis are the usual considerations. If tuberculosis is the cause of FUO, a decrease in the magnitude or total subsistence of fever will occur within three weeks of institution of at least two antituberculous medications, one of which should be isoniazid.

Presumed endocarditis should be treated for two weeks with penicillin and an aminoglycoside. If a good clinical response is obtained, these antibiotics should be continued for a further two weeks. Such patients should always have a Q fever titer; chronic Q fever nearly always means endocarditis. Echocardiograms should be repeated at weekly intervals looking for vegetations. Many patients with endocarditis never have the vegetations visualized echocardiographically, and old vegetations cannot be distinguished from new ones.

Since the treatment for vasculitis depends upon histologic type, it is best to obtain a tissue diagnosis and not treat empirically.

ANNOTATED BIBLIOGRAPHY

Bujak TS, Aptekar RG, Decker JL, Wolff SM. Juvenile rheumatoid arthritis presenting in the adult as fever of unknown origin. Medicine 1973;52:431–444.
Describes an important diagnostic entity to be considered in all adults with fever, joint symptoms, evanescent rash, lymphadenopathy, splenomegaly, myocarditis, pericarditis, and pneumonitis in various combinations.

Esposito AL, Gleckman RA. Fever of unknown origin in the elderly. J Am Geriatr Soc, 1978;26:298–505.
All cases of FUO in patients over age 65 years published in 1961–1978 are reviewed. Temporal arteritis is a very important cause of FUO in this group of patients.

Esposito AL, Gleckman RA. A diagnostic approach to the adult with fever of unknown origin. Arch Intern Med, 1979;139:575–79.
Outlines the approach to FUO in both the ambulatory and the hospitalized patient.

Gleckman RA, Crowley A, Esposito A. Fever of unknown origin: a view from the community hospital. Am J Med Sci 1977;274:21–25.
High percentage in the undiagnosed category, none of whom lost over two pounds per week during hospitalization.

Kluger MJ. Fever. Pediatrics 1980;66:720–724.
A review of the pathophysiology of fever.

Larson EB, Featherstone JH, Petersdorf RG. Fever of undetermined origin: diagnosis and follow-up of 105 cases, 1970–1980. Medicine 1982;61:269–292.
Contrasts patients with FUO in the 1970s with those reported in earlier studies, and notes that malignancy has supplanted infection as the most common disease category.

Murray HW, Ellis GC, Blumenthal DS, Sas TA. Fever and pulmonary thromboembolism. Am J Med 1979;67:232–235.
Describes the course of fever in pulmonary throm-

boembolism and shows that prolonged fever can be an indication of reembolization.

Murray HW, Tuazon CU, Guerrero IC, Claudio MS, Alling DW, Sheagram JN. Urinary temperature: a clue to early diagnosis of factitious fever. N Engl J Med 1977;296:23–24.

Using the normogram in this article, the oral temperature can be determined from urinary temperature, making this measurement valuable in diagnosing factitious fever.

Petersdorf RG, Beeson PB. Fever of unexplained origin. Report on 100 cases. Medicine 1961;40:1–30.

The original article to define FUO.

Pizza PA, Lovejoy FH, Smith DH. Prolonged fever in children: review of 100 cases. Pediatrics 1975;55:468–473.

Highlights the difference in FUO in children — they are not the same as adults.

Simon HB, Wolff SM. Granulomatous hepatitis and prolonged fever of unknown origin. A study of 13 patients. Medicine 1973;52:1–21.

Describes an illness of unknown etiology characterized by hepatic granulomata, prolonged FUO, chills, sweats, arthralgia, myalgia, asthenia, weight loss, and abdominal pain.

Youngs EJ, Fainstein V, Musher D. Drug-induced fever: cases seen in the evaluation of unexplained fever in a general hospital population. Rev Infect Dis 1982:4:69–77.

A good overview of drug-induced fever.

22 INFECTIONS IN THE IMMUNOCOMPROMISED HOST

Lionel A. Mandell and Ronald Feld

From a functional point of view, a compromised host is any patient whose normal defense mechanisms are impaired, making that person more susceptible to infection (see Chapter 2 for a description of normal defense mechanisms against infection). Predisposing conditions run the gamut from esoteric entities such as congenital immunodeficiency diseases to more common problems such as aspiration by an alcoholic. It is obviously not possible in this chapter to discuss in detail all aspects of infection in the compromised host. What we attempt to do is to cover some of those conditions likely to be seen by the average physician. The first part of this chapter deals with conditions not primarily due to neoplasms, and the second half focuses on infections in the patient with cancer.

In contrast with many other chapters in this book, where the standard format of etiology, pathophysiology, and clinical manifestations, and so on are employed, the organization is somewhat different because of the diverse nature of the conditions. We consider factors predisposing to infection, the organisms causing the infection, and diagnosis and treatment. The subsection on AIDS uses the standard format.

There is a wide variety of conditions and illnesses that suppress normal defenses and allow infections to develop. Frequently, these infections are due to pathogens that one encounters in other noncompromised hosts, but they may be caused by organisms that do not usually result in disease in patients whose defenses are intact. These are referred to as opportunistic infections.

FACTORS THAT PREDISPOSE TO INFECTION

Many factors predispose to infection:

1. Congenital
   Immunodeficiency syndromes (severe combined immunodeficiency syndromes, Wiskott-Aldrich syndrome, ataxia telangiectasia, chronic mucocutaneous candidiasis, congenital neutropenia)
   Sickle cell anemia
2. Acquired
   Splenectomy
   Diabetes mellitus
   Alcoholism
   Rheumatic diseases
   Uremia
   Malnutrition
   Drugs
   Transplantations

If one considers the various defense mechanisms available to deal with infection, such as surface and mechanical factors, inflammation, humoral and cell-mediated immunity, disease processes can be found in which any one or all of these are impaired.

Congenital

Congenital Immunodeficiency Syndromes

Congenital immunodeficiency syndromes represent a varied and fascinating group of disorders that primarily affect the pediatric population. As such, it is given only passing mention here but in the annotated references, the reader can find an excellent review of this area. Defects can be found involving virtually any of the defenses listed above. For example, abnormalities of the classic and alternate complement pathways, of neutrophil function and isolated or combined B and T cell dysfunction.

Sickle Cell Anemia

Sickle cell anemia affects approximately 0.15% to 0.2% of black children in the United States. The disease is due to a specific biochemical defect but the major cause of morbidity and mortality is bacterial infection, usually from encapsulated organisms such as *Salmonella* and *Pneumococcus*. Several mechanisms have been postulated to explain the increased prevalence of infection in patients with sickle cell disease.

Because of recurrent splenic infarcts, the spleen is eventually replaced by fibrotic tissue. Infection appears to be related to the development of functional asplenia. Once this occurs, the filtering mechanisms of the spleen are no longer able to clear organisms presented to them. Not only is the phagocytic function impaired, but opsonization is compromised. A possible defect in opsonization involving the alternate complement pathway and fixation of C3b to antigen may predispose to infection as well.

Vasoocclusive phenomena produce areas of ischemic and infarcted tissue that are more readily infected than healthy tissue. Because of local conditions within such areas, neutrophil function is impaired, resulting in decreased clearance of organisms that might settle out in these areas.

Acquired

Splenectomy

A spleen may be removed for a variety of reasons — traumatic rupture, staging procedure in lymphoma, etc. As pointed out, removal of the spleen whether functionally or anatomically, predisposes the patient to infection. In addition to the factors discussed above, three more issues appear to play a role in predisposition to infection in splenectomized patients as opposed to those with sickle cell anemia. These include loss of local splenic production of IgM antibody against bloodborne antigens; loss of an opsonizing tetrapeptide called tuftsin which is manufactured in the spleen; and a deficiency of properidin necessary for activation of the alternate complement pathway. The reasons for such differences are not well understood.

Diabetes Mellitus

One often hears that diabetics are more likely to develop infection than nondiabetics. While this is true for poorly controlled diabetics, infections are often related to patients' poor general state of health and may not necessarily be due to impairment of host defenses that results from the diabetes per se.

A great many studies have been carried out to determine whether or not specific defects can be found in defense mechanisms of diabetic patients. In many cases, however, due to differences in methodology and study design, conflicting data were found. One is also faced with the problem of trying to determine whether clinical significance can be attributed to any of the defects found, and this is often difficult at best.

Most of the studies have focused on polymorphonuclear neutrophils. It appears that neutrophils from diabetic patients have impaired chemotaxis, although the exact reason for this is not known. It was thought originally that it might be related to acidosis, but defects have been reported in nonacidotic diabetics and it is felt that it is probably due to an inherent abnormality in the neutrophil. With regard to phagocytosis, there is impairment of ingestion related to serum hyperosmolarity, but no convincing evidence exists that microbicidal activity is impaired. Metabolic studies have shown impaired anaerobic glycolysis, again likely related to an intrinsic cell defect.

Function of B cells in the diabetic is intact, but some problems with T cell function have been noted, including depressed delayed-type hypersensitivity and altered lymphocyte transformation. Complement function and opsonizing activity are normal.

What are probably more important in the diabetic in terms of predisposition to infection are problems of compromised circulatory function and neuropathy. These factors singly or in combination are largely responsible for foot infections, and neuropathy which can lead to impaired bladder emptying may result in infection as well.

Alcoholism

Alcoholism is a form of disease with both social and physical ramifications. Alcoholics suffer a twofold to threefold greater mortality than their nonalcoholic counterparts, as well as increased morbidity; part of this is due to infection. Obviously the inebriated host, like anyone with an impaired level of consciousness, is more likely to aspirate. This fact coupled with increased oropharyngeal carriage of gram-negative organisms, particularly *Klebsiella*, and possibly impaired clearance of organisms by pulmonary alveolar macrophages make them more likely to develop pneumonia. Both quantitative and qualitative defects in polymorphonuclear neutrophils have been described. Leukopenia may be due to several mechanisms: a direct toxic effect of alcohol on granulocyte production, folate deficiency secondary to malnutrition, and hypersplenism. The data are somewhat confusing and at times contradictory regarding qualitative defects. In animal as well as some human studies, neutrophil mobilization was impaired. It is felt that this may be due to problems in granulocyte adherence to the vascular endothelium and the presence of chemotactic inhibitors in the serum. Phagocytosis and microbicidal activity appear to be unaffected, but alcohol may have deleterious effects on serum bactericidal activity, particularly against certain gram-negative bacilli.

In patients with cirrhosis, hyperglobulinemia in the form of a polyclonal gammopathy (IgG, IgA, and IgM) can be found. Several explanations for this have been offered. With liver damage, its reticuloendothelial function is disturbed and so bacteria normally cleared by the liver present a chronic antigenic challenge to the spleen. This, coupled with a possible defect in T cell suppressor function, allows B cell stimulation to go on unchecked. The clinical relevance of such elevated levels is not clear, and it may not be significant in terms of infection.

Defects in cell-mediated immunity have been documented in some alcoholics, particularly with respect to T cell responsiveness to challenge by new antigens. Whether or not these are due to the alcohol or associated nutritional problems is unclear.

Rheumatic Diseases

Of the rheumatic diseases, those that have been investigated most intensively with regard to host defense mechanisms are systemic lupus erythematosus (SLE), rheumatoid arthritis, and Felty's syndrome.

Systemic Lupus Erythematosus. With active SLE, neutropenia (fewer than 3000/cu mm) may occur, possibly as a result of IgG antigranulocyte antibodies or suppression of granulopoiesis. Data on neutrophil function are somewhat confusing. Chemotaxis is abnormal because of impaired generation of chemotactic factors by serum of these patients and chemotactic inhibitors present in their serum. Also, some studies suggest that intrinsic defects in cell function may result in defective migration. Serum inhibitors of phagocytosis have also been described. In addition to these defects, opsonization may be impaired secondary to hypocomplementemia.

No definite B cell problems seem to exist, but impaired cell-mediated immunity as reflected by anergy, and defective mitogen responses can be found with active disease.

Rheumatoid Arthritis. In rheumatoid arthritis, although peripheral blood polymorphs have impaired chemotaxis, their phagocytic activity is normal. This is in contrast to cells from synovial fluid in which phagocytosis is impaired, implying that something in the synovial fluid of these patients is able to impede ingestion by the polymorphonuclear neutrophils.

Felty's Syndrome. Felty's syndrome is in fact a subtype of rheumatoid arthritis and consists of a triad of rheumatoid arthritis, splenomegaly, and neutropenia. Several reasons for the neutropenia have been given, including increased margination, decreased production, increased destruction of cells, and the presence of granulocyte-specific antinuclear antibodies.

It is important to note that not all patients with Felty's syndrome are subject to recurrent infections and that the absolute granulocyte count does not distinguish between patients at risk versus those not at increased risk. Chemotactic defects were found in most patients studied, but impaired neutrophil bactericidal activity was only found in those with recurrent infection. This has been attributed to the presence of smaller phagolysosomes in their cells, since reduction and ingestion of nitroblue tetrazolium were normal.

Uremia

Infection is a major cause of morbidity and mortality in uremic patients. Predisposition to infection in this group is probably a multifactorial problem since they have some impairment of host defenses, are subjected to many procedures, and often are debilitated. With respect to specific defects, those undergoing dialysis often have transient, short-lived neutropenia, probably due to activation of complement and sequestration of cells in the pulmonary vasculature. Since the neutropenia only lasts a few hours, however, it probably does not play a role in predisposition to infection. Defects have been reported in neutrophil chemotaxis, and conflicting results on phagocytosis and microbicidal activity exist. Although cell-mediated immunity is impaired, immunoglobulin levels are usually normal. Antibody response to primary immunization may be blunted, however.

Malnutrition

In most of North American and Western European medical practice, malnutrition is usually not a primary problem but is associated with other severe illnesses or conditions such as malignancy and other debilitating diseases. In patients with severe protein-calorie malnutrition, protein synthesis is impaired, resulting in problems with the integrity of surface defenses such as skin and mucous membranes. This is compounded by secretory IgA deficiencies in the gut so that bacteria normally colonizing the colon may gain access to the systemic circulation. There is a defect in the early chemotactic response of neutrophil function, but phagocytosis is usually normal. Cells of the fixed-tissue monocyte macrophage type, however, have impaired phagocytic activity. Most complement components are low and this can be associated with defective opsonizing activity. Cell-mediated immunity is impaired as well.

Drugs

It has been well recognized for years that certain drugs particularly those used in the treatment of neoplastic diseases and glucocorticosteroids, can adversely affect host defenses. Recently, a good deal of experimental data have been published regarding the effects of antimicrobial agents on the immune system.

Numerous effects have been noted with the first two categories. Drugs such as methotrexate and cyclophosphamide can cause transient pancytopenia with attendant impairment of neutrophil, B, and T cell function. Also, turnover times for cell reproduction are impaired so that cells with rapid renewal rates such as those lining the intestinal tract are interfered with. This is also classically seen with radiation exposure as well.

Steroids are known to cause transient lymphopenia and monocytopenia, with more selective effects noted on T cell subpopulations. Functional effects are noted as well, including altered monocyte and neutrophil microbicidal activity and impaired cell-mediated immunity.

Many effects of antibiotics have been reported, but these are largely based on in vitro experiments and it is difficult to know how relevant they are clinically. Some of the reported adverse effects include inhibition of chemotaxis, phagocytosis, lymphocyte transformation, and delayed hypersensitivity. A more direct effect well known to clinicans is the problem of superinfection occurring as the result of alterations of normal human flora in patients receiving long-term antimicrobial therapy.

Transplantations

Patients undergoing organ or marrow transplantation are at risk of serious infection. The defects in host resistance in such patients are due not to the transplant itself but to the regimens used to suppress rejection of the graft. Depending on the type of transplant, various regimens are used, but generally they include agents that are both immunosuppressive and cytotoxic. If marrow transplants are used as a model, the host is rendered neutropenic and lymphopenic as well, and virtually all aspects of host defenses (surface barriers, inflammation, humoral and cell-mediated immunity) are impaired.

Surgical and burn patients also represent hosts whose normal defense mechanisms may be compromised to various degrees. They are discussed in Chapters 23 and 24 respectively.

ORGANISMS THAT CAUSE INFECTION

The organisms that cause infection depend largely upon the type of immunologic deficit found in a given host. Selected examples are listed in Table 22.1.

Diagnosis

The diagnosis of infection in the compromised host depends upon a careful and detailed history, physical examination, and laboratory assessment. It is always dangerous in such patients to jump to conclusions or make assumptions based on poorly gathered or sparse information. For example, the patient with sickle cell anemia and bone pain may have a bone infarct and not necessarily *Salmonella* osteomyelitis. A patient with rheumatoid arthritis with exacerbation of joint pain may have septic arthritis and not just a flare-up of disease in one joint. One must be careful to take nothing for granted and realize that particularly in cases where neutrophil counts are low, classic signs and symptoms of inflammation may not be present or may be blunted to such a degree that one fails to think of infection. This is usually not a problem in most of the conditions discussed so far, but is a major issue in patients with cancer who undergo chemotherapy, as discussed in the last half of this chapter.

A detailed and chronologic description of the presenting complaint is the first step. One must also ascertain the status of the underlying disease, any therapy currently in use, as well as other medications and concurrent or past illnesses. It is also important to find out about travel, hobbies, occupation and any family history of disease.

A complete and thorough physical examination is

TABLE 22.1. Selected Examples of Host Defense Defects and Associated Pathogens

Defects	*Pathogens*
Neutrophils	
Chemotaxis	Bacteria (*Staphylococcus aureus, Streptococcus pyogenes*)
Phagocytosis	Bacteria (*Pseudomonas aeruginosa*) Fungi (*Candida albicans*)
Microbicidal activity	Bacteria (*S. aureus, Salmonella* sp.)
Complement	Bacteria (*S. aureus, Nesseria gonorrhoeae*)
Antibody	
IgG	Encapsulated bacteria (*S. pneumoniae, Hemophilus influenzae*)
IgA	*Giardia lamblia*
T cells	Bacteria (*Listeria monocytogenes*) *Mycobacteria tuberculosis* (typical and atypical) Herpesviruses Protozoa (*Toxoplasma gondii, Pneumocystis carinii*)

essential but may not be as rewarding as the history.

It is important when considering laboratory tests not to order an all-inclusive battery of tests and hope that something will come back positive. If careful thought is given to the information obtained from the history and physical examination and what infections or disease processes are likely to account for symptoms, sensible use can be made of the laboratory. With judicious use of serologic and skin testing procedures, and culturing and staining of appropriate tissues or body fluids, a proper diagnosis can often be made. In cases where unusual or fastidious organisms are suspected, the clinician should always discuss the problem and suspected pathogens with the microbiologist so that appropriate cultures using selective media can be prepared.

If a diagnosis is particularly difficult, radiologic techniques such as gallium and technetium scanning and computerized transaxial tomography may help in localizing a site of involvement; then biopsy may provide the answer.

Treatment

In any compromised host, treatment can be divided into that aimed specifically at the infection itself and that aimed at correction of the host defect. In most instances, particularly in nonneutropenic cases, bacterial infection in compromised hosts is dealt with no differently than in other patients, although one must occasionally resort to empiric use of antibiotics before culture results are available if the clinical condition warrants it. One can then change if necessary once final culture and sensitivity results are available. Treatments of fungal, viral, and mycobacterial infections are dealt with in the treatment part of the last half of this chapter.

One must manage each patient individually. If protein-calorie malnutrition is obvious, hyperalimentation can be instituted. Diabetics have to be brought under control, patients with uremia may require dialysis, and those with sickle cell crises can be treated with hydration and analgesia. Most of the observed abnormalities in cases of systemic lupus erythematosus are associated with active disease, and even though it may seem somewhat contradictory to give drugs such as steroids, which may themselves predispose to infection, patients must be treated for their underlying disease. In the long run, this is the best way to deal with their infection.

Prevention

Control of the underlying disease process provides the best chance of preventing infection. In the case of patients with functional or anatomic asplenia, the pneumococcal vaccine should be given.

In all cases where one is dealing with a compromised host, the physician must instruct patients as to possible signs and symptoms that might indicate the development of infection, and urge them to contact the responsible physician as soon as possible.

AIDS

Over the past four years, what appears to be a new disease manifesting as a life-threatening, opportunistic infection and/or malignancy has been described. The acronym AIDS stands for acquired immunodeficiency syndrome, and since 1981 close to 6000 cases have been reported.

According to the Centers for Disease Control, AIDS

is defined as "a disease at least moderately predictive of a defect in cell-mediated immunity occurring in a person with no known cause for diminished resistance to that disease." One can see that this is really a working definition and may need to be changed as more is learned about the disease, its cause, and one hopes, its cure.

Etiology and Epidemiology

It appears that AIDS is caused by a virus called Human T cell Lymphotropic Virus III (HTLV-III).

Of the cases reported to date, approximately 70% to 75% occur in homosexual or bisexual males, approximately 15% in intravenous drug abusers, 5% to 6% in Haitians living in the United States or Canada, and 1% in patients with hemophilia A who are heterosexual and do not use intravenous drugs. A small group comprising approximately 5% of the total is made up of infants or partners of persons with AIDS, patients who have received blood transfusions, and prostitutes.

Pathogenesis

At present the exact pathogenetic mechanisms are not understood. Presumably, however, once the HTLV-III gains entry into the body, the immune system is affected. Ultimately, the result is an acquired defect in cell-mediated immunity. This is compatible with known models of infection and resultant transient immunosuppression, and is seen, for example, with cytomegalovirus, Epstein-Barr virus, and measles infections. If the HTLV-III agent causes immunologic dysfunction, this may lead to impairment of host defenses, resulting in opportunistic infection and/or malignancy. A characteristic feature of the altered cellular immune function is a decrease in the ratio of helper/inducer T cells to suppressor/cytotoxic T cells. In addition to this, one can find lymphopenia, anergy, and impaired natural killer-cell activity.

What is fascinating now are data showing similar alterations in ratios of T helper and suppressor cells in some asymptomatic homosexual males and some in otherwise healthy patients with hemophilia A treated with commercial clotting factor concentrates. The significance of such findings is not known at present, but they may imply that if these immune deficiencies are in fact markers of the disease, it may exist in a subclinical form in some patients while in others it goes on to a full-blown syndrome with obvious clinical findings.

Clinical Manifestations

The clinical manifestations of AIDS are varied and depend to a great extent on the nature of the opportunistic infection and/or malignancy present in the host. Up to 30% of patients with AIDS had a prior syndrome of fatigue, fever, malaise, and generalized lymphadenopathy for several months. Referred to as the gay lymphadenopathy syndrome, this may represent a prodrome of the disease. Conversely, however, patients with this syndrome have not necessarily gone on to develop full-blown AIDS.

Pneumocystis carinii pneumonia is the most common of the opportunistic infections, occurring in approximately 50% of patients. Other infections as mentioned by the Centers for Disease Control in their working definition include: "pneumonia, meningitis or encephalitis due to one or more of the following: aspergillosis, candidiasis, cryptococcosis, cytomegalovirus, nocardiosis, strongyloidiasis, toxoplasmosis, zygomycosis or atypical mycobacteriosis (species other than tuberculosis or lepra); esophagitis due to candidiasis, cytomegalovirus or herpes simplex virus; progressive multifocal leukoencephalopathy; chronic enterocolitis (more than four weeks) due to cryptosporidiosis; or unusually extensive mucocutaneous herpes simplex of more than five weeks duration." The malignant diseases include Kaposi's sarcoma, undifferentiated non-Hodgkin's lymphoma, Burkitt's lymphoma, cloacogenic carcinoma, and carcinoma of the tongue in nonsmokers.

Diagnosis

Unfortunately, at present there are no generally available, clinically useful laboratory tests that reliably determine whether or not a patient has AIDS. As indicated at the beginning of this section, the definition of AIDS is a working one and as such may be subject to change as more is learned about the disease. Conditions that might result in immunodeficiency and that should be absent in order to make the diagnosis include malnutrition, treatment with immunosuppressive or cytotoxic drugs, preexisting neoplasms, recent viral infections, particularly measles, mumps, and mononucleosis, and age greater than 60 years.

Treatment

There is no specific treatment for AIDS. Depending on the type of infection or tumor present, therapy is aimed at that particular condition, for example, trimethoprim/sulfamethoxazole or pentamidine isethionate for *Pneumocystis carinii* pneumonia. Interferon is also being evaluated for use in certain cases.

Prognosis

The prognosis unfortunately is not good. Overall mortality rates for *Pneumocystis carinii* pneumonia are 47%, for Kaposi's sarcoma 21%, and for persons with both, 68%. Those with opportunistic infections with neither Kaposi's sarcoma nor *Pneumocystis carinii* pneumonia have mortality rates of 48%.

Prevention

Current recommendations to avoid the spread of AIDS include avoiding sexual contact with persons either known or suspected to have AIDS and refusal to allow members of high-risk groups to be blood donors. A rational and understanding approach is required by both the medical and lay communities to avoid panic and to avoid stigmatizing groups unnecessarily. Work is also being carried on in several centers to develop a vaccine against the causative virus.

INFECTION IN PERSONS WITH CANCER

Infection is the leading proximate cause of death in patients with leukemia, lymphoma, and most solid tumors. As well as being a complication of both the tumor and its treatment, infections are also found to be a complication in surgical staging procedures in some malignancies such as Hodgkin's disease. Since the treatment of malignancy is rapidly improving, it is essential that a thorough understanding of the pathogenesis and therapy of life-threatening complications of such treatment are understood by physicians caring for these patients.

A partial list of the pathogens found in this population is as follows:

1. Bacteria
   - *Klebsiella pneumoniae*
   - *Escherichia coli*
   - *Pseudomonas aeruginosa*
   - *Serratia marcescens*
   - *Enterobacter* sp.
   - *Aeromonas hydrophila*
   - *Salmonella* sp.
   - *Staphylococcus aureus*
   - *Clostridium perfringens*
   - *Listeria monocytogenes*
   - *Nocardia asteroides*
2. Fungi
   - *Candida* sp.
   - *Aspergillus* sp.
   - *Cryptococcus neoformans*
   - *Mucor* sp.
3. Protozoa
   - *Toxoplasma gondii*
   - *Pneumocystis carinii*
4. Viruses
   - Herpes simplex
   - Varicella zoster
   - Cytomegalovirus
   - Hepatitis B

The most common causes of both fatal and nonfatal infections are gram-negative bacilli and *S. aureus*. *Klebsiella pneumoniae, E. coli* and *P. aeruginosa* are particularly common pathogens in the gram negative group. Therefore one should not immediately suspect less common organisms such as fungi, viruses, and protozoa since they usually occur in patients with certain specific, predisposing factors, for example, those receiving long-term immunosuppressive agents or broad-spectrum antibiotics.

Patients with different malignancies may be at risk from different organisms, as shown in Table 22.2.

Factors that Predispose to Infections

Common factors are as follows:

1. Granulocytopenia and granulocyte dysfunction
2. Immunosuppression (cell-mediated and humoral)
3. Chemotherapy
4. Obstruction of natural body passages
5. Treatment with broad-spectrum antibiotics
6. Standard causes of nosocomial infection

TABLE 22.2. Infectious Agents and Types of Cancer

			Neoplasms		
Pathogens	*Acute Leukemia*	*Chronic Lymphocytic Leukemia*	*Hodgkin's and non-Hodgkin's Lymphomas*	*Multiple Myeloma*	*Solid Tumors*
Bacteria					
Gram-negative bacilli	+ +	+	+	+ +	+ +
Anaerobes	0	0	+	0	+ +
Pneumococci	0	+ +	+	0	+ +
Staphylococci	+	0	+	+	+
Tuberculosis	+	0	+	0	+
Nocardia	+	+	+ +	0	+
Fungi					
Candida sp.	+ +	0	+	0	+
Aspergillus sp.	+ +	+	+	+	+
Cryptococcus sp.	+	+ +	+ +	0	0
Phycomycetes sp.	+ +	+	+	0	0
Viruses					
Varicella zoster	+	+	+ +	+	+
Herpes simplex	+	+	+ +	0	+
Protozoa					
Pneumocystis carinii	+ + +	+	+	0	+

+ + = marked association, + = definite association; 0 = no or rare association.
+ + + = particularly childhood acute lymphoblastic leukemia.

7. Splenectomy

Most of these result from defects in normal host defence mechanisms.

Granulocytopenia

Granulocytopenia is a major predisposing factor to infection in persons with cancer. The frequency of infection is directly related to the absolute granulocyte count. Bodey and his colleagues observed years ago that the frequency of infections increased as granulocyte counts dropped below 1000 per μl. Many investigators today consider 500 granulocytes per μl a far more significant level for predisposition to infection. Very low counts (below 100/μl) are particularly dangerous as they are associated with a major increase in gram-negative bacteremia. There also appears to be increased risk for infection with rapidly dropping blood counts. In addition, low granulocyte counts make the treatment of infection more difficult. Some patients with malignancies have adequate total granulocyte counts but have defects in their function. Some of these abnormalities include chemotaxis, phagocytosis, and microbial killing, as may occur in chronic myelogenous leukemia. These patients obviously are at risk from infection.

Immunosuppression

Cellular immunity can be impaired by treatment with agents such as corticosteroids and other drugs. In patients with Hodgkin's disease, defects in cellular immunity exist even prior to treatment. Patients with multiple myeloma, because of the increase in abnormal gamma globulin, are predisposed to infection with encapsulated organisms such as *S. pneumoniae* or *H. influenzae*, as they lack opsonizing activity against these bacteria.

Chemotherapy

Chemotherapy can cause infection by a number of mechanisms. These agents are often immunosuppressive, and in addition often cause granulocytopenia. They may affect the mucous membranes, causing mucositis, which may also predispose to infection. In many cases, combinations of chemotherapeutic agents are used to treat patients with malignant disease and these differ in their ability to predispose to infection.

Obstruction of Natural Passages

Partial or complete obstruction of a body orifice or passage can lead to infection due to stasis of body fluids and overgrowth of resulting organisms. Among the most frequent forms of obstruction are those of the urinary tract caused by prostatic, ovarian, cervical, or rectal carcinoma that lead to urinary tract infection. Obstruction of the main bronchus can occur in carcinoma of the lung and often results in susceptibility to pneumonia. Ascending cholangitis, due to neoplastic obstruction of the biliary tract, can also predispose to infection at this site.

Treatment with Broad-spectrum Antibiotics

Although broad-spectrum antibiotics are used to treat a proved or suspected infection, in fact, they can predispose to other infections as alluded to in the first part of this chapter.

Causes of Nosocomial Infection

Patients with cancer are susceptible to infection just as other hospitalized patients are. They may be at risk due to contaminated intravenous fluids, intravenous and urinary catheters, respirators, and the like. In addition, since they may have Ommaya reservoirs inserted to treat carcinomatous meningitis, this may act as a nidus for infection. The numerous blood product transfusions that they receive may be associated with an increased occurrence of hepatitis.

Most infections in patients with cancer are caused by organisms that colonize at or near the site where infections ultimately develop, as has been well-established by a number of groups doing repeated surveillance cultures. Colonization may be present when the patient arrives in hospital or may be acquired from the environment. This knowledge has led to attempts at suppression of the colonizing process so as to prevent infection from occurring. In addition, invasive procedures may create a pathway along which organisms can travel and result in infection.

Diagnosis

Certain areas of the body must be examined very carefully in this population, particularly in patients who are neutropenic from either treatment or disease. The clinician must also always keep in mind that in neutropenic patients, the classic findings of inflammation and infection may be absent.

The throat should be carefully examined since it may reveal evidence of thrush, which could be a hint that a serious fungal infection may be the cause of fever. The skin must also be examined for specific lesions. Ecthyma gangrenosum, initially thought to be diagnostic of *Pseudomonas* septicemia, has more recently been described with other gram-negative organisms such as *K. pneumoniae, E. coli,* and *Aeromonas*. Tissue from the lesion can be taken for biopsy and organisms can actually be seen and often cultured. Small, nodular lesions on the skin have been described, which if biopsied, reveal evidence of disseminated *Candida* infection. Other fungi can also cause skin involvement on rare occasions. Evidence of viral infection due to herpes simplex or varicella zoster is often found only in the skin and can be either localized or widespread. Areas such as skin folds, particularly in the axillary and inguinal regions, should be checked for carbuncles and ecthyma gangrenosum, and lesions that are found should be biopsied and cultured if possible. If viral infections are suspected, electron microscopy can also be helpful.

The perirectal area is frequently infected, particularly in patients with acute leukemia. When these patients are neutropenic, an abscess is often not demonstrable and only an area of erythema is present; however, this can lead to gram-negative septicemia. Examination of the eyes is often forgotten. Fungal infections particularly systemic candidiasis may be associated with infiltrates in the choroid. The abdomen and pelvis should be particularly well-examined in patients with gynecologic or gastrointestinal malignancies, as both sites can be sources of abscesses or perforations leading to systemic infection. The central nervous system is much less of a problem in this population, but can be associated with unusual infection, such as toxoplasmosis and herpes zoster encephalitis, and therefore must be carefully examined. Devices such as intravenous catheters, surgical drains, and/or Ommaya reservoirs must be carefully examined as possible sources of infection.

Standard investigations carried out in febrile patients, particularly those who are neutropenic are as follows:

1. Hemoglobin, white blood cell count, differential, and platelet count
2. Urinalysis and microscopic examination of urine
3. Baseline renal function and electrolytes
4. Cultures of blood, throat, sputum (if available), urine, skin lesions, and other appropriate sites
5. Posteroanterior and lateral x-ray views of the chest
6. Liver and spleen scans and computerized tomographic scans if abscesses are suspected

These tests should be done prior to empiric therapy even though the results will not be immediately available.

Many different organisms can cause pulmonary infiltrates in patients with lung tumor. In addition, there are several other causes of infiltrates in such patients, such as congestive heart failure, chemotherapy, tumor, irradiation, and pulmonary hemorrhage, to name a few. It is clear that pulmonary infection is the most frequent cause of fatal infection in the compromised host. Therefore an organized approach to the patient with a pulmonary infiltrate and cancer is absolutely essential.

Certainly, a chest x-ray must be obtained and if cavitation or other unusual findings are noted, tomograms may also be indicated. The radiologic picture will not be diagnostic of a particular etiology, although an experienced radiologist can narrow down the differential diagnoses to a reasonable number of possibilities. The rate of onset of the infiltrate may be helpful in diagnosis. Rapid onset tends to suggest a conventional bacterial infection (if an infectious cause is found), while subacute onset implies a viral or fungal origin as well as a less common etiology such as *Pneumocystis carinii*. A more chronic course over many weeks suggests a fungal, nocardial, or tuberculous infection.

Sputum cultures should be obtained if possible but, as often happens, particularly when patients are neutropenic, this may be difficult. If necessary, one can consider a transtracheal aspiration. This procedure can be associated with significant morbidity, particularly in patients with thrombocytopenia, and therefore is not frequently done in this population. Transbronchial lung biopsy may be a useful procedure. If all these techniques fail, open lung biopsy should be considered. In the hands of an experienced thoracic surgeon, this procedure causes little morbidity and almost no mortality. The results usually clarify the diagnosis, although there are always certain cases in which the pathology is said to be nonspecific.

TREATMENT

Bacterial Infections in Neutropenic Patients

In patients who are neutropenic (fewer than 1000 neutrophils/μl), death from infection can occur very rapidly (24 to 48 hours) if appropriate antibiotic treatment is not instituted. A site of infection may not be found in these patients, partly because an inflammatory response may not be possible without polymorphs. A pneumonia, for example, may be present with only a few rales heard on examination and a negative chest x-ray. Infections in these patients are most frequently caused by Enterobacteriaceae, *P. aeruginosa*, or *S. aureus*. It has therefore become customary to use a combination of antibiotics rather than a single agent as empiric therapy in febrile, neutropenic patients. More than two or three drugs, however, is probably not necessary. Choice of antibiotics is somewhat variable but usually includes at least two of an aminoglycoside, a cephalosporin or an antipseudomonal beta-lactam. The most frequently used agents are as follows: aminoglycosides — tobramycin and amikacin; cephalosporin — cefazolin; and antipseudomonals — ticarcillin and piperacillin. Examples of some commonly used regimens currently in use include ticarcillin plus tobramycin, cefazolin plus tobramycin, and piperacillin plus amikacin. Several third-generation cephalosporins have recently become available as well. These agents have a much broader spectrum of activity with, in some cases, reasonable coverage of *P. aeruginosa*. It is possible that some of these agents combined with antipseudomonal drugs may replace aminoglycosides or in some situations, where the third-generation cephalosporin is very active against *Pseudomonas*, there may actually be a place for single-drug therapy. At present, most of these agents are experimental and their efficacy in treatment of neutropenic patients has not been definitively established.

Patients with documented infections such as pneumonia or bacteremia should be treated for a minimum of 10 to 14 days. If infection is not documented either clinically or microbiologically, but the patient becomes afebrile, there is some debate as to just how long to continue antibiotic treatment. Current evidence suggests that treatment should continue until the granulocyte count is over 500/μl.

If the patient remains febrile longer than 7 to 10 days and especially if there is evidence of clinical deterioration, consideration should be given to empiric antifungal therapy with amphotericin B.

Granulocyte transfusions do not appear to play any role either prophylactically or therapeutically. This may, however, change if harvesting techniques can be improved so that larger numbers of cells can be given with each transfusion. This would apply primarily to their use in treatment of documented infection, rather than prevention.

Prophylactic Antibiotics in Neutropenic Patients

The use of oral, nonabsorbable antibiotics such as neomycin sulfate, gentamicin sulfate, and vancomycin hydrochloride has been found to reduce the infection rate, fatalities from infection, and febrile episodes during induction therapy in adult acute leukemia. Often, oral nystatin is used in an attempt to prevent fungal infection. These agents have been shown to be of value in controlled studies, even without the use of protected environment units. The value of laminar air-flow rooms is less well established. They are very difficult and expensive to use. Controlled trials have suggested that reverse isolation in this population probably has little value.

Recently, the use of a simple regimen consisting of prophylactic oral trimethoprim/sulfamethoxazole (TMP/SMZ) has been found by some investigators to be useful during induction therapy of acute leukemia in adults. This combination has also been found to be excellent prophylaxis against infection due to *Pneumocystis carinii* in childhood leukemia. There is still controversy, however, as to whether or not it has been established as a beneficial approach in adults, since the results of controlled trials at present appear to differ. The combination is certainly well tolerated, although possibly, development of resistant organisms may pose problems in the future. Fungal superinfections may also occur; nalidixic acid is being studied as a prophylactic agent.

Patients with Adequate Neutrophils

In general, patients who are febrile but have adequate neutrophils (over 1000/μl) should be investigated but not treated until an etiologic diagnosis is made, unless they are very ill. In this situation, appropriate empiric antibiotic therapy may be necessary. Similar antibiotic combinations, such as aminoglycosides and cephalosporins, are often chosen for these patients. Appropriate antibiotics can be added or substituted based on culture results.

Treatment of Unusual Infections

Tuberculosis

Tuberculosis appears to be somewhat more common in persons with cancer, particularly those with head and neck or lung tumors. Atypical mycobacterial organisms may be seen in a higher percentage of mycobacterial infections in the cancer population than in the healthy population. Standard therapy with two or three agents should be initiated when the diagnosis is made or strongly suspected. The general approach, including dosage and duration of treatment, is the same as for all cases of tuberculosis. Some patients at potentially high risk for developing this infection while receiving chemotherapy may be treated prophylactically with isoniazid.

Nocardia asteroides

The organism *N. asteroides* is a gram-positive, nonmotile, frequently acid-fast bacterium. The respiratory tract is the usual site of entry. Involvement of a lymphocutaneous site is not uncommon and spread to the brain can also occur, particularly in the compromised host. Although occasionally sputum cultures may be positive, often invasive procedures are necessary to make the diagnosis. A combination of pulmonary infiltrate and central nervous system disease or skin infection in the compromised host should prompt a vigorous search for this organism.

In addition to the usual supportive care necessary for the treatment of respiratory infections, the antibiotic of choice is a sulfonamide. Six to 10 gm per day are required and should be continued for at least three months and perhaps for the life of the patient, since relapses frequently occur. Other antibiotics show in vitro activity but have not been well studied clinically. Surgical intervention may be necessary for brain abscesses.

Fungal Infections

The most frequently seen fungal infections in persons with cancer are those caused by *Candida* sp., *Aspergillus* sp., and *Mucor* sp. Their diagnosis is often difficult premortem. Generally, they occur in a setting of long-term, broad-spectrum antibiotic or steroid therapy, often, when the malignancy, such as acute leukemia, is in a state of relapse.

Candida *Infections.* Thrush is extremely common and easily identified, although white lesions on the tongue or buccal mucosa may be due to many other causes and should be cultured. When this organism invades the upper gastrointestinal tract, it produces a characteristic cobblestone appearance radiologically. Systemic candidiasis is often suspected when classic lesions are seen on the skin or during a funduscopic examination. It is difficult to evaluate the significance of culture results from blood or other sites. The use of serology is controversial, although newer methods are being developed for detection of *Candida* antigens. Systemic infections, such as pneumonia, are extremely difficult to diagnose, with a recent study suggesting that probably only a tissue diagnosis is reliable.

Aspergillus *Infections.* *Aspergillus* infections usually involve the lungs but often go on to widespread infection of the skin and central nervous system. There is no typical radiologic appearance since a classic aspergilloma or fungus ball is not typical. Invasive aspergillosis can occur as an acute event, particularly in patients with acute leukemia. A positive sputum culture in patients with underlying malignancy, particularly acute leukemia, is frequently felt to be diagnostic, even though this organism can be found in some normal hosts. Small epidemics due to environmental contamination have been well documented at a number of institutions. When the source has been removed, often the infections stop occurring.

Phycomycetes. Mucormycosis is a very rare infection and classically occurs in the diabetic with associated sinusitis. This infection can cause an acute pneumonitis or even a widely disseminated infection in patients with cancer. It is most commonly seen in persons with hematologic malignancies but also occurs in patients with solid tumors. Most studies have shown premortem cultures to be negative. Usually the infection arises in the lung.

Cryptococcosis. A relatively rare type of fungal infection even in the cancer patient is that caused by *Cryptococcus neoformans*. The infection can either be localized to the lung or central nervous system or can be disseminated. It is most commonly found in patients with an underlying malignancy, particularly Hodgkin's disease, but is still unusual. The organism is usually found in soil contaminated by pigeon and chicken droppings. When infection does occur, it usually is present in the central nervous system with meningitis, but can involve the lungs, with hemoptysis or other respiratory symptoms. Occasionally, a diagnosis can be made by sputum culture. In the case of meningitis, the organism may be seen in cerebrospinal fluid when stained with India ink. Detection of cryptococcal antigen in the serum or cerebrospinal fluid is diagnostic.

Treatment of Fungal Infections

Fungal infections are extremely difficult to treat and only a few agents are commonly used for systemic infections. These include amphotericin B, 5-fluorocytosine, miconazole, and more recently, oral ketoconazole. Nystatin may be used for oral or vaginal infections. Nystatin, clotrimazole, and miconazole can all be used topically as well.

Amphotericin B. The treatment of fungal infections previously described usually includes the most active antifungal agent, amphotericin B. This drug is given as a test dose of 1 mg, followed by increasing daily doses. Our general practice is to give no more than 50 mg per day, although some authors suggest higher dosages are more beneficial, particularly with alternate-day regimens. The drug should be given over four to six hours, although some report that it is safe to give it over as little as two hours. In the case of *Candida* infections, as little as two weeks may be sufficient for systemic infection, and a 10-mg daily dose for five days is often enough for *Candida* esophagitis. For other systemic fungal infections, including some not mentioned, such as histoplasmosis, sporotrichosis, and coccidioidomycosis, longer periods of therapy are necessary, with total doses of 1 to 3 gm and sometimes more being required for eradication of these organisms. Intrathecal or intraventricular administration of amphotericin (through an Ommaya reservoir) can also be carried out for the treatment of central nervous system infections, using very low dosages of this agent. This medication is associated with some toxicity including nausea and vomiting, hypotension, fever, phlebitis, hypokalemia, and nephrotoxicity, to mention a few. In our hands, most of the patients have tolerated the drug quite well and with premedication with acetaminophen and diphenhydramine, therapy can be continued without much problem.

Fear of toxicity often results in a delay in instituting therapy, with a fatal outcome occurring in some instances. Recently, earlier diagnosis and aggressive treatment have resulted in cures of some of these infections. As previously mentioned, this agent is often used when patients with neutropenia continue to be febrile despite an adequate trial of antibacterial drugs. This is an empiric approach and has yet to be proved to have definite value.

Flucytosine. This agent was initially thought to be a useful antifungal agent but the rapid development of resistance when it is employed alone has limited its use. It seems to act at least additively and perhaps synergistically with amphotericin B against some fungi, particularly *Cryptococcus,* and is often used in combination when treating this central nervous system infection. A controlled trial has shown the combination to be superior to amphotericin B alone. It also may permit a slightly lower dose of amphotericin B to be administered.

Flucytosine is usually given orally in a dosage of 150 mg per kg per day (lowered to 100 mg/kg/day when used in combination with amphotericin B) in divided doses. Its potential to cause myelosuppression, particularly in patients with renal dysfunction, is its most significant toxicity.

Miconazole. Miconazole has a wide spectrum of antifungal activity in vitro. It has been marketed in the United States in intravenous form and is available in a topical form in many other countries, including Canada. It is quite useful in the treatment of coccidioidomycosis, but its value in other systemic fungal infections such as those due to candidal and cryptococcal organisms is much less well defined, although some data suggest it may be a second choice in situations where either amphotericin has failed or is clearly contraindicated. It also has a number of side effects, including nausea and vomiting, hyponatremia, hypertriglyceridemia (due to its vehicle), as well as others less frequently seen, such as hematologic and hepatic enzyme changes.

Ketoconazole. This agent has recently been marketed in the United States as a 200-mg tablet, to be given in a dosage of one to three tablets daily. Higher doses are being investigated. This drug has a broad spectrum of activity, with good oral absorption and very little toxicity. Its disadvantages are that it does not get into the cerebrospinal fluid and is not active against a number of organisms frequently seen in patients with cancer, such as *Aspergillus* and *Mucor.* Several imidazole derivatives being produced by the pharmaceutical industry may prove to be of value.

Protozoal Infections

The two protozoa that most frequently cause infection in patients with cancer are *Toxoplasma gondii* and *Pneumocystis carinii.*

Toxoplasmosis. Toxoplasma infection is not particularly common in cancer patients, but when it does occur, in approximately 50% of cases it causes encephalitis. Its diagnosis is usually made by serology and occasionally by biopsy. Treatment of this infection in the compromised host includes pyrimethamine, 25 mg three times a day for one week, and 25 mg per day for at least a further three weeks, plus sulfadiazine in a loading dose of 4 gm, followed by 1 gm four times a day.

Pneumocystis carinii. This organism usually causes interstitial pneumonia, particularly in the pediatric age group with acute leukemia, and is often seen in these children when their disease is in complete remission. The diagnosis can occasionally be made by sputum examination or transtracheal aspiration, but most often requires either a transbronchial or open lung biopsy. Treatment of this infection in the past consisted of pentamidine isethionate, 4 mg per kg intramuscularly per day for 10 days to 2 weeks. This drug has been quite toxic and not very active, particularly in the adult population. The use of trimethoprim/sulfamethoxazole in very high dosage has been effective against this infection, both in children and in adults, and is now the drug of first choice. In cases of treatment failure, however, pentamidine isethionate can still be used. As previously mentioned, trimethoprim/sulfamethoxazole can be used prophylactically in groups at high risk of developing this infection.

Viral Infections

The most common viral infections affecting patients with cancer are those caused by the herpes group of DNA viruses. This includes varicella zoster, herpes simplex, and cytomegalovirus.

Varicella Zoster. Varicella (chicken pox) can frequently be a disseminated infection in pediatric immunosuppressed patients and is occasionally seen in adults. Herpes zoster is much more frequent in adults but can occur in children. It often causes a localized dermatome distribution, but can disseminate and involve major organs. Lymphomas, particularly Hodgkin's disease, are the malignancies most frequently associated with this infection but, in fact, virtually every neoplastic disease has some slight predisposition to this problem.

The diagnosis is often made on clinical grounds when the classic dermatomal lesions associated with pain are seen. It can be proved by biopsy of the lesion with immediate electron microscopy, which will at least determine whether or not it is a herpesvirus infection. A specific diagnosis may be available when culture results are complete. Serology may also be helpful.

Treatment of localized infection includes analgesics and soothing topical medication, such as calamine lotion. When it disseminates, however, there may be a place for systemic antiviral therapy. More recently, there has been some evidence that early antiviral therapy may reduce the incidence of postherpetic neuralgia, increase the rapidity of healing, and reduce the frequency of dissemination.

Adenine arabinoside (ara-A) is of value in localized herpes zoster as previously mentioned, and probably has some benefit in disseminated disease. Treatment consists of 10 to 15 mg per kg per day, given over 12 hours in a large fluid volume because of its relative insolubility. Studies are under way on a more soluble derivative (ara-A monophosphate) that theoretically can be given intramuscularly or by rapid intravenous injection, and would appear to be as active as ara-A in preliminary studies. A much more active agent has recently become available (acyclovir). It appears in preliminary testing in vitro to be at least as good as ara-A and probably superior. Controlled trials have been completed that clearly show this agent to have activity against most herpesviruses as compared to placebo. It has also been compared to ara-A in double blind trials, but the results are not available. Acyclovir appears to be relatively nontoxic and very active.

Varicella-immune globulin or zoster-immune plasma may be useful in preventing or modifying the effect of herpes zoster or chicken pox in the pediatric age group. Recently, the use of a live varicella vaccine has been tried in Japan, and a large North American trial is under way, but no results are available. Human leukocyte interferon or other forms of interferon may also have some value in this infection, but experience is very limited.

Herpes Simplex. This organism causes local infections in the oral and genitourinary areas. In addition, in the compromised host, it can cause disseminated infection or multiple lesions on the skin in a manner that mimics herpes zoster. Recurrent herpes simplex in the mouth can be a problem in persons with cancer but herpes simplex encephalitis, a potentially rapidly fatal infection, does not seem to be found with increased frequency in the compromised host.

Encephalitis is usually treated with 20 mg per kg of adenine arabinoside for approximately 10 days. Its therapeutic value in other herpes simplex infections has not been established. Acyclovir also appears to be useful in this population, but the details of the ongoing studies are not yet available.

Cytomegalovirus. This organism is only rarely found in cancer patients, except those with acute leukemia who undergo bone marrow transplantation. In this situation it is often the cause of a pulmonary infiltrate that goes on to be fatal. Diagnosis of this organism can be made by serology, although open lung biopsy may be necessary. No available antiviral agent has been found to be therapeutically effective in this infection.

Other Viral Infections. Progressive multifocal leukoencephalopathy appears to be caused by a papovavirus and is an infrequent cause of central nervous system infection. It is usually insidious in onset with gradual progression for a few months in most cases. Biopsy of brain tissue is necessary to make the diagnosis. Unfortunately, at present there is no proven therapy for this disease, although some people feel cytosine arabinoside may have some activity.

Hepatitis is relatively frequently seen in persons with cancer. These patients often receive many transfusions and are therefore at particular risk for hepatitis B as well as the non-A, and non-B form of disease. The diagnosis of hepatitis B can usually be made by radioimmunoassay detection of the hepatitis B surface antigen. There is no proved specific form of treatment for this infection.

Other Unusual Infections

Strongyloidiasis is caused by the intestinal threadworm, *Strongyloides stercoralis.* Although relatively benign in the general population in whom it causes occasional symptoms of epigastric discomfort, this infection can progress to a fatal outcome in the compromised host. Patients can develop diffuse pneumonitis, eosinophilia, and variable gastrointestinal syndromes. The disease occurs in individuals with lymphomas, leukemias, and solid tumors. Patients with intact host defenses still have potential for accelerated autoinfection, and therefore it has been recommended that every patient with *Strongyloides* infestation should be treated. This usually includes thiabendazole, 25 mg per kg twice daily, or mebendazole, 100 mg twice daily for 7 to 14 days. This is much longer than is used generally (three days), but there is little danger of drug toxicity. Patients with repeat episodes of infection may benefit from thiabendazole, 25 mg per kg two to three days every month.

ANNOTATED BIBLIOGRAPHY

Allen JC. Infection and the compromised host. Clinical correlations and therapeutic approaches, 2nd edition. Baltimore: Williams & Wilkins, 1981.
A smaller text dealing with selected types of compromised hosts, such as the alcoholic or diabetic patient. Well written but not as detailed or comprehensive as Grieco's text.

Fauci AS, et al. Acquired immunodeficiency syndrome: epidemiologic, clinical, immunologic and therapeutic considerations. Ann Intern Med 1984;100:92–106
A comprehensive review of this syndrome focusing on the epidemiology, clinical manifestations, immunologic abnormalities, and treatment.

Grieco H, ed. Infections in the abnormal host. Yorke Medical Books, 1980.
A detailed and comprehensive textbook dealing with virtually all aspects of infection in immunocompromised hosts. The book is divided into three major sections: host defenses, infections associated with the abnormal host, and management.

Hill HR. Infections complicating congenital immunodeficiency syndromes. In Rubin RH, Young LS eds., Clinical approach to infection in the compromised host. New York: Plenum Press, 1981:417–46.
An excellent review of the major congential immunodeficiency syndromes and the diagnosis and management of infection in these patients.

Pizzo PA. Empiric antibiotic and antifungal therapy for cancer patients with prolonged fever and granulocytopenia. Am J Med 1982;72:101–111.
Essentially a continuation of the 1979 study with an attempt to determine the role of empiric antifungal therapy. The results suggest that such empiric therapy may be useful in patients who remain febrile and granuocytopenic despite seven days of antibacterial therapy.

Pizzo PA. Antimicrobial prophylaxis in the immunosuppressed cancer patient. In Remington JS, Swartz MN, eds. Current clinical topics in infectious diseases. New York: McGraw-Hill, 1983:153–185.
An excellent review of the issues involved in designing prophylactic regimens for patients with cancer. The literature dealing with this area is reviewed in detail and the strengths and weaknesses of the various studies are discussed.

Pizzo PA, et al. Duration of empiric antibiotic therapy in granulocytopenic patients with cancer. Am J Med 1979;67:194–200.
A well-designed, randomized clinical study that examines how long one should continue antibacterial drugs in granulocytopenic patients who have become afebrile. The study concludes that patients with a fever of unknown origin who become afebrile and remain granulocytopenic should be treated until the cell count improves ($>500/mm^3$).

Symposium on infectious complications of neoplastic disease. Part II. Am J Med 1984;76:631–684.
A series of review papers on various topics dealing with infection in cancer.

Young LS. The role of granulocyte transfusions in treating and preventing infection. Cancer Treat Rep 1983;67:109–111. Schiffer CA. Granulocyte transfusion therapy. Cancer Treat Rep 1983;67:113–119.
Two excellent summaries of issues involved in white blood cell transfusions.

23 POSTOPERATIVE INFECTION

John M.A. Bohnen and Jonathan L. Meakins

The management of postoperative infections is a problem as old as surgery itself. Before Lister's time, most infections after operation were due to gram-positive bacteria such as staphylococci and streptococci, derived from the hospital environment (exogenous) and not the patient's own endogenous flora. With the emphasis on asepsis and antisepsis that began in the late nineteenth century, exogenous infections have decreased, though they may still end in disaster. The more common endogenous infections involve bacteria from the skin or mucosa-lined tracts, and usually result from surgery in which previously sterile tissue is exposed to the contaminated contents of hollow organs.

If the first important step was asepsis, the next was an appreciation of the local biology in the establishment of an infection at surgery. From the late 1950s, Miles and others described the events associated with bacterial lodgement in tissue. It was then found that antibiotics would prevent wound infections only if given before or soon after the first incision was made.

The third important event, in the 1960s, was the classification of operative wounds based on the degree of bacterial contamination (Table 23.1). This improved the evaluation of preventive and therapeutic measures, and promoted surgeons' acceptance of wound infection surveillance. Finally, greater attention has been paid recently to host defenses to prevent infections by identifying and correcting abnormalities in such conditions as malnutrition, trauma, and cancer. The types of postoperative infection are listed as follows:

1. At operative site
   - Wound infection
   - Deep infection
   - Regional extension of infection from wound (cellulitis, fasciitis, lymphangitis), or deep operative site such as peritonitis
2. Distant from operative site
   - Metastatic
   - Primary infection elsewhere (pneumonia, intravenous catheter sepsis)
3. Blood stream
   - Bacteremia
   - Septicemia

Wound and deep infections at the operative site, and primary infections distant from the operative site are the most common.

GENERAL PRINCIPLES

Microbial Etiology

Infections in clean cases (Table 23.1) usually involve exogenous organisms or endogenous skin bacteria; *Staphylococcus aureus* is still the most common offender in clean cases (endemic cases) and is usually endogenous. Epidemics of clean wound or remote site infections, whether they involve staphylococci, streptococci, or enteric organisms, are usually exogenous. Careful search will often identify the common source (person or equipment) from which the organism is being disseminated.

Endogenous bacteria are usually responsible for infections in clean-contaminated, contaminated, and so-called dirty operations. The oropharynx, stomach, biliary tree, small and large intestines, and other mucosa-lined surfaces all have characteristic and different flora. The species involved in a postoperative infection depend on the operative site. The choice of prophylactic antibiotics should be a reflection of the expected pathogens.

Fungal and protozoal (e.g., pneumocystis) infections infrequently occur postoperatively, but are more

TABLE 23.1. Classification of Operations by Degree of Contamination

Type of Surgery	*Rate of Wound Infection (%)* Reported	Ideal
Clean	1–5	< 1
Nontraumatic		
No inflammation encountered		
No break in technique		
Alimentary, respiratory, genitourinary tracts not entered		
Clean-contaminated	3–12	< 3
Alimentary, respiratory, or genitourinary tract entered, without significant spillage or inflammation		
Minor break in sterile technique		
Contaminated	10–20	< 7
Gross spillage from gastrointestinal tract		
Entrance of inflamed respiratory, genitourinary, or biliary tract; no pus present		
Fresh traumatic wound		
Major break in technique		
Dirty and infected	25–40	<10*
Perforated viscus		
Old or clinically infected traumatic wound		
Inflammation with pus		

*Selected wounds not closed primarily.

common in immunosuppressed patients or those receiving prolonged therapy with several antibiotics. Viral infections such as posttransfusion hepatitis may also occur; however, most infections after surgery are bacterial.

Pathophysiology

Factors leading to infection after surgery are preoperative, operative, or postoperative. In the last two categories especially, many are preventable.

Preoperative factors can be divided into those that were previously present in the patient and those that are a result of some clinical action. Patient-related conditions that are associated with an increased chance of subsequent infection are malnutrition, cancer and other diseases that impair immunity, old age, obesity, skin test anergy, remote infection or bacterial colonization, immunosuppressive medications, and fluid volume depletion. These features are usually a result of the underlying disease for which the surgery was indicated. With the exception of malnutrition and volume depletion, conditions associated with alterations in host defenses are not yet amenable to correction before surgery.

Preoperative considerations relating to clinical management are the type of ward and length of hospitalization before surgery (a long stay and open, multibed wards are associated with increased wound infection), and the preparation of the patient for surgery. Preparation involves the correction, if possible, of patient-related factors and the use of prophylactic antimicrobial agents (discussed under Chemoprophylaxis, Chapter 7). Inadequate skin antisepsis and the shaving (rather than clipping) of skin hair at the operative site have been shown repeatedly to increase the chance of wound infection.

Good operative technique, which will prevent many infections, is described in surgical texts. It involves delicate handling of tissue, anatomic dissection, meticulous hemostasis, removal of any dead tissue, and the use of drains when appropriate. Blood and devitalized tissue act as culture media for the growth of bacteria, and in their presence, fewer bacteria are required to produce infection. The longer an operation is, the more likely a subsequent infection will occur. Foreign material left in situ increases the infection risk; thus as little as possible should be left behind, and materials that promote inflammation (such as silk) should generally be avoided. Examples of foreign bodies intentionally inserted are sutures, artificial joints, vascular grafts, and prosthetic heart valves. Failure to eradicate an infection involving a foreign body with medical treatment alone may necessitate removal of the inserted material.

The important intraoperative factor over which the surgeon may or may not have control is the degree of bacterial contamination (Table 23.1). A perfectly executed operation for a ruptured colon still carries a high risk of wound infection and intraabdominal abscess because of the severe initial contamination of sterile tissue.

Postoperative factors tend to be more important in leading to infections remote from the operative site. Invasive diagnostic and therapeutic procedures such as intravascular and urinary catheters break down epithelial barriers to sepsis. Postoperatively, patients are often immobilized by pain and sedation. This may lead to pulmonary infections and decubitus ulcers. The hospital milieu is a factor, especially in critically ill patients. Proximity to other patients with infection, poor hand washing by ward personnel, and the presence of virulent nosocomial bacterial strains all make infection more likely in a given patient. Cross-infection was first controlled by Semmelweiss and the efficacy of hand washing was firmly established. The concurrent development of Lister's concepts of antisepsis provided the basis of hospital infection control.

During an operation and in the first three hours postoperatively, a battle is being waged between the patient and the bacteria at the operative site. The events during this time usually determine whether an infection develops, even if sepsis is not clinically evident until days or weeks later. The occurrence of an infection depends on the presence of the causative factors described above. Of utmost importance are the magnitude of the bacterial contamination and the state of host's defenses.

Once an infection is established, the local and systemic consequences give rise to the clinical picture. Locally, the presence of bacteria and surgical trauma cause acute inflammation, with an influx of fluid and white blood cells. If the bacteria are not contained locally, there may be extension regionally as in cellulitis, lymphangitis, and lymphadenitis, or systemically with bacteremia and septicemia.

Systemic consequences of established infection may occur with local, spreading, and generalized infection. Fever and hypercatabolism are common effects of postoperative infection, and malnutrition often results; other metabolic changes such as hyperglycemia can occur.

Multisystem organ failure is frequently seen when there is postoperative sepsis. Why this occurs is a subject of much research. Such patients have weakened host defenses and are at risk for further sepsis. The end of the vicious cycle of organ failure after surgical sepsis is usually death. Surgical drainage of a focus of infection in the presence of organ failure may reverse the patient's downhill course, however. Any patient with unexplained failure of one or more organ systems postoperatively should be assumed to harbor a focus of infection until proved otherwise.

Clinical Manifestations

The signs and symptoms of postoperative infection are those of acute local inflammation and systemic manifestations including fever and leukocytosis. Fever is commonly present with postoperative infections, although there are other causes of fever in this setting (Table 23.2). Furthermore, the absence of fever does not rule out an infection, especially in immunosuppressed and elderly patients.

Systemic manifestations of infection include jaundice, renal insufficiency, respiratory distress, gastrointestinal bleeding, ileus, coagulopathy, hyperglycemia, hypotension, and abnormal mentation. These systemic effects are most commonly associated with deep infection. Wound infections are usually treated before severe organ dysfunction supervenes.

Diagnosis

Laboratory investigations that may be indicated include a complete blood count, Gram's stain and culture

TABLE 23.2. Causes of Postoperative Fever

Common		*Uncommon*	
Infectious	*Noninfectious*	*Infectious*	*Noninfectious*
Urinary tract infection	Physiologic response to surgery	Parotitis	Thyroid storm
Pneumonia	Atelectasis	Endocarditis	Myocardial infarction
Intravascular catheter sepsis	Aspiration pneumonitis	Infected decubitus ulcer	Malignant hyperthermia
Deep operative infection	Pulmonary embolus	Transfusion-related infection	Acalculous cholecystitis
Operative wound infection	Deep vein thrombosis	Antibiotic-associated infection	Adrenal insufficiency
Infected prosthesis	Drugs	Unrelated infection	
	Transfusion		
	Allograft rejection		

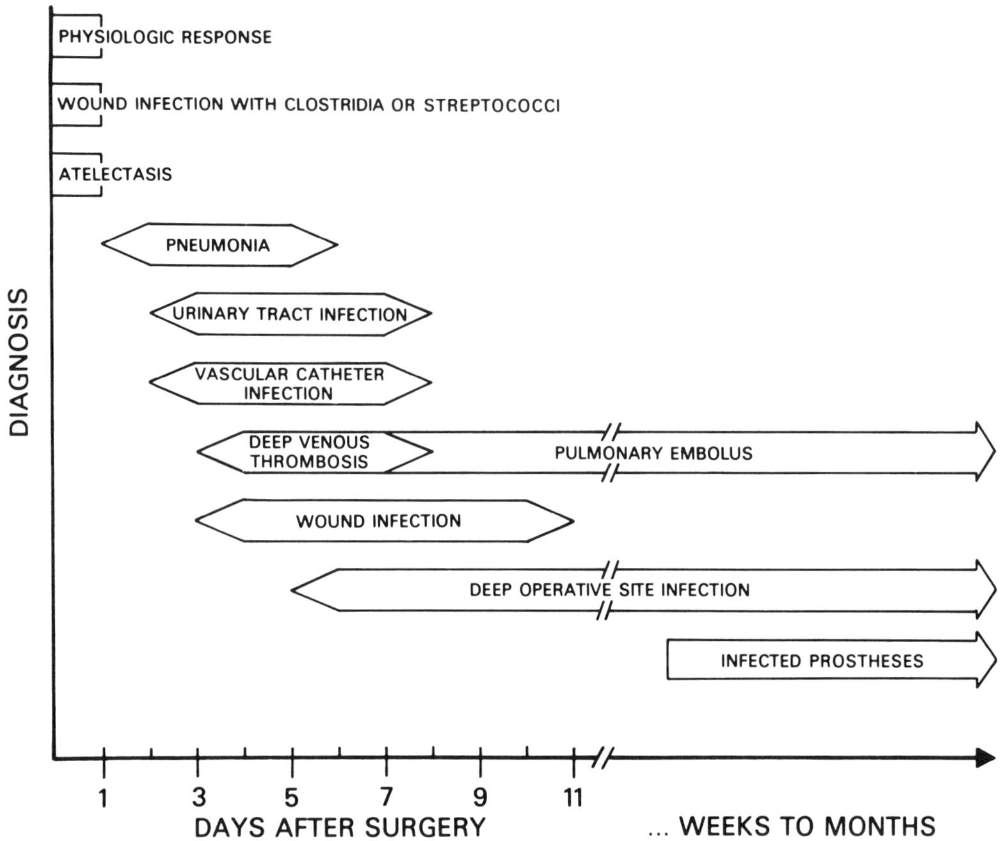

FIGURE 23.1. The postoperative timing of events producing fever, not all of which are infectious.

of pus or purulent material, and blood cultures in cases of severe sepsis or when sepsis is suspected but cannot be demonstrated by other means. Serum biochemistry measurements (e.g., bilirubin, creatinine) may clarify the diagnosis of organ failure. Diagnostic imaging such as x-rays, computerized tomographic (CT) scans, sonograms, and isotopic scans may be useful in the diagnosis of deep infections in the head, thorax, and abdomen.

Treatment

The therapy of an established infection after surgery primarily involves drainage of a purulent focus and removal of the source of infection, either by operation or percutaneous cannula. The adjunctive use of antibiotics, which depends on the severity of the infection, is a matter of clinical judgment. The drug(s) should be chosen on the basis of the likeliest pathogens for a given type of infection, and altered if necessary on the basis of Gram's stain and culture and sensitivity results.

Prophylaxis

As in any disease, the best treatment is prevention, which in this case means avoiding the causative factors mentioned above. The practice of asepsis and antisepsis develops appropriate operating room attitudes and behavior. These activities create the appearance of a ritual that often puzzles and irritates medical students and nonsurgeons. Such rituals are an integral part of the surgical conscience and are effective in preventing postoperative infections. Planning the correct operation and meticulous, quick surgery are of equally great importance.

Another preventive measure is the proper use of prophylactic antimicrobial agents, which have been demonstrated to decrease the frequency of wound and sometimes deep infections in selected instances. In general, preoperative antibiotics are indicated either in clean cases in which infections would be disastrous (e.g., vascular prostheses) or contaminated cases in which infections are common (e.g., colon surgery). (See Chapter 7 for detailed discussion.)

Infections after surgery may be divided into two categories: those that may occur after any kind of operation and those that are fairly specific to a given type of surgery.

INFECTIONS COMMON TO ALL TYPES OF OPERATIONS

Wound Infection

Wound infection is a common (but decreasing) complication that may result in disability, prolongation of hospital stay, significant social and financial costs, and very occasionally, death. The frequency of wound infection is very dependent upon the degree of contamination. Following clean cases, the rate is now about 1% whereas when all types of cases are examined, the infection rate is slightly less than 5%.

Etiology

Bacterial pathogens involved in wound infections depend to a large extent on the type of operation. Infections in clean operations usually result from *S. aureus,* which is the organism most commonly cultured from all infected wounds, occurring in 20% to 25% of cases. These bacteria are most often endogenous from skin or nose, but occasionally come from the operating room staff. Wound infections with group A streptococci are uncommon, but may be very serious. Attending staff are also checked to see if any members are colonized or infected with the organism. *Escherichia coli* is the second most common organism, and as a group, the gram-negative facultative rods are the most common cause of wound infections. These are usually endogenous bacteria, include *Proteus, Enterobacter,* and *Klebsiella* species, and generally come from the gastrointestinal tract. *Pseudomonas* organisms may come from the gut or from the hospital environment. Anaerobes, especially *Bacteroides* spp., often accompany gram-negative facultative rods in wound infections. Infections with clostridial species usually result from dirty traumatic wounds, amputations of ischemic limbs, or contamination of wounds with feces.

Pathophysiology

See the discussion of pathophysiology under General Principles. Clostridial wound infections are a special case in that they are likely to occur in wounds with poor blood supply, local anoxia, and dead tissue.

Clinical Manifestations

Although most wound infections are diagnosed between the fourth and eighth days postoperatively, one out of ten become evident only after the patient has left hospital. The usual signs and symptoms are fever plus the signs of local acute inflammation: pain, swelling, heat, and redness. Occasionally, such an infection will cause a discharge of pus or wound disruption.

In staphylococcal disease, the infection usually becomes a localized abscess containing creamy pus four to six days after surgery. Streptococcal infections arise earlier, often within 24 hours of surgery, and do not usually form much pus; rather, cellulitis with lymphangitis is the typical picture. If not recognized or adequately treated, rapid progression to fasciitis, gangrene, and septicemia is possible. High fever and chills are usually present. The other type of wound infection, potentially catastrophic, that may occur on the first day postoperatively is caused by *Clostridia* species. With these organisms, cellulitis, fasciitis, and/or myonecrosis may result, usually with gas formation. Gas may be produced by other anaerobes as well. Anaerobic wound infection may in particular occur late in the clinical course, with minimal local findings, low-grade fever, but upon drainage, a large, tissue-destroying abscess is found. Infections with gram-negative facultative organisms may develop several days later than staphylococcal infections and with less obvious local signs. In fact, systemic sepsis with bacteremia may be the initial clinical picture in these infections, before local signs are apparent.

Diagnosis

The most important diagnostic measure is frequent examination of the wound, looking for inflammation and absence of a normal wound ridge. The diagnosis is confirmed by opening the wound (drainage), which is the first step in treatment. Gram's stain and culture should be carried out on pus, or if there is no pus, on a wound swab. A foul odor on drainage suggests that anaerobes are present. It must also be pointed out that the infected wound may be the tip of an iceberg; a larger or more serious infection may lie in the operative site deeper in the wound.

Treatment

The treatment of a wound infection consists of immediate opening of the wound, upon which pus usually escapes and the pain at the site is relieved. Skin sutures are removed and the wound is packed loosely with saline- or antiseptic-soaked dressings. Dressings should be changed several times a day and the wound inspected regularly. Antimicrobial agents are not usually indicated unless there is regional or distant spread, marked systemic manifestations, the patient is immunodepressed, or there is fear of infecting with a bacteremia an implanted prosthesis such as a heart valve, vascular graft, or artificial joint. When intravenous antimicrobial agents are indicated, a staphylococcal infection requires a penicillinase-resistant penicillin (e.g. cloxacillin) or penicillin G (if susceptible), or a cephalosporin (such as cefazolin). In antibiotics are needed for an infection with gram-negative rods, usually an aminoglycoside is administered; if anaerobes are also present, clindamycin or metronidazole should be added to the antimicrobial regimen.

The treatment of a clostridial wound infection requires extensive debridement, usually in the operating room, with particular attention to necrotic tissue. High-dose parenteral penicillin with metronidazole, clindamycin, or chloramphenicol is essential. Hyperbaric oxygen therapy has been advocated by some, but is of less importance and should never cause a delay in surgical debridement.

The treatment of streptococcal wound infection is wound drainage and debridement of devitalized tissue. High-dose intravenous penicillin is indicated in these cases. Gram's stain and culture should be performed, but even in the absence of microscopic confirmation, penicillin should be administered for any wound infection that occurs on the first day after surgery.

Staphylococcus aureus and group A streptococci are highly pathogenic organisms that can produce disease in healthy patients undergoing surgery. These bacteria survive well on the skin of patients and hospital personnel, facilitating cross-infection. Although isolating patients with wound sepsis has gone somewhat out of fashion, it should be done for those with infections with gram-positive pathogens.

Prognosis

After treatment the usual complication of a wound infection is simply an unsightly scar. Wound dehiscence and incisional hernia are serious consequences that may require further surgery (repair).

Prophylaxis

Preventive measures such as good operative technique and prophylactic antibiotics (see Chapter 7) have been discussed. Skin hair should be clipped immediately before operation rather than shaved. The patient's skin and operators' hands must be made as close to sterile as possible, using iodine, an iodophor, or chlorhexidine; a five-minute scrub of the operating team's hands is adequate. Great care must be taken in gowning, gloving, and the use of masks, as well as draping the patient. Sterile adhesive skin drapes are costly and of no proved value.

Delayed primary closure is an effective method of preventing wound infection. Sometimes the operative field is so heavily contaminated that infection is likely even in the presence of otherwise careful wound management. In these cases the risk of infection is greatly lessened by closing the fascia, leaving the skin and subcutaneous tissue open at the end of the operation, and packing them with sterile dressings. Five days later, if the wound appears uninfected and has healthy granulation tissue, it can then be closed (delayed primary closure). If the wound has poor granulation tissue, appears soupy or infected, it is allowed to heal by secondary intention.

Possibly the most interesting preventive measure against wound infection is peer group pressure. It has been shown that if all surgeons are informed of their own wound infection rate plus that of the whole surgical service, the overall rate of infections will decrease. Dissemination of this information should be the function of the hospital infection control committee and the surgeons' representative.

Over the last ten years, there has been a significant decrease in the prevalence of wound infections and a consequent reduction in the number of incisional hernias. Important factors contributing to this change have been the proper use of prophylactic antibiotics, delayed primary closure, surveillance, and peer pressure.

Pneumonia

Pneumonia is also a common postoperative infection. In present times, it is now a more frequent postoperative complication than wound infection. See also Chapter 12.

Etiology

As with other nosocomial pneumonias, about half the cases are caused by gram-negative aerobic rods. Aerobic gram-positive cocci and anaerobes are also commonly involved.

Pathophysiology

The evolution of pneumonia in postoperative thoracic and abdominal surgery starts with atelectasis secondary to pain, immobilization, and/or oversedation. If the inadequate ventilation is not corrected, bronchopneumonia will often result. Other factors contributing to postoperative pneumonia include aspiration of oropharyngeal secretions or gastric contents secondary to sedation or neurologic impairment, preexisting lung disease, and contamination of ventilatory equipment.

Clinical Manifestations and Diagnosis

Pneumonia may develop at any time after an operation, and is one of the most common causes of fever in the first three postoperative days. Diagnosis is established by clinical and radiographic examination, and Gram's stain and culture of sputum (not saliva). What appears to be a severe pneumonia may in fact be the adult respiratory distress syndrome, which is part of the syndrome of multiple organ failure; if this is suspected, remote sites of sepsis must be searched for.

Treatment

See Chapter 12.

Prognosis

Respiratory insufficiency, septicemia, and local septic sequelae such as lung abscess may occur after postoperative pneumonia. The mortality is not known but may be high if complications occur.

Prophylaxis

Early ambulation after operation and avoidance of other predisposing factors are important. Prophylactic antibiotics are not indicated.

Urinary Tract Infection

Etiology and Pathophysiology

Gram-negative aerobic bacilli are the usual pathogens with postoperative as with other urinary infections. Excluding infections secondary to operation on the genitourinary tract, postoperative urine infections are usually associated with urethral catheterization.

Clinical Manifestations and Diagnosis

Urinary infection is a common cause of fever at any time after surgery. Pain in the flank or pubic region, dysuria, urinary frequency, and chills, are other manifestations. Bacteriologic diagnosis is usually made by the finding of 10^8 or more organisms per liter of urine (midstream); however, if pyuria or urinary symptoms are present, or if an indwelling catheter is used for specimen collection, less than 10^8 bacteria per liter may be significant.

Treatment

Treatment, when possible, is removal of the catheter. The culture is repeated in a few days. Systemic antimicrobial therapy will never sterilize the urine if a catheter is in place; if the catheter cannot be removed, antibiotics should only be given for signs of renal infection, systemic sepsis, or symptomatic lower tract disease. If a catheter is not present, treatment is as for other causes of urinary tract infection (see Chapter 16).

Prognosis

These infections are rarely lethal, but are important, as the potential for septicemia and renal abscess is always present and discharge from hospital is delayed.

Prophylaxis

Urinary infections after nonurinary tract surgery are generally preventable. Many can be avoided by strict attention to the proper technique of starting and maintaining a closed drainage system. Even proper technique will be followed by infections usually within seven days, so patients should only be catheterized when necessary, and if possible with only a single catheterization (in and out). Condom catheters should be used in males if incontinence is the problem. Patients who have early postoperative urine retention should be encouraged to void in as private and relaxed an environment as possible so as to avoid catheterization. Spatial dispersal of ward patients with urinary catheters will help prevent patient-to-patient spread of established infections.

Vascular Catheter Infections

Infections associated with vascular catheters are the most frequent complications after surgery.

Etiology and Pathophysiology

Cannula site infections are generally caused by skin organisms that track along the catheter. *Staphylococcus aureus* and *S. epidermidis* are the most commonly implicated pathogens. In parenteral nutrition (central) line infections, *Candida* species are especially important. The frequency is higher with cutdowns than with percutaneously inserted lines.

Clinical Manifestations and Diagnosis

These infections may occur at any time after surgery, with fever and the signs of acute inflammation. Inspection and gentle milking of the cannula site may reveal pus.

Treatment

The vascular catheter should be removed promptly; the presence of pus demands surgical drainage of the site. Exactly how long to treat such conditions with antibiotics is not well established. If the patient appears ill but there is no evidence of established infection elsewhere, a seven-day course may be sufficient. If the pathogen was *S. aureus,* a 14-day course may be needed. For line-associated candidemia with no evidence of metastatic spread, a two-week course of amphotericin B is usually given.

Prognosis

Bacteremia usually occurs, often associated with septicemia. The response to removal of the cannula is often dramatic. If initial or previous surgery has included the insertion of a vascular or cardiac prosthesis, these infections may be particularly serious.

Prophylaxis

As with urinary catheters, these infections are almost completely preventable: avoidance of unnecessary usage and rigorous adherence to sterile techniques of insertion and care are essential. Cutdowns should be avoided as a relic of the past. In addition to wound assessment, part of the daily postoperative evaluation of patients is examination of the veins immediately proximal to intravenous catheter sites. All peripheral intravenous catheters should be changed every 48 hours. In particular, the intravenous started in the operating room should be replaced on the first postoperative day.

Antibiotic-associated Colitis

Etiology and Pathophysiology

Antibiotic-associated colitis, also called pseudomembranous colitis, results from toxins produced by *Clostridium difficile*. Clindamycin, lincomycin, and ampicillin are most often implicated, but virtually every antibiotic has been reported to cause this syndrome. See also Chapter 14.

Clinical Manifestations and Diagnosis

Diarrhea may be mild to fulminant and is accompanied by a yellowish pseudomembrane seen at sigmoidoscopy or colonoscopy. Identification of the toxin in stool confirms the diagnosis.

Treatment

Early diagnosis is important; a patient who develops diarrhea while taking antibiotics should be carefully watched and the drug stopped if diarrhea becomes moderately severe. Treatment includes withdrawal of the causative drug and if necessary, administration of vancomycin or metronidazole.

Prognosis

The prognosis is generally favorable, but death may occur in severe cases, usually secondary to toxic megacolon.

Prophylaxis

This preventable complication is a strong reason for the rational use of antibiotics for as short a time as possible.

Acute Parotitis

Etiology

Acute, purulent inflammation of the parotid gland(s), once common, is now a rare postoperative complication. *Staphylococcus aureus* is the most common pathogen, but streptococci and gram-negative rods may be responsible in the hospitalized patient.

Pathophysiology

Dehydration, poor oral hygiene, old age, and debility secondary to disease are the most important predisposing factors to acute parotitis. In chronic care units and geriatric homes, where these factors are often present, the condition is a common problem.

Clinical Manifestations and Diagnosis

Acute parotitis may occur hours to weeks after surgery. The diagnosis is based on the clinical picture of diffuse acute inflammation in one or both glands. The patient is usually very ill.

Treatment

Initial therapy includes intravenous fluids and an intravenous antistaphylococcal agent; low-dose irradiation therapy reduces pain if given early. If there is not significant improvement by the third day of antibiotic treatment, operative drainage of the parotid glands is indicated.

Prognosis

Because impaired host defenses and severe underlying diseases are often present, death occurs in up to 20% of patients with this complication.

Prophylaxis

Good hydration and mouth care are the most important preventive measures.

Infections Secondary to Blood Transfusion

Etiology

Infections secondary to blood therapy may be bacterial, viral, fungal, or protozoal. Viral infections are the most common and bacterial the most serious. Bacterial infections are usually caused by gram-negative rods.

Pathophysiology

Contaminated blood or its components is the cause. Viral infections are uncommon in areas where blood donation is entirely voluntary, not paid, and efficacy of screening tests is good. Bacterial contamination is rare but may result if blood components are left at room temperature (e.g., hanging at the bedside) for more than three hours, or if a leak in the system occurs.

Clinical Manifestations and Diagnosis

Infections with the hepatitis viruses (B or non-A, non-B) and cytomegalovirus manifest themselves weeks to months after operation, and may vary from subclinical to fulminant conditions. Posttransfusion viral hepatitis must be considered in any patient who develops jaundice weeks after an operation. Serology establishes the diagnosis.

Bacterial contamination of transfused blood causes high fever, chills, and often vascular collapse during or immediately after transfusion. Culture of the transfusate will reveal the pathogen.

Treatment

When signs of bacterial infection are present, the transfusion should be stopped immediately, Gram's stain and culture of the transfusate performed, and broad-spectrum antibiotics given parenterally.

Prognosis

Viral infections are usually self-limited but may become chronic and associated with a poor prognosis. Bacterial infections are fatal if not treated in time.

Prophylaxis

Screening of donated blood significantly reduces viral hepatitis. An important bedside practice is a three-hour limit on the duration of any single unit of transfusion.

INFECTIONS SPECIFIC TO THE SITE OF OPERATION

Infections After Abdominal Surgery

Etiology

Surgery inside the abdomen usually involves the gastrointestinal tract or hepatobiliary tree. The endogenous flora includes many bacterial species, especially gram-negative anaerobes (notably *Bacteroides* spp.), coliforms, streptococci, and clostridia. Bacterial counts are higher in stool than anywhere else in the body.

Pathophysiology

Sepsis can occur because of preoperative, intraoperative, or postoperative contamination, or a combination of the three. Whether or not infection does occur depends on the degree of bacterial challenge and the manner in which the peritoneum localizes the invading organisms. Strong local host defenses will result in no infection at all, or one or more well-defined abscesses. If local peritoneal defenses are less adequate in relation to the bacterial challenge, peritonitis will occur, possibly associated with septicemia. Thus the peritoneum acts as a first line of defense against bloodstream invasion. Even if local defenses are such that the infection

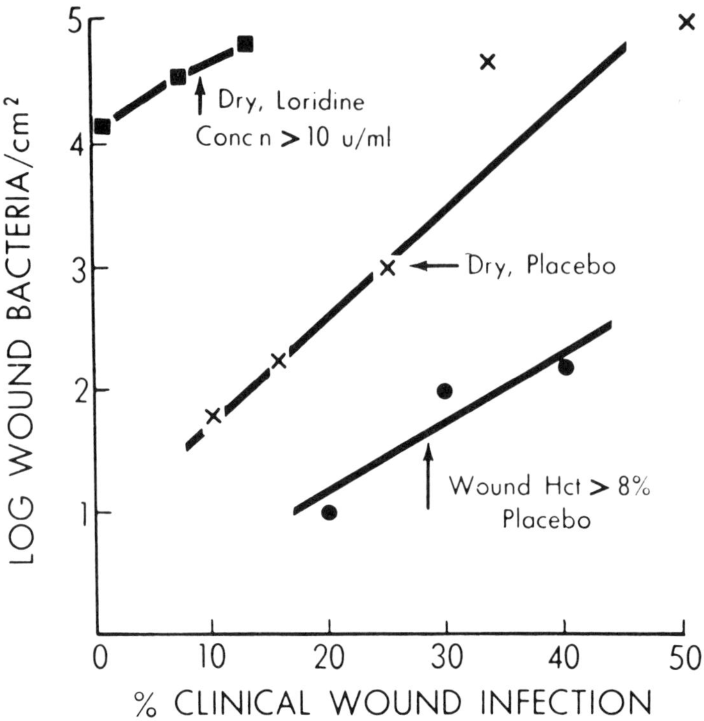

FIGURE 23.2. Coliform bacteria in midline abdominal incisions. The frequency of clinical wound infection is related to the logarithm of the number of coliform bacteria in the dry wound at surgical closure. Relatively bloody wounds become infected more frequently than do dry wounds at similar levels of bacterial contamination. Dry wounds with high levels of cephaloridine are more resistant to clinically apparent infections than are similarly contaminated, placebo-treated, dry wounds. Reproduced by permission of the authors and publisher: Polk HC Jr, Lopez-Mayor JF. Postoperative wound infection: a prospective study of determinant factors and prevention. Surgery 1969;66:97–103.

is walled off into discrete abscess cavities, the undrained abscesses themselves have serious consequences. They do this in three ways: (1) invasion and pressure on adjacent structures, (2) rupture, with subsequent diffuse peritonitis, and (3) their tendency to produce multisystem organ failure (see under General Principles).

Postoperative peritoneal sepsis is more likely to complicate emergency surgery, in which gross peritoneal contamination often occurs, than elective gastrointestinal surgery. Infection after surgery may be a continuation of sepsis that had existed preoperatively, or it can result from a postoperative event such as a leaking anastomosis. The latter phenomenon usually occurs within the first week of the operation.

Peritonitis may be anatomically limited to one or more regions of the peritoneal cavity, or it may be generalized. Local peritonitis has the potential either to become generalized or become walled off as an abscess. Abcesses are most commonly located near the site of initial contamination and in parts of the abdomen that are dependent, such as the pelvis. They can be found in intraperitoneal, retroperitoneal, or visceral (liver, spleen, etc.) sites.

Clinical Manifestations and Diagnosis

The clinical features of intraabdominal sepsis after laparotomy are not necessarily the same as in patients who have not had an operation; this is especially true of sepsis in the first postoperative week, although abscesses may occur years after operation. In the first week after abdominal surgery, the usual warning signs of pain and tenderness are difficult to interpret because of analgesics and because the operative site itself is painful. The classic signs of guarding and rebound tenderness may be absent. An abscess may cause a palpable mass, but more often the pus-filled cavity is too small or the bowels too distended with gas for a mass to be felt. The exception is a pelvic abscess, which is usually palpable by rectal or vaginal examination.

Some of the other usual indicators of intraabdominal sepsis such as fever, leukocytosis, and paralytic ileus are common after uncomplicated gastrointestinal surgery, and their true significance may be missed in a patient with an abscess. Although these traditional signs are still very important, a high index of suspicion after operations with severe contamination is of equal value. Furthermore, both in postoperative peritonitis and abscesses, the initial signs may be those of remote organ failure.

Multiple organ failure after abdominal surgery should promote an urgent and thorough search for one or more foci of sepsis. Imaging techniques such as computerized tomography (CT), ultrasound, and isotopic scans enable accurate diagnosis, but if radiologic and clinical examinations are unrewarding, diagnostic laparotomy may be indicated.

Treatment

Postoperative peritonitis is treated by fluid resuscitation, antibiotics, and laparotomy, with the goals of cleaning out the peritoneal cavity and preventing further contamination by exteriorization of dehisced anastomoses or other defects of the gastrointestinal tract. Antimicrobial agents should be administered parenterally to provide coverage of most gastrointestinal organisms. Which antibiotic regimen(s) is/are best is a widely debated issue but coverage of both aerobic and anerobic bacteria is essential. Various combinations of aminoglycosides with or without penicillin, ampicillin or a cephalosporin combined with clindamycin or metronidazole have been tested. However, whether a single cephalosporin such as cefoxitin, or double or triple therapy is used, the mortality rate is still high.

The treatment of postoperative intraabdominal abscesses is undergoing a change. Whereas ten years ago virtually all were treated by surgical drainage, now it appears that many can be managed by percutaneous catheter drainage under CT or ultrasound guidance. Surgery is still indicated if other pathologic processes (such as gallstones, dehisced anastomosis, multiple abscesses) exist, or if an abscess is anatomically inaccessible to the needle. A short course of antibiotics is usually indicated at the time of abscess drainage and may be continued as a therapeutic course depending upon the individual case. Again, controversy confounds the selection of the "best" antimicrobial regimen.

Prognosis

Postoperative intraabdominal infection results in significant patient disability and cost, and high mortality. Over half of all cases of peritonitis and one-third of those with abscesses after abdominal surgery have a lethal outcome, and peritonitis due to feces continues to have a mortality rate of about 75%.

Prophylaxis

Preoperative antibiotics are indicated in many types of surgery of the alimentary tract and biliary tree (see Chapter 7, Table 7.5). High-risk biliary operations include those done on diabetics, persons over age 70 years, patients with jaundice, and those with acute cholecystitis or cholangitis and common duct stones. In operations on the colon, preoperative antimicrobials should be accompanied by complete mechanical cleansing of the bowel, without which antibiotics would be ineffective.

Operative technique is more important than antibiotics in preventing sepsis. Inside the operating room there are many measures designed to prevent anastomotic breakdown and other causes of sepsis. Important among these is the avoidance of creating an anastomosis with tissues that are already severely inflamed, under tension, or with marginal blood supply.

Infections After Splenectomy

Local infections after splenectomy are common and usually occur in the first postoperative month. Disseminated overwhelming postsplenectomy sepsis is uncommon but is life-threatening.

Etiology

The local infections are wound sepsis and subphrenic abscess, both of which usually involve gastrointestinal organisms. Overwhelming postsplenectomy sepsis is most likely due to *Streptococcus pneumoniae,* although other encapsulated organisms (e.g., *Hemophilus influenzae, Neisseria meningitidis*) are dangerous to the asplenic host.

Pathophysiology

Local infections generally result from contamination by gastrointestinal contents, usually when splenectomy is associated with other operative procedures. Overwhelming postsplenectomy sepsis occurs after about 2% of elective splenectomies for an underlying disease in children, and less than 1% in adults and in children with splenectomy for trauma. Removal of the spleen causes several defects in the immune response and impairment in bacterial clearance from the blood stream.

Clinical Manifestations and Diagnosis

Clinically, in overwhelming postsplenectomy sepsis there is sudden onset of nausea, vomiting, and confusion, which may progress to death in hours, usually with DIC in spite of massive doses of penicillin. The source of the infection is usually obscure. Blood cultures are positive for pneumococci, which can often be seen directly on the peripheral blood smear.

Treatment

Very high doses of intravenous penicillin are required for *S. pneumoniae* or *N. meninigitidis*. For *H. influenzae* ampicillin and chloramphenicol should be given until susceptibility tests are known. Rarely, sepsis with gram-negative enteric organisms requires other antimicrobial agents.

Prognosis

Since the mortality rate is over 50% much research is being directed toward prevention of this complication.

Prophylaxis

Prevention is the most important measure. Splenectomy is now avoided by surgeons where possible, especially in children. New techniques of partial splenectomy are being evaluated for trauma and elective resections. Daily oral penicillin prophylaxis has been given to infants and children for up to five years after surgery, when the risk of overwhelming sepsis is highest. During and after this time, patients should be instructed to carry penicillin with them at all times, and commence therapy at the first general sign of any infection, such as fever. Immunoprophylaxis with pneumococcal vaccine should be given to all patients over 2 years of age after splenectomy. Although its value has not been firmly established, this appears to be beneficial, and side effects are mild and uncommon.

Infections After Urinary Tract Surgery

Four types of infection may occur after urologic procedures (not including transplantation): bacteremia (with or without septicemia), urinary tract infection, deep local infection, and wound infection.

Etiology

In open clean surgery of the kidney or prostate, *S. aureus* is the most common infective agent. In patients with pre-existing urinary tract infection, with operation or instrumentation, the gram negative rods (eg. *E. coli, Proteus* spp.) are the usual pathogens.

Pathophysiology

Sepsis after urologic surgery is infrequent if the urine is sterile at the time of operation. In the presence of infected urine, however, an operation is contaminated (Table 23.1) and therefore has a greater chance of infection.

Bacteremia may occur after any urinary tract operation or instrumentation if bacteriuria is present. In open operations of the kidney and prostate, drains are commonly used so that extravasated urine can be removed, and local or systemic infection will be unlikely. After cystoscopy and transurethral endoscopic surgery, however, drains cannot be placed; if perforation of the urinary tract and extravasation of contaminated or infected urine occur, a local infection or bacteremia is quite likely. Urinary tract infection may be caused by any urologic operation or procedure, especially when followed by prolonged catheterization.

Deep infection in the perirenal region is usually a result of contamination with infected urine; the same is true of wound infection.

Clinical Manifestations and Diagnosis

Septicemia is accompanied by fever, chills, and positive blood cultures. If urinary extravasation is suspected, it should be confirmed radiographically where possible. Urinary tract infection may occur as cystitis, prostatitis, epididymitis, or less commonly, pyelonephritis. Epididymitis causes severe unilateral or bilateral scrotal pain. Urine cultures confirm the diagnosis of urinary tract infection. Deep infections such as perinephric abscess cause pain, tenderness, and sometimes a palpable mass, but urine cultures may be negative.

Treatment

Bacteremia is treated parenterally with a penicillin, cephalosporin, or an aminoglycoside, depending on the pathogen. If cystitis occurs in the presence of a urinary catheter, antibiotics are usually only indicated if fever, chills, kidney infection, or epididymitis occurs. The catheter should be removed as soon as possible. If cystitis develops when no catheter is present, antibiotics are indicated; the choice of drug depends on culture and sensitivity results. Acute epididymitis requires antibiotics, scrotal support, and ice packs.

Wound and deep local infections require the same treatment as infections after other abdominal operations (see page 365).

Prognosis

The results of infection after urinary tract surgery vary from minor inconvenience and increased cost to infrequent septicemia and death.

Prophylaxis

When bacteriuria is present, perioperative antimicrobial therapy is warranted and if possible, a full course of antibiotic treatment should be given before surgery. One should not operate on the genitourinary tract in the presence of infected urine; when necessary, specific prophylactic antibiotics are indicated. The use of prophylactic antibiotics when urine is sterile is controversial and its value is unproved.

Infections After Kidney Transplantation

Etiology

Infections after kidney transplantation are considered separately because they include opportunistic infections commonly found in immunosuppressed patients. In the early posttransplantation period, most infections are bacterial and are similar to those after any surgery: wound, pulmonary, urinary, and intravenous sites. It is later in their course that unusual pathogens or infections appear. Bacterial opportunistic infections include legionnaires' disease, *Salmonella* infections, tuberculosis, nocardiosis, and listerial infection. Opportunistic fungi include *Candida, Torulopsis, Aspergillus,* and *Cryptococcus* organisms. *Pneumocystis carinii* is a common protozoal pathogen in these patients, and viral infections (cytomegalovirus and other herpesviruses are common). Cytomegalovirus infections may appear early, mimic rejection, and make management with immunosuppressive drugs difficult.

Pathophysiology

Immunosuppression secondary to medications is the main cause of infection; uremia may also contribute. In addition to the opportunistic infections mentioned above, infections common to other urinary tract operations are also frequent, especially if technical complications such as bleeding or anastomotic leakage occur.

Clinical Manifestations and Diagnosis

The clinical picture of infection after transplantation is usually muted due to immunosuppressive therapy and depends on the microbial etiology. Diagnosis is often difficult and may require invasive procedures. A common triad associated with cytomegalovirus infections is fever, hepatitis, and leukopenia.

Treatment

Treatment depends on the pathogen. It is usually necessary to adjust immunosuppression doses or to discontinue immunosuppressive agents; this may in turn endanger the transplanted kidney, but if necessary the kidney is sacrificed to control the infection. See Chapter 22.

Prognosis

Most infections in transplant recipients must be considered serious, both to the patient and the graft. Graft removal is now being carried out earlier when the patient's life is jeopardized by a serious infection.

Prophylaxis

Preventive measures include careful preoperative screening of patients for remote sites of infection (e.g., dental caries), prophylactic antibiotics, and good operative technique.

Infections After Gynecologic and Obstetric Surgery

Etiology

The cervicovaginal flora is comprised of various aerobic and anaerobic organisms that are potential pathogens in pelvic surgery. These include various streptococcal species (group B, enterococci), staphylococci (*S. aureus* and coagulase-negative staphylococci), gram-negative rods (*E. coli, Proteus* spp.), and peptostreptococci, peptococci, *Bacteroides, Fusobacteria,* and *Clostridia* species.

Pathophysiology

Because the vagina normally harbors abundant bacteria and cannot be completely sterilized prior to surgery, operations on the female genital tract with exposure to the vaginal mucosa carry a 10% to 30% prevalence of subsequent infection.

Infections after hysterectomy are slightly more common when the vaginal rather than abdominal route of excision is used. Abdominal wound infections after hysterectomy are similar in frequency and characteristics to those of other clean-contaminated abdominal operations. Deep infections that can occur include cellulitis or abscess of the remaining vaginal cuff, pelvic cellulitis or abscess, septic thrombophlebitis, and ovarian abscess.

The presence of endogenous vaginal flora plus devitalized tissue and blood cause vaginal cuff infection. If vaginal cuff sepsis is treated late or if infection is severe, spread may occur to the general pelvic or peritoneal cavity, resulting in cellulitis or an abscess. Pelvic sepsis that is still not adequately treated may then spread further to cause salpingo-oophoritis, tubo-ovarian abscess, or septic thrombophlebitis. The last may cause septic pulmonary emboli.

A solitary ovarian abscess may occur, apart from other pelvic infection, if an ovary becomes disrupted and contaminated at the initial operation.

Puerperal sepsis refers to any postpartum genital tract infection. The same types of infection occur as those after hysterectomy, but with the important difference that the initial bacterial proliferation and invasion occur in the endometrium rather than the vaginal cuff. Puerperal sepsis is more common with cesarean than with vaginal delivery. Other risk factors are rupture of the amniotic membranes more than 48 hours before delivery, chorioamnionitis, prolonged labor, genital tract trauma, and retained placental fragments. It is controversial whether or not fetal heart monitoring is a causative factor.

Clinical Manifestations and Diagnosis

Vaginal cuff infection, whether cellulitis or localized abscess, is the most common cause of fever beginning the third day after hysterectomy. In addition to fever, the patient develops local pain, especially on defecation. Pelvic examination is quite painful; separation of the sutured edges of the vaginal cuff reveals a foul-smelling exudate that should be Gram's stained and cultured. Pelvic abscess should be suspected if fever or paralytic ileus persists despite initial drainage of a vaginal cuff infection. The clinical features and diagnosis of a solitary ovarian abscess are similar to those of a pelvic abscess.

The first signs of puerperal sepsis are fever and chills followed by foul lochia, a boggy tender uterus, and local pain. Any postpartum fever should be assumed to be endometritis until proved otherwise, although fever may result from urinary tract infection.

In pelvic infections, computerized tomography or ultrasound are particularly helpful in diagnosis.

Treatment

Vaginal cuff infection is treated by opening the edges of the vaginal stump to provide drainage. Antibiotic therapy is required to cover both the aerobic and anaerobic flora; various combinations of aminoglycoside, penicillin, or cephalosporin with metronidazole or clindamycin are effective. Pelvic abscess requires drainage, which can be done per vaginam but sometimes requires a laparotomy. For salpingo-oophoritis and tubo-ovarian abscesses, removal of the ovaries and fallopian tubes may be necessary. A solitary ovarian abscess is treated by excision of the ovary.

Suppurative thrombophlebitis is initially treated with heparin and antibiotics. If septic emboli occur despite this therapy, surgical ligation of the inferior vena cava and ovarian veins may be necessary.

The treatment of puerperal sepsis is urgent. Cervical dilatation and removal of any retained placental fragments should allow drainage of necrotic or purulent material from the uterus; a sample should be sent for culture and sensitivity. Broad-spectrum parenteral antibiotics as noted above are required. Life-threatening infection unresponsive to these measures may require hysterectomy and bilateral salpingo-oophorectomy.

Prognosis

While most of these infections are well controlled, postpartum endometritis and suppurative thrombophlebitis are occasionally life-threatening.

Prophylaxis

Preoperative prophylactic antimicrobial agents have been shown to decrease the frequency of infections after hysterectomy. Prevention also requires careful attention to antiseptic preparation of the vagina at the time of operation.

Prevention of postpartum infection requires aseptic obstetric technique and avoidance of potentiating factors. In high-risk patients, a prophylactic cephalosporin should be administered intravenously as soon as the cord is clamped to avoid exposing the infant to the drug.

Infections After Chest Surgery

The most important infections after surgery of the esophagus and lungs are pleural empyema and mediastinitis. Infections after cardiac surgery are considered separately, and pneumonia was discussed previously.

Etiology

Virtually any bacterial species can be involved, and polymicrobial infection is common. In mediastinitis, a synergistic infection with anaerobes and aerobes from the oropharyngeal flora is particularly virulent.

Pathophysiology

Empyema (purulent infection of the pleural space) may occur if the pleural cavity becomes contaminated as a result of pulmonary or esophageal surgery. Empyema secondary to esophageal procedures occurs after a leaking anastomosis or perforation (Boerhaave's syndrome or by instrument) of the esophagus. Infection caused by esophageal contents begins in the mediastinum and extends into one or both pleural cavities. Empyema after pulmonary operation results from contamination of blood or residual air space, or from a leaking closure of a bronchial stump. The latter is an example of a bronchopleural fistula.

A pleural empyema may be loculated to a part of the pleura or may occupy the whole space. Initially, an empyema contains thin fluid with a low number of inflammatory cells, but soon develops a thick, purulent exudate.

Acute mediastinitis is an uncommon but serious infection. The mediastinum contains soft tissue fascial planes that offer little resistance to the spread of infection. Postoperative mediastinitis is usually a result of esophageal instrumentation or anastomotic breakdown. Occasionally, mediastinitis complicates a sternal wound infection (see under Infections After Cardiac Surgery).

Clinical Manifestations and Diagnosis

The clinical picture of thoracic empyema is that of the underlying problem leading to the pleural infection, fever, and the physical and radiographic signs of pleural fluid accumulation. Diagnosis is established at thoracentesis by the aspiration of pus, which should undergo Gram's stain and culture.

The patient with mediastinitis secondary to instrumental perforation of the esophagus complains of severe midchest pain, dysphagia, and shortness of breath. High fever usually develops rapidly. Pleural effusion may occur; the fluid may be serous, or purulent if intrapleural rupture has occurred. Subcutaneous emphysema may be felt, and tissue emphysema, widening of the mediastinum, and pneumothorax may be evident on chest x-ray. The clinical signs of mediastinitis secondary to a leaking esophageal anastomosis have a more gradual onset, but eventually resemble that of instrumental perforation. Diagnosis may by more difficult because of factors such as analgesics and ventilatory support after thoracotomy. In doubtful cases of esophageal rupture or dehiscence, chest x-ray after a swallow of contrast material may be diagnostic.

Treatment

Tretment of an empyema requires drainage of the pleura, reexpansion of the involved lung, and antibiotics based on susceptibility data. The first two of these goals can usually be achieved by tube thoracostomy. Occasionally, operation is required for a chronic empyema.

Acute mediastinitis requires urgent surgical drainage and debridement, prevention of further contamination by one of a variety of operative techniques, and antibiotic coverage, which usually includes a penicillin or a cephalosporin. Mediastinitis in patients who may have been colonized with gram-negative aerobes in the oropharynx is usually also covered with an aminoglycoside.

Prognosis

Acute mediastinitis is often fatal, especially if diagnosed late in its course. Empyema has a much better prognosis.

Prophylaxis

The issue of prophylactic antibiotics in esophageal and pulmonary surgery has not been resolved. A cephalosporin should be given to patients with impaired host defenses or for potential or actual gross intraoperative contamination.

Infections After Cardiac Surgery

The most frequently used incision in heart operations is the median sternotomy. Sternal infection (sternal osteomyelitis) occurs in about 2% of cases but is higher in reoperative surgery. The other important infection is prosthetic valve endocarditis (PVE), which occurs in about 1% of prosthetic valve insertions. It is discussed in Chapter 10.

Etiology

Although staphylococcal species (*S. aureus* and coagulase-negative staphylococci) and gram-negative rods are most common, virtually any organism can cause sternal osteomyelitis.

Pathophysiology

Factors leading to sternal infection are similar to those of other types of wound sepsis. Osteomyelitis of the sternum is a serious complication because anastomoses in the heart and aorta can become secondarily involved by spread of the infection, and prosthetic valves may become seeded by bacteria shed into the blood stream.

Clinical Manifestations and Diagnosis

Clinically, the patient with sternal osteomyelitis may be acutely ill with anterior mediastinitis and sternal dehiscence, or the infection may take a slower, chronic course. Local tenderness and fever are usually present. Needle aspiration or spontaneous drainage of the sternal wound may reveal pus, which should be examined microscopically and cultured.

Antibiotic treatment of sternal osteomyelitis should be based on a bacteriologic diagnosis if possible. Otherwise a cephalosporin or antistaphylococcal penicillin is indicated. Wound debridement and irrigation are important in early infections. In infections that arise more than one month postoperatively, the sternum will not heal with these measures, and resection of the entire sternum is usually necessary.

Prognosis

Sternal osteomyelitis has up to 20% mortality.

Prophylaxis

Prevention of sternal wound infections requires meticulous preoperative skin sterilization and operative technique. Antibiotic prophylaxis with a cephalosporin or antistaphylococcal penicillin is also indicated and has been shown significantly to reduce the frequency of wound infections.

Vascular Graft Infection

Etiology

Graft infection is most commonly caused by *S. aureus*, but numerous organisms have been implicated. Contamination from the patient's skin at the time of surgery is the usual route, although organisms may seed out from a bacteremia.

Pathophysiology

Although some cases occur within days of surgery, infection may not be evident until months or years have passed. Many of these later infections result from hematogenous seeding.

Other factors that predispose to graft sepsis are vascular reconstruction for trauma, especially if intestinal contents have spilled; combination of the vascular operation with some other contaminated elective procedure; a break in aseptic operative technique; and preexisting infection in the artery to be reconstructed. Reconstruction requiring groin incisions has a higher infection rate.

An infected prosthetic graft may thrombose or leak at the anastomosis. If the latter occurs, a false aneurysm, which is a pulsating hematoma, will be formed; this often results in hemorrhage into adjacent structures such as the gut (aortoenteric fistula). Systemic sepsis and septic emboli are other known complications.

Clinical Manifestations and Diagnosis

If the infected segment is superficial it will probably cause a purulent draining sinus. If it is deep, one of the complications mentioned above is the initial feature. A false aneurysm forms a pulsatile mass that is usually palpable when superficial or large. A patient with a previously inserted prosthetic graft who develops gastrointestinal bleeding should be presumed to have a graft-enteric fistula until proved otherwise. Aortoenteric fistula secondary to graft sepsis usually results in a few episodes of relatively minor upper gastrointestinal bleeding, followed, if untreated, by massive exsanguinating hemorrhage.

The diagnosis of graft infection is made by a combination of previously mentioned clinical factors. Positive blood cultures and history of predisposing factors are helpful.

Treatment

Treatment of established infection consists of removal of the entire infected graft, a two-week course of intravenous antibiotics followed by several months of oral antibiotics, and a new vascular reconstruction that avoids the infected region. In practice, therapeutic success is difficult to achieve.

Prognosis
Hemorrhage, systemic sepsis, and amputation often result, and the mortality rate is about 50%.

Prophylaxis
Preventive measures include rigorously aseptic operative technique and skin preparation, plus prophylaxis with a cephalosporin. A patient with a prosthetic graft in situ should receive antimicrobial prophylaxis before procedures such as sigmoidoscopy that may result in bacteremia.

Infections After Orthopedic Procedures

Etiology
Although staphylococcal species are most common, many types of organism can cause postoperative infection after bone and joint surgery. See also Chapter 18.

Pathophysiology
Infections after orthopedic procedures are classified as superficial or deep, depending on their relationship to the fascial layer. Superficial infections can be considered as wound infections previously discussed, and are not described further except to say that they may be the first manifestations of deep infections.

Deep postoperative skeletal infections occur in less than 1% of elective reconstructions in adults, but have a five times higher prevalence after surgery for open traumatic fractures. Although the use of aseptic techniques and prophylactic antibiotics has made sepsis uncommon after elective procedures, once infection is present it is extremely difficult to eradicate because of the foreign material that is so often used. The frequency of infection after reconstruction for trauma varies with the amount of contamination and degree to which devitalized tissue was debrided.

Clinical Manifestations and Diagnosis
The clinical features of deep skeletal infections vary with the type of procedure. If elective reconstruction was performed without antibiotic prophylaxis or insertion of foreign material, infection usually arises within two weeks of operation, with fever and local inflammatory signs. Infection after trauma usually occurs within days of the operation. If prosthetic material was inserted and perioperative antibiotics given, as for a total hip replacement, infection may occur early, but usually becomes established months to years after operation, and causes joint pain but few signs of sepsis.

The diagnosis may be obvious in acute cases, but low-grade, chronic infections are very difficult to diagnose. Plain radiographs, arthrography, and needle aspiration of material for culture may be helpful, but in some cases operative exploration is necessary to establish the cause of a patient's chronic pain.

Treatment
Treatment of established infection requires antimicrobial therapy plus drainage and soft tissue debridement. If no foreign implant is present this is usually sufficient. A chronically infected foreign implant usually requires removal. See also Chapter 18.

Prognosis
Deep infections, although not usually lethal, are associated with significant morbidity.

Prophylaxis
The frequency of infection can be reduced by several measures. Unidirectional air flow and other technical advances in operating room procedure, as well as strict attention to the details of aseptic technique have resulted in a lowering of the rate of infection. Prophylactic antibiotics that cover staphylococci reduce the chance of deep infection in the presence of foreign material.

Infections After Intracranial Operations

The most common postoperative infections seen in neurosurgical practice are those after insertion of cerebrospinal fluid shunts for the treatment of hydrocephalus. Infection occurs in up to 15% of such cases; this complication is described in Chapter 9. Excluding cerebrospinal fluid shunting procedures, the frequency of postcraniotomy infection is about 5%, including wound infections.

Etiology
In procedures not involving shunts, *S. aureus* is the most commonly implicated organism, but gram-negative rods are frequent as well.

Pathophysiology
Suppurative infections after nonshunt surgery of the brain can occur in extradural, subdural, or intracerebral locations. Pus may be well localized into a walled-off abscess or may fill a potential space with fluid, as in a subdural empyema. Complicated, prolonged surgical

procedures requiring intracranial pressure monitoring are associated with a much higher frequency of infection.

Clinical Manifestations and Diagnosis

Clinical manifestations in nonshunt cases result from the effects of a space-occupying lesion and the presence of sepsis. The diagnosis is established by clinical examination and imaging techniques such as computerized tomography and angiography.

Treatment

Subdural empyema requires urgent surgical drainage and antibiotics. A brain abscess requires initiation of antibiotic therapy followed, if necessary, by surgical drainage or excision. Extradural collections require drainage and appropriate antibiotic therapy.

Prognosis

Suppurative intracranial infections are lethal in up to 25% to 50% of cases. The poor prognosis is usually related to the severity of the underlying neurologic disease.

Prophylaxis

The role of prophylactic antimicrobial agents in intracranial procedures not involving shunts is still unresolved and at present their use is not recommended. Widespread use of prophylactic agents in patients undergoing neurosurgical procedures has resulted in serious outbreaks of nosocomial infections.

Conclusion

Postoperative infection is still a very common cause of morbidity and mortality. The most important aspect of control is maintenance of the surgical conscience. Careful surveillance is essential. The very knowledge that a certain complication is frequent or hazardous leads to preventive measures. Improvements in prevention and therapy are also occurring because our understanding of the biology of infection is deepening. The augmentation of local and systemic host defenses should provide a significant breakthrough in the near future.

ANNOTATED BIBLIOGRAPHY

Bohnen J, Boulanger M, Meakins JL, McLean APH: Prognosis in generalized peritonitis: relation to cause and risk factors. Arch Surg 1983;118:285–290.
Postoperative peritonitis is shown to be more lethal than other types of peritonitis; it is associated with difficulty in diagnosis and delay in treatment.

Burke JF. The effective period of preventive antibiotic action in experimental incisions and dermal lesions. Surgery 1961;50:161–168.
This classic paper and that by Miles et al. give the scientific basis for the use of preincisional antibiotics for preventing wound infections.

Cruse PJE, Foord R. The epidemiology of wound infection: a ten-year prospective study of 62,939 wounds. Surg Clin North Am 1980;60:27–40.
This is an enormous collection of data regarding determinants of wound infection, in particular those related to the operating room.

Dougherty SH, Simmons RL. Infections in bionic man: the pathobiology of infections in prosthetic devices. Curr Probl Surg 1982;19(5,6):218–319.
This two-part monograph lucidly describes an increasingly common postoperative problem.

Fry DE, Pearlstein L, Fulton RL, Polk HC Jr. Multiple-system organ failure: the role of uncontrolled infection. Arch Surg 1980;115:136–140.
Multiple-system failure is found to be due to sepsis and is an important cause of death after surgery.

Miles AA, Miles EM, Burke J. The value and duration of defence reactions of the skin to the primary lodgement of bacteria. Br J Exp Pathol 1957;38:79–96.

Polk HC Jr, Lopez-Mayor JF. Postoperative wound infection: a prospective study of determinant factors and prevention. Surgery 1969;66:97–103.
The authors' study demonstrates clinical efficacy of prophylactic antibiotics as well as biologic principles.

Simmons RL, Howard RJ, ed. Surgical infectious diseases. New York: Appleton-Century-Crofts, 1982.
This authoritative yet readable text covers all aspects of infections related to surgical practice, including postoperative infections. Subjects are discussed in depth, and complete, current reference lists are provided.

24 INFECTIONS IN BURN PATIENTS

Stephan J. Landis

Skin is the major structure separating the human internal environment from the outside world. It not only retains body fluids and heat, but provides a protective barrier against microbial invasion. In the severely burned patient, this protective barrier is destroyed. As a result, major problems in temperature control and fluid balance occur, and the patient is predisposed to infection.

Initial evaluation of the burn patient requires a measurement of the surface area burned and depth of burn. The partial-thickness burn, or first- or second-degree injury, involves destruction of local skin tissues for various depths from epidermis into dermis, sparing dermal appendages, such as papillae, sweat glands, and hair follicles. The full-thickness burn or third-degree injury, involves destruction of epidermis, dermis, and dermal appendages.

ETIOLOGY

The bacteriology of the burn wound has changed dramatically over the last 30 years. In the 1950s, beta-hemolytic streptococci and *Staphylococcus aureus* accounted for a large percentage of infections. With the advent of new topical and systemic antibiotics and improved burn wound management, aerobic gram-negative organisms such as *Pseudomonas, Enterobacter,* and *Proteus* species have played an increasingly greater causative role. *Staphylococcus aureus* and *Pseudomonas* species are generally the predominant organisms seen in burn wounds. Occasionally, specific strains of other gram-negative organisms may predominate, including the following:

1. Common
   S. aureus
   P. aeruginosa
2. Less common
   Pseudomonas pyocyanea
   Serratia marcesens
   Klebsiella pneumoniae
   Enterobacter sp.
   Proteus sp.
   Candida sp.

Anaerobic organisms such as *Bacteroides* species are sometimes isolated, but rarely cause wound sepsis. The virulence of *P. aeruginosa* is due to its production of endotoxin, hemolysins, exotoxins, and protease enzymes, and it is likely that these bacterial factors are the major determinants for the establishment of *Pseudomonas* infection in the early burn period.

EPIDEMIOLOGY

Colonization of burn wounds with bacteria occurs primarily as a result of cross-contamination among patients. Members of the hospital ward staff or the patients themselves are usually the vehicles for transmission of the organism. Air-borne transmission occurs infrequently. Autoinoculation of burn wounds can occur with flora from the patient's own oral, respiratory, or gastrointestinal tract. This last route, however, is probably less important than direct cross-contamination.

PATHOPHYSIOLOGY

In the partial-thickness burn, dermal appendages remain intact from which the wound can reepithelialize spontaneously. The local vascular circulation usually reestablishes itself within 24 to 48 hours. Extravascular fluid at the junction of burn and viable tissue is in dynamic equilibrium with the systemic circulation. If a deep partial-thickness wound dries out or becomes infected, thrombosis of capillaries and venules may occur, causing the partial-thickness burn to become a full-thickness injury.

Spontaneous reepithelialization usually does not occur in full-thickness injuries. Microangiographic studies have shown these burns to be virtually avascular. Neovascularization by means of the ingrowth of new blood vessels from granulation tissue takes about three weeks. It is this full-thickness injury, by virtue of its slow healing, that is particularly at risk of infection.

The skin is sterile immediately after a burn. Within 24 to 48 hours, bacteria start to grow in the wound and colonization begins. The first microorganisms to appear are diphtheroid and *Staphylococcus* species that have escaped thermal destruction at the bases of hair follicles or skin glands. They proliferate rapidly on dead skin (eschar) and in the rich extravascular fluid that has accumulated on the wound surface. Organisms such as aerobic gram-negative bacilli begin colonization only after the first week postinjury. Deeper penetration of the eschar occurs and spread to the lymphatics may result; however, the clinical boundary between colonization and infection is not always clear. If bacterial numbers continue to increase, destruction of the underlying viable tissue occurs. Burn wound sepsis or invasive infection is defined as "presence of, and invasion through, the burn wound of bacteria in numbers reaching 10^5 or greater per gram of tissue." The risks of bacteremia and mortality increase significantly with burn wound sepsis.

In recent years, there has been considerable interest in the immune response of the burn patient. A number of factors may adversely affect this response, including drugs and anesthetic agents, poor nutritional status, and shock. Transient decreases in levels of serum immunoglobulin and complement as well as altered neutrophil and T cell function have been documented. The relevance of these findings, however, is at this point still uncertain.

CLINICAL MANIFESTATIONS

The following clinical features may indicate sepsis in the severely burned individual: hyperpyrexia and occasionally hypothermia, confusion, perspiration, weight loss, productive cough, tachypnea, tachycardia, and adynamic ileus or acute dilatation of the stomach. The signs of invasive burn wound infection include:

1. Conversion of a partial-thickness burn to full-thickness injury
2. Unexpectedly rapid eschar separation with evidence of pus
3. Advancing violaceous wound margin
4. Fat necrosis
5. Vesicular lesions in healed or healing burn wounds
6. Degeneration of granulation tissue

DIAGNOSIS

Since burn wound sepsis tends to be focal, making a clinical diagnosis of invasive infection can be difficult. Bacteremia is not always present since extravascular sites of infection are primarily involved. The likelihood of bacteremia or septicemia increases as the total area of burn wound invasion increases. Bacteremia is less likely to occur if invasive infection involves less than 20% of the total burn wound area.

Surveillance cultures of the burn surface provide only qualitative bacteriologic information and do not correlate with the presence of sepsis. Quantitative information must be obtained with biopsy. This involves a punch biopsy of the subeschar region looking for evidence of invasion of viable tissue. Isolation of organisms in numbers greater than 10^5 per gm of tissue is considered evidence of wound sepsis. The specific biopsy site is important and the predictive value of this technique increases with several punch biopsies. Histologic criteria of invasive infection include:

1. Increased inflammatory response in adjacent viable tissue
2. Invasion of microorganisms into the viable subeschar tissue
3. Presence of microorganisms in blood vessels
4. Ischemic necrosis of injured tissue
5. Presence of foreign body giant cells

ASSOCIATED INFECTIONS

Apart from wound sepsis, severely burned patients are at greater risk of developing other infections.

Pneumonia is the second most common cause of death. Inhalational burn injury causes sloughing of bronchial mucosal linings, thereby predisposing the patient to pneumonia. Prolonged intubation, poor cough reflex, and inadequate nutrition can also lead to nosocomial pneumonia. A tracheostomy performed through burned tissue, or even normal tissue, increases the risk of introducing microorganisms into the lower respiratory tract. Urinary tract infection, resulting from prolonged bladder catheterization, is a frequent occurrence.

In the early postburn period, intravascular catheter lines are required for monitoring purposes and for the delivery of fluids and nutrition. Prolonged cannulation can lead to suppurative thrombophlebitis in about 4% of severely burned individuals. Signs of local inflammation occur in only 35% of cases. It may be manifested either by fever of undetermined etiology, or positive blood cultures from an unrecognized source.

Viral infections such as herpes simplex or cytomegalovirus are uncommon. Invasive fungal infection usually occurs as a preterminal event. *Candida* species colonize about one-third of all burn wounds, but account for only 6% of invasive infection. The successful treatment of invasive fungal infection requires aggressive wound debridement combined with systemic antifungal drugs, such as amphotericin B and flucytosine where appropriate. The mortality rate is, nevertheless, still high. The best preventive measures against this complication include early excision and closure of the wound.

PREVENTION

The bacteria-controlled nursing unit is a self-contained area in which the patient resides. It acts as a form of protective and reverse isolation, thereby reducing problems of cross-contamination. Whether this form of patient isolation is superior to early burn wound excision, meticulous nursing care, and judicious use of topical antimicrobial agents has never been tested in a controlled manner.

ANTIMICROBIAL MANAGEMENT

Appropriate use of topical and systemic antibiotics is critical to the management of infection in the burn patient. Topical agents, while not eradicating bacteria, reduce or control the numbers of organisms in the tissue. In established sepsis, bacteria are present in numbers as high as 10^8 organisms per gram of tissue. Effective topical therapy may keep these counts in the range of 10^3 to 10^4 per gram of tissue. Topical therapy must be adapted to the needs of the individual patient and the physician must be prepared to change the agent if and when required. No single drug is universally effective in a given burn population. Appropriate management requires close monitoring of clinical, laboratory, and bacteriologic values, and realization that different topical antimicrobial agents vary in their chemical properties, side effects, and ability to penetrate the wound. Commonly used topical agents are as follows:

1. Silver nitrate, 0.5% solution
2. Mafenide acetate, 10% in water-miscible base
3. Silver sulfadiazine, 1% cream
4. Cerium nitrate-silver sulfadiazine, 2.2% cerium nitrate solution added to 1% silver sulfadiazine cream
5. Chlorhexidine, 0.2% to 0.5% solution
6. Povidone-iodine, 10% solution in water-miscible base
7. Topical gentamicin, 0.1% cream or ointment

Silver nitrate, 0.5% solution, applied every two hours controls bacterial growth within the burn wound. Its mechanism of action is unknown, but it has a wide spectrum of activity against major pathogens including *Pseudomonas* and *Staphylococcus* species. Acquired resistance is unknown. The main drawbacks to its use include minimal penetration into the deeper tissues of the burn wound, precipitation of silver salts on the wound surface, and leeching out of electrolytes from extracellular fluids by the distilled water vehicle used to carry the silver nitrate.

Mafenide, a methylated sulfonamide, has been available for many years. It has a broad spectrum of activity, being effective against both gram-positive and gram-negative organisms. It actively penetrates into the subeschar tissues in effective concentrations. In the wound, mafenide undergoes deamination by amine oxidase, which limits its systemic activity. Unfortunately, the metabolic product of mafenide has strong carbonic anhydrase-inhibiting properties, thereby interfering with the buffering capacity of the renal tubule. Increased acid loads to the kidney result in tachypnea and/or hyperpnea, which can exhaust some patients, and metabolic acidosis may then develop. With the availability of less toxic topical agents, side effects such as inhibition of carbonic anhydrase and pain on local application have limited the use of mafenide.

Unlike silver nitrate, silver sulfadiazine (SSD) actively penetrates into deeper tissues. Silver sulfadiazine is a complex formed by the reaction between sulfadiazine and silver nitrate, and in tissues it dissociates, with the sulfadiazine being the more active antimicrobial agent. The mechanism of action of SSD is thought to be due to its binding with bacterial DNA and RNA. Bacteria initially sensitive to silver nitrate or sulfadiazine are usually sensitive to SSD; however, staphylococcal species appear to grow in larger numbers in the burn wound if the wound is treated with SSD alone rather than with a combination of topical agents. The addition of cerium, forming a cerium nitrate-silver sulfadiazine mixture, can modify burn wound flora by eliminating *P. aeruginosa*. In one study of 60 patients with major burns, however, no clear superiority was found over those treated with silver sulfadiazine alone.

Silver sulfadiazine is applied as a 1% cream twice daily. An important advantage of this agent is the lack of local pain or discomfort on application. Rarely, crystalluria, skin rash, or leukopenia may preclude its use.

Chlorhexidine has been used as a general antiseptic for years and as a topical agent, 0.2% to 0.5% solution, in burns with relatively few side effects. It is active against many bacteria especially gram-negative bacilli (including *P. aeruginosa*) and systemic absorption is minimal. It does not cause pain or electrolyte imbalance.

Povidone-iodine solution has had limited use as a topical agent because of serious drawbacks, including pain on application and emergence of resistant gram-negative organisms, particularly *Pseudomonas*.

Topical gentamicin was initially designed to combat *Pseudomonas* burn wound sepsis. Unfortunately, resistant strains of *P. aeruginosa* developed rapidly when topical gentamicin was used exclusively. As a result, it was withdrawn from the commercial market. In cases of burn wound sepsis caused by sensitive *Pseudomonas* species, however, it is still effective when used sparingly. It is applied as a 0.1% cream or ointment directly to the burn wound. Application is painless and systemic toxicity is minimal when prolonged use is avoided.

In the treatment of presumed or suspected infection, it is best to select agents that offer a broad spectrum of activity coupled with minimal toxicity to treat known colonizing organisms or those known to cause infection in that particular burn unit (Figure 24.1). Since *S. aureus* and/or *P. aeruginosa* are frequently present in burn wounds, cloxacillin and/or tobramycin may be required. If the patient is penicillin-allergic or if a methicillin-resistant *S. aureus* is present, vancomycin is indicated. Occasionally, a gentamicin- or tobramycin-resistant strain of *Pseudomonas* will require amikacin as the aminoglycoside of choice. Narrow-spectrum antibiotic treatment should be instituted when a specific pathogen is isolated.

Aminoglycosides, particularly gentamicin, appear to have shortened serum half-lives in younger patients, necessitating administration at more frequent intervals such as every four to six hours, with close monitoring of serum drug levels and renal function. Subeschar administration of antibiotics is a debatable mode of treatment, and improved efficacy over the intravenous route of administration has never been conclusively demonstrated.

Treatment must be tailored to the patient's clinical response and culture results. The most effective and least toxic regimen for the specific organism recovered should be used for no longer than two weeks if clinical response has been satisfactory.

In addition to antibiotics, intensive nutritional support may improve host defense and accelerate healing. Early excision of the burn wound with grafting and closure is the best preventive measure against colonization and infection.

PROGNOSIS

At the Cincinnati Unit of the Shriners' Burn Institute, overall mortality rates fell from 14% in 1970 to 10% in 1978. During this same period, the septic mortality rates fell from 9% to 4%. Invasive burn wound infection remains the primary cause of death from sepsis.

The use of topical antimicrobial agents, early burn wound excision, and meticulous nursing care probably account for the reduction in septic burn deaths in the 1970s.

Burns involving more than 60% to 70% of the body's surface area still carry a bad prognosis, no matter what the patient's age. In the elderly, even relatively confined burns of 5% to 10% may be lethal.

PROPHYLAXIS

Routine prophylactic administration of penicillin in the immediate post burn period is no longer justified. Cellulitis caused by beta-hemolytic streptococci is now uncommon, and the use of prophylactic penicillin during the first week postburn may contribute to colonization with gram-negative organisms.

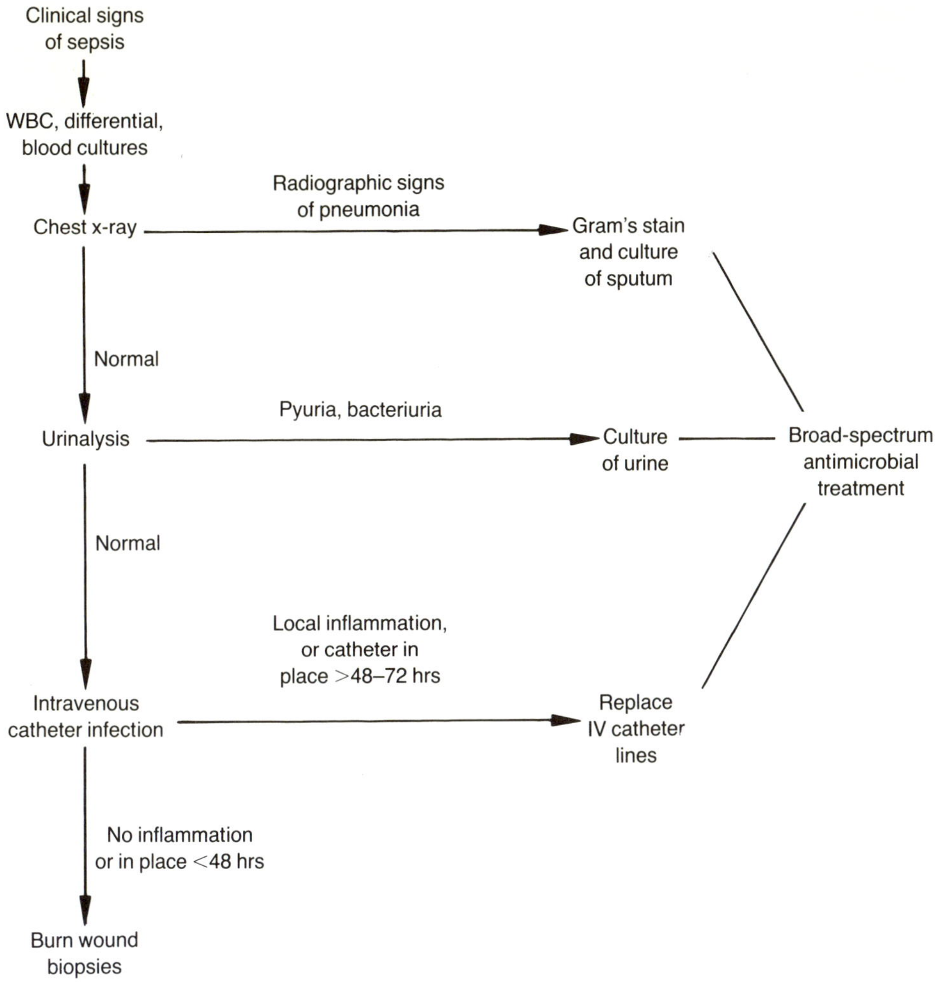

FIGURE 24.1. Flow diagram illustrates steps in management of septic burns. While awaiting results of hematologic and microbial cultures, parenteral administration of broad-spectrum antibiotics is indicated. When the infecting pathogen is isolated, more narrow-spectrum anitmicrobial therapy should be instituted.

Antimicrobial prophylaxis is indicated only during autografting and burn wound excision. Potentially serious bacteremias can be minimized during manipulation of the eschar that occurs during the procedure. In this situation, it is important to know the antimicrobial sensitivities of the microflora colonizing the wound and to use the appropriate prophylactic agent. There is no value in continuing prophylactic antibiotics longer than 48 hours after surgery.

ANNOTATED BIBLIOGRAPHY

Artz CP, Moncrief JA, Pruitt BA Jr. Burns: a team approach. Philadelphia: WB Saunders, 1979.
This comprehensive textbook serves as a useful resource to different groups of health care workers involved in the care of burn patients.

Durtschi MB, Orgain C, Counts GW, Heimbach DM. A prospective study of prophylactic penicillin in

acutely burned hospitalized patients. J Trauma 1982;22(1):11–14.
Routine administration of prophylactic penicillin protects against neither cellulitis nor burn wound infection.

Howard RJ. Effect of burn injury, mechanical trauma, and operation on immune defenses. Surg Clin North Am 1979;59:2:199–211.
Abnormalities of immunologic factors of severely burned patients are highlighted. The difficulties of sorting out the effects of burn injury, surgery, and anesthesia on the humoral and cellular immune systems are described.

MacMillan BG. Infections following burn injury. Surg Clin North Am 1980;60(1):185–196.
The experience of the Cincinnati Unit of the Shriners' Burns Institute is described with respect to overall prognosis of burn wound infection, and surgical excisional procedures of burn wounds.

Moncrief JA. Topical therapy for control of bacteria in the burn wound. World J Surg 1978;2:151–165.
A well-organized review of burn wound sepsis and topical antibiotics commonly used in the management of burns.

Volenec FJ, Clark BM, Mani MM, Humphrey LJ. Burn wound biopsy bacterial quantitation: a statistical analysis. Am J Surg 1979;138:695–697.
Quantitative bacteriologic monitoring using the wound biopsy technique provides an objective assessment of invasive burn wound infection.

25 SEPTIC SHOCK

Michael R. Achong

Shock is a clinical syndrome in which the supply of blood to the tissues is inadequate to meet their metabolic needs. The most common causes of this syndrome are hypovolemia, acute cardiac failure, and sepsis. The feature that distinguishes septic shock from shock due to other causes is the occurrence of the syndrome without preceding loss of intravascular fluid or damage to a specific organ such as the heart. Certain infections can result in the shock syndrome by precipitating (1) loss of intravascular volume (severe gastroenteritis); (2) impairment of cardiac function (acute valvular insufficiency in infective endocarditis); (3) decreased arteriolar tone (anaphylaxis due to rupture of an echinococcus cyst). The syndrome of septic shock described in this chapter is that seen as a complication particularly of gram-negative bacteremia.

ETIOLOGY

Shock may occur with a wide variety of bacterial, fungal, viral, rickettsial, and parasitic infections, particularly when there is blood stream invasion; however, bacterial infection is the most common underlying problem. In about two-thirds of patients, septic shock results as a complication of bacteremia with endotoxin-containing gram-negative bacilli so that the terms gram-negative shock, endotoxin shock, and septic shock are often used interchangeably. The organisms that most commonly cause bacteremia are as follows:

1. Gram-negative bacteria
   - *Escherichia coli*
   - *Klebsiella, Enterobacter, Serratia* spp.
   - *Pseudomonas aeruginosa*
   - *Proteus* spp.
   - *Neisseria meningitidis*
   - *Bacteroides fragilis*
2. Gram-positive bacteria
   - *Staphylococcus aureus*
   - *Streptococcus pneumoniae*
   - Other streptococci
   - *Clostridia* spp.

Gram-positive bacteremia has been incriminated in up to one-third of patients with septic shock. In the United States, the shock syndrome occurring mainly in menstruating women using tampons (toxic shock syndrome) has been widely publicized. Toxin-producing strains of *S. aureus* have been isolated from the vagina of the majority of these patients. The most common sources of infection in septic shock are as follows: urinary tract, lung, colon and peritoneal cavity, biliary tract, wound infections, site of intravascular cannulation, and female genital tract. Certain sites are frequently associated with particular bacteria: *E. coli* and the biliary tract, *B. fragilis* and the colon and female genital tract, *S. pneumoniae* and the lung, *S. aureus* from soft tissue or wound infections, and *P. aeruginosa* from burns. Polymicrobial bacteremia may account for up to 10% of all recognized bacteremias and usually originates from the gastrointestinal or genitourinary tract.

EPIDEMIOLOGY

Gram-negative bacteremia with septic shock was an uncommon problem in the preantibiotic era. It occurred mainly in outpatients, affecting most often older men with prostatic obstruction, young women with septic abortions, and patients with hepatobiliary disease. Over the past 40 years, several changes have taken place: broad-spectrum antibiotics have become available; medical and surgical advances have prolonged the life of elderly, debilitated patients; the aggressive use of cytotoxic and immunosuppressive drug therapy results in immunocompromised hosts; and the increasing use of indwelling urethral and venous catheters and respirators disrupts some of the normal mechanical barriers to infection. As a result, the spectrum of underlying disease in septic shock has greatly expanded, and the frequency of nosocomial gram-negative bacteremia is not only steadily increasing, but the condition occurs with organisms that are often resistant to several antibiotics. In recent surveys of hospitals in the United States, the incidence of bacteremia varied from 34 per 10,000 hospital admissions in community hospitals to 127 episodes per 10,000 hospital admissions in teaching and referral hospitals. Shock developed in about 10% of bacteremic patients in the community hospitals compared to about 44% of those in teaching hospitals. Such differences between community and teaching hospitals probably reflect the nature and severity of the underlying diseases in patients referred to these respective hospitals.

Gram-negative bacteremia may occur at any age, but neonates and the elderly are especially susceptible. Over age 50 years, most of those who develop gram-negative bacteremia are males, while from age 20 to 50 years, most are females. The age-sex distribution probably reflects the increased prevalence of urinary tract infections in women during the childbearing years and increased frequency of these conditions in older men, in whom prostatic obstruction is common.

Septic shock usually occurs in the setting of a breakdown of the body's normal protective mechanical barriers and impairment of host defenses against infection, as follows:

1. Breakdown of normal mechanical barriers
   - Urinary tract catheter
   - Tracheostomy, mechanical ventilation
   - Peripheral and central venous catheters
   - Intraarterial catheters
   - Extensive burns
2. Impaired resistance to infection
   - Neutropenia
   - Corticosteroid, cytotoxic drug therapy
   - Radiotherapy
   - Malignant disease
   - Cirrhosis
   - Diabetes mellitus
   - Alcoholism
3. Recent invasive procedures
   - Drainage of infected tissues
   - Genitourinary procedures
   - Colonic operations

In about one-third of patients, an invasive procedure such as drainage of infected tissues or manipulation of the gastrointestinal or genitourinary tracts precedes the development of shock by less than 24 hours. Recognition of this clinical setting is very important in suggesting the diagnosis.

PATHOPHYSIOLOGY

The exact mechanisms by which the infection and its attendant bacteremia trigger the hemodynamic changes culminating in the shock syndrome are still unclear. The lipid component (lipid A) of endotoxin, a complex lipopolysaccharide in the cell wall of gram-negative bacteria, is thought to be the major factor that initiates a number of events that result ultimately in the shock syndrome (Figure 25.1). Several effects of endotoxin have been described.

Endotoxin activates Hageman factor (factor XII) of the intrinsic coagulation system, which in turn initiates several events. The activated Hageman factor produces complex changes and interactions among the coagulation and fibrinolytic systems. These effects are manifested as ischemic organ damage due to widespread fibrin deposition (disseminated intravascular coagulation) and bleeding as a result of fibrinolysis, as well as the consumption of clotting factors and platelets. Activated Hageman factor also triggers enzymatic reactions in the kinin system, resulting in the formation of bradykinin. This potent vasodilator has been incriminated as a major cause of hypotension seen in the shock syndrome.

Endotoxin is capable of activating both the classic and alternative complement pathways. Chemotactic substances produced by these reactions can cause leukocytes to aggregate as well as to stick to endothelial surfaces. The local release of humoral substances such as prostaglandins and lysosomal enzymes causes endothelial damage and increased vascular permeability. Such changes in the lung are thought to be responsible for the development of the adult respiratory distress syndrome (ARDS or shock lung). Activation of the complement pathway may also trigger the release of histamine from mast cells, which in turn contributes to the hypotension.

Although much attention has been given to the role of endotoxins in the pathogenesis of septic shock, it is important to realize that shock can result from infection with a wide variety of microorganisms, many of which do not contain endotoxin, implying that other mecha-

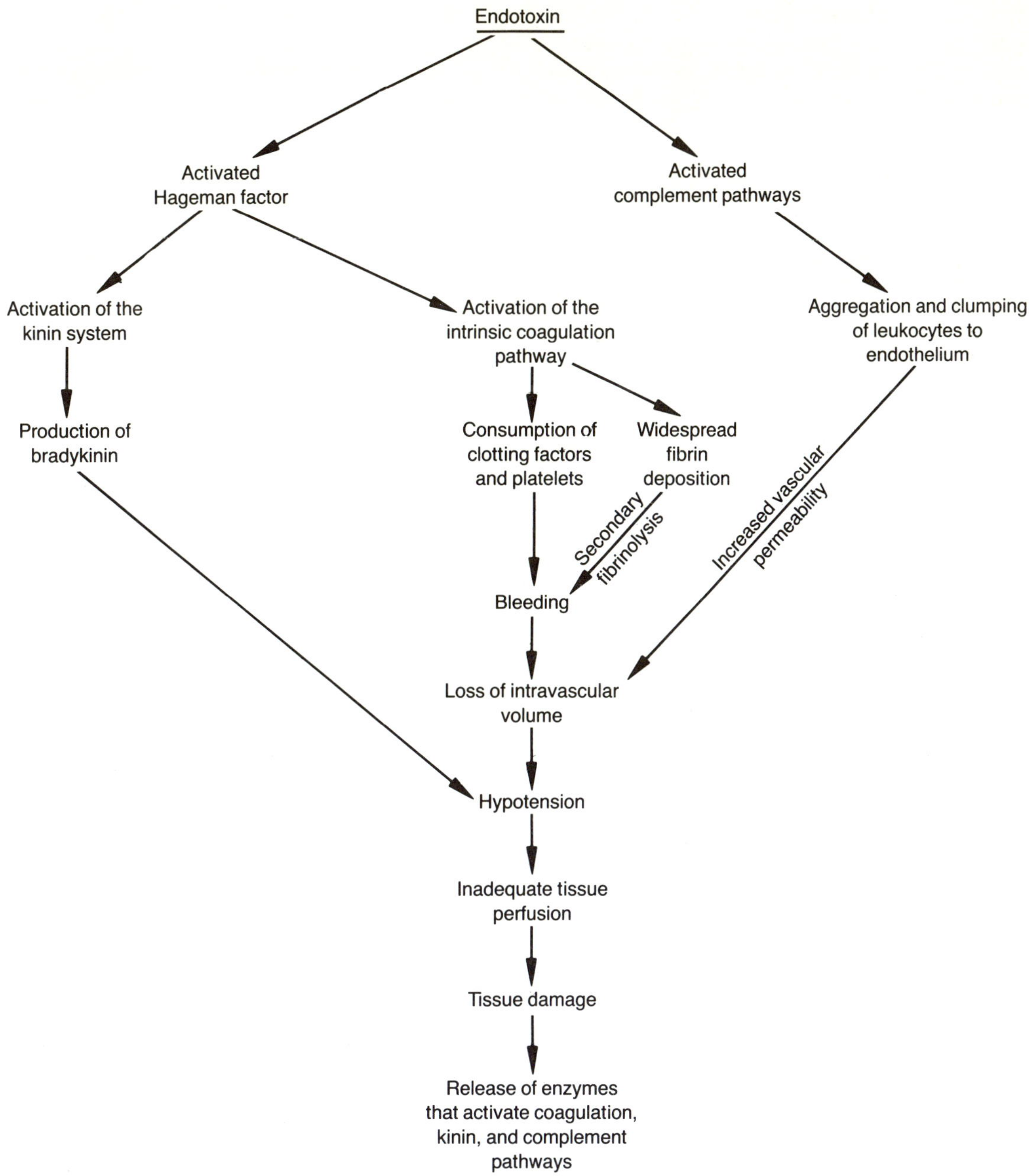

FIGURE 25.1. Proposed mechanisms of endotoxin-mediated shock.

nisms such as extracellular bacterial toxins may be involved in its pathogenesis. Apart from bradykinin and histamine, other vasoactive substances such as prostaglandins and endorphins are being actively investigated as causes for the early hemodynamic changes in septic shock. Subsequently, reflex changes in the sympathetic nervous system add vasoconstriction and tachycardia to the clinical picture.

The result of all these changes is inadequate tissue perfusion, widespread ischemic damage, anaerobic tissue metabolism and lactic acidemia. The release of enzymes from damaged cells may add to the activation of coagulation, complement, and kinin systems, which in turn contributes to further tissue damage. Interruption of this vicious cycle may be the reason why early treatment of bacteremia and elimination of the underlying focus of infection may prevent the full-blown shock syndrome.

CLINICAL MANIFESTATIONS

The fully developed syndrome of septic shock is not difficult to recognize. Typically, the appearance is that of a patient with marked systemic toxicity, fever, cool and moist extremities, hypotension, and oliguria. The diagnostic issue at this stage is whether the syndrome in a particular patient is due to sepsis, hypovolemia, or myocardial infarction. In some patients, the syndrome of so-called warm shock is seen initially. This includes warm, dry skin, mild hypotension, increased pulse volume, tachycardia, and respiratory alkalosis. If appropriate treatment is not started, some patients develop the full-blown syndrome of cold shock, in which peripheral vascular resistance is increased and cardiac output is decreased.

The clinical features of septic shock are quite varied and several points are noteworthy:

1. It is usually impossible to determine the microbial cause of the bacteremia on clinical findings alone. It has been suggested that in shock due to gram-negative bacteremia, there is likely to be marked peripheral vasoconstriction and decreased cardiac output, but such a distinction between gram-positive and gram-negative bacteremia is unreliable.
2. Bacteremia typically begins with a chill followed by fever; however, the febrile response to bacteremia may be blunted, particularly in elderly, debilitated patients, persons with impaired renal function, and those receiving corticosteroids. Paradoxically, hypothermia is sometimes an early feature of bacteremia.
3. Hypotension in the shock syndrome may be defined as a systolic blood pressure of less than 90 mm Hg, or a decrease of more than 50 mm Hg in the systolic pressure of a previously hypertensive individual. Shock is not synonymous with arterial hypotension, however, and the diagnosis should not be based solely on the level of arterial blood pressure, but should take into consideration signs of inadequate perfusion of organs such as the brain and kidney.
4. Some of the early features of the shock syndrome may be subtle and nonspecific. Changes in mental status such as drowsiness, apathy, or agitation may be features suggestive of bacteremia. Tachypnea and subsequent respiratory alkalosis is often a valuable early clue. Nonspecific gastrointestinal symptoms such as nausea, vomiting, and diarrhea may also be part of the syndrome. Septic shock should be considered in any elderly patient who has developed an otherwise unexplained acute confusional state, tachypnea, or hypotension.
5. A particular focus of infection may be so prominent that the associated bacteremia is not appreciated. For example, the dramatic features of fecal peritonitis may overshadow the accompanying bacteremia, while in pneumococcal pneumonia, about one-quarter of patients have an associated bacteremia. In contrast, the focus of infection may not be clinically evident in febrile neutropenic patients with bacteremia. Occasionally, sepsis may cause remote gastrointestinal hemorrhage, organ dysfunction such as respiratory failure, renal failure, cholestatic jaundice, or a bleeding diathesis.
6. A variety of skin lesions may be seen in patients with bacteremia and septic shock. Ecthyma gangrenosum consists of tender lesions with a vesicular or necrotic ulcerated center surrounded by an erythematous base. While these lesions are suggestive of *Pseudomonas* bacteremia, they may be seen with bacteremia caused by other organisms as well. Petechial lesions may reflect a vasculitis caused by meningococcemia or thrombocytopenia precipitated by the bacteremia.
7. Retinal hemorrhages and cotton wool spots have been observed in about one-quarter of bacteremic patients unassociated with diabetes mellitus, hypertension, or leukemia.
8. The transition from the clinical features of bacte-

remia to those of shock may be sudden and dramatic or insidious. Sometimes, bacteremia may be unrecognized until shock occurs, or shock may be unrecognized until oliguria, metabolic acidosis, or coagulation abnormalities appear. Two situations deserve special mention because of the fulminant and often fatal nature of septicemia: (a) bacteremia, usually with *S. pneumoniae,* in patients who are anatomically or functionally asplenic and (b) acute meningococcemia, which can be a rapidly fatal disease in previously healthy individuals.

LABORATORY DIAGNOSIS

It is important that appropriate specimens for Gram's stain and culture be obtained before antimicrobial therapy is started. Cultures and microscopic examination of blood, urine, sputum, wound drainage, and intravenous catheter tips can be obtained rapidly even in the most urgent situations. Ideally, three sets of blood samples should be taken to provide the maximum yield of positive cultures prior to starting antimicrobial therapy. In neonates, a single specimen may be satisfactory. The intervals between blood sample collections are determined by clinical circumstances and the urgency to initiate antimicrobial therapy. Examination of a Gram's stain of the patient's buffy coat granulocytes for intracellular bacteria may be helpful in patients with heavy bacteremia as in asplenic patients or those with staphylococcal sepsis.

The leukocyte count is usually increased, with greater numbers of immature polymorphonuclear leukocytes (shift to the left); but in some fulminant infections the leukocyte count may be normal or markedly decreased. Examination of the peripheral blood smear may also be helpful. Although not specific for bacteremia, the presence in the neutrophils of toxic granulation, vacuolization of the cytoplasm, or Döhle bodies in a patient with shock may suggest infection as a possible cause. A complete blood count is helpful in establishing the hemoglobin concentration early on and thrombocytopenia may be detected in up to 60% of patients with bacteremia. If there is extensive bleeding from sites of intravenous cannulation, disseminated intravascular coagulation (DIC) must be suspected. It is characterized by a decrease in plasma fibrinogen concentration, platelet count, and clotting factors, particularly factors V and VII, together with the presence of fibrin split products in the peripheral blood.

Arterial blood gases are important to detect hypoxemia and acid-base abnormalities. Respiratory alkalosis may be found early in septic shock when tachypnea is prominent. If shock proceeds uncorrected, serum lactate concentration increases (normal range 0.5 to 2.0 mM) and frank metabolic acidosis develops.

The blood urea nitrogen and serum creatinine concentrations are important indices of renal function, which, if impaired, would affect the dosages of some of the antibiotics employed. Abnormalities of liver function tests may be found even when the liver is not directly involved in the infectious process. Hypophosphatemia may be a nonspecific feature of bacteremia.

An electrocardiogram may be useful in pointing to acute myocardial infarction as the cause of shock. It may also reveal ischemic damage to the heart as a result of prolonged hypotension and decreased coronary artery perfusion. A chest x-ray is particularly important in patients with respiratory distress; diffuse parenchymal infiltrates in the presence of progressive hypoxemia and respiratory distress suggest the development of the adult respiratory distress syndrome.

TREATMENT

Treatment should be aimed at correcting the underlying cause of septic shock and improving tissue perfusion. Early institution of therapy is essential since the events are frequently irreversible by the time the full-blown syndrome is evident. A management plan is outlined as follows:

1. Elimination of infection
   - Antibiotics
   - Drainage of abscess, removal of source of infection
2. Enhancing tissue perfusion
   - Fluids
   - Inotropic agents
3. High-dose intravenous steroids
4. Correction of acid-base disorders
5. Ventilatory support
   - Oxygen
   - Mechanical ventilation
6. Attention to associated problems
   - Thrombocytopenia, DIC
   - Renal failure
   - Stress ulcers of the gastrointestinal tract
   - Poor nutritional status

TABLE 25.1. Initial Choice of Second Antibiotic To Be Given with an Aminoglycoside

Suspected Source of Infection	*Organisms To Be Specifically Affected by Second Antibiotic*		*Second Antibiotic*
Colon, female genital tract	*Bacteroides fragilis*		Clindamycin, 600 mg IV q6h
		or	cefoxitin, 2 gm IV q4h
		or	chloramphenicol, 1 gm IV q6h
		or	metronidazole, 500 mg IV q8h
Urinary tract	*S. faecalis*		Ampicillin, 2 gm IV q4h
Pneumonia			
Hospital-acquired	*Klebsiella* sp.		Cephalothin, 2 gm IV q4h
In neutropenic patients	*P. aeruginosa*		Carbenicillin, 5 gm IV q4h
		or	ticarcillin, 3 gm IV q4h
Skin, soft tissue	*S. aureus*		Cloxacillin, 2 gm IV q4h
Unknown source in neutropenic patient; burns	*P. aeruginosa*		Carbenicillin, 5 gm IV q4h
		or	ticarcillin, 3 gm IV q4h

Elimination of Infection

Both antimicrobial therapy and prompt removal of any source of infection are essential. If intravascular catheters are in place at the time bacteremia is diagnosed, they should be removed, cultured, and replaced aseptically at least 24 hours later, if possible, or under antibiotic coverage.

In patients in whom a site of infection and the causative bacteria have been previously recognized, it may be reasonably assumed that bacteremia is due to the same organism, and antibiotic therapy should be selected accordingly. Otherwise, the initial choice of antibiotics should be a combination of agents that would be effective against the possible pathogens. Arguments in favor of combination therapy include a broader spectrum of antimicrobial coverage and possible additive or synergistic activity against the offending bacteria. Furthermore, the development of resistant organisms may be delayed, particularly to drugs such as carbenicillin or ticarcillin. An aminoglycoside such as gentamicin or tobramycin should be part of most if not all combinations, since aminoglycoside-sensitive gram-negative aerobic bacteria are responsible for most cases of septic shock. If one suspects infection with an organism that might be resistant to gentamicin or tobramycin, amikacin should be used. The usual dosage of gentamicin or tobramycin is 1.0 mg per kg body weight every eight hours. For amikacin, the usual dosage is 15 mg per kg body weight every 24 hours divided into two or three doses given at equal intervals. With rapidly changing renal function, the appropriate dosage of aminoglycoside can be chosen only by obtaining blood for determination of serum aminoglycoside concentrations just prior to a dose (trough concentration) and about 30 minutes after the end of intravenous infusion (peak concentration). The choice of a second antibiotic depends mainly on the suspected or established source of the infection (Table 25.1). The new third-generation cephalosporins such as cefotaxime and moxalactam may have a role to play as initial therapy for suspected bacteremia in nonneutropenic patients, particularly if the organisms responsible for nosocomial infections are resistant to aminoglycosides.

Long periods of therapy with several antibiotics may have certain disadvantages, such as superinfection and increased risk of adverse drug effects. For these reasons, one should modify the choice of antibiotics as soon as culture results are known. The adverse effects of antibiotics can be recognized earlier if the physician is aware of the potential toxicity of the drugs being used. The duration of antibiotic therapy depends mainly upon the nature of the underlying illness and the source of bacteremia. Relatively shorter courses of antimicrobial therapy are acceptable when the source of bacteremia can be quickly removed and the local infection cured; for example, in patients with a stone obstructing the urinary tract and those with infected sites of intravascular cannulation. Another guideline is that therapy should be continued for at least five days after the patient has become afebrile, but this should not be adhered to slavishly.

Enhancing Tissue Perfusion

An effective circulating volume should be maintained by judicious use of parenteral fluids. There is debate as to whether the fluids should be crystalloid such as normal saline or colloid such as fresh-frozen plasma or albumin. The most frequently used crystalloid solution is normal saline, which is 0.9% saline and contains 154 mEq sodium and chloride per liter.

The adequacy of fluid replacement can be assessed by the clinical signs of improving tissue perfusion, such as clearing sensorium, adequate urine output (greater than 30 ml/hour), and a stable arterial blood pressure with a systolic value greater than 100 mm Hg. Close supervision is necessary for early detection of pulmonary edema. If available, measurement of either right or left heart filling pressures with a central venous catheter and a flow-directed pulmonary artery catheter (Swan-Ganz), respectively, would allow a better assessment of the heart's capacity to handle the fluid volume administered without the development of pulmonary edema. A useful technique of fluid challenge is to give pulses of 200 ml intravenously over ten minutes and observe the response both clinically and in the central venous or pulmonary artery wedge pressure. Usually, pulmonary edema will not develop when the pulmonary artery wedge pressure is kept at or below 18 mm Hg.

If aggressive volume replacement does not improve tissue perfusion, a trial of an inotropic agent such as dopamine is worthwhile, although there is no evidence that such therapy improves the overall outlook for patients with septic shock. Apart from its inotropic effect, dopamine produces dilatation selectively in renal and mesenteric vessels. Dopamine is given by continuous intravenous infusion; the starting dosage is 2 μg per kg body weight per minute, but may be increased every 15 minutes until the systolic blood pressure exceeds 100 mm Hg and urine output exceeds 30 ml per hour. Dosages greater than 15 μg per kg body weight per minute should be avoided, since they cause generalized vasoconstriction as a result of alpha-adrenergic receptor stimulation. Some have advocated the use of digoxin in patients with septic shock who fail to respond to volume replacement, but there is no controlled clinical trial to support this routinely.

Corticosteroids

The value of corticosteroids in septic shock still remains a controversial topic and a detailed discussion of the issue is beyond the scope of this chapter. If used, therapy should be with very large doses of a glucocorticoid for not longer than 24 hours. Schumer has suggested the following regimen: methylprednisolone, 30 mg per kg body weight, or dexamethasone, 3 mg per kg body weight. The drug is diluted in 100 ml saline and infused intravenously over 20 minutes. The first dose is given as soon as the diagnosis is made and repeated only once, about four hours later. Such short courses of corticosteroid therapy are usually not harmful, but rapid intravenous injections of dexamethasone have been incriminated in the production of cardiac arrhythmias.

Correction of Acid-Base Disorders

Metabolic acidosis is usually due to inadequate tissue perfusion with the accumulation of lactic acid, so that rational treatment should be aimed at improving tissue perfusion. Severe degrees of acidemia can depress cardiac function and affect the action of catecholamines, however. An arterial blood pH that persists below 7.2 may be reversed by small (50 mEq) intravenous doses of sodium bicarbonate. Administration of excessive amounts of sodium bicarbonate carries the risk of sodium overload and the development of alkalosis that impairs oxygen release to the tissues.

Ventilatory Support

Arterial hypoxemia is a feature of septic shock in some patients, possibly because of intrapulmonary arteriovenous shunting or alveolocapillary block to oxygen transfer in shock lung. Attempts should be made to maintain the arterial blood PO_2 above 60 mm Hg. Oxygen through a face mask may be sufficient, but if not, intermittent positive-pressure ventilation should be started without delay. The addition of positive end-expiratory pressure may be helpful in some patients with shock lung.

Associated Problems

Specific problems such as disseminated intravascular coagulation and renal failure due to acute tubular necrosis or glomerular dysfunction require special attention. Stress ulceration of the upper gastrointestinal tract may result in bleeding that may compound the problem of inadequate tissue perfusion. Some advocate the routine prophylactic use of cimetidine in all seriously ill patients and this would include patients with septic shock. Alternatively, hourly intragastric instillation of antacids may be used. The need for parenteral nutritional support should be considered early, particularly in situations where sepsis is not relieved promptly, oral feeding is not feasible, and the underlying illness has produced severe debilitation.

PROGNOSIS

The more serious the underlying disease, the higher the mortality rate of any complicating bacteremia: for example, elderly patients with fecal peritonitis have a much higher mortality rate compared with younger patients with urinary tract obstruction. Polymicrobial bacteremia also seems to carry an increased risk. *P. aeruginosa* is associated with the highest mortality rate of all gram-negative bacteremias. This reflects, at least in part, the relative resistance of *Pseudomonas* species to antibiotics and the association of *P. aeruginosa* with neutropenia and conditions such as extensive burns that are by themselves associated with a higher mortality. The mortality rates of other forms of gram-negative bacteremia reflect the severity of the host's underlying disease and extent of impairment of the host defense mechanisms.

When shock occurs in the course of bacteremia, the mortality rate is greatly increased and may be as high as 50%. Early diagnosis and prompt initiation of appropriate antimicrobial therapy are crucial to improving the prognosis.

PROPHYLAXIS

The prevention of septic shock is based on minimizing the risk of nosocomial bacteremia by paying special attention to intravascular or urinary catheters and mechanical ventilators. Medical personnel should be encouraged to wash their hands after examining each patient. Prompt recognition and early treatment of bacteremia with appropriate antibiotics are also preventive.

ANNOTATED BIBLIOGRAPHY

Bryant RE, Hood AF, Hood CE, Koenig MG. Factors affecting mortality of gram-negative rod bacteremia. Arch Intern Med 1971;127:120–128.
Poor prognostic factors were shock, azotemia, *Pseudomonas aeruginosa* bacteremia, and low or normal temperature during bacteremia.

Kreger BE, Craven DE, Carling PC, McCabe WR. Gram-negative bacteremia. III. Reassessment of etiology, epidemiology and ecology in 612 patients. Am J Med 1980;68:332–343.

Kreger BE, Craven DE, McCabe WR. Gram-negative bacteremia. IV. Reevaluation of clinical features and treatment in 612 patients. Am J Med 1980;68:344–355.
These two papers describe the problem of gram-negative bacteremia seen in a teaching hospital.

Rietchel ET, Schade U, Jensen M, Wollenweber H-W, Luderitz O, Greisman SG. Bacterial endotoxins: chemical structure, biological activity and role in septicemia. Scand J Infect Dis 1982;Suppl 31:8–21.
A review of the role of endotoxin in septic shock.

Scheckler WE. Septicemia in a community hospital 1970 through 1973. JAMA 1977;237:1938–1941.
A good study of bacteremia and septic shock in patients in a community hospital.

Schumer W. Steroids in the treatment of clinical septic shock. Ann Surg 1976;184:333–341.
The most widely quoted paper supporting the use of steroids in the treatment of septic shock, but has several methodologic deficiencies.

Sheagren JN. Septic shock and corticosteroids. N Engl J Med 1981;305:456–458.
A discussion of the shortcomings of the available studies on the value of corticosteroids in septic shock.

Shine KI, Kuhn M, Young LS, Tillisch JH. Aspects of the management of shock. Ann Intern Med 1980; 93:723–734.

This overview includes a useful discussion of the controversial aspects of the management of septic shock.

Todd JK. Toxic shock syndrome: a perspective through the looking glass. Ann Intern Med 1982;96(part 2):839–842.

An introductory article to a recent symposium on the toxic shock syndrome.

Young LS, Martin WJ, Meyer RD, Weinstein RJ, Anderson ET. Gram-negative rod bacteremia: microbiologic, immunologic and therapeutic considerations. Ann Intern Med 1977;86:456–471.

A superb overview of gram-negative bacteremia.

26 NOSOCOMIAL INFECTIONS

Peter Phillips and Anthony W. Chow

Nosocomial (hospital-acquired) infection is defined as infection that is neither present nor incubating at the time of hospital admission. When the incubation period is unknown, an infection is generally considered nosocomial if it becomes apparent 48 hours or more after the patient is hospitalized. All other infections are designated as community-acquired. Reports from the National Nosocomial Infections Study (NNIS) of the Centers for Disease Control indicate that the mean rate of nosocomial infections among patients discharged from acute care facilities in the United States has been relatively constant over the past several years, with an annual incidence of approximately 3.3% (Table 26.1). Hospital-acquired infections have a major impact on both patient well-being and health care costs, and in the past few years, more attention has been paid to the important questions of epidemiology and prevention that relate to these diseases. Physician awareness of the risks, modes of spread, and preventive measures for the common nosocomial infections is essential in order to minimize the infectious complications of hospital care.

Although there continue to be new developments in the spectrum of nosocomial pathogens, the problem of hospital-acquired infections is not a new one. In 1843, Oliver Wendell Holmes drew attention to the contagiousness of puerperal fever. A reduction in maternal mortality from this complication was reported a few years later, attending the practice of hand washing with calcium chloride solution in obstetrical practice. Joseph Lister was responsible for the first effective attack on wound infection in 1865 when he introduced antiseptics to the management of orthopedic wounds.

The majority of nosocomial infections involve surgical wounds, respiratory tract, urinary tract, or primary bacteremia (Table 26.2). In the last decade, nosocomial bacteremia has occurred with increasing frequency on all hospital services, while wound infections have been more frequent on obstetrical services; the latter observation may in part be due to an increased delivery rate by cesarean section. Hospital-acquired pneumonia, although less common than infections involving the urinary tract or wounds, is more likely to result in a fatal outcome.

ETIOLOGY

Since the late 1960s, gram-negative bacilli have continued to be the predominant nosocomial pathogens (Table 26.3). The commonly encountered organisms are *Escherichia coli, Pseudomonas aeruginosa, Klebsiella, Proteus, Providencia,* and *Serratia. Staphylococcus aureus,* group D streptococci, and *Candida* are common gram-positive nosocomial isolates. Important viral and protozoal agents include hepatitis B virus, rubella, cytomegalovirus, herpes simplex, herpes zoster, influenza, *Toxoplasma gondii,* and *Pneumocystis carinii.*

Until relatively recently, a number of other nosocomial pathogens have either escaped detection by standard culture techniques or have not been appreciated as being pathogenic in a given setting. *Legionella pneumophila* was overlooked in the past because of its failure to stain well on Gram's stain or to grow on standard media. It is the cause of legionellosis, both as a sporadic disease and in the form of epidemics in the hospital setting as well as the community. Renal disease, immunosuppressive therapy, and malignancy appear to be the most important predisposing conditions. *Mycobacterium chelonei* and *M. fortuitum* have been responsible for a variety of infectious complications that occur after cardiac surgery, including wound infec-

TABLE 26.1. Number of Nosocomial Infections by Service and Category of Reporting Hospitals

	Service						
Category of Reporting Hospital	*Medicine*	*Surgery*	*Obstetrics*	*Gynecology*	*Pediatrics*	*Newborn Nursery*	*All Services*
Community	2.4	3.5	1.6	2.1	0.7	0.9	2.5
Community-teaching	3.5	4.5	1.5	3.0	0.4	0.9	3.1
Federal	4.0	3.8	3.8	7.7	1.2	1.1	3.7
Municipal or county	3.9	5.8	3.2	4.5	3.4	2.0	4.1
University	4.8	5.9	2.9	2.9	3.2	1.6	4.4
All hospitals	3.4	4.6	2.1	2.9	1.6	1.2	3.3

Numbers per 100 patients discharged.

Modified from Centers for Disease Control National Nosocomial Infections Study Report, Annual Summary 1979. US Dept HEW, Public Health Service. Atlanta: Centers for Disease Control, 1982:6.

TABLE 26.2. Percentage of Various Nosocomial Infections by Hospital Service

	Service						
Type of Infection	*Medicine*	*Surgery*	*Obstetrics*	*Gynecology*	*Pediatrics*	*Newborn Nursery*	*All Services*
Urinary tract	53	38	21	51	13	5	40
Surgical wounds	2	30	50	36	11	4	22
Respiratory tract	21	17	3	5	21	11	16
Skin and subcutaneous tissues	6	4	2	2	18	38	6
Primary bacteremia	7	4	1	1	11	10	5
Other	11	7	23	5	26	32	11
Totals	100	100	100	100	100	100	100

Modified from Centers for Disease Control National Nosocomial Infections Study Report, Annual Summary 1979. US Dept HEW, Public Health Service. Atlanta: Centers for Disease Control, 1982:7.

tion, sternal osteomyelitis, pericarditis, and endocarditis. Although considered to be rapid growers, these atypical mycobacteria still require two to five days to form visible colonies on appropriate media, and may be missed by standard culture techniques. Another group of recently recognized potential pathogens responsible for a variety of nosocomial infections including endocarditis are the diphtheroids. Diphtheroids are members of the *Corynebacterium* genus. They are normally abundant on the skin and mucous membranes, are usually sensitive to antibiotics, and seldom cause infection. The ones designated group JK bacteria have been most frequently implicated in nosocomial infections. They are motile and biochemically distinct from other well-recognized members of the *Corynebacterium* genus. Infections related to defective epithelial barriers, prosthetic devices, and the postoperative period are characteristic of these organisms, and vancomycin is the treatment of choice.

Antibiotic-induced enterocolitis in the 1950s was frequently attributed to *S. aureus,* but today *Clostridium difficile* is the pathogen most often responsible. Animal experiments support the possibility of cross-infection with *C. difficile,* therefore suggesting the possible usefulness of special precautions for hospitalized patients with pseudomembranous colitis.

TABLE 26.3. Percentage of Isolate Frequency of Selected Pathogens in Various Nosocomial Infections

Pathogen	Type of Infection: Urinary Tract	Surgical Wounds	Respiratory Tract	Skin and Subcutaneous Tissue	Primary Bacteremia	Other	All Types
Escherichia coli	32	13	7	7	14	8	18
Staphylococcus aureus	2	15	10	30	14	12	10
Group D streptococci	14	9	1	6	7	6	9
Pseudomonas sp.	13	6	11	7	6	6	9
Klebsiella sp.	9	5	11	4	14	5	8
Proteus-Providencia sp.	9	6	5	5	2	4	7
Enterobacter sp.	4	4	6	3	6	2	4
Candida sp.	4	1	2	5	5	8	3
Staphylococcus epidermidis	3	5	1	7	8	5	4
Other	10	36	46	26	24	44	28
Totals	100	100	100	100	100	100	100

Modified from Centers for Disease Control National Nosocomial Infections Study Report, Annual Summary 1979. US Dept HEW, Public Health Service. Atlanta: Centers for Disease Control, 1982:11.

The spectrum of disease related to *Chlamydia trachomatis* has been extended to include conjunctivitis and pneumonia, occasionally acquired by infants after vaginal delivery from colonized mothers. Antibiotic prophylaxis has been effective for prevention of chlamydial conjunctivitis but not for the pneumonia, which typically occurs 3 to 11 weeks postnatally.

As a result of effective screening of blood donors for hepatitis B virus, non-A, non-B hepatitis has emerged as the most frequent cause of nosocomial hepatitis related to blood transfusion.

EPIDEMIOLOGY

Host Factors

The increased susceptibility of the hospitalized patient to infection stems from one or more of the following factors: underlying disease, invasive diagnostic or therapeutic procedures, therapy with irradiation or immunosuppressive drugs, and exposure to the sometimes formidable hospital microflora. Several underlying diseases are associated with altered host defenses and some of these are summarized in Table 26.4. Devices used in the management of ill patients such as endotracheal tubes, intravenous and urinary catheters are known to dramatically increase the incidence of hospital acquired infection. Less well recognized has been the association of sinusitis with the use of nasotracheal and nasogastric tubes. In this setting, the development of unexplained fever may be the first clue to the presence of sinusitis.

Microbial Factors

Antibiotic therapy has been accompanied by the emergence of a variety of resistant organisms. Multiple-drug resistance is defined as resistance to two or more antibiotics to which the bacterium is usually sensitive. Bacteria may become resistant by spontaneous chromosomal mutation and subsequent selection from other sensitive organisms in the presence of antibiotic therapy. Another way in which a bacterium develops resistance is through the acquisition of extrachromosomal genetic material, known as a resistance plasmid or R factor, that codes for an enzyme active against certain antibiotics. Plasmid-mediated resistance has generally been less of a problem in the community than in the hospital setting. Nevertheless, it has been well documented with *Salmonella, Shigella, E. coli, Neisseria*

TABLE 26.4. Altered Host Factors and Predisposing Conditions for Nosocomial Infections

Altered Host Factor	*Predisposing Conditions*
Anatomic barriers to infection	Surgery, burns or other trauma, invasive diagnostic procedures, urinary and intravenous catheters, prosthetic devices, antimetabolites and irradiation
Protection by colonization with normal flora	Hospitalization; antimicrobial therapy and disinfectants; coma, acidosis, azotemia, hypotension
Leukocyte function and the inflammatory response	Diabetic ketoacidosis and uremia, granulocytopenia and other diseases of hematopoietic system, antimetabolites, corticosteroids, irradiation
Humoral immunity	Multiple myeloma, chronic myelogenous leukemia; nephrotic syndrome; immunosuppressive therapy
Cellular immunity	Hodgkin's lymphoma, advanced malignancies, extremes of age and chronic debilitation, cytotoxic drugs and immunosuppressive therapy

gonorrhoeae, Hemophilus influenzae, and *Streptococcus pneumoniae* infections.

Any hospitalized patient, either colonized or infected with drug-resistant bacteria, most likely acquired the organisms in one of four ways: (1) direct person-to-person spread by the hands of hospital personnel; (2) indirect spread from reservoirs in the hospital environment, particularly equipment used in patient care such as urine-measuring devices; (3) during a previous hospital admission, since which time the patient harbored the resistant organisms; and (4) through resistance developed during a course of antibiotic treatment.

Modes of Transmission

At one time, there was considerable interest in the hospital environment and its role in causing nosocomial infections. This was attended by the frequent use of routine surveillance cultures and attempts to purge hospitals of perennial pathogens by disinfecting walls, floors, sinks, and so on. These efforts proved to have little impact upon the problem, partly because the sources of infection have sometimes remained obscure. However, surveillance cultures have been useful in some outbreaks; Legionellosis and disease caused by groups JK of the *corynebacterium* genus are examples.

Endogenous versus Exogenous Infections

Nosocomial infections may be endogenous or exogenous. An infection with an organism that is usually part of a patient's own microflora is considered to be endogenous. An example would be a granulocytopenic patient who develops septicemia with an organism originating from normal bowel flora, such as *E. coli.*

An exogenous nosocomial infection is one in which the offending organism is acquired from the hospital environment. *Staphylococcus aureus* and *Streptococcus pyogenes* are often transmitted from other patients or hospital personnel and usually cause an exogenous infection. Similarly, *Enterobacter agglomerans, Serratia* sp., *Pseudomonas* sp., and *Flavobacterium* sp., which are usually not constituents of the normal human flora, generally result in exogenous infection. These bacteria are extremely hardy and may survive and proliferate in moist environments such as nebulizers, respiratory support equipment, isolette humidifiers, intravenous solutions, and even certain antiseptic agents. Often patients may first become colonized with one or more organisms from the hospital flora and then develop clinical infection with these recently acquired organisms.

Endemic versus Epidemic Infections

Endemic nosocomial infections occur with a given frequency in a particular hospital setting. Their epidemiology tends to be less well characterized than epidemic hospital infections, which often have a definable reservoir and mode of spread. Endemic nosocomial infections are frequently influenced by specific host factors such as granulocytopenia and immunosuppression, which may be difficult to control, whereas epidemic infections are often the result of exogenous and environmental factors. This point was exemplified by the 1970 outbreak of septicemia involving hundreds of patients across the United States that resulted from the distribution of contaminated intravenous fluids from one manufacturer. Although hospital epidemics attract considerable attention, they are much less important in terms of prevalence than endemic infections.

Except for outbreaks of varicella zoster or *Aspergillus,* there is little evidence that air-borne spread plays a significant role in the transmission of most nosocomial pathogens. Hospital epidemics are most often caused by *S. aureus* (19%), *Salmonella* (13%), organisms of the genus *Klebsiella* (12%), hepatitis B virus (8%), *Pseudomonas* strains (6%), enteropathogenic *E. coli* (5%), and group A streptococci (5%). Between 1956 and 1979, gastroenteritis was the infection most frequently investigated among hospital outbreaks (21%) and was most often caused by *Salmonella* or enteropathogenic *E. coli*. Gram-negative bacteremias and epidemics of cutaneous infection are also commonly investigated; the latter usually due to staphylococci, streptococci, and varicella.

Outbreaks of nosocomial infections must be carefully distinguished from pseudoepidemics, the latter are usually related to errors in processing microbiologic specimens such as contamination during collection, transport, or laboratory manipulation. Other pseudoepidemics have resulted from failure to distinguish between community-acquired and hospital-acquired infection, and changes made in the methods, intensity, or analysis of surveillance. Occasionally, laboratories switching to more sensitive culture techniques may be responsible for apparent epidemics.

COMMON NOSOCOMIAL INFECTIONS

Surgical Wound Infection

Specific rates of surgical wound infection vary depending on the type of operation performed and the nature of the surgical service. "Dirty" or contaminated wounds increase the risk of infection by at least tenfold compared to clean or clean-contaminated wounds. Although several risk factors are present, the important major variables as determined by well-controlled, prospective studies include the extent of contamination at operation, age of the patient, duration of the operation, use of drains, and length of preoperative hospitalization. The presence of a foreign body, necrotic tissue, hematoma, and general debilitation secondary to malnutrition or underlying disease are important predisposing factors to development of infection.

Most surgical wound infections derive from microorganisms of endogenous origin introduced into the wound during the operation. These contaminants come either from the patient's own skin or from deeper sites transected during surgery such as the tracheobronchial tree, bowel, or genitourinary tract. Wound infections are much more frequent when the patient has a coexisting infection at some other site.

Extrinsic contamination or air-borne transmission of organisms responsible for surgical wound infection is much less common. The *S. aureus* and group A betahemolytic streptococci are the most important agents that may be extrinsically introduced by human carriers. Less common are surgical infections linked to inanimate or environmental sources of contamination. These include (1) many aerobic gram-negative bacilli such as *Pseudomonas, Klebsiella, Enterobacter,* or *Serratia* species, which have been traced to contaminated disinfectants, shaving brushes, or local anesthetics; (2) *Aspergillus* species from contaminated ventilation systems; and (3) atypical mycobacteria or saprophytic fungi from contaminated prosthetic devices (intraocular lenses or porcine heart valves).

Pneumonia

Hospital-acquired pneumonia most often encountered in the intensive care unit is usually caused by gram-negative bacilli and is associated with a high mortality rate. Important risk factors include the severity of the underlying illness, antibiotic treatment, and respiratory tract instrumentation. The ability of gram-negative organisms to adhere to the oropharyngeal epithelial cells is low in healthy individuals but increases in ill patients, thereby facilitating colonization of the upper respiratory tract. A bedridden existence and respiratory disease appear to be the two best predictors of colonization of the oropharynx with gram-negative bacilli. Once colonization is established, these organisms may cause pulmonary infection if the lung defense mechanisms are inadequate to deal with the small inocula of mouth flora that readily gain access to the lower respiratory tract. In addition to impairment of the cough reflex and mucociliary transport, experimental evidence suggests that pulmonary bacterial defenses become compromised in the presence of acidosis, hypoxia, and edema.

Unlike adult nosocomial pneumonias in which

gram-negative organisms predominate, viruses are most important in the pediatric population. Another major feature of pediatric pneumonia is that no significant differences exist among respiratory isolates causing infection in the hospital and in the community. In order of importance, the most frequent pathogens in pediatric patients are respiratory syncytial virus, influenza, and parainfluenza viruses. Viral outbreaks on pediatric wards are often difficult to control, frequently involve both patients and staff, and may result in severe disease among children with underlying medical problems.

Urinary Tract Infection

Urinary tract infections occur in approximately 2 patients per 100 admissions. *Escherichia coli* accounts for about 50%. Other gram-negative organisms such as *Proteus* spp., *Klebsiella, P. aeruginosa, Enterobacter,* and *Serratia* are common as well. Gram-positive pathogens have generally been less important, although *S. epidermidis,* enterococci, and yeasts accounted for as many as one-third of all hospital-acquired urinary infections in one recent series. One can expect to see bacteremia much more frequently when the urinary tract is infected with *Serratia* or *Klebsiella.* Bacteremia and death are noted mainly in persons over 50 years of age, and the risk of infection increases with the duration of urinary catheterization.

In the patient with an indwelling urinary catheter, neither antibiotic prophylaxis prior to development of bacteriuria nor antibiotic treatment of asymptomatic bacteriuria has been efficacious in preventing infection; in addition the indiscriminate use of antibiotics only encourages the development of resistant organisms. Antibiotic therapy should be reserved for catheterized patients who manifest fever and other overt signs or symptoms of urinary tract infection. Although unproven, antibiotics may be beneficial in the catheterized patient with bacteriuria if there is a co-existent immune disorder, pre-existing renal disease or if catheter removal is anticipated within a few days.

Bacteremia

Most nosocomial bacteremias are secondary, resulting from urinary tract infection, pneumonia, wound or intraabdominal infection. This group accounts for most of the endemic bacteremias. Primary bacteremia occurs when the source is clinically unrecognized, but such infections often originate from intravascular devices. Most hospital epidemics of bacteremia are considered primary and should be suspected when blood cultures yield organisms such as *Pseudomonas cepacia, Pseudomonas maltophilia, Flavobacterium* organisms, or *Enterobacter agglomerans,* all of which are rarely encountered in secondary bacteremias. Most cases of primary bacteremia have occurred in patients with compromised immunity; those who have undergone recent invasive intravascular procedures or insertion of an intravascular device; or who have been sequestered in a special area such as an intensive care unit, where the likelihood of contamination with hospital flora is particularly high. Although the mortality rate associated with nosocomial bacteremia approaches 50%, there is room for optimism with regard to prevention. This is particularly true for primary bacteremias, which are more likely to result from hospital or physician practices and are therefore more amenable to intervention. Hospital epidemics of primary bacteremia should be distinguished from pseudobacteremia, which is the result of contamination of blood culture collection devices rather than a true infection.

NOSOCOMIAL INFECTIONS IN HOSPITAL EMPLOYEES

Certain hospital personnel are repeatedly exposed to blood or blood products and are therefore particularly at risk for hepatitis B infection. These include operating room personnel, emergency room and ambulance staff, intravenous teams, laboratory staff, and workers in blood bank, autopsy, oncology, nephrology, and hepatology units. The availability of hepatitis B immune globulin (HBIG) and the recently developed hepatitis B vaccine are important in the prevention of hepatitis B in this high-risk group. Nosocomial transmission among hospital employees has been demonstrated with non-A, non-B hepatitis, but not with hepatitis A virus (HAV). The latter is not a significant nosocomial pathogen, probably due to the fact that low numbers of viral particles are shed in the stools of patients hospitalized with this infection. Active virus shedding in stools occurs primarily in the preclinical phase of hepatitis A infection and is minimal by the time clinical manifestations develop.

Many pediatric hospitals have adopted a policy of

determining the immune status of their staff with respect to rubella, and keeping nonimmune individuals away from areas where the risk of contracting rubella is particularly high. Such a policy has not been applied to the problem of potential hospital acquisition of cytomegalovirus by pregnant employees. Also, epidemic respiratory viruses in pediatric patients often infect both the staff and other patients.

The incidence of nosocomial tuberculosis in physicians during the years of training is in the order of 1% per year in the United States. Active tuberculosis subsequently develops in approximately 10% of those who initially contract primary infection.

PREVENTION

Despite the lack of clear-cut evidence of benefit, numerous precautions have been recommended and widely adopted in an attempt to minimize hospital-acquired infections. There is certainly the suggestion that simply heightening physician awareness is an important measure in controlling the problem. By altering physician behavior with regard to prescription practice of antibiotics and indiscriminate use of invasive diagnostic and therapeutic procedures, a significant reduction in hospital-acquired infection may be realized.

Control of nosocomial infections has relied primarily on immunization, chemoprophylaxis, and isolation of infected patients. Immunoprophylaxis with zoster-immune globulin has been effective in modifying or preventing disease in immunocompromised patients exposed to varicella. Active immunization against hepatitis B virus has recently been proved both safe and effective. Lack of identifiable markers for non-A, non-B hepatitis has hampered efforts to develop effective active or passive immunization against this infection. A vaccine with antigenic specificity for the lipopolysaccharide common to gram-negative bacteria is under investigation and may prove useful for prevention of nosocomial gram-negative infections in those at particular risk.

Chemoprophylaxis is useful where there is an increased risk of infection extending for a short period of time, such as hours or days. Only in this situation can one hope to inhibit a wide variety of potentially patho-

TABLE 26.5. Hospital Isolation, Precaution, and Control Measure Guidelines in Selected Conditions Leading to Potential Nosocomial Infection

		Control Measures						
Selected Conditions	*Type of Isolation or Precaution*	*Private Room*	*Gown*	*Mask*	*Gloves*	*Dressing and Secreta*	*Excreta and Soiled Articles*	*Blood*
Burn wound	WSP*		(+)†	(+)	(+)	+‡		
Diarrhea, acute (infectious etiology suspected)	EP§		(+)		(+)		+	
Diphtheria (pharyngeal and cutaneous)	SI//	+	(+)	+	(+)	+		
Furunculosis (staphylococcal)	WSP		(+)	(+)	(+)	+		
Gas gangrene (caused by *Clostridium perfringens*)	WSP				(+)	+		
Hepatitis, viral (type A, B, or unspecified)	EP, BP**		+		+		+	+
Hepatitis B antigen carrier	BP							+
Herpes simplex (disseminated neonatal vesicular disease)	SI	+	(+)		(+)	+	+	

TABLE 26.5. (continued)

		Control Measures						
Selected Conditions	*Type of Isolation or Precaution*	*Private Room*	*Gown*	*Mask*	*Gloves*	*Dressing and Secreta*	*Excreta and Soiled Articles*	*Blood*
Herpes zoster								
Disseminated	SI	+	(+)	+	(+)	+	+	
Localized	WSP		(+)		(+)	+		
Malaria	BP							+
Meningitis, meningococcal	RI††	+		+				
Meningococcemia	RI	+		+				
Mumps	RI	+		+		+		
Pertussis	RI	+		+		+		
Plague								
Bubonic	WSP		(+)	(+)	(+)	+		
Pneumonic	SI	+	+	+	+	+		
Pneumonia								
S. aureus	SI	+	(+)	+	(+)	+		
Group A streptococci	SI	+	(+)	+	(+)	+		
Rabies	SI	+			(+)	+		
Rubella (german measles)	RI	+		+		+		
*(congenital syndrome)	SI	+	(+)	+		+	+	
Rubeola (including encephalitis)	RI	+		+		+		
Salmonellosis	EP		(+)		(+)		+	
Shigellosis	EP		(+)		(+)		+	
Tuberculosis (pulmonary, suspected, or sputum-positive)	RI	+		+		+		
Vaccinia, generalized (eczema vaccinatum)	SI	+	+	+	+	+		
Varicella	SI	+	+	+	+	+		

Adapted from Yoshikawa TT, Chow AW, Guze LB. Infectious diseases — diagnosis and management. Boston: Houghton Mifflin, 1980:268–270.

*Wound and skin precautions.

†Recommended during direct contact with patient.

‡Recommended.

§Enteric precautions.

//Strict isolation.

**Blood precautions.

††Respiratory isolation.

genic organisms. Prophylaxis on a long-term basis has only been effective when dealing with one particular organism that does not have a tendency to develop resistance. Penicillin prophylaxis against the group A beta-hemolytic streptococcus in patients with a history of rheumatic fever is such an example. Patients with chronic conditions associated with an increased incidence of infectious complications, unless the complications are readily reversible, are unlikely to benefit from chemoprophylaxis. Examples of this situation include patients with malignancy, diabetes mellitus, congestive heart failure, indwelling catheters, prostheses, and drainage tubes. A more detailed discussion of chemoprophylaxis can be found in Chapter 7.

Isolation procedures often involve considerable expense, may be psychologically stressful for the patient, and may at times compromise overall patient care. Despite these negative aspects, such measures when stringently applied may be important for effective control of certain hospital infections (Table 26.5). An extreme example of this is the total protected environment (TPE). The exogenous organisms in the environment are diminished by measures such as use of laminar air-flow rooms and high-efficiency particulate air filters. The patient's endogenous flora are reduced through the use of presterilized foods, nonabsorbable antibiotics for suppression of gut flora, and topical applications of antibiotics or antiseptics to mucocutaneous surfaces. Although expensive and awkward, TPE has been effective in reducing serious infections in severely immunocompromised patients such as recipients of bone marrow transplantation. Decontamination is usually not achieved until 1 to 3 weeks after the above measures have been instituted, so that such drastic steps are not indicated in patients whose granulocytopenic immunocompromised state is expected to be less than 25 days in duration.

INVESTIGATION AND CONTROL OF HOSPITAL OUTBREAKS

Investigation and corrective measures must be undertaken whenever evidence suggests that cross-infection among hospitalized patients has occurred (Figure 26.1).

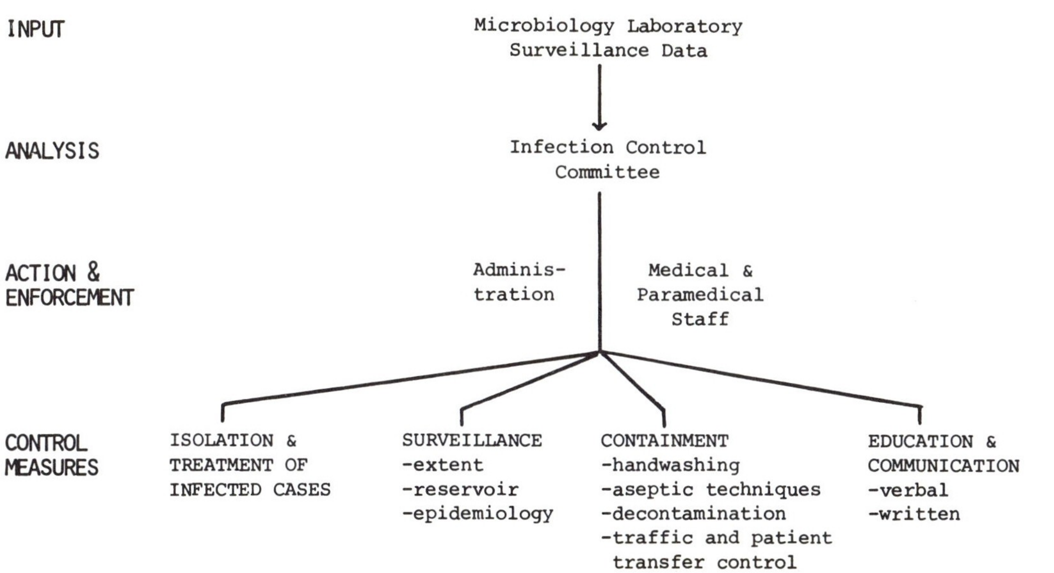

FIGURE 26.1. Approach to investigation and control of hospital outbreaks. Reproduced with permission from Yoshikawa TT, Chow AW, Guze LB. Infectious diseases — diagnosis and management, Boston: Houghton Mifflin, 1980:271.

Epidemiologic investigation relies almost entirely on fact gathering. Evidence for cross-infection depends on compatible clinical and epidemiologic findings and on laboratory confirmation that the same strain of microorganism has been transmitted from one individual to another. Antibiogram patterns, phage typing, serotyping, and other biotyping facilities can be most helpful in this regard. The index case should be identified and the extent of the outbreak determined. Risk factors, particularly those common to all infected patients, must be elucidated. If a particular risk factor or common reservoir of infection is suspected, it is useful to perform a case-control study to verify the significance of the suspected factor. Once the nature and significance of a particular suspected risk factor or common reservoir have been confirmed, a rational plan of action for control and prevention may be formulated. The prompt and effective implementation of such control measures often requires the close cooperation and active support of a multidisciplined infection-control team.

Outbreaks of several drug-resistant bacteria may be the result of R plasmid transfer among various species of bacteria. If bacteria of different species exhibit identical multiple-drug-resistance patterns, one should suspect a plasmid outbreak. Confirmation may be obtained by demonstrating identical plasmid DNA patterns with gel electrophoresis. Measures useful for the control of such outbreaks include: (1) restricting or rotating antibiotics, since it appears that maintaining plasmid-mediated resistance requires "antibiotic pressure"; (2) careful dosing of antibiotics to minimize the chance of subinhibitory antibiotic levels that may select for a resistant microbial subpopulation (secondary to chromosomal mutations); and (3) barrier-type antibiotic resistance precautions that have been shown to be useful in certain situations. Such precautions include emphasis on hand washing or gloving prior to contact with patients or patient secretions and excretions, segregation of patients with drainage tubes or indwelling urinary catheters, and careful disposal and handling of contaminated utensils such as urinals and bedpans.

ANNOTATED BIBLIOGRAPHY

Centers for Disease Control. National nosocomial infections study report annual summary, 1979. Atlanta: Centers for Disease Control, 1982.

Annual incidences of nosocomial infections reported from 82 hospitals cooperating with the Centers for Disease Control in the National Nosocomial Infections Study are summarized by type, service, site, and pathogen.

Chow AW. Nosocomial infections. In: Yoshikawa TT, Chow AW, Guze LB, eds. Infectious diseases — diagnosis and management. Boston: Houghton Mifflin, 1980:268–271.

A brief overview of nosocomial infections is succinctly presented.

Fraser DW. Bacteria newly recognized as nosocomial pathogens. Am J Med 1981;70:432–438.

Recently recognized nosocomial pathogens are reviewed and their clinical as well as microbiologic characteristics are highlighted.

Hall CB. Nosocomial viral respiratory infections — perennial weeds on pediatric wards. Am J Med 1981;70:670–675.

The epidemic respiratory viruses of nosocomial importance on pediatric wards are emphasized, with a lucid discussion of their hospital epidemiology and methods of control.

Jackson GG. Considerations of antibiotic prophylaxis in nonsurgical high-risk patients. Am J Med 1981;70:467–473.

The rationale and risk-benefit considerations for use of antibiotic prophylaxis in nonsurgical high-risk patients are critically reviewed and the need for proper assessment of efficacy and efficiency of prophylaxis is further amplified.

LaForce FM. Hospital-acquired gram-negative pneumonias: an overview. Am J Med 1981;70:664–669.

An overview of the current knowledge of epidemiology, pathogenesis, and risk factors of nosocomial gram-negative pneumonias is succinctly presented, with a brief discussion of future directions in the development of new preventive measures.

Maki DG. Nosocomial bacteremia. Am J Med 1981; 70:719–732.

The epidemiology and risk factors of both epidemic and endemic nosocomial bacteremias are summarized, with helpful suggestions for surveillance technique and preventive measures.

Stamm WE, Weinstein RA, Dixon RE. Comparison of endemic and epidemic nosocomial infections. Am J Med 1981;70:393–397.

Characteristics differentiating epidemic and endemic nosocomial infections are compared, and the predictability of mode of transmission in a given epidemic by careful site-pathogen analysis and application of this knowledge for establishing initial control measures are emphasized.

Tulby JL, Friedland GH, Baldini LM, Goldmann DA. Complications of intravenous therapy with steel needles and Teflon catheters. Am J Med 1981; 70:702–706.

The risk-benefits of intravenous therapy with steel needles versus Teflon catheters are compared in a prospective study; helpful considerations for minimizing complications from intravenous therapy are presented.

Turck M, Stamm W. Nosocomial infection of the urinary tract. Am J Med 1981;70:651–654.

Difficulties in effective treatment and prevention of nosocomial urinary tract infections are highlighted and the need for better understanding of pathogenesis and assessment of risk factors is underscored.

Weinstein RA, Kabins SA. Strategies for prevention and control of multiple drug-resistant nosocomial infection. Am J Med 1981;70:449–454.

Newer approaches to prevention and control of several drug-resistant nosocomial infections are outlined. The application and usefulness of barrier-type antibiotic resistance precautions for containment of such outbreaks are clearly presented.

27 PARASITIC INFECTIONS

Jay S. Keystone

Although many microbial creatures, including bacteria, viruses, and fungi, often exist in a parasitic relationship with their respective hosts, historically, the team parasite has come to be associated with metazoa (multicelled organisms called helminths) and protozoa (single-celled organisms) (Figure 27.1).

It is helpful to remember that helminths (worms) are classified as roundworms (nematodes) and flatworms. The latter are further subdivided into segmented tapeworms (cestodes) and unsegmented flukes (trematodes). Protozoa are classified according to their locomotory organelle or attachment site to the host cell. Some protozoa propel themselves by flagella *(Giardia lamblia),* others by extending pseudopodia *(Entamoeba histolytica),* and still others by cilia *(Balantidium coli).* Those without a specific locomotor organelle *(Plasmodia* sp. and *Toxoplasma gondii)* have an apical complex that functions in the attachment of the organism to the host cell.

Diagnosis and management of parasitic infections requires a basic understanding of the organisms' epidemiology and pathophysiology. Most parasites have a complex life cycle that involves either a period of incubation in the soil or development in a specific intermediate host such as an insect, mammal, or snail. Therefore transmission of many parasites in North America is not possible because of high standards of hygiene and sanitation and lack of appropriate insect vectors or specific intermediate hosts. The obvious exceptions to this rule are intestinal protozoa and a few helminths that are infective at the time of passage in the stool.

Helminths and protozoa differ in several major respects. Being multicellular, worms are usually visible to the naked eye, whereas protozoa can only be seen with the aid of a microscope. Helminths tend to have a finite life span and with few exceptions, do not multiply in the human host. Protozoa, on the other hand, may persist for the lifetime of the host in which they live. Eosinophilia is associated with helminthic but rarely with protozoan infections.

An important principle to note about helminth infections is that worm burden is determined by the degree of exposure to infective ova or larvae, since helminths do not multiply in the host. Furthermore, the extent of tissue damage and hence human morbidity is directly proportional to worm burden. On the basis of these principles, one can understand why a reduction in worm number without parasitologic cure may produce an acceptable therapeutic result. Since most antihelminthics reduce worm burden by over 90%, repeated courses of therapy would be of little benefit to the patient.

PROTOZOAL DISEASE

Intestinal Protozoa

Intestinal protozoa are the most common cause of parasitic infection encountered by North American physicians. Although increased travel to and immigration from developing countries undoubtedly have increased the pool of these infections, changing lifestyles probably account for the high endemicity of intestinal protozoa in some North American populations. Fecal-oral transmission by male homosexuals, day-care nursery children, and institutionalized, mentally retarded patients have produced rates of infection from 5% to 80% within these specific groups.

With most intestinal protozoal infections, the diagnosis is confirmed or excluded by examination of stool

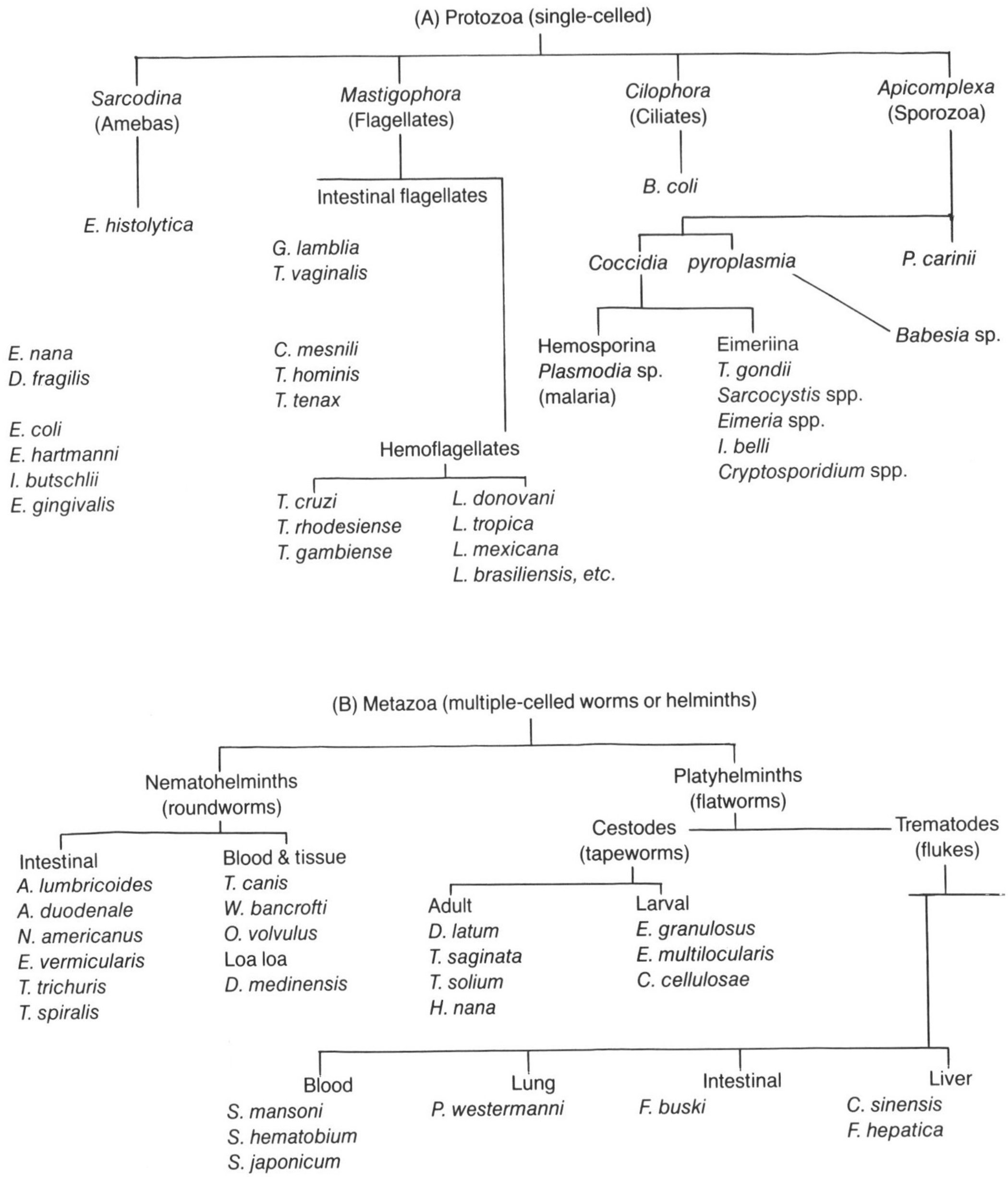

FIGURE 27.1. Life trees of protozoa (A) and metazoa (B).

specimens. Since intestinal protozoa are excreted intermittently, several (at least three) specimens are needed to exclude infection. Stools must be examined in the fresh state (within 12 hours of passage) or collected in preservatives such as polyvinyl alcohol or sodium acetate formalin. Examination of fresh stool offers little advantage over preserved samples; however, it does enable the technologist to detect characteristic motility of vegetative forms. Most laboratories examine a direct smear and prepare a concentrate using a sedimentation (formalin ether) or flotation (zinc sulfate) technique. Examination of a permanently stained smear (using iron hematoxylin, Lawless, or trichrome) is the most sensitive method to detect intestinal protozoa and enables one to visualize the nuclear detail necessary for identification of these organisms. Unfortunately, many laboratories do not have the expertise to prepare and examine permanently stained smears.

When testing for intestinal parasites, it is important to ensure that the patient has not received orally or by rectum substances that would interfere with stool examination, such as barium, antacids, antibiotics, cathartics, and bismuth. In such cases, examinations should be postponed for 7 to 10 days.

Amebiasis

Etiology. Amebiasis is an infection with *Entamoeba histolytica,* a large bowel intestinal protozoan that has a noninfective vegetative form (trophozoite) and an infective cyst form. Uninuclear trophozoites, measuring 20 to 30 μ, feed on bacteria and cellular debris in the large bowel, especially the sigmoid colon and cecum. As they pass down into unfavorable conditions, they develop into 10 to 20 μ quadrinucleate cysts. When passed in the feces, contamination of the environment (food, water) or fingers may occur. Cysts may remain viable outside of the host for several months, particularly at low temperatures. After ingestion by a new host, the organisms excyst in the small bowel. Each cyst gives rise to four new trophozoites and the cycle repeats itself.

Pathophysiology. Most of the time, *E. histolytica* acts as a commensal and does not damage the bowel mucosa. Recent isoenzyme studies suggest that most strains of *E. histolytica* are non-pathogenic and will not invade tissue or produce symptoms in humans. Pathogenic strains, on the other hand, under the influence of immunosuppression and/or other unknown factors, may invade the large bowel mucosa, classically producing discrete, flask-shaped ulcers. From the bowel, the organism usually spreads hematogenously to the liver, where an abscess can develop, usually in the right lobe. Spread to other viscera such as lung or brain is rare.

Clinical Manifestations. Patients with intestinal amebiasis are generally asymptomatic. When tissue invasion occurs, intermittent diarrhea alternating with constipation is common. Amebic dysentery is rare. It is characterized by the insidious onset of tenesmus, urgency, lower abdominal cramping, bloody diarrhea, and low-grade fever. Rarely, an inflammatory mass (ameboma) may develop in the colon, usually in the cecum or sigmoid colon.

Amebic liver abscess is the most frequent manifestation of extraintestinal amebiasis. It is characterized by high fever, right upper quadrant pain, shoulder tip pain, and nonproductive cough. On physical examination, elevation of the right hemidiaphragm, tender hepatomegaly, and a small right pleural effusion may be present. The patient is often cachectic and pale.

Diagnosis. The diagnosis of intestinal amebiasis requires examination of several stool specimens. When invasive bowel disease is suspected, sigmoidoscopy with ulcer scrapings or biopsy may be necessary. The presence of trophozoites that contain ingested red cells (hematophagous trophozoites) in stool or scrapings is pathognomonic of invasive disease. The diagnosis of an amebic liver abscess may be suggested by elevation of the right hemidiaphragm on chest x-ray and further supported by ultrasound, radionuclide or computerized tomographic scanning. Amebic serology (indirect hemagglutination — or IHA; enzyme-linked immunoabsorbent assay — ELISA; indirect fluorescent autibody — IFA) is specific and positive in 85% of cases of amebic colitis and 95% of cases of amebic liver abscess. Since intestinal amebas cannot be detected in most individuals with an amebic liver abscess, serology plays an important role in diagnosis. It is usually unnecessary to aspirate the abscess for diagnostic (or therapeutic) purposes. Classically, amebic pus is odorless, reddish brown (anchovy sauce), and contains no inflammatory cells.

Treatment. Patients who are asymptomatic passers of *E. histolytica* cysts or trophozoites require lumen-acting agents such as diiodohydroxyquin, 650 mg orally three times a day for 20 days; diloxanide furoate, 500 mg three times a day for 10 days; or diphetarsone, 500 mg three times a day for 10 days. Invasive amebiasis (colitis or abscess) must be treated with a tissue-acting drug such as oral metronidazole, 750 mg three times a day for 5–10 days, plus a lumen-acting agent. Metronidazole, even in high dose, when given alone frequently fails to clear amebas from the gut lumen. The mortality rates for invasive intestinal and hepatic amebiasis range from less than 1% in uncomplicated cases to 40% where peritonitis or pericarditis are present.

Nonpathogenic Amebiasis

The nonpathogens *Entamoeba coli, Endolimax nana, Entamoeba hartmanni, Dientamoeba fragilis* (really a flagellate), and *Iodamoeba bütschlii* should be considered as markers for more virulent organisms, stimulating the physician to search harder for potential pathogens such as *E. histolytica* or *Giardia lamblia;* however, *D. fragilis* has been associated with an irritable bowel-like syndrome. *Dientamoeba fragilis* is also associated with pinworm infection. Asymptomatic individuals who are infected with nonpathogens do not require treatment. Tetracycline or diiodohydroxyquin (or diphetarsone, an emergency drug available in Canada) are effective for the treatment of *D. fragilis*.

Giardiasis

Etiology. Giardiasis is an infection with *G. lamblia,* a small bowel flagellated protozoan. The infection is ubiquitous and has a worldwide distribution. In North America, the beaver and dog may serve as important reservoirs. Giardiasis is the most common cause of water-borne outbreaks of diarrhea in the United States. It is an important cause of traveler's diarrhea, particularly in those who visit Leningrad. Food-borne transmission of *G. lamblia* is rare. In North America, high-risk groups for person-to-person transmission include day-care nursery children, male homosexuals, and institutionalized, mentally retarded individuals. Patients with adult-onset combined variable hypogammaglobulinemia are quite susceptible to giardiasis.

Pathophysiology. Pear-shaped trophozoites of *G. lamblia,* measuring 15 by 9 μ are found in the upper small bowel where they attach by ventral sucking discs to the gut mucosa. Invasion of the mucosa has been documented, but is distinctly rare. The exact mechanism by which this parasite produces its damage to bowel mucosa is unknown. As trophozoites move down the intestine and encounter unfavorable conditions, flagellae are lost, nuclear division occurs, and quadrinucleate cysts are produced. Cysts are infective at the time of passage in the feces, whereas trophozoites desiccate rapidly in the environment. Cysts can survive for up to one month in water at 21°C and two months at 8°C. After ingestion of cysts, two trophozoites are released per cyst during excystation in the upper small bowel. Trophozoites multiply by binary fission.

Clinical Manifestations. Most individuals with giardiasis are asymptomatic. When illness does occur, the incubation period is one to three weeks. Symptoms and infection often resolve spontaneously within several weeks and months respectively. Symptomatic disease is characterized by an acute or chronic diarrheal illness associated with marked fatigue, bloating, borborygmi, flatulence, nausea, and pain in the middle to upper abdomen. Lactose intolerance is a common finding. Severe infection may lead to a malabsorption syndrome that is clinically indistinguishable from tropical sprue.

Diagnosis. The diagnosis of giardiasis often can be made on stool examination; usually several specimens are needed because of the intermittency of cyst excretion. When stools are negative, examination of small bowel contents using a nasogastric tube or enterotest capsule (string test) may be necessary. Biopsy of small bowel tissue with an impression smear is the most sensitive diagnostic method.

Treatment. Metronidazole, 2 gm orally once daily for three days, or 250 mg orally three times a day for five to seven days; atabrine, 100 mg by mouth three times a day for seven days; or furazolidone, 100 mg four times a day for seven days, may be used for the treatment of symptomatic giardiasis. Some authors advocate a trial of drug therapy in suspected cases where the parasite cannot be detected by routine methods. Symptomatic patients should temporarily be fed a lactose-free diet.

Prognosis. The natural course of untreated giardiasis usually is one of spontaneous resolution. Occasionally, a progressive and persistent malabsorption syndrome may develop.

Follow-up stools should be examined one to two weeks after therapy has been completed. Except for food handlers, asymptomatic individuals need not be treated.

Nonpathogenic Flagellates

Trichomonas hominis, Enteromonas hominis, and *Chilomastix mesnili* are flagellated commensals of the large bowel that have not been associated with clinical disease in humans. Infections with these organisms do not require therapy, even in symptomatic individuals.

Other intestinal protozoa not covered in this chapter include several rare zoonotic infections that can lead to serious gastrointestinal disease in humans: *Balantidium coli, Isospora hominis* or *belli,* and *Cryptosporidia* species.

Genital Tract Protozoa

Trichomoniasis

Trichomoniasis is a sexually transmitted infection of the genitourinary tract of males and females caused by the flagellated protozoan *T. vaginalis*. This 13 by 7 μ piriform parasite exists only in the trophozoite form and is found in the urethra and vagina of females and the urethra, epididymis, and prostate of males. It is found most frequently in women 30 to 50 years of age and is one of the most common infectious causes of leukorrhea.

Clinical Manifestations. Infections in males are almost always asymptomatic. When symptoms occur, epididymitis and prostatitis are usual. Females complain of a malodorous, yellowish vaginal discharge associated with vaginal pruritus. Dysuria, frequency, and dyspareunia may accompany the vaginitis.

Diagnosis. The diagnosis of trichomoniasis is made by a hanging-drop preparation or culture of the vaginal discharge. Organisms may sometimes be found by examination of urine and prostatic fluid.

Treatment. Metronidazole, (2 gm once in females or 250 mg three times each day for 7 days in males or females) by the oral route is the treatment of choice for women. Sexual partners should be treated concomitantly with the index case regardless of whether the parasite can be detected in such contacts.

Prognosis. The symptoms of untreated trichomoniasis often resolve spontaneously even though the parasite persists for long periods, producing an asymptomatic carrier state.

Blood and Tissue Protozoa

Malaria

Etiology. Malaria is a protozoal infection of the blood with *Plasmodia* species: *P. vivax, P. falciparum, P. ovale,* and *P. malariae*. On a worldwide basis, *P. vivax* and *P. falciparum* are the most common species. *Plasmodium vivax* is the usual species of malaria imported into North America with *P. falciparum, P. malariae,* and *P. ovale* malaria occurring in decreasing order of frequency. Malaria is endemic in tropical and subtropical climates and follows the distribution of the *Anopheles* mosquito. In addition to direct contact with the mosquito, malaria can be transmitted by blood transfusion, parenteral inoculation, and placental leak during delivery. The placenta serves as an effective barrier to malaria while the fetus is in utero.

Pathophysiology. The malaria life cycle begins with the blood meal of the female *Anopheles* mosquito, during which infective forms (sporozoites) are inoculated into the host circulation (Figure 27.2). These forms are taken up rapidly by the liver where they develop and multiply within hepatocytes (hepatic schizonts). The liver (exoerythrocytic) phase usually takes two to four weeks but may take up to a year to complete. In *P. vivax* and *P. ovale* only, dormant forms known as hypnozoites may produce late relapses for up to three years after the initial infection. When hepatic schizonts rupture, the parasites that are released enter red cells and initiate the erythrocytic cycle. Once inside the red cell, the parasite develops through a trophozoite stage and multiplies to produce a red cell schizont. When the mature schizont and red cell rupture, the released parasites (now called merozoites) invade new red cells to repeat the cycle.

In the red cell, some merozoites develop into sexual forms (gametocytes), which may be ingested by a mosquito during its blood meal. Further development of the sexual forms in the mosquito leads to the production of infective sporozoites that concentrate in the mosquito salivary glands. With the mosquito's next meal, the malaria cycle is completed.

Clinical Manifestations. Uncomplicated malaria is characterized by periodic fever, headache, myalgia,

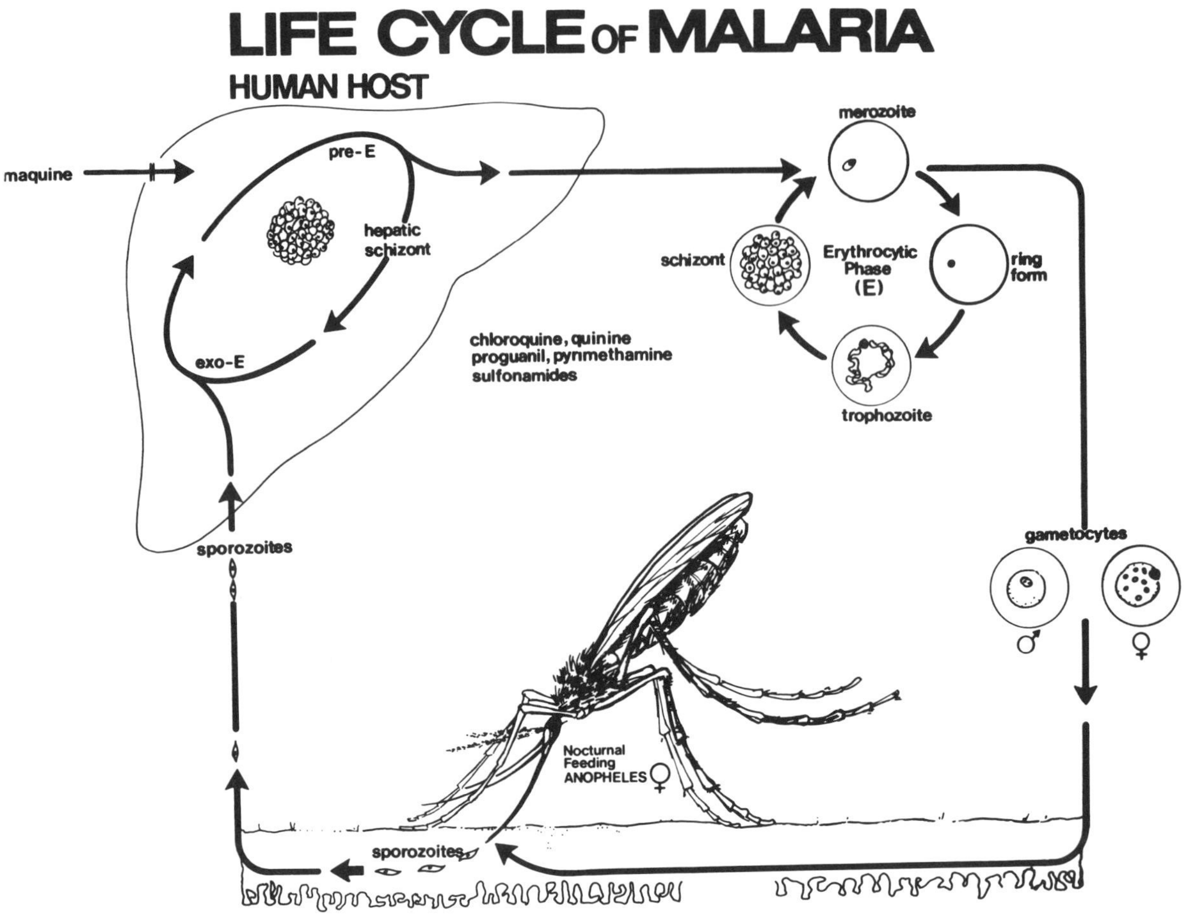

FIGURE 27.2. Life cycle of malaria.

malaise, and hepatosplenomegaly. The periodicity of fever corresponds with the erythrocytic cycle, specifically, with the release of merozoites from ruptured red blood cells. Since *P. vivax* and *P. ovale* take 48 hours to complete the erythrocytic cycle, and *P. malariae* takes 72 hours, fevers associated with these species occur every 48 and 72 hours respectively. In *P. falciparum,* asynchronous fever spikes are the rule, and periodic 48-hour fevers the exception. With all malaria species, several days of asynchronous fever often precede the establishment of a periodic pattern, particularly in non-immune individuals.

In heavy infections with *P. falciparum* only, anemia, jaundice, renal insufficiency, adult respiratory distress syndrome, hemoglobinuria (black water fever), diarrhea, adrenal insufficiency, and coma may occur. Chronic *P. malariae* infections in children occasionally produce an immune complex nephritis manifested by the nephrotic syndrome. Massive splenomegaly in association with intravascular volume overload (tropical splenomegaly syndrome) can result from an aberrant response to any malaria species.

Diagnosis. The most common laboratory finding in malaria is immune-mediated pancytopenia. Malaria is diagnosed by thick blood film whereas the species is determined by means of a thin film. Where there is a high index of suspicion, serial thick films should be taken six to eight hours apart. Serology is helpful retrospectively and in the diagnosis of the tropical spleno-

TABLE 27.1. Treatment of Malaria

Drug of Choice	*Adult Dose*	*Pediatric Dose*
Uncomplicated attack (all *Plasmodia* except chloroquine-resistant *P. falciparum*)		
Chloroquine phosphate	600 mg base (1 gm) then 300 mg base in 6 hrs; then 300 mg base/d × 2 d	10 mg base/kg (max. 600 mg base), then 5 mg base/kg in 6 hrs, then 5 mg base/kg/d × 2 d
Prevention of relapsed (*P. vivax* and *P. ovale* only) add		
Primaquine phosphate (check G6PD level)	15 mg base/d × 14 d	0.3 mg base/kg/d × 14 d
Treatment of severe illness (all *Plasmodia,* except chloroquine-resistant *P. falciparum* see below)		
Quinine dihydrochloride	600 mg in 300 ml normal saline IV over 2 hrs; repeat in 6–8 hrs if oral therapy still cannot be started (max. 1800 mg/d)	25 mg/kg/d; administer half of dose in 2 hrs, then rest 6–8 hrs later if oral dose cannot be started (max. 1800 mg/d)
Treatment of uncomplicated attack (chloroquine-resistant *P. falciparum*)		
Quinine sulfate	650 mg tid × 3–7 d	25 mg/kg/d in 3 doses × 3–7 d
plus		
A. pyrimethamine/sulfadoxine	3 tablets	
or		
B. pyrimethamine	25 mg bid × 3 d	<10 kg: 6.25 mg/d 10–20 kg: 12.5 mg/d 20–40 kg: 25 mg/d × 3 d
plus		
sulfadiazine	500 mg qid × 5 d	100–200 mg/kg/d in 4 doses × 5 d (max. 2 gm/d)
or		
C. tetracycline	250 mg qid × 7 d	5 mg/kg qid × 7 d
Treatment of severe illness (chloroquine-resistant *P. falciparum*):		
As for severe illness with other *Plasmodia* plus one of the regimens A–C when the patient is able to start oral therapy.		

megaly and quartan malaria nephrotic syndromes. Babesiosis, endemic on Nantucket Island, Massachusetts is a rare tick-borne protozoal infection with *Babesia microti,* which may be extremely difficult to distinguish microscopically from *P. falciparum* malaria.

Treatment. Chloroquine phosphate, (1 gm to start, 500 mg in 6 hours, then 250 mg twice a day for two days) is the drug of choice for the treatment of all but chloroquine-resistant *P. falciparum* malaria (Table 27.1). Drug-resistant *P. falciparum* malaria is now firmly established in South America, East Africa, and Southeast Asia. In these areas, a rapidly acting schizonticide, quinine, 650 mg by mouth every eight hours for three to seven days, must be combined with tetracycline (250 mg by mouth q.i.d. for 7 days) or pyrimethamine/ sulfadoxine (Fansidar), (3 tablets as a single dose). In *P. vivax* and *P. ovale* malaria, primaquine, (15 mg daily for 14 days) must be added to eradicate the dormant liver forms (hypnozoites), thereby preventing late relapses (Figure 27.1). Primaquine is a strong oxidant and therefore is contraindicated in individuals with G6PD deficiency. Inadequately treated malaria (*P. malariae*) may relapse up to 30 years after the primary infection.

Prognosis. Untreated *P. falciparum* malaria in nonimmune individuals is often fatal; other species give rise to a self-limited illness that may take weeks or months to resolve. Resolution occurs gradually with increasing symptom-free intervals between attacks and decreasing severity of subsequent attacks. In semiimmune individuals who have acquired some degree of immunity, infections with all species are self-limited unless a decrease in host defenses occurs.

Prophylaxis. Chemoprophylaxis should be administered to all travelers to areas where malaria is endemic. Antimalarials are started two weeks prior to entering an endemic area in order to get the traveler in the habit of taking the medication and to enable the physician to change the agent should side effects occur (Table 27.2). It is crucial to remember that, with the exception of primaquine, antimalarial drugs act on the erythrocytic cycle and do not usually prevent the hepatic phase from occurring. For this reason, travelers are instructed to continue taking antimalarials for six to eight weeks after departure from the tropics so that drug will be in the circulation to eradicate parasites released from the liver during that period. For travelers with extensive exposure to *P. vivax* malaria, primaquine, 15 mg daily for 14 days is recommended on return from endemic areas to prevent late relapses from dormant hypnozoites.

Toxoplasmosis

Etiology. Toxoplasmosis is caused by *Toxoplasma gondii,* a small (3 by 5μ) obligate intracellular protozoan. Toxoplasmosis has worldwide distribution. In Ontario, Canada, for example one-third of the population have antibodies to toxoplasmosis, with a peak prevalence of 50% in those over 45 years of age. Congenital toxoplasmosis occurs in approximately 1:1000 live births.

Pathophysiology. After the cat, the definitive host, acquires the infection by ingesting tissue cysts from raw meat or oocysts from another cat, a sexual cycle occurs in small bowel epithelial cells. On completion of this phase, cats excrete infective oocysts in stools for approximately two weeks. When humans or other mammals (pigs, sheep, goats, cattle, etc.) ingest oocysts, the organisms penetrate the gut to enter the circulation where they invade reticuloendothelial, muscle, and other tissue cells. Common target organs include the eye, brain, heart, lymph nodes, and striated muscle. In these cells, tissue cysts are formed, containing thousands of zoites that are viable for the lifetime of the host.

In addition to infection by ingestion of oocysts from cat feces or tissue cysts from poorly cooked or raw meat, humans can be infected by placental transfer of maternal toxoplasmosis, organ transplantation, or leukocyte transfusions, and in the laboratory by tachyzoites.

Clinical Manifestations. Most infections are asymptomatic or unrecognized. Clinical toxoplasmosis takes several forms: (1) congenital toxoplasmosis (2) chorioretinitis, (3) acquired toxoplasmosis in the immunocompetent host, and (4) acquired or reactivated toxoplasmosis in the immunosuppressed host. Congenital toxoplasmosis occurs when the fetus is infected in utero and is the result of an active maternal infection during pregnancy. Over all, the risk of fetal morbidity or mortality with maternal toxoplasmosis is between 10% and 40%. From first to third trimester, the risk of infection rises while the risk of serious disease (i.e., fetal morbidity) decreases. Most maternal infections are asymptomatic. Maternal infection confers lifelong immunity and hence there is no risk of congenital toxoplasmosis for subsequent pregnancies. Approximately 10% to 15% of infected newborns will be symptomatic at birth. Seventy percent of these children have a neurologic syndrome consisting of chorioretinitis, cerebral calcifications, seizures, hydrocephaly or microcephaly, and mental retardation. Thirty percent have systemic symptoms mimicking the rubella syndrome.

Chorioretinitis, usually of congenital origin, is one of the most common infectious causes of blindness in North America. With onset in the second or third decade of life, one or both eyes may be involved, and relapses are common.

Acquired toxoplasmosis in the immunocompetent host is usually asymptomatic or a mild, self-limited, flulike illness. It is generally a mononucleosis-like syndrome consisting of fever, pharyngitis, cervical lymphadenopathy, rash, and hepatosplenomegaly. Myocarditis and pneumonitis occur rarely.

In the immunosuppressed host, disseminated infection may produce life-threatening encephalitis, brain abscess, pneumonitis, or myocarditis.

Diagnosis. Although it is possible to diagnose toxoplasmosis by direct isolation of the organism from tissue (e.g., cord blood, placenta), serology is the most practical diagnostic test. Lymph node histology is frequently suggestive but not diagnostic. The most common serologic tests in use are the ELISA and IFA

TABLE 27.2. Malaria Chemoprophylaxis

Drug of Choice	*Adult Dose*	*Pediatric Dose*
All *Plasmodia* except chloroquine-resistant *P. falciparum* (start 1–2 wks before departure and continue for 6–8 wks after last exposure)		
Chloroquine phosphate	500 mg (300 mg base) weekly	<50 kg: 5 mg base/kg 1 × weekly
Chloroquine-resistant *P. falciparum* malaria* (start 1–2 wks before departure and continue for 6–8 wks after last exposure) Chloroquine PLUS		
A. pyrimethamine/sulfadoxine (fansidar)	25 mg pyrimethamine and 500 mg sulfadoxine (1 tablet) weekly	6–11 mo: 1/8 tablet 1–3 yr: 1/4 tablet 4–8 yr: 1/2 tablet 9–12 yr: 3/4 tablet (weekly)
or		
B. pyrimethamine/dapsone (maloprim)	12.5 mg pyrimethamine and 100 mg dapsone (1 tablet weekly)	
Extensive *P. vivax* exposure — on completion of chloroquine chemoprophylaxis add		
Primaquine phosphate†	15 mg base (1 tablet) daily × 14 d	0.3 mg base/kg/d × 14 d

* Distribution of chloroquine-resistant *P. falciparum* reported in Morbidity, Mortality Weekly Review (CDC, Atlanta).
†Check G6PD level.

methods for detecting IgG and IgM antibodies. Seroconversion, a fourfold rise in IgG antibody, and the presence of IgM antibodies are diagnostic of a recent infection. Since IgG antibodies may remain elevated for many years, and single high titer cannot distinguish recent from past infections. Two points concerning serodiagnosis are worth noting: (1) *Toxoplasma* chorioretinitis is a clinical diagnosis since antibody titers do not change during active retinal inflammation; and (2) IFA-IgM antibodies in the newborn are frequently undetectable because of passive transfer of maternal IgG, which interferes with IgM determination. However, the ELISA test is very sensitive in detecting IgM antibodies in the newborn.

Treatment. Treatment with a four- to six-week course of pyrimethamine and sulfadiazine should be instituted in congenital toxoplasmosis and infections in the immunocompromised host. Dosages for these drugs are as follows. For infants, pyrimethamine, 1 mg per kg per day (maximum of 25 mg/day); and sulfadiazine, 100 to 200 mg per kg per day. For adults; 25 mgm per day of pyrimethamine and 2–6 gm per day of sulfadiazine. Loading doses of both drugs can be given as well. The addition of clindamycin, 300 mg four times a day for four weeks, may improve the results of treatment for chorioretinitis, although no controlled studies of its use have been published. In fact, there is little evidence to show that drug therapy has a beneficial effect on chorioretinitis. Systemic steroid therapy has been useful in cases of severe chorioretinitis (under cover of antibiotic therapy). Abortion should be considered for maternal toxoplasmois acquired in the first trimester. Spiramycin therapy, 2 to 4 gm per day for three to four weeks, for infections detected in the second and third trimesters is advisable.

Prognosis. Toxoplasmosis in the immunocompetent host is a self-limited infection. In the immunosuppressed host, however, untreated infections are often fatal. Recent studies of small numbers of patients suggest that the majority of normal-appearing newborns of mothers with maternal toxoplasmosis later develop chorioretinitis, mental retardation, or other defects. The natural history of *Toxoplasma* chorioretinitis is one of relapses and remission with eventual spontaneous resolution.

Prevention. Precautions against toxoplasmosis may be taken by eating well-cooked meat, avoiding contact with cats or cat litter (especially during pregnancy), and by keeping cats out of childrens' play areas or sandboxes.

Leishmaniasis-Cutaneous

Cutaneous leishmaniasis is an infection with *Leishmania tropica* (Old World), *L. brasiliensis, L. mexicana,* and probably others (New World).

Etiology. The infection is widely distributed in India, the Middle East, Africa, the Mediterranean, Mexico, and most of Central and South America. Wild rodents, dogs, and other animals can act as reservoir hosts. Transmission usually occurs by the bite of an infected female sandfly *(Plebotomus)*. The disease is generally more common in rural than urban areas. In the New World, persons working in forested areas are at increased risk.

Pathophysiology. The flagellated promastigote form of the parasite is injected into or contaminates the wound during the bite of an infected sandfly. The parasite loses its flagellum, becoming an amastigote, and enters tissue macrophages where it replicates. It may then rupture the cell and spread locally, or spread to distant sites (espundia). A granulomatous inflammatory response usually occurs, resulting in the typical clinical findings and eventually, healing with scarring ensues. Anergy may result in diffuse cutaneous leishmaniasis (DCL), while a rigorous cell-mediated response may produce the recidiva form.

Espundia (mucocutaneous leishmaniasis) is associated with late, distant metastasis to the nose or oropharynx.

Clinical Manifestations. After a few days to one or two months, a nodule appears on the skin (there may be several lesions) and progresses to ulceration. It is an indolent ulcer with a violaceous rolled edge, which may take several months to a year to heal. The disease is transmissible as long as the ulcer is present. Healing occurs with a cigarette-paper-thin, depressed scar.

Mucocutaneous and diffuse forms are progressive if untreated.

Diagnosis. The diagnosis may be suggested by a positive skin test (Montenegro delayed-hypersensitivity skin test) or positive serology (IFA). It is confirmed by finding the parasite in stained smears of aspirates or scrapings from the edge of the ulcer, or by seeing them in a biopsy specimen. *Leishmania* may also be cultured using a suitable medium.

Treatment. Stibogluconate sodium (Pentostam®), 10–20 mg per kg per day intramuscularly or intravenously for 10 days may be useful for cutaneous ulceration. Treatment may have to be repeated, Local heat may increase the rate of healing.

In espundia and DCL, pentamidine, 2 to 4 mg per kg per day intramuscularly or intravenously for 15 days, and amphotericin B are alternative drugs that may be effective.

Prognosis. Cutaneous leishmaniasis tends to self-heal and is associated with little morbidity except for scarring. Espundia may be fatal when involvement of the oral mucosa leads to aspiration or starvation.

Leishmaniasis-Visceral

Visceral leishmaniasis (kala azar) is a chronic systemic infection caused by *L. donovani.*

Etiology. Kala azar occurs focally in India, the Middle East, Africa, the Mediterranean, and Central and South America. Transmission is through the bite of an infected female sandfly. Reservoirs include dogs, rodents, and humans. Humans are the only known reservoir in India.

Pathophysiology. A cutaneous phase occurs as above, but undergoes spontaneous healing in about a month. At the time of the local lesion the parasite is either contained and killed, resulting in cure and immunity, or parasitemia occurs, resulting in dissemination and progressive disease. The parasite invades macrophages, but is not killed, and thereby is able to spread throughout the reticuloendothelial system.

Clinical Manifestations. Fever, lymphadenopathy, and hepatosplenomegaly characterize this infection. The fever may be of sudden or gradual onset, is prolonged and irregular and alternates with periods of normal temperature. There is progressive weakness and wasting.

Diagnosis. The diagnosis of kala azar is made by demonstrating the intracellular amastigotes (Leishman-Donovan bodies) in stained smears of spleen, bone marrow, liver, lymph nodes or blood. The parasite can also be cultured. Pancytopenia and marked elevation of gammaglobulins are the rule. Leishmania serology is usually positive.

Treatment. Due to the poor condition of the patient, nutritional and hematologic support may be necessary prior to specific chemotherapy. Therapy is as outlined above with Pentostam® (6 days for Indian form and 30 days for all others) or pentamidine may be used. Treatment may have to be repeated.

Prognosis. Recovery from cutaneous leishmaniasis does not confer immunity against kala azar. Outcome depends on the general condition of the patient. Bacterial infection as a cause of death is common. Some patients develop post-kala azar dermal leishmanoid after an apparent cure. Untreated cases are usually fatal.

Trypanosomiasis

Etiology. African sleeping sickness is caused by the hemoflagellate *Trypanosoma brucei gambiense* (West African form) and *T. b. rhodesiense* (East African form). It is confined to tropical Africa corresponding to the distribution of the tsetse fly. The Western African form occurs along waterways (riverine) and humans are the major reservoir. The East African form occurs over wider, dry savanna; bushbuck, antelope, and cattle serve as reservoirs.

The disease is transmitted by the bite of a tsetse fly, which gets the parasite from an infected animal or human. Mechanical transmission can occur through the bite of other blood sucking insects. Congenital infection is also possible.

Pathophysiology. After transmission of the organism by the bite of the tsetse fly, a chancre may appear in about five days at the site where the parasite replicates extracellularly. After 10 days or so, systemic spread occurs. It is likely that the central nervous system is invaded at this time. The incubation period for *T. b. rhodesiense* may be as short as two weeks. It is usually longer for *T. b. gambiense* and may vary from months to years.

Subsequently, waves of parasitemia occur, with each peak yielding trypanosomes bearing different surface antigens (antigenic variation), at seven- to ten-day intervals.

Upon entering the extracellular brain substance, the parasite induces a local inflammatory response characterized by a mononuclear cell infiltrate and perivascular cuffing. The immune response to *T. b. rhodesiense* is usually more vigorous than to *T. b. gambiense,* and hence the clinical signs and symptoms are more acute.

Clinical Manifestations. A chancre may or may not be present at the site of the original bite. Fever occurs preceding each peak of parasitemia and is associated with an intense headache, somnolence, lymph node swelling (especially the posterior cervical nodes — Winterbottom's sign), and splenic swelling. A peculiar peripheral neuropathy may be seen with hyperesthesia and delayed response to painful stimuli (Kerandel's sign).

The Gambian form is usually insidious and progresses slowly to psychosis, somnolence, and coma. Death usually results from secondary bacterial infection. The Rhodesian form may be acute and rapidly fatal as a result of myocarditis or encephalitis.

Diagnosis. Anemia and thrombocytopenia occur. Indirectly the diagnosis suggested by an elevation (8 to 16 times) of serum or cerebral spinal fluid IgM. An antibody rise by fluorescent antibody or complement fixation technique may be demonstrated but has a low sensitivity due to antigenic variation.

The characteristic movement of the parasite may be seen directly using a wet preparation of blood or CSF, or in stained thick and thin films. Concentration techniques greatly enhance the yield. In addition, in vitro cultivation and animal inoculation may be used to confirm the diagnosis.

Treatment. Suramin is the drug of choice early in the infection. A test dose of 100 to 200 mg is followed by 20 mg per kg per day (maximum 1 gm) intravenously on days 1, 3, 7, 14, and 21. Pentamidine, 4 mg per kg per day intramuscularly for 10 days, is an alternative drug in the early phase.

When central nervous system involvement occurs, melarsoprol (MEL-B, 3.6% solution), 3.6 mg per kg per day intravenously for three to four doses is given and repeated after a week interval for a total of three courses (maximum adult dose 40 ml). Either suramin or pentamidine may be used concurrently.

Prognosis. Untreated infections are frequently fatal. With treatment prior to CNS involvement, the prognosis is good. Later in the illness, recovery is less likely to be complete. Severe wasting and malnutrition are common in the affected patients. Secondary bacterial infections are frequent at this stage of the disease.

Chagas' Disease

Etiology. Chagas' disease is caused by *T. cruzi,* which is transmitted during the feeding of the reduviid bug by the bug's fecal contamination of the bite wound or the mucous membranes. Congenital transmission and transmission by blood transfusion are also possible. The infection occurs in rural areas from Mexico to Central and South America and the disease is highly endemic in Brazil. Approximately 40 million people are at risk of the infection, and 7 million have the disease. Wild animals (armadillo, opossum) have been found to be reservoirs, as have the domestic guinea pig, cat, and dog.

Pathophysiology. The flagellate form (trypomastigote) is passed in the feces of the infected vector. It then gains entry to the human host through the wound or by being rubbed into a mucous membrane, such as the conjunctiva. On entering a host cell, it replicates as the amastigote form. The cell becomes filled with parasites and eventually ruptures, resulting in infection of additional cells and a local mononuclear cell infiltrate. The parasite has a predilection for cardiac muscle and the nerve plexus of the gut. Inflammation with fibrosis eventually damages the cardiac muscle and the innervation to the esophagus and bowel. There is no evidence for immune complex deposition or antigenic variation with *T. cruzi*.

Clinical Manifestations. The acute disease is seen more commonly in children and is associated with local swelling at the site where the parasites replicate (chagoma). If the face is involved, conjunctivitis (Romaña's sign) may be seen. Fever and hepatosplenomegaly occur acutely. Occasionally acute myocarditis or encephalitis may develop.

Chronic damage follows after many years. Cardiac enlargement with ventricular aneurysm formation, heart block, and dysrhythmias are late sequelae. Megaesophagus and megacolon are associated with dysphagia and incomplete evacuation of the bowel, respectively. Most infected people have no clinical disease, however.

Diagnosis. During the acute phase the parasite may be demonstrated in sites of local swelling or in lymph nodes by aspiration or on biopsy. When the patient is febrile, it may be found in the blood. In the chronic stages the parasite may be difficult to find. Serology (Macado-Guierro complement fixation) can be useful. Animal inoculation, in vitro culture, and xenodiagnosis increase the diagnostic yield. The latter refers to examination of reduviid bug fecal contents for organisms following the feeding of uninfected bugs on patients suspected of having the disease.

Treatment. Nifurtimox, (available in the U.S. from the Parasitic Diseases Division, Center for Infectious Diseases, CDC, Atlanta, Georgia) 5 mg per kg per day orally, (in divided doses) increased by 2 mg per kg per day every two weeks to a maximum of 15 to 17 mg per kg per day, is given for 90 to 120 days.

Prognosis. In the early phases, with treatment, prognosis is felt to be good. In the late symptomatic stage the disease is usually fatal. Sudden death in cases of cardiomyopathy is not uncommon in persons 15 to 30 years of age.

Prevention. Improved housing construction to prevent colonization of the mud brickwork by the insect vector has a significant effect on transmission. Adding 25 ml gentian violet, 0.5%, to 500 ml of blood for 24 hours prior to transfusion also prevents transmission.

METAZOAN INFECTIONS (HELMINTHS OR WORMS)

Nematodes are unsegmented roundworms that vary in size from several millimeters to 80 cm or more. The three basic types of nematode life cycles require soil, no intermediate host, or an intermediate host for completion.

Intestinal Nematodes

Ascariasis

Etiology. Ascariasis (roundworm) is an infection with *Ascaris lumbricoides,* a geohelminth that measures 15 to 35 cm in length and has the width of a lead pencil. *Ascaris* has a life span of approximately one and a half years. It has a worldwide distribution but is seen mostly in the tropics or subtropics where eggs can incubate readily in the soil under appropriate conditions of heat, shade, and moisture. It is estimated that almost one-quarter of the world's population is infected with this worm.

Pathophysiology. The worm is found in the small bowel where it maintains its position by muscular action against the forces of peristalsis. Fertilized eggs excreted in the stool become infectious within two to three weeks of incubation in the soil. Humans are infected by ingesting eggs in contaminated water, food, or soil. In the small bowel, larvae are released from the eggs and penetrate the bowel mucosa. They are carried hematogeneously to the heart and lungs where they penetrate the alveoli and migrate up the respiratory tree to the pharynx. Larvae are then swallowed and complete their development to adult worms in the small bowel. The time from egg ingestion to egg production is about three months.

Clinical Manifestations. Most individuals with ascariasis are asymptomatic, particularly if the infection is light. During the migratory larval phase, transient pulmonary infiltrates, asthma, and eosinophilia may be seen (Löffler's syndrome). Nausea, anorexia, and abdominal pain may occur, but for the most part adult worms produce few gastrointestinal symptoms unless complications arise. *Ascaris* worms have the unfortunate habit of migrating within the gut lumen when stimulated by drugs or anesthetics. Such worms can mechanically obstruct the pancreatic and biliary ducts as well as the appendiceal lumen. In children, large numbers of worms may coil into a ball to produce partial or complete intestinal obstruction. Ascarids have been known to crawl out the mouth, nose, or even the middle ear via the eustachian tube.

Diagnosis. Diagnosis is made by finding characteristic eggs on stool examination, finding an adult worm in stool, or seeing a wormlike filling defect on a contrast study of the small bowel. Eosinophilia is a feature of larval migration only, and subsides with adult worm development.

Treatment. Piperazine citrate, 75 mg per kg (maximum 3.5 gm) a day for two days; pyrantel pamoate, 11 mg per kg (maximum 1 gm) in a single dose; and mebendazole, 100 mg twice a day for three days, are very safe and effective drugs for the treatment of ascariasis. *Ascaris* should always be eradicated first when numerous parasitic infections are treated because of its propensity to wander with drug exposure. Since a single worm may obstruct a duct lumen, ascariasis should be treated to cure.

Prognosis. As with most of the intestinal worms, the natural history of ascariasis is one of spontaneous cure. This coincides with the completion of the worm's natural life span.

Enterobiasis

Etiology. Enterobiasis (oxyuriasis, pinworm, threadworm) is an infection with *Enterobius vermicularis,* a small (2 to 13 mm) roundworm that lives for only two to four weeks. Although it has a worldwide distribution, enterobiasis is most prevalent in temperate climates. It is the most common helminth infection in North America.

Pathophysiology. Adult worms that inhabit the cecum migrate to the perianal skin at night where females lay their eggs and soon die. Within six hours of deposition, eggs become infectious. With the stimulus of pruritus ani, fecally contaminated fingers carry infective eggs to the mouth. Ingested eggs release larvae that mature to adults in the gut within 45 days. Infection also may be acquired by ingestion or inhalation of contaminated fomites such as dust, since eggs can live outside the host for up to 10 days under optimal conditions.

Clinical Manifestations. Clinically, enterobiasis is characterized by pruritus ani and visible white worms in the stool or perianal region. Abdominal pain, anorexia, and vomiting are rare. In young females, recurrent urinary tract infections, vaginitis, and eneuresis are well documented but uncommon complications of enterobiasis. Many infected individuals remain asymptomatic.

Diagnosis. Diagnosis is made by carrying out several cellulose acetate tests to detect eggs or worms on the perianal surface. At least five tests are needed to rule out the diagnosis, and they should be done on consecutive mornings before the patient has bathed. Stools rarely contain pinworm eggs. Eosinophilia is very common.

Treatment. Pyrantel pamoate, 11 mg per kg (maximum 1 gm) in a single dose; pyrvinium pamoate, 5 mg per kg (maximum 350 mg) in a single dose; or mebendazole, 100 mg in a single dose, are very effective and safe treatments for enterobiasis. The medication should be repeated in two weeks. Ancillary measures such as keeping the finger nails short, wearing pajamas to sleep, daily change of underwear, clean bed linen, and the like are necessary only with recurrence of the infection. Recurrences are more commonly associated with new exogenous infections than autoinfection by the patient.

Hookworm

Etiology. Hookworm (ancylostomiasis) is an infection with *Necator americanus* or *Ancylostoma duodenale.*

These small bowel intestinal nematodes measure 1 to 1.5 cm in length and live four to five years. Hookworm is distributed in tropical and subtropical regions where sanitation is poor and human excrement is used as fertilizer.

Pathophysiology. Hookworm eggs passed in feces are not infectious until they incubate in soil for one to two weeks. Infectious larvae that hatch may penetrate the buccal mucosa on ingestion (*A. duodenale* only), but usually enter the unbroken skin of the foot when it comes in contact with fecally contaminated soil. Larvae then migrate through the circulation to the lungs where they enter the alveoli and move up the respiratory tree to the pharynx. Larvae are swallowed and complete their development to adult worms in the small bowel. From larval penetration to egg production by adults takes approximately two months.

Clinical Manifestations. Local erythema, macules, or papules develop at the site of dermal penetration. This is known as "ground itch." Larval migration through the lungs produces a transient Löffler's syndrome. Adult worm attachment and subsequent injury to small bowel mucosa produces anorexia, peptic ulcer-like symptoms, and chronic intestinal blood loss that leads to anemia. Hookworm infection is the most common cause of iron-deficiency anemia in the world.

Diagnosis. The diagnosis may be suspected by the presence of a mild to moderate eosinophilia and confirmed by finding characteristic eggs in the stool. The eggs of *N. americanus* are identical to those of *A. duodenale*.

Treatment. Treatment is unnecessary in asymptomatic individuals who are not anemic. Treatment with pyrantel pamoate, 11 mg per kgm (maximum 1 gm) daily for three days, or mebendazole, 100 mg twice a day for three days, is usually effective.

Strongyloidiasis

Etiology. Strongyloidiasis is an infection with *Strongyloides stercoralis,* a small bowel nematode measuring 2.5 mm in length, with an undetermined life span. Strongyloidiasis has a worldwide distribution identical to that of ascariasis, trichuriasis, or hookworm infections.

Pathophysiology. Its complex life cycle involves both free-living and parasitic forms. Humans acquire the infection when the unbroken skin comes in contact with fecally contaminated soil. Infective (filariform) larvae in the soil penetrate host skin to migrate through the circulation to the lungs. There they enter the alveoli and move up the respiratory tree to the pharynx. The larvae are then swallowed and complete their development to adult worms in the small bowel mucosa. Eggs deposited in the mucosa by female worms hatch and release rhabditiform larvae that enter the gut lumen. From skin penetration to excretion of larvae takes approximately one month. Completion of the cycle can occur in the following ways: (1) excreted rhabditiform larvae develop into infective filariform larvae in the soil; (2) excreted rhabditiform larvae develop into free-living adult worms in the soil and in turn, produce infective filariform larvae; and (3) in the intestine, rhabditiform larvae may be transformed into filariform larvae that penetrate the colonic mucosa (endoautoinfection) or the perianal or perineal skin (exoautoinfection).

Clinical Manifestations. At the site of perianal skin penetration, larval migration may occur intradermally to produce a pruritic, serpiginous rash that migrates rapidly across the buttocks (cutaneous larva migrans). Larva migrans is seen also at the site of skin penetration of dog or cat hookworms. The rash from *Strongyloides* may recur indefinitely, whereas zoonotic infections are self-limited.

The initial pulmonary larval migration may give rise to a transient Löffler's syndrome. Peptic ulcer-like symptoms, diarrhea, or protein-losing enteropathy may result from the inflammatory response to adult worms and penetrating larvae in the gut mucosa. In the immunocompromised host, loss of cell-mediated immunity allows for precocious development and migration of filariform larvae. Consequently, large numbers of worms and larvae are produced. The clinical features of this hyperinfection syndrome or disseminated strongyloidiasis include hemorrhagic bronchopneumonia, gram-negative bacteremia, bacterial meningitis or peritonitis, paralytic ileus, septic shock, and death.

Diagnosis. Although strongyloidiasis may be diagnosed by finding larvae (usually rhabditiform, except in the hyperinfection syndrome) in concentrated stool samples, examination of small bowel contents by duodenal aspirate, Enterotest (string test), or small bowel biopsy may be necessary. In the hyperinfection syndrome, filariform larvae often are seen in the sputum. Moderate to marked eosinophilia is common except in the hyperinfection syndrome, where it is usually absent. *Strongyloides* serology (ELISA) appears to be fairly sensitive and specific.

Treatment. Strongyloidiasis should be treated until cure is achieved with oral thiabendazole, 25 mg/kg twice daily (maximum 3 gm) for two days, because of the potential for dissemination. In the hyperinfection syndrome in the immunosuppressed host, treatment should be prolonged for 5–7 days. The infection may persist for the lifetime of the host because of autoinfection. Topical thiabendazole 15% solution in a water-soluble base is the treatment of choice for zoonotic cutaneous larva migrans.

Trichuriasis

Etiology. Trichuriasis or whipworm is an infection with *Trichuris trichiura,* a large bowel nematode that measures 2.5 by 5.0 cm in length and has a life span of approximately seven years. Next to *Ascaris,* this is the most common intestinal helminth infection of humans. It has the same distribution as ascariasis and hookworm infections.

Pathophysiology. Eggs excreted in the stool must incubate in warm, moist soil for two to three weeks before becoming infectious to humans. Infection is acquired by ingesting embryonated eggs from soil or fecally contaminated food or water. Ingested eggs hatch in the small bowel and released larvae develop into adults in the large bowel (usually the cecum). From egg ingestion to egg production by adults takes one to three months.

Clinical Manifestations. Lightly infected individuals invariably are asymptomatic. Moderate infections produce lower abdominal pain, diarrhea, and flatulence. In very heavy infections, bloody diarrhea, weight loss, anemia, and rectal prolapse may occur.

Diagnosis. The diagnosis of trichuriasis is made by finding characteristic eggs in the stool. Adult worms may be visualized on proctoscopic examination and occasionally are passed with stool. Mild eosinophilia is common.

Treatment. Treatment of asymptomatic individuals is unnecessary. Where treatment is required, mebendazole, 100 mg twice a day for three days, is the drug of choice. Diphetarsone, (500 mg three times a day for 10 days) a restricted, emergency drug available in Canada, also is very effective.

Blood and Tissue Nematodes

Toxocariasis

Etiology. Toxocariasis (visceral larva migrans) is a human infection with the dog *(Toxocara canis)* or cat *(Toxocara cati)* roundworm. *Toxocara canis* is by far the most common infecting organism. Up to 80% of puppies less than six months of age are infected as a result of transplacental migration of larvae from infected bitches to fetal pups. Lactating bitches also may shed infective larvae into the feces because of reactivation of a dormant infection during pregnancy.

Pathophysiology. Roundworm eggs shed in dog feces are not infectious until they have undergone a two- to seven-week period of incubation in the soil. Humans are infected by ingesting embryonated eggs present in soil or contaminated hands, food, or fomites. Ingested eggs hatch in the small bowel and larvae penetrate the gut mucosa to enter first the portal and later the systemic circulation. Larvae then leave the circulation to migrate aimlessly in tissue, with a predisposition for lung, liver, brain, and eyes. Many become dormant and can remain viable for years. Clinical manifestations result from mechanical damage or the inflammatory response to migrating larvae.

Clinical Manifestations. Most infections are asymptomatic or unrecognized. Infection is most common in children 1 to 4 years of age who have pica. Symptomatic infections are characterized by cough, wheezing, fever, malaise, weight loss, and hepatosplenomegaly. Seizures occur rarely. In older children (10 to 15 years), unilateral loss of vision or eye pain may result from a retinal granuloma or endophthalmitis. The eye lesion must be distinguished from retinoblastoma.

Diagnosis. Nonspecific diagnostic features include marked eosinophilia, leukocytosis, hypergammaglobulinemia (especially IgE), elevated anti-A and anti-B titers, and pulmonary infiltrates on chest x-ray. *Toxocara*

(ELISA) serology is highly sensitive and specific. Liver biopsy detects larvae in less than 25% of patients.

Treatment. Toxocariasis is generally a benign, self-limited infection except for the ocular manifestations. Steroids may be helpful in serious illness. Thiabendazole, 25 mg per kg twice a day (maximum 3 gm per day) for five days, or diethylcarbamazine, 2 mg per kg three times a day for 28 days, are of questionable benefit.

Trichinosis

Etiology. Although strictly speaking, *Trichinella spiralis* is an intestinal nematode, it is included with the discussion of blood and tissue nematodes because the major clinical pathology results from larval migration through host tissue. It is a small, threadlike worm, measuring 1 to 3 mm, with a life span of several weeks. Trichinosis has a worldwide distribution. In North America, domestic pigs are the main source of human infection, with bear meat a less frequent source.

Pathophysiology. Humans are infected when raw or poorly cooked meat containing *Trichinella* larval cysts is ingested. Worm development takes place in the duodenal mucosa. Within five days, infective larvae are released from adult worms. Larvae travel hematogenously to skeletal muscle where they encyst or are destroyed by the host's inflammatory response. Encysted larvae may live for the lifetime of the host. The human is a dead-end host since the cycle usually ends with human infection. In nature, the cycle is maintained by carnivorous rodents or other mammals feeding on infected animals.

Clinical Manifestations. Within 48 hours of ingestion of infected meat, worm development in the duodenum causes transient diarrhea, abdominal pain, and vomiting. Between days 14 and 28, during larval invasion of muscle, the host's inflammatory response produces the classic symptoms of trichinosis: fever, cough, chest pain, myalgia, facial and periorbital edema, rash, and splinter hemorrhages. Severe infections may lead to congestive heart failure, CNS manifestations, and death. Muscle stiffness and fatigue may persist for weeks or months during convalescence.

Diagnosis. Nonspecific diagnostic findings include marked eosinophilia, leukocytosis, pulmonary infiltrates, and electrocardiographic changes of myocarditis. *Trichinella* antibodies (CFT, ELISA) are detectable between the second and fourth weeks, and muscle biopsy is positive after the fourth week.

Treatment. Nonsteroidal antiinflammatory agents may be useful in mild infections, whereas steroids should be used in severe infections. Mebendazole 200–400 mg three times a day for 3 days, then 400–500 mg three times a day for 10 days or thiabendazole, 25 mg per kg twice a day (maximum 3.0 gm per day) for five to seven days are effective in killing adult worms, but have not been tested in controlled studies against the migrating or encysted larvae in humans. Stringent regulations governing the cooking of swill before it is fed to swine, a decline in home processing of pork sausages, meat inspection, and deep freezing of pork have led to a dramatic reduction of trichinosis in North America.

Prognosis. Except in very heavy infections, death from trichinosis is rare. Essentially, the infection is self-limited, although symptoms may persist for many weeks or months.

Lymphatic Filariasis

Etiology. Lymphatic filariasis is caused by an infection with a nematode that develops and remains in the lymphatics of the host. These threadlike worms are 80 to 100 mm long by 0.25 mm (the males being about half this size) and are transmitted by the bite of a mosquito (*Anopheles, Culex,* or *Aedes*).

Wuchereria bancrofti is present in most equatorial countries of tropical Africa, Asia, the Pacific Islands, the West Indies, and the northern part of South America. *Brugia malayi* is confined to Asia and *B. timori* is found in Indonesia.

The adults may live for 5–8 years producing microfilariae that may be found in the blood stream and live there for three to six months. It is the circulating microfilariae that infect the mosquito. Man is the reservoir, except for *B. malayi,* which is a zoonosis (cats, other primates).

Pathophysiology. The living worms cause blockage of lymph flow and leakage of lymph into the tissues. When the adult forms die and degenerate, local inflammation occurs, resulting in damage and fibrosis of the lymphatics. Long-standing lymphedema results in hyperplasia and fibrosis in the affected tissues.

Clinical Manifestations. In the acute phase, fever, lymphadenitis, lymphangitis, orchitis, and epididymitis may occur in the absence of microfilaremia. Of the thousands of servicemen exposed in the South Pacific during World War II, none subsequently developed elephantiasis. This illustrates the point that in helminth infections disease is related to worm burden, which is usually accumulated over many years.

Chronic lymphatic damage results in hard, nonpitting edema of the lower limb *B. malayi* and *W. bancrofti).* Similar changes occur in the scrotum, upper limbs, and breasts with *W. bancrofti.* Chyluria may result from the rupture of lymph varices into any portion of the urinary tract.

The affected skin, which becomes thickened and verrucous, is predisposed to secondary bacterial infection, which further damages the lymphatics.

Diagnosis. Direct diagnosis is made by finding the microfilara in stained thick blood films. Blood should be taken between 11:00 P.M. or 2:00 A.M. for the nocturnally periodic forms, or between 10:00 A.M. to 4:00 P.M. for the subperiodic forms (*W. bancrofti* in the South Pacific). Concentration techniques enhance the yield. Indirect diagnosis may be supported in the appropriate clinical setting by an eosinophilia or positive serology (CFT, IFA). However, filaria serology is notoriously non-specific and cross-reacts with many other nematode infections. Microfilaremia may be provoked by a single dose of diethylcarbamizine, 50 mg, but should not be used in areas endemic for onchocerciasis or loiasis.

Treatment. Diethylcarbamizine at a maintenance dose of 2 to 3 mg per kg orally three times a day for 21 days (gradually increase to maintain a dose over 5 to 7 days), is very effective at clearing microfilaremia, but is much less effective against the adult forms. Severe reactions due to microfilarial death may occur, but these can be controlled with steroids.

Prognosis. Prognosis is excellent if therapy is instituted prior to the development of lymphatic fibrosis, which is irreversible. Corrective surgery may be possible for cases with severe involvement of the limbs or scrotum.

Subcutaneous Filariasis

Etiology. The adult organisms that cause subcutaneous filariasis are found in the subcutaneous tissues while the microfilaria can be found in blood *(Loa loa),* on skin *(Onchocerca volvulus),* or deposited outside of the host through an ulcer on the skin (*Dracunculus medinensis).* Blood-sucking arthopods transmit *L. loa* (*Chrysops* — deer fly) and *O. volvulus* (*Simulium* — black fly), but *D. medinensis* is transmitted by the ingestion of an infected crustacean *(Cyclops)* found in water.

Loiasis (eye worm, Calabar swelling) is distributed in West and Central Africa. Onchocerciasis (river blindness) is found scattered through West, East, and Central Africa as well as Central America and the northern parts of South America. Dracunculiasis (guinea worm) is located throughout India and West and Central Africa, as well as in foci in the Middle East and Pakistan.

Pathophysiology. Loiasis is characterized by migration of the adult worm through subcutaneous or deep tissues of the body. This results in well-localized and transient swelling that are several centimeters in size.

Onchocerciasis is associated with nontender nodules typically over bony prominences. These nodules are stable and occur singly or may be multiple. The adults are found within these fibrous nodules in a coiled, tangled mass. There is very little pathology associated with the nodules, although abscesses may form or pressure on a bone may cause erosion. The skin microfilariae are associated with acute inflammation. This results initially in lichenification and then atrophy of the skin. The most serious damage occurs in the eye, which early manifests as conjunctivitis, but may progress through the stages of punctate keratitis, sclerosing keratitis (blindness), iritis (second-degree glaucoma, blindness), and chorioretinitis with optic atrophy.

In dracunculiasis, the adult female migrates through the host's body, maturing for 8 to 10 months after being infected. At the appropriate time, and when stimulated by the presence of water, the gravid uterus is protruded through a blister in the host's skin (usually on the lower limb) and the first-stage larvae are discharged. This usually occurs aseptically, but occasionally the worm enters a joint space or becomes secondarily infected along its tract. When this happens, an intense inflammatory reaction occurs. Occasionally the adult worm dies and is found as a calcified cord palpable under the skin of the host.

Clinical Manifestations. Loiasis classically produces fugitive swelling. Occasionally an adult will migrate across the bulbar conjunctiva of the eye, causing painful conjunctivitis.

Cutaneous nodules, chronic pruritic dermatitis, and ocular damage are characteristic of onchocerciasis.

Guinea worm infection is often asymptomatic until the adult female produces a blister on the host's skin to discharge her uterine contents. Local pain and pruritus occur and nonspecific constitutional symptoms may be seen. Bacterial infection of the open wound may result in crippling sequelae.

Diagnosis. The microfilariae of *Loa loa* may be demonstrated in a blood film as with lymphatic filariasis. The microfilariae may be distinguished from those of other species by morphologic characteristics. The adult worm extracted from the eye or seen in a skin biopsy can be diagnostic. Eosinophilia is often present.

Microfilaria in onchocerciasis may be seen on examination of the eye with a slit lamp, but the preferred method of detection is by doing skin snips or a skin biopsy. Adult forms may be found in excized nodules. In the Mazotti reaction, 25 mg of diethylcarbamazine orally produces an intensely pruritic rash that is characteristic of this infection.

The diagnosis of acute dracunculiasis is based on the clinical picture. The larva can be identified or the adult can be extracted from the wound.

Treatment. Treatment of loiasis is the same as for the lymphatic filariasis. Rarely encephalopathy can occur during therapy with a heavy infection due to death of organisms and resultant inflamation.

Diethylcarbamazine is useful in treating onchocerciasis, 25 mg per day for two days, increasing by 1 mg per kg per day, to a maximum dosage of 9 mg per kg per day for 21 days. For ocular involvement, suramin may be used; after a test dose of 100 mg intravenously 1 gm intravenously is given weekly for five weeks. Severe allergic reactions may be precipitated by therapy, resulting in additional eye damage. Patients should be protected with antihistamines, and steroids may also occasionally be needed. Nodulectomy may decrease microfilaremia. Diethylcarbamazine is microfilaricidal but has no effect on the adult worm. Recent studies suggest that mebendazole, b.i.d., might sterilize adult worms leading to symptomatic cure.

Niridazole, 25 mg per kg per day (maximum 1.5 gm/day) in three divided doses for seven days; or metronidazole, 250 to 500 mg orally three times a day for seven days, may be used in guinea worm infections. Both of these agents have antiinflammatory actions.

Prognosis. Loiasis is a nonfatal infection that usually responds to therapy. Onchocerciasis is one of the leading causes of blindness in the world today. Therapy before eye damage occurs may prevent this devastating complication.

Guinea worm has a good prognosis as long as there is no joint involvement or septic cellulitis.

Adult Cestodes

Tapeworms

Etiology. Tapeworms are segmented flatworms that live in the small bowel, attached to the wall of the intestine by specialized suckers or hooklets located on the head (scolex). Each mature segment (proglottid) has both male and female sexual organs for laying fertile eggs. The five important tapeworms in humans include: beef *(Taenia saginata)*, pork *(T. solium)*, fish *(Diphyllobothrium latum)*, dwarf *(Hymenolepis nana)*, and dog *(Echinococcus granulosus)* (Table 27.3). Adult tapeworms vary in size from 2 cm *(H. nana)*, to 7 meters *(D. latum)*. In between are *Taenia* species, which measure 3 meters. Tapeworm life span can be as short as several months *(H. nana)* to over 20 years *(T. solium, T. saginata*, and *D. lata)*.

Pathophysiology. Adult worms live in the small bowel of the definitive host (usually human) and release large numbers of eggs daily. Ova passed in feces survive in soil or water until they are ingested by an intermediate host (cattle, pig, fish) in whom larval development takes place. The cycle is completed when a human consumes the uncooked flesh of the infected intermediate host. The ingested larval form then matures in the intestine to an adult worm over several months.

This general cycle does not apply to *H. nana*, in which eggs excreted in the stool are infective to humans at the time of passage, allowing for direct fecal-oral transmission. Internal auto-infection (see strongyloidiasis) may also occur. This organism does have a wild cycle, in which the rodent acts as the definitive host and a flea as the intermediate host.

Clinical Manifestations. Adult tapeworm infections usually are asymptomatic although abdominal pain, diarrhea, nausea, and anorexia can occur. Most infected individuals harbor only one worm. Pruritus ani is associated with the passage of motile *Taenia* segments. Since vitamin B_{12} is adsorbed to the surface of

TABLE 27.3. Tapeworms of Humans

Tapeworm	*Geographic Distribution*	*Intermediate Host(s)*	*Definitive Host*
T. saginata	Worldwide	Cattle	Humans
T. solium	India, Mexico, S. America, S. Africa, Asia, S.E. Asia	Pigs	Humans
D. latum	N. America, Scandinavia	First: crustacean (*Cyclops*) Second: freshwater fish	Humans and fish-eating mammals
H. nana	Worldwide	None or flea	Human or rodent
E. granulosus	N. America, S. America, Europe, Africa, Oceania	Sheep, cattle, deer, moose	Dog, wolf

D. latum, megaloblastic anemia may occur (rarely in the North American strains). The psychologic effects of passing enormous worm segments by rectum far outweigh any pathologic effects on the human host.

Diagnosis. Tapeworms are diagnosed by food history and the identification of characteristic proglottids or ova in the stool. Since eggs of *Taenia saginata* are indistinguishable from those of *T. solium*, species identification requires examination of worm proglottids. Eosinophilia is not usually present.

Treatment. All tapeworms except *H. nana* can be eradicated with a single dose of niclosamide (2 grams - chewed in a single dose). To treat *H. nana*, six days of drug therapy are required (2 grams on day 1 and ½ gram daily for 5 days). Follow-up stools should be examined three months after treatment. Since the eggs of *T. solium* are infective to humans, treatment should be followed by a purge, and stool precautions should be instituted. Praziquantel is a good alternate drug for the treatment of all human tapeworms.

Larval Cestodes

Cysticercosis

Cysticercosis is an infection with the larval form of *T. solium* known as *Cysticercus cellulosae*.

Pathophysiology. Cysticercosis results when a human ingests *T. solium* eggs that have contaminated the environment. Autoinfection occurs externally, when a person ingests eggs from his or her own tapeworm or internally, when eggs are regurgitated into the stomach and duodenum. Eggs activated by bile salts and gastric acid release hexocanth embryos that penetrate the gut wall and migrate hematogenously to the brain, eye, muscle, and subcutaneous tissue. In tissue, a larval cyst (bladder worm) develops that varies in size from 0.5 to 5 cm. A host inflammatory response only occurs with cyst death, usually four to five years after the onset of infection.

Clinical Manifestations. Clinical manifestations of cysticercosis depend upon the location of the parasite larvae. Most individuals remain asymptomatic. Brain infections commonly produce seizures and occasionally focal neurologic signs. Obstructive hydrocephalus may result from a cyst that blocks the third ventricle or from basal meningitis, which occurs in the racemose form. Painless, subcutaneous nodules may develop in the skin. Visual disturbances result from eye involvement.

Diagnosis. A history of pork tapeworm infection and/or travel to endemic areas is helpful in diagnosis. Indirect evidence of infection includes eosinophilia (uncommon), soft tissue calcifications in muscles and brain, and the presence of *Cysticercus* antibodies. *Cysticercus* serology (IHA, IFA) is positive in 50% of patients with seizure disorders, 70% of those with basal meningitis, and 95% of those with increased intracranial pressure. Over all, serology is positive in 85% of infected persons. Cross-reacting antibodies are seen in individuals with hydatid disease. A definitive diagnosis can be made by excisional biopsy of the affected tissue.

Treatment. In most cases, symptomatic therapy (e.g., anticonvulsants) suffice. Praziquantel, a new broad-spectrum antihelminthic, is effective in eliminating uncalcified cerebral and subcutaneous cysts. In cerebral cysticercosis, steroid therapy should be given concomitantly with praziquantel; the dose of the latter is 50 mg/kg daily for 10 days. Surgical therapy may be required to create a shunt in an individual with hydrocephalus or excise an area of scar tissue in the brain that is acting as a focus for uncontrolled seizures.

Prognosis. Untreated cysticercosis often resolves spontaneously unless obstructive hydrocephalus or the racemose form is present. Such cases are frequently fatal unless therapeutic intervention is undertaken.

Echinococcosis

Echinococcosis (hydatid disease) is a zoonotic infection with the larval form of *E. granulosus* or *E. multilocularis* in humans.

Etiology. Two geographic forms of cystic hydatid disease are found in nature. The pastoral or domestic variety is seen wherever sheep and cattle (the intermediate hosts) are found in association with dogs: North and East Africa, South America, southern and eastern Europe, Australia, and New Zealand. The sylvatic variety is found in Canada and Alaska wherever moose, caribou, and reindeer (the intermediate hosts) are found in association with hunting dogs or wolves. This latter variety is called *E. granulosus,* var. *Canadensis*. Both forms are acquired by man's close association with canines (e.g., skinning wolves) or ingestion of food and water contaminated with canine feces.

Pathophysiology. The general life cycle begins with the excretion of *E. granulosus* (canine tapeworm) eggs in the feces of the definitive host (a canine) and their subsequent ingestion by a ruminant intermediate host. The ingested eggs hatch in the intestine and release a larval stage that penetrates the gut mucosa to enter the portal circulation. When larvae lodge in the liver, lung, brain, or other tissues, they develop into viable, expanding, fluid-filled, cystic masses. The cycle is completed when the intermediate host dies and the viscera that contain larval cysts are ingested by a canine. The human is a dead-end, accidental, intermediate host who is infected when he ingests canine feces containing *E. granulosus* eggs. Ingestion of the infected intermediate host will not produce an adult worm in humans.

The clinical manifestations of hydatid disease result from the mechanical effects of a space-occupying cystic mass and the allergic effects of cyst-fluid antigen that leaks into the circulation. The cyst wall is made up of three layers. The innermost is a single-celled, germinal membrane surrounded by a thick, laminated membrane. Both of these are parasite derived. The outer wall, the pericyst, is the result of the host's inflammatory response. Budding internally from the germinal membrane and lying free in the cyst fluid are protoscolices and daughter cysts. Each scolice has the capacity to generate a new cyst if released into the circulation or peritoneal cavity. Alternatively, the scolice can differentiate into an adult tapeworm if ingested by a canine.

Clinical Manifestations. Pastoral hydatid cysts, usually solitary, are located (in decreasing order of frequency) in the right lobe of the liver, lung, kidney, brain, spleen, and bone. In the Canadian variant, the lung is most commonly affected. Symptoms and signs are dependent on which organ is affected. Liver involvement usually leads to right upper quadrant pain and hepatomegaly, whereas lung involvement may produce cough, hemoptysis, and pleural effusion. A hydatid cyst grows very slowly (0.5 to 1 cm a year) and therefore presents clinically many years after the infection is acquired. A sudden leak of cyst fluid may evoke a picture of mild urticaria or full-blown anaphylaxis. Many patients, particularly those with the Canadian variant, remain asymptomatic, and the disease is identified on routine x-ray or physical examination.

Diagnosis. Most helpful in the diagnosis of hydatid disease is an epidemiologic history of exposure to canine host in an endemic area. Ultrasonography, radionuclide, or computerized tomographic (CT) scanning usually demonstrates a cystic lesion in the liver that may be difficult to distinguish from a congenital cyst, abscess, or necrotic mass.

Liver hydatids frequently have a calcified pericyst that can be detected on plain x-ray films of the abdomen. Pulmonary cysts usually present as a large coin lesion without calcification. Scolices may be found in the sputum of individuals who are infected with pulmonary hydatids that have ruptured into the bronchial tree.

Serology (IHA or ELISA) is positive in 80% of liver hydatids, but only 40% of lung hydatids. Serologic cross-reactions occur with cysticercosis, cirrhosis, and collagen-vascular disease. The immediate skin test response to cyst antigen (Casoni test) has many false positive reactions, and therefore reliance on it for diagnosis is not recommended. Biopsy of a hydatid cyst is contraindicated because leakage of cyst fluid might provoke anaphylaxis or lead to the development of new cysts in the peritoneal cavity.

Treatment. Asymptomatic hydatids of the *Canadensis* variety do not require treatment because they rarely lead to complications. Surgical therapy is the treatment of choice for pastoral hydatid disease. Usually, liver cysts are evacuated and the germinal layer destroyed with a scolicidal agent such as hibitane, 3% saline, or cetrimide. Formalin is no longer recommended as a scolicidal agent. Pulmonary hydatids often can be removed intact by excision. Inoperable or recurrent disease may be treated with high-dose mebendazole, 50–200 mg per kg per day, for three months or more. Chemotherapy will lead to clinical improvement in approximately two-thirds of cases. Although studies of the natural history of untreated human infections have not been carried out, data from animal studies suggest that one third or more cysts die spontaneously.

Alveolar or Malignant Hydatid

Etiology. *Echinococcus multilocularis* parasite is seen throughout the Arctic, in Western Europe, and in Russia. In this form of hydatid disease, silver or red foxes act as definitive hosts, and voles and lemmings as intermediate hosts. Humans are infected accidentally when fox feces containing *E. multilocularis* ova are ingested.

Pathophysiology. This is a very slow growing parasite that buds exogenously from the germinal membrane, forming an invading, solid mass very different from the localized, fluid-filled cyst of *E. granulosus.*

Clinical Manifestations. Clinically, alveolar hydatid disease causes pain or a mass in the right upper quadrant. Uniformly, the liver is involved and metastases occur frequently to lung and brain. Essentially, this parasite behaves like a malignant tumor.

Diagnosis. Diagnosis is suspected by positive serology and the presence of pathognomonic "Swiss cheese" calcification in the liver. Confirmation of the diagnosis can be made by needle biopsy without risk of seeding the "tumor" into the surrounding tissues.

Treatment. Where possible, cure can be achieved by total excision of the parasitic mass. High-dose mebendazole, 50 mg per kg per day, administered indefinitely, may slow parasite growth but will not eradicate it. Untreated persons die within 10 to 20 years of diagnosis, perhaps considerably sooner.

Trematodes

Trematodes (flukes) are unsegmented flat worms measuring 1 to 8 cm in length. Except for *Fasciola hepatica,* they are not indigenous to North America because the snail (intermediate host) is absent from our environment.

The five important trematodes of humans have a similar life cycle. Eggs, excreted in stool, urine, or sputum (depending on the species of fluke), must come into contact with fresh water, where they hatch into short-lived, free-swimming larvae known as miracidia. Miracidia are ingested by or penetrate a snail intermediate host (specific for the genus and species of fluke) where further development and multiplication take place. Several weeks later, different short-lived (24 to 48 hours), free-swimming larvae known as cercariae emerge from the snail. In the blood fluke (*Schistosoma* species) life cycle, no further intermediate host is required, and cercariae penetrate the skin of the human host in whom the adult worm develops. For the remaining trematodes, a second intermediate host is required. Cercariae must penetrate the flesh of fish *(Clonorchis sinensis)* or crustaceans *(Paragonimus westermani),* settle on the surface of grass *(F. hepatica)* or water chestnuts *(Fasciolopsis buski),* where encystment into thick-walled metacercariae occurs. When man ingests one of the above second intermediate hosts, adult worms develop in an organ system specific for the fluke: liver — *Clonorchis sinensis* and *Fasciola hepatica;* lung — *Paragonimus westermani;* intestine — *Fasciolopsis buski;* and veins of the bowel or bladder — *Schistosoma* species.

Schistosomiasis

Etiology. Schistosomiasis is an infection with *Schistosoma* species, also known as blood flukes. Three major species infect humans, each with a different geographic distribution: *S. mansoni* in the Caribbean, South America, Africa, and the Middle East; *S. haematobium* in Africa and the Middle East; and *S. japonicum* in Southeast Asia. It is estimated that over 200 million people are infected with *Schistosoma* parasites.

Pathophysiology. Humans acquire the infection when they come in contact with cercariae in slow-moving fresh water. After penetrating the skin, cercariae develop into larval schistosomules that first migrate through the lungs and then reach the portal veins of the liver where adult worms develop in two to three months. Each species of adult worm migrates against portal flow to lodge in the superior mesenteric vein — *S. japonicum;* the inferior mesenteric vein — *S. mansoni;* and the venous plexus of the bladder — *S. hematobium*. These worms, measuring 1 to 3 cm in length, are paired, in copula, for a life span of up to 25 years. Two-thirds of the eggs released by the female worm are carried by the circulation to liver or lung, while the rest penetrate bowel or bladder mucosa to be excreted in the stool and urine respectively. Eggs embedded in tissue provoke a cell-mediated immune response resulting in granuloma formation followed by fibrosis. Thus in schistosomiasis, it is the host response to the egg, and not the adult worms, that is responsible for tissue pathology.

Clinical Manifestations. Most individuals with schistosomiasis are asymptomatic. When symptoms do occur, the disease occurs in three phases:

1. Cercarial penetration of the skin elicits an inflammatory response consisting of a papular, pruritic, self-limited urticarial rash known as cercarial dermatitis or swimmer's itch. This entity is seen commonly in North America when humans have contact with bird schistosomiasis.
2. Acute schistosomiasis (Katayama disease) coincides with egg deposition four to eight weeks after infection. It is a self-limited serum sickness-like illness consisting of fever, cough, abdominal pain, rash, arthralgia, and marked eosinophilia. This syndrome occurs infrequently, but is most commonly associated with *S. japonicum* infections.
3. Chronic schistosomiasis, resulting from a granulomatous response to egg antigen, is clinically noticeable only in individuals who are heavily infected. In *S. mansoni* and *S. japonicum* infections, egg deposition in the liver leads to presinusoidal portal hypertension with preservation of hepatocellular function. Egg deposition in the bowel produces mucosal polyps and ulceration, which may give rise to abdominal pain, diarrhea, and rectal bleeding. When portasystemic anastomoses occur, eggs that reach the lungs may produce an endarteritis and pulmonary hypertension. Ectopic worm pairs in the cerebral circulation, especially *S. japonicum,* may give rise to headache, seizures, and focal neurologic signs, when egg granuloma develop in brain tissue.

   In *S. haematobium* infections, egg deposition at the distal end of the ureters can lead to ureteric obstruction with subsequent hydronephrosis. Involvement of the bladder (especially the trigone) produces trigonitis and bladder polyps. Clinically, patients complain of frequency, dysuria, or most often, painless terminal hematuria. Squamous cell carcinoma of the bladder is associated with *S. haematobium* infection and occurs in the 20- to 40-year age group.

Diagnosis. To consider the diagnosis of schistosomiasis, an individual must have had contact with fresh water in an area known to be endemic for the infection. Schistosomiasis is most often diagnosed by finding eggs in stool or midday urine. In light infections, biopsy of rectal or bladder tissue may be necessary. Calcification of the bladder wall in heavy *S. haematobium* infections can be detected by pelvic x-rays. Liver biopsy may be helpful when egg production has ceased. Eosinophilia is common but not uniformly present. The presence of antibodies to schistosomes (IFA) is suggestive but not diagnostic of human schistosomiasis since seropositivity also occurs with cercarial dermatitis secondary to bird schistosomiasis.

Treatment. The recent introduction of safe and effective antischistosome agents has revolutionized the treatment of schistosomiasis. The drugs of choice for *S. mansoni, S. haematobium,* and *S. japonicum* are oxamniquine, metrifonate, and praziquantel, respectively. The dose of each drug is as follows: oxamniquine, 15 to 60 mg per kg over one to two days, depending on geographic area in which it is acquired; metrifonate, 10 mg per kg every two weeks for three doses and praziquantel, 40 to 60 mg per kg in one day. Praziquantel is effective against all species and therefore, some authors consider this to be the drug of choice for all schistosome infections. Since dead eggs may be excreted for years after successful eradication of adult worms, only individuals who excrete viable eggs (as determined by morphology and miracidia hatching) need to be treated. Excretion of viable eggs beyond three months after treatment indicates reinfection or drug failure.

Prognosis. Untreated light infections are not likely to harm the host, whereas a heavy infection, if left untreated will in time produce the chronic sequelae outlined above.

Clonorchiasis

Etiology. Clonorchiasis is an infection with *Clonorchis sinensis* (the Oriental liver fluke), which measures 1 to 2 cm in length and has a life span of almost 25 years. Clonorchiasis is endemic to several countries in Southeast Asia. The animal reservoir for the infection includes many carnivores such as dogs, rodents, and pigs. Up to 20% of Hong Kong Chinese are infected with this parasite.

Pathophysiology. Humans are infected by eating uncooked fresh-water fish or food contaminated with metacercariae from utensils used to cut infected fish. In the duodenum, larvae that are released from ingested metacercariae migrate up the common bile duct to develop into adult worms in the biliary tree. Egg excretion in the stool begins several months after onset of infection.

Clinical Manifestations. All but the heaviest infections are asymptomatic. Inflammation of the bile ducts in response to adult worms leads to bile duct dilatation, stone formation, and subsequent cholangitis. Such complicated infections cause right upper quadrant pain, hepatomegaly, and jaundice. Biliary cirrhosis and cholangiocarcinoma have been associated with clonorchiasis.

Diagnosis. A history of eating poorly cooked fish in an endemic area is an important clue to the diagnosis of clonorchiasis. The presence of typical eggs in the stool or duodenal aspirate confirms the diagnosis. Eosinophilia is not a feature of this infection.

Treatment. Praziquantel, 25 mg per kg three times a day for one day, is the drug of choice for clonorchiasis.

MEDICAL PROBLEMS IN RETURNING TRAVELERS

With the influx of immigrants from underdeveloped countries into developed countries, and an increase in the number of North Americans traveling abroad, physicians must have a heightened awareness of medical problems unique to these two patient populations.

The diagnosis of tropical or exotic diseases begins with the question, *Unde venis?* (Where have you been?). A complete geographic history should be followed by a detailed exposure history, during which the physician should ascertain whether the patient has been exposed to a number of infectious agents. For example, it must be determined if the patient has been drinking untreated water (giardiasis, cholera, shigellosis), walking without shoes (hookworm, strongyloidiasis), eating uncooked meat or fish (trichinosis, tapeworm), drinking unpasteurized milk (brucellosis, tuberculosis), or swimming in fresh water, lakes, or rivers in an area endemic for schistosomiasis.

Fever

Fever in an individual returning from a malarious area is a medical emergency and is always considered to be malaria until proved otherwise. Where expertise is not available locally to make a diagnosis of malaria, patients should be referred elsewhere, or blood samples sent to a laboratory experienced in diagnosing malaria. A thick blood film concentrates the parasites and is the method of choice for making the diagnosis. Thin films, containing fewer parasites, are used to determine the species found on thick films. With the recent dramatic increase in chloroquine-resistant strains of *Plasmodium falciparum* malaria, it is most important to ascertain both the infecting species and the area of the world in which the infection was acquired.

Since *P. falciparum* malaria can kill within several days of onset of illness, time is of the essence in making a correct parasitologic diagnosis. In descending order of frequency, other causes of fever in travelers or immigrants include viral influenza, hepatitis prodrome, typhoid fever, arbovirus infections (dengue), tuberculosis, and amebic liver abscess. Travelers are not immune to the usual causes of fever, including pneumonia and urinary tract infection.

A note of caution must be interjected here about the African hemorrhagic fevers (Lassa, Marburg, and Ebola viruses). These viral infections, which are transmitted by the parenteral and aerosol route, have a high mortality. Since their clinical signs and symptoms cannot be distinguished from those of most other febrile illnesses, the epidemiologic history plays a major role in determining whether one should consider them in the differential diagnosis of fever in a patient returning from the tropics.

In anyone who develops fever within 21 days of departure from a rural area of Africa, particularly if the individual has been in contact with ill persons, viral hemorrhagic fever should be considered. In such cases, the patient must be placed in strict isolation; no blood tests should be performed and all biologic specimens should be held until the local medical or health officer has been consulted. To end this topic on a cheery note, there has been no secondary spread of these infections to individuals who have been in contact with index cases outside of Africa.

Eosinophilia

Parasitic infections are an important cause of tissue and peripheral blood eosinophilia. The diagnosis is often straightforward, but at times presents a difficult diagnostic challenge.

Most hematology laboratories accept as normal eosinophil counts less than 450 per cu mm. The criterion for eosinophilia is the absolute count and not the percentage of eosinophils. It is not necessary to order absolute eosinophil counts, since a reasonable estimate can be obtained by multiplying the total white count by the percentage of eosinophils. There is some merit in the classification of eosinophilia by degree: fewer than 1000 eosinophils per cu mm is considered to be mild eosinophilia; between 1000 and 3000 per cu mm moderate, and greater than 3000 per cu mm, marked eosinophilia. Table 27.4 lists a number of selected parasitic infections and the degree of eosinophilia usually seen in clinical practice.

There are two important rules regarding the relationship of eosinophilia to parasitic infection. With few exceptions (toxoplasmosis and isosporosis), protozoal infections such as malaria, giardiasis, amebiasis, and so on do not produce blood eosinophilia. Even in toxoplasmosis, eosinophilia is seen in less than 15% of cases. Second, the degree of eosinophilia usually depends upon the degree of tissue invasion by the parasite. For example, pure lumen-dwelling parasites that do not invade tissue (pinworms, tapeworms, adult roundworms, and Chinese liver flukes) are rarely associated with eosinophilia. On the other hand, parasites that have a larval migration phase through tissue, such as *T. canis* (visceral larva migrans) and *Trichinella spiralis,* are associated with marked eosinophilia. Finally, allergic states (with the exception of drug reactions) rarely produce eosinophilia much above 1000 cells per cu mm.

TABLE 27.4. Degree of Eosinophilia in Selected Parasitic Infections

None	*Mild to Moderate (450/cu mm–3000/cu mm)*	*Marked (>3000/cu mm)*
Pinworm	Hookworm	Trichinosis
Adult roundworm	Strongyloidiasis	Toxocariasis
Tapeworm	Migrating roundworm larvae	Filariasis†
Hydatid disease*	Schistosomiasis	
Oriental liver fluke	Whipworm	
Protozoal infections		

*Eosinophilia seen in approximately 25% of cases.
†Eosinophilia quite variable and often absent in late stages.

Since many helminth infections have a long prepatent period, eosinophilia may develop before larvae or eggs appear in the blood or excreta respectively. In such cases, examinations of these biological specimens for ova and parasites should be repeated several months after a patient's return from the tropics. Where repeated investigations do not yield an answer to a patient's eosinophilia, a thorough epidemiologic history (travel plus exposure) combined with knowledge of the geography of disease distribution usually points one in the direction of a correct diagnosis. For example, the patient from Guyana with marked eosinophilia probably has Bancroftian filariasis and night blood samples must be drawn to confirm the diagnosis; while the East Asian from Uganda who swam in Lake Victoria needs a rectal biopsy to rule out schistosomiasis. Unfortunately, there is no single reference source that will provide the physician with a handy guide to the geography of disease distribution.

Diarrhea

Diarrhea is the most common problem facing physicians who care for returning travelers. Up to 50% of travelers to the tropics suffer tourista or traveler's diarrhea. Typically, the condition is characterized by an abrupt-onset illness, beginning within the first week after arrival and consisting of abdominal cramps, watery

TABLE 27.5. Diarrhea in Returning Travelers

	Small Bowel Diarrhea	*Large Bowel Diarrhea*
Selected pathogens	Enterotoxigenic *E. coli*	*E. coli* (invasive)
	Vibrio cholerae	*Shigella*
	Rotavirus	*Entamoeba histolytica*
	Giardia lamblia	
Leukocytes and blood in stool	Very rare	Very common

diarrhea, flatulence, and fatigue. The symptoms tend to resolve spontaneously within a few days, although in some instances, diarrhea may persist for weeks. Several studies have shown that the major cause of traveler's diarrhea is enterotoxin-producing strains of *E. coli*. Unfortunately, clinical laboratories do not yet have the facilities to diagnose these strains. Less common causes of traveler's diarrhea include *Shigella* spp., *Salmonella* spp., *G. lamblia, E. histolytica, Campylobacter* spp. and rotavirus.

In making a presumptive etiologic diagnosis in patients with infectious diarrhea, it is often helpful to separate diarrhea involving the small intestine from that of the large bowel (Table 27.5). Organisms that cause small bowel diarrhea usually produce watery diarrhea in large volume, vomiting, and diffuse, poorly localized periumbilical pain. Large bowel pathogens produce an illness characterized by small volumes of often bloody or mucoid diarrhea associated with tenesmus. Microscopic examination of stool usually reveals abundant erythrocytes and leukocytes in large but not small bowel diarrheas. *Salmonella* and *Campylobacter* organisms do not fit into the above schema since they may produce features of both types of diarrhea.

Most of the pathogens listed in Table 27.5 are associated with a self-limited illness that usually resolves within several days or weeks of the traveler's return from the tropics. There is, however, a small group in whom diarrhea tends to persist. Chronic diarrhea or other intestinal complaints in these persons most frequently are caused by a postinfectious irritable bowel syndrome which may persist for months or years after the bowel has been insulted by an often undetermined infectious agent. Virtually all age groups are affected and the premorbid bowel appearance is often one of perfect normalcy. The addition of dietary fiber is most helpful in producing symptomatic relief for these individuals.

Another important cause for chronic gastrointestinal symptoms in returning travelers is lactose intolerance. Any infection of the small bowel (especially giardiasis) may aggravate preexisting, subclinical lactase deficiency or cause transient lactose intolerance. For this reason, milk products should be the first foods eliminated from the diet of symptomatic patients and the last to be added after recovery. Lactose intolerance may only be one manifestation of a global malabsorption syndrome, which in returning travelers may be caused by giardiasis, tropical sprue, strongyloidiasis, capillariasis, or tuberculosis.

The approach to medical problems in immigrants and returning travelers, more than in any other branch of medicine, hinges upon thorough knowledge of geographic medicine, infectious disease epidemiology and natural history of disease. With this information, one is capable of determining if and when an individual might have been exposed to an infection and whether it is likely that such an infection is responsible for the clinical or laboratory findings. A well-known tropical disease expert is fond of characterizing his subspecialty in the following words: "Epidemiology is everything" . . . and so it is.

Treatment

The cornerstone of treatment in diarrheal diseases, including those in travelers, is rehydration with appropriate fluids and electrolytes (Figure 27.3). Most patients can be rehydrated by the oral route using fruit juices, table salt, and a glucose or sucrose containing substance. Sugar is an important element in this solution because its absorption across the intestinal mucosa is linked with sodium, so that water follows in a passive manner.

Milk and dairy products should be avoided during the acute episode, especially in children, since associated lactose deficiency is a common result of small bowel injury from many different intestinal pathogens. Beverages containing alcohol or caffeine and theophylline such as tea, coffee, and cola drinks tend to increase intestinal motility and potentiate abdominal cramps and diarrhea.

Synthetic narcotic analogs such as loperamide (Imodium®), 2 tablets promptly and 1 after each loose bowel movement to a maximum of 8 per day, and di-

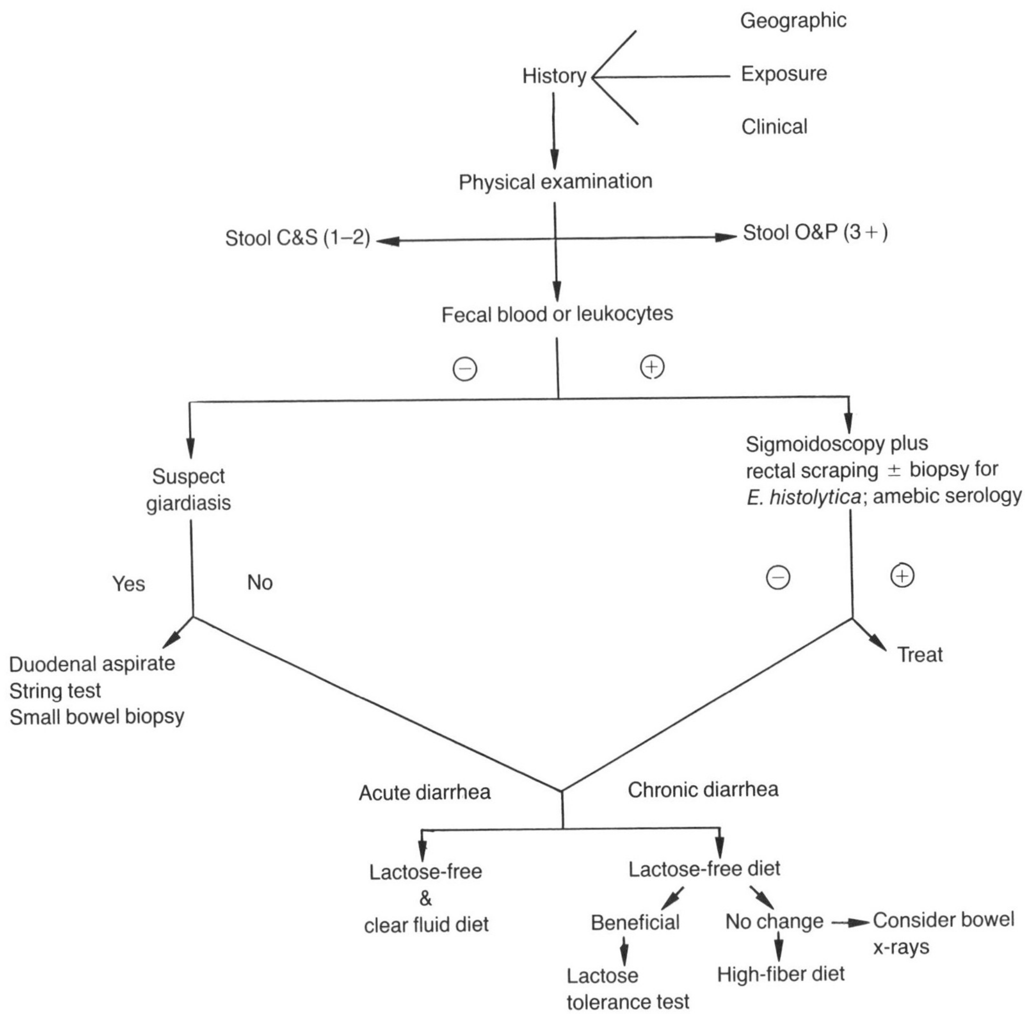

FIGURE 27.3. Management of diarrhea in returning travelers.

phenoxylate (Lomotil), 2 tablets three or four times a day, are very useful antimotility agents for symptomatic relief. These drugs must be used with caution, however. In severe amebic or bacillary dysentery, this family of drugs can enhance symptoms, prolong fecal excretion of the pathogen, and even provoke toxic megacolon. They should not be used in traveler's diarrhea associated with dysentery, high fever, severe diarrhea, or systemic toxicity.

Where local medical attention is not available, travelers may shorten the course of their illness by taking any one of the following preparations, which have been tested and found to be useful: (1) bismuth subsalicylate (Pepto-Bismol) taken orally in 30- to 60-ml doses every half-hour for eight doses; (2) double-strength TMP/SMZ, 160 mg TMP and 800 mg SMZ, or 200 mg of trimethoprim alone, taken twice daily for five days; or (3) bicozamycin orally, 500-mg tablets four times daily for three days. As a general rule, however, antibiotics should not be used for the typical case of traveler's diarrhea, which usually is short lived and resolves spontaneously without specific treatment. Rather than medicating themselves with antibiotics, travelers with more severe symptoms such as bloody diarrhea or systemic toxicity should be encouraged to seek medical attention for a definitive diagnosis.

Prevention

Prevention of traveler's diarrhea (most commonly caused by toxigenic *E. coli*) is often a matter of common sense with respect to precautionary measures concerning food and fluid intake. They include avoidance of untreated tap water, ice cubes, salads, unpeeled fruits and vegetables, custards and cream desserts, unpasteurized dairy products, items from street vendors, and buffet foods that are left to stand at room temperature or are reheated. Bottled water, canned or bottled carbonated beverages, hot drinks, or halide-treated water should be the sources of fluids for travelers to the tropics.

Prophylactic Drugs. Pepto-Bismol, which contains bismuth subsalicylate as the active ingredient, is an over-the-counter preparation that has been shown to be effective in both prophylaxis and treatment of traveler's diarrhea. The prophylactic dosage, 60 ml four times a day, or one 240-ml bottle per day is impractical and inconvenient. It should be noted that large doses of bismuth subsalicylate can lead to toxic serum concentrations of salicylate in patients already taking large doses of salicylates for arthritis.

A single dose of doxycycline, a long-acting tetracycline, taken on the day of travel and followed by one 100-mg capsule during travel and for several days after return, has been shown to prevent traveler's diarrhea. Some strains of enterotoxigenic *E. coli* and many tropical strains of *Salmonella* and *Shigella* are resistant to tetracyclines, however. These agents also can cause photosensitivity reactions and are contraindicated for pregnant women or children under 12 years of age.

A recent study indicates that one tablet of double-strength trimethoprim/sulfamethoxazole (TMP/SMZ), 160 mg TMP and 800 mg SMZ daily, can prevent traveler's diarrhea caused by a variety of enteric pathogens. As with doxycycline, the drug should be continued for several days after departure from the tropics.

In spite of the availability of the above drugs for prevention of traveler's diarrhea, most tropical disease consultants would not recommend their widespread use because they induce antibiotic resistance, increase susceptibility of the host to resistant pathogens, and cause several side effects. The use of antibiotic prophylaxis might be considered in the following circumstances: (1) for short-term visits (three weeks or less); (2) for travelers who have experienced previous episodes of severe diarrhea; (3) for the military, athletes, or business persons who require uninterrupted use of their time; (4) for individuals with diabetes mellitus, renal stones, or inflammatory bowel disease whose condition would be worsened by severe diarrhea and dehydration; and (5) for individuals who are more susceptible to enteric pathogens because of gastric resection, achlorhydria, or antacid therapy.

ANNOTATED BIBLIOGRAPHY

Adams EB, MacLeod IN. Invasive amebiasis, Parts I and II. Medicine 1977;56:315–323, 325–334.

A complete overview of amebiasis and its complications based on extensive experience by the Amebiasis Research Unit in Durban, South Africa.

Centers for Disease Control. Health information for international travel. Washington, DC: U.S. Government Printing Office, 1982.

A highly recommended, annually updated monograph that outlines vaccination requirements, antimalarial recommendations, and other health information for international travel. The vaccination and antimalarial recommendations are listed by country.

Centers for Disease Control. Prevention of malaria in travelers. 1982;31:1–28. Supplement to MMWR, U.S. Department of Health and Human Services, Atlanta, Georgia.

A complete current guide to the use of antimalarials for international travel.

Claquin P, Keystone JS. Malaria. Medicine North America 1st series, No. 9, p. 1001-1007.

Concise, practical review of the pathophysiology and clinical aspects of malaria with emphasis on drugs for treatment and prevention of malaria.

Drugs for the treatment of parasitic infections in the handbook of antimicrobial therapy. New York: Medical Letter of Drugs and Therapeutics, 1982:86–102.

Complete listing of currently available antiparasitic drugs of choice and dosage (adult and pediatric) as recommended by United States consultants.

Gorbach SL, Hoskins DW. Traveler's diarrhea. DM (Oct) 27:1–44, 1980.
An excellent, complete monograph on the etiology, diagnosis, management, and prevention of traveler's diarrhea.

MacLean JD. Medical problems imported from the tropics. Modern Med Can 1980;35:1536–1543.
Well-organized, good overview of medical problems facing practitioners who care for international travelers.

Markell EK, Voge M. Medical parasitology. 5th ed. Philadelphia: WB. Saunders, 1981.
A well-written, up-to-date textbook of parasitology containing basic information on epidemiologic, clinical, diagnostic, and management aspects of parasitic infections.

Marsden PD. Intestinal parasites. In: Marsden PD (ed). Clinics in gastroenterology. Vol. 7. Philadelphia: WB Saunders, 1978.
An excellent, well-written many-authored monograph covering all of the clinically important intestinal parasites. Some treatment regimes may be out of date.

Shafer N. Toxoplasmosis. NY State J Med 1049–1061, 1975.
Very good review of the epidemiologic, clinical, diagnostic, and therapeutic aspects of toxoplasmosis.

Smith JW, Wolfe S. Giardiasis. Ann Rev Med. 1980;31:373–383.
Good, detailed review of giardiasis.

Warren KS, Mahmoud AAF, eds. Geographic medicine for the practitioner. Chicago: University of Chicago Press, 1978.
Brief, concise review of selected tropical and parasitic diseases contains a good algorithmic approach to diagnosis and management.

INDEX